# Diagnosis and Treatment of
# SYMPTOMS of the
# RESPIRATORY TRACT

Edited by

**Richard S. Irwin, MD**

**Frederick J. Curley, MD**

**Ronald F. Grossman, MD**

# Diagnosis and Treatment of
# SYMPTOMS of the
# RESPIRATORY TRACT

Edited by

## Richard S. Irwin, MD

*Professor of Medicine*
*University of Massachusetts Medical School;*
*Director, Division of Pulmonary, Allergy, and Critical Care Medicine*
*Department of Medicine*
*University of Massachusetts Medical Center*
*Worcester, Massachusetts, USA*

## Frederick J. Curley, MD

*Associate Professor of Medicine*
*University of Massachusetts Medical School*
*Worcester, Massachusetts, USA*

## Ronald F. Grossman, MD

*Professor of Medicine*
*University of Toronto;*
*Head, Division of Respiratory Medicine*
*Mount Sinai Hospital*
*Toronto, Ontario, Canada*

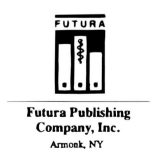

**Futura Publishing**
**Company, Inc.**
Armonk, NY

**Library of Congress Cataloging-in-Publication Data**
Diagnosis and treatment of symptoms of the respiratory tract edited by
  Richard S. Irwin, Frederick J. Curley, Ronald F. Grossman.
      p.  cm.
    Includes bibliographical references and index.
    ISBN 0-87993-657-6
    1. Respiratory organs—Diseases.  2. Pulmonary manifestations of
general diseases.  3. Symptomatology.  I. Irwin, Richard S.
II. Curley, Frederick J.  III. Grossman, Ronald F.
    [DNLM:  1. Respiratory Tract Diseases—diagnosis.  2. Respiratory
Tract Diseases—therapy.    WF 143 D536   1997]
RC732.D53   1997
616.2—dc21
DNLM/DLC
for Library of Congress                                     97-10812
                                                                CIP

Copyright 1997
Futura Publishing Company, Inc.

135 Bedford Road
Armonk, New York 10504-0418
LC #: 97-10812
ISBN: 0-87993-657-6

Every effort has been made to ensure that the information in this book is as up to date
and as accurate as possible at the time of publication. However, due to the constant
developments in medicine, neither the author, nor the editor, nor the publisher can
accept any legal or any other responsibility for any errors or omissions that may occur.

Printed in the United States of America.

This book is printed on acid-free paper.

# ❖ ❖ Dedication ❖ ❖

*To our families:*

*Diane, Rachel, Sara, Jamie, Rebecca, John, Andrew, Kate, Patrick, Timothy, Michael, Nancy, Suzanne, and Jonathan*

❖ ❖ ❖ ❖ ❖ ❖ ❖

# Contributors

**Meyer Balter, MD**
Assistant Professor of Medicine, University of Toronto; Director of Asthma Education Clinic, Mount Sinai Hospital; Toronto, Ontario, Canada

**Lipa Bodner, DMD**
Associate Professor and Head, Oral and Maxillofacial Surgery Unit, Soroka Medical Center, Ben-Gurion University of Negev, Beer-Sheva, Israel

**Jerry S. Chapnik, MD**
Associate Professor of Otolaryngology, Department of Otolaryngology and Cosmetic Facial Surgery, University of Toronto, Mount Sinai Hospital, Toronto, Ontario, Canada

**Philip Cole, MD**
Professor, Department of Otolaryngology, University of Toronto, Toronto, Ontario, Canada

**Kris Conrad, MD**
Assistant Professor of Medicine, University of Toronto, Toronto, Ontario, Canada

**Frederick J. Curley, MD**
Associate Professor of Medicine, University of Massachusetts Medical School, Worcester, MA, USA

**Dan M. Fliss, MD**
Associate Professor of Otolaryngology, Director, Head and Neck Surgical Oncology Unit, Soroka Medical Center, Ben-Gurion University of the Negev, Beer-Sheva, Israel; Department of Otolaryngology, University of Toronto, Mount Sinai Hospital, Toronto, Ontario, Canada

**Jeremy L. Freeman, MD**
Professor of Otolaryngology, University of Toronto, Mount Sinai Hospital, Toronto, Ontario, Canada

**David R. Goldfarb, MD**
Lecturer, University of Toronto, Mount Sinai Hospital, Toronto, Ontario, Canada; Director, North Toronto Snoring and Laser Center, Richmond Hill, Ontario, Canada

**Allan S. Gordon, MD**
Associate Professor of Medicine, Assistant Dean of Development, University of Toronto; Chief and Co-director, Craniofacial Pain Research Unit, Mount Sinai Hospital, Toronto, Ontario, Canada

**Ronald F. Grossman, MD**
Professor of Medicine, University of Toronto; Head, Division of Respiratory Medicine, Mount Sinai Hospital, Toronto, Ontario, Canada

**Helen M. Hollingsworth, MD**
Associate Professor of Medicine, Boston University School of Medicine, Pulmonary Center, Boston University Medical Center, Boston, MA, USA

**Martin Hyde, MD**
Professor, Department of Otolaryngology, Preventive Medicine and Biostatistics, University of Toronto; Director, Research and Development, Otologic Function Unit, Mount Sinai Hospital, Toronto, Ontario, Canada

**Richard S. Irwin, MD**
Professor of Medicine, University of Massachusetts Medical School; Director, Division of Pulmonary, Allergy and Critical Care Medicine, Department of Medicine, University of Massachusetts Medical Center, Worcester, MA, USA

**Stephen E. Lapinsky, MD**
Assistant Professor of Medicine, University of Toronto; Staff Physician, Division of Respirology, Mount Sinai Hospital, Toronto, Ontario, Canada

**J. Mark Madison, MD**
Associate Professor of Medicine and Physiology, University of Massachusetts Medical School; Director, Pulmonary Diagnostic Laboratories, University of Massachusetts Medical Center, Worcester, MA, USA

**Martyn Mendelsohn, MD**
Visiting Medical Officer, Department of Otolaryngology, Head and Neck Surgery, Royal Prince Alfred Hospital, Sydney, Australia

**David Mock, DDS**
Professor, Faculty of Dentistry, University of Toronto; Dentist-in-Chief, Co-director, Craniofacial Pain Research Unit, Department of Dentistry, Mount Sinai Hospital, Toronto, Ontario, Canada

**Arnold Noyek, MD**
Professor of Otolaryngology, Professor of Medical Imaging, University of Toronto; Executive Director, Isabel Silverman CISEPO Program, Otolaryngologist-in-Chief, Mount Sinai Hospital, Toronto, Ontario, Canada

**Blake C. Papsin, MD, MSC**
Assistant Professor of Otolaryngology, University of Toronto, Mount Sinai Hospital, Toronto, Ontario, Canada

**Renato Roithmann, MD**
Former Clinical Research Fellow, Department of Otolaryngology, University of Toronto, Mount Sinai Hospital, Toronto, Ontario, Canada; Brazilian Representative on the International Committee on Objective Assessment of the Nasal Airway, CISEPO Consultant, Brazil

**Yehudak Roth, MD**
Director, The Institute of Nose and Sinus Therapy and Clinical Investigations, Department of Otolaryngology-Head & Neck Surgery, The Edith Wolfson Medical Center, Holon, Israel; The Saul A. Silverman Family Foundation Nasal Airflow Laboratory, Department of Otolaryngology, Mount Sinai Hospital, Unversity of Toronto, Toronto, Ontario, Canada; Canada-International Scientific Exchange Program (CISEPO); Consultant on Biomedical Technologies

**Oren P. Schaefer, MD**
Assistant Professor of Medicine, University of Massachusetts Medical School, Worcester, MA, USA

**Nicholas A. Smyrnios, MD**
Assistant Professor of Medicine, University of Massachusetts Medical School; Director of the Medical Intensive Care Unit, Division of Pulmonary, Allergy and Critical Care Medicine, Department of Medicine, University of Massachusetts Medical Center, Worcester, MA USA

**Mark M. Wilson, MD**
Assistant Professor of Medicine,University of Massachusetts Medical School; Associate Director, Medical Intensive Care Unit, University of Massachusetts Medical Center, Worcester, MA, USA

**Ian J. Witterick, MD**
Assistant Professor, University of Toronto, Mount Sinai Hospital, Toronto, Ontario, Canada

# Preface

Respiratory symptoms are among the most common reasons for which patients seek medical care. Yet, there has not been an attempt in the medical literature to approach the management of all of these symptoms in a comprehensive, systematic manner. This book was written to fill what we perceived was a void and a need.

The National Ambulatory Medical Care Survey published in 1993 by the U.S. Department of Health and Human Services[1] showed that respiratory system-related symptoms were the most common symptoms for which patients made office visits in 1991, accounting for approximately 20% of the total. Other common system-related symptoms are shown in Table I. This survey summarized data from an estimated 669.7 million patient visits to nonfederally employed, office-based physicians during the 12-month period from January 1991 through December 1991.

This survey also revealed that five respiratory complaints were among the 12 most common symptoms for which patients sought medical care (Table II).[1] Cough was first; symptoms referable to the throat, second; headache/pain in head, eighth; nasal congestion, eleventh; and nasal discharge, twelfth.

Although patients with respiratory diseases usually seek medical attention complaining of a symptom, textbooks of the respiratory system (and for that matter, all systems) have been disease-oriented rather than symptom-oriented. Even though disease-oriented scholarly works are important, we do not believe that this focus accurately reflects the patient/physician interaction. Patients complain of symptoms, not diseases, and physicians primarily determine the disease that is causing the patient's problem by taking a history that begins with the patient's chief complaint.[2]

Even though research regarding the management of respiratory symptoms has been modest and predominantly limited to cough and dyspnea, it has shown that when these symptoms have been evaluated and treated in a systematic manner they can be successfully diagnosed and treated in most cases.[3-12] On the other hand, when these symptoms, as well as others, have not appeared to have been managed in such a systematic fashion, their causes have not been determined in the majority[13] and they have remained persistently troublesome to the patient.

By utilizing what we have learned about managing cough and dyspnea, and applying this management framework to other respiratory symptoms, we and our contributors hope that this book has filled the void left by other scholarly works and has allowed for all respiratory symptoms to be successfully diagnosed and treated in a consistent manner by all health care practitioners. It has been written with the intent to deal systematically and comprehensively with chest pain, cough, dyspnea, hemoptysis, wheeze, nasal obstruction/rhinorrhea/postnasal drip, hoarseness, sneeze, epistaxis, hiccough, facial pain and headache, snoring, anosmia, halitosis, sore throat, and globus sensation. By virtue of the fact that the individual chapters reflect the existing literature, they vary in length and breadth.

The management strategy that we have used throughout this book is as follows: (1) understand the basic anatomy and physiology that relate to each symptom; (2) determine the intrinsic and extrinsic influences that can cause the symptom; (3) evaluate first for the most common diseases that cause the symptom; (4) identify a limited number of diagnostic tests that in combination with the history and physical examination can identify the common causes while screening for the less common causes; (5) develop an effective and cost-efficient rationale for treating the specific causes of the symptom; and (6) apply nonspecific treatments only when specific therapy is not available.

**Table I**

Spectrum/Frequency of Symptoms by System for Which Patients Sought Medical Care in the Office Setting in the United States in 1991

| Reason for Visit | % of Sxs |
|---|---|
| Sxs referable to the respiratory system | 19.8% |
| Sxs referable to the musculoskeletal system | 19.7% |
| Sxs of a general nature | 11.4% |
| Sxs referable to the skin, hair, and nails | 11.3% |
| Sxs referable to the eyes and ears | 11.2% |
| Sxs referable to the genitourinary system | 8.1% |
| Sxs referable to the digestive system | 7.0% |
| Sxs referable to the nervous system | 5.4% |
| Sxs referable to psychological/mental disorders | 4.7% |
| Sxs referable to the cardiovascular/lymphatic system | 0.8% |

Sxs = symptoms; % = percent.
Adapted from Schappert SM. National ambulatory medical care survey: 1991: Summary. In *Vital and Health Statistics* (No. 230) U.S. Department of Health and Human Services, March 29, 1993, p. 7.

The strategy to manage each of the symptoms of the respiratory tract applies to students of the health sciences, and to all who care for patients from nurse practitioners, physician assistants, and physicians in training to primary care specialists, allergists, otolaryngologists, and pulmonologists. While the book is meant to be clinically oriented and useful from a management standpoint, it is based upon sound, scientific principles.

**Table II**

Spectrum/Relative Frequency of Symptoms of Which Patients Sought Medical Care in the Office Setting in the United States in 1991

| Reason for Visit | Relative Frequency |
|---|---|
| Cough | 1 |
| Symptoms referable to the throat | 2 |
| Earache or ear infection | 3 |
| Back symptoms | 4 |
| Skin rash | 5 |
| Stomach pain, cramps, and spasms | 6 |
| Fever | 7 |
| Headache/pain in head | 8 |
| Vision dysfunctions | 9 |
| Knee symptoms | 10 |
| Nasal congestion | 11 |
| Head cold/nasal discharge | 12 |
| Neck symptoms | 13 |
| Depression | 14 |

Adapted from Schappert SM. National and ambulatory medical care survey: 1991: Summary. In *Vital and Health Statistics* (No. 230) U.S. Department of Health and Human Services, March 29, 1993, p. 7.

We are indebted to many who have helped in the production of this book. Our administrative assistants, Karol Lempicki and Adele Orlans, and Cynthia French, Coordinator of our division's clinical programs at the University of Massachusetts Medical Center, helped us manage busy professional lives and carve out the substantial time needed to write and edit. Steven Korn and Jacques Strauss at Futura Publishing Company provided encouragement and support throughout the entire 1-year process. Our families provided unfailing love and support. To these, and the many others who offered help, encouragement, and advice, we are deeply grateful.

*R.S. Irwin, MD*
*F.J. Curley, MD*
*R.F. Grossman, MD*

## References

1. Schappert SM. National ambulatory medical care survey: 1991: Summary. In: *Vital and Health Statistics*. No. 230. U.S. Department of Health and Human Services, March 29, 1993: 1–20.
2. Peterson MC, Holbrook JH, Hales DV, Smith NL, Staker LV. Contributions of the history, physical examination, and laboratory investigation in making medical diagnoses. West J Med 1992; 156: 163–165.
3. Irwin RS, Corrao WM, Pratter MR. Chronic persistent cough in the adult: the spectrum and frequency of causes and successful outcome of specific therapy. Am Rev Respir Dis 1981; 123: 413–417.
4. Irwin RS, Curley FJ, French CL. Chronic cough: the spectrum and frequency of causes, key components of the diagnostic evaluation, and outcome of specific therapy. Am Rev Respir Dis 1990; 141: 640–647.
5. Poe RH, Israel RH, Utell MJ, et al. Chronic cough: bronchoscopy or pulmonary function testing? Am Rev Respir Dis 1982; 126: 160–162.
6. Poe RH, Harder RV, Israel RH, et al. Chronic persistent cough: experience in diagnosis and outcome using an anatomic diagnostic protocol. Chest 1989; 95: 723–728.
7. Holinger LD, Sanders AD. Chronic cough in infants and children: an update. Laryngoscope 1991; 101: 596–605.
8. Pratter MR, Bartter T, Akers S, et al. An algorithmic approach to chronic cough. Ann Intern Med 1993; 119: 977–983.
9. Hoffstein V. Persistent cough in nonsmokers. Can Respir J 1994; 1: 40–47.
10. Pratter MR, Curley FJ, Dubois J, et al. Cause and evaluation of chronic dyspnea in a pulmonary disease clinic. Arch Intern Med 1989; 149: 2277–2282.
11. DePaso WJ, Winterbauer RJ, Lusk JA, et al. Chronic dyspnea unexplained by history, physical examination, chest roentgenogram, and spirometry: analysis of a seven-year experience. Chest 1991; 100: 1293–1299.
12. Martinez FJ, Stanopoulos I, Acero R, et al. Graded comprehensive cardiopulmonary exercise testing in the evaluation of dyspnea unexplained by routine evaluation. Chest 1994; 105: 168–174.
13. Kroenke K, Mangelsdorff AD. Common symptoms in ambulatory care: incidence, evaluation, therapy, and outcome. Am J Med 1989; 86: 262–266.

# Table of Contents

# Cough

Richard S. Irwin, M.D.

## Introduction

The sound of a cough is easy to identify by the human ear. The initial cough sound is formed by a compression phase followed by an expiratory phase and most resembles mechanisms used to form plosive phonemes in speech.[1] Phoneme refers to one of the sounds that make up a language. Plosive phonemes (sounds) result from a complete closure of the vocal tract, a build up of pressure, and a sudden release of air.

Healthy people rarely cough during wakeful hours and especially during sleep and when they do, it is essentially devoid of any clinical significance. For instance, in a lecture room, a group of 100 healthy people will cough on average only 2.5 times per minute.[2] Presumably, those few "healthy" individuals who coughed had the common cold. The lesser frequency of cough during sleep compared to wakefulness in normals as well as in patients with chronic bronchitis and emphysema is likely due to higher thresholds to coughing stimuli during sleep.[3] However, when cough is present and persistent, it can assume great clinical significance. Cough may be an important defense mechanism that helps clear excessive secretions and foreign material from the airway; it can be an important factor in the spread of infection; and it is one of the most common symptoms for which patients seek medical attention and spend health care dollars.

In a national medical care survey in the United States in 1991, cough was the most common complaint for which patients sought medical attention and the second most common reason for a general medical examination.[4] Moreover, the common cold, the most common condition that afflicts mankind, is almost always accompanied by cough (Figure 1).[5] Referrals of patients with persistently troublesome chronic cough of unknown causes have been shown to account for 10% to 38% of a pulmonologist's outpatient practice.[6,7]

Treatment of cough is responsible for a substantial amount of health care dollars. For instance, in 1981, more than 800 nonprescription and nearly 100 prescription remedies promising relief of cough were available to be purchased by Americans.[8] The expenditure for the over-the-counter cough suppressant drugs designed to modify rather than eliminate cough has been estimated to exceed $1 billion annually.[8a]

Why do patients with cough seek medical attention so frequently and spend

From Irwin RS, Curley FJ, Grossman RF (eds): Diagnosis and Treatment of Symptoms of the Respiratory Tract. Armonk, New York, Futura Publishing Company, Inc., © 1997.

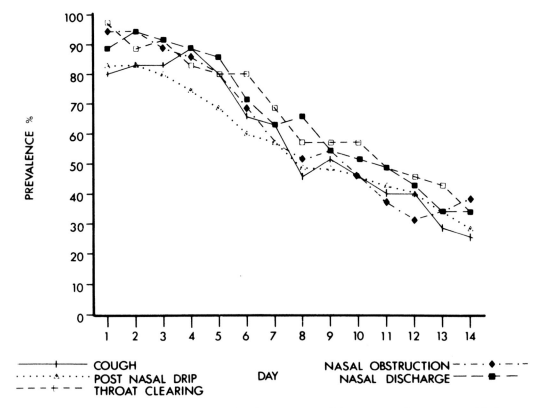

**Figure 1.** The prevalences of the five cardinal symptoms of the untreated common cold. (Reproduced with permission from Curley FJ, Irwin RS, Pratter MR, et al. Am Rev Respir Dis 1988; 138: 305–311.)

so much money for cough medications? They do so because cough can substantially and significantly affect their quality of life in adverse ways.[9] The more common reasons why patients with chronic cough seek medical attention appear in Table I. Based upon these findings, it is inappropriate to minimize a patient's complaint of cough and/or advise them to "live with it" as is too frequently done.[7]

The purpose of this chapter is to comprehensively review the anatomic, physiologic, and etiologic aspects of cough, as well as mechanisms whereby cough may be ineffective or even harmful. A systematic, diagnostic approach of evaluating patients with cough is presented and treatment discussed. Lastly, the use of voluntary coughing as a means of providing cardiopulmonary resuscitation will also be reviewed.

## Anatomy of the Cough Reflex

Each cough involves a complex reflex arc. The reflex begins with stimulation of a receptor. Impulses from these receptors are conducted to a central area by way of afferent nerves. The function of this central area is to receive these impulses and to produce a cough by passing impulses down appropriate efferent nervous pathways to the diaphragm and laryngeal, thoracic, and abdominal musculature. Like any reflex, once started, it proceeds according to a fixed pattern. The receptors, afferents, "cough center," and efferents will be discussed individually (Figure 2). It must be noted that the anatomy of the cough reflex presented has been constructed from clinical observations in case reports in humans as well as from animal

**Table I**
Reasons Why Patients with Chronic
Cough Seek Medical Attention

| Reason(s) | Frequency (%) |
|---|---|
| Something's wrong | 98 |
| Exhaustion | 57 |
| Self-conscious | 55 |
| Insomnia | 45 |
| Lifestyle change | 45 |
| Musculoskeletal pain | 44 |
| Hoarseness | 43 |
| Excessive perspiration | 42 |
| Urinary incontinence | 39 |
| Dizziness | 38 |
| Fear of cancer | 33 |
| Headache | 32 |
| Fear of AIDS or tuberculosis | 28 |
| Retching | 21 |
| Vomiting | 18 |
| Nausea | 16 |
| Anorexia | 15 |
| Syncope/near-syncope | 5 |

Lifestyle change includes curtailing speaking on the telephone, not going to church or the symphony, no longer singing in the church choir, and not going out socially for fear of becoming incontinent of feces as well as urine. Urinary incontinence is most common in women but may also occur in men who have undergone prior transurethral prostatectomy; it can be so frequent and severe that patients have to wear diapers. Musculoskeletal pain most commonly originates from muscle trauma but may also be due to rib fractures. (Modified from Irwin RS, Curley FJ. The treatment of cough: a comprehensive review. Chest 1991; 99:1477–1484.)

studies; therefore, it may not be anatomically exact. For instance, cough receptors have been placed in the upper respiratory tract even though they have not been identified there; and the trigeminal, glossopharyngeal, and phrenic nerves have been included as afferent nerves subserving the cough reflex along with the vagus nerve even though there are no experimental data to support this.

## Laryngeal and Tracheobronchial Receptors

Histologic studies of the respiratory tract in both animals and humans[10–14] have revealed nerve endings within the epithelium of the larynx, trachea, and bronchi. They have been found to be most numerous on the posterior wall of the trachea, at the carinae and at points of bronchial branching of large airways, and less numerous in the more distal smaller airways; none have been found beyond the respiratory bronchioles.

In animals, irritation of receptive areas in the lower respiratory tract by mechanical, chemical, thermal, and electrical stimuli have all been reported to cause cough.[15] In humans, experimental evidence suggests that two types of receptors, mechanical and chemical, are clinically important.[16–21] Mechanical receptors, those sensitive to touch and displacement, are concentrated in the larynx, trachea, and carinae and become progressively less numerous more distally in the tracheobronchial tree. Their location and function correlate with the clinical observations that patients undergoing bronchoscopy cough vigorously when the larynx and central airways are touched,[22] but patients undergoing transbronchoscopic lung biopsy cough less commonly when the more distal airways and lung parenchyma are biopsied. Chemical receptors, those sensitive primarily to noxious gases and fumes, are concentrated more in the larynx and bronchi than in the trachea. Although both mechanical and chemical receptors become less sensitive when subjected to continuous stimulation, the mechanical receptors adapt more rapidly.[17,18] Adaptation of mechanical receptors is seen frequently in patients who are able to tolerate prolonged endotracheal intubation without anesthesia.

Many studies point to the receptors for cough belonging to the general group of rapidly adapting irritant receptors found in the mucosa of the larynx and tracheobronchial tree.[23–25] Once activated, they cause rapidly adapting impulses in an irregular pattern to be conducted in the relatively fast-velocity vagal-myelinated nerve fibers. While rapidly adapting irritant receptors appear to be primarily responsible for coughing, other receptors such as the slowly adapting lung stretch

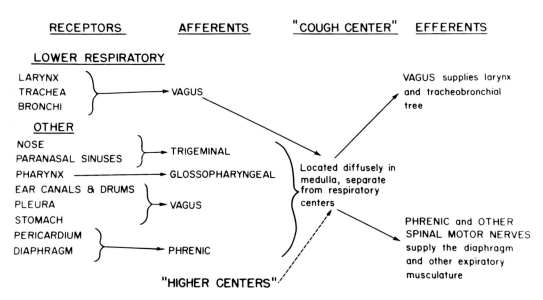

**Figure 2.** Anatomy of cough reflex. This schema represents an amalgamation of clinical observations in humans and histological and physiological results in experimental animal studies. (Reproduced with permission from Irwin RS, Rosen MJ, Braman SS. Arch Intern Med 1977; 137: 1186–1191. Copyright 1977, American Medical Association.)

receptors may also interact. Although these latter receptors do not respond directly to chemical and mechanical triggers, they appear to be activated by the deep initial breath of a cough and enhance cough by making the expiratory effort more forceful.[26] While C-fiber receptors with nonmyelinated vagal afferent fibers are activated by similar triggers as the rapidly adapting receptors, they do not appear to participate directly in cough. Indeed, in experimental animals, they inhibit cough.[27]

## All Other Receptors

Outside of the lower respiratory tract, cough receptors have been demonstrated histologically only in the pharynx.[15] However, it is inferred that they must exist in other sites since mechanical stimulation of the external auditory canals and eardrums, paranasal sinuses, pharynx, diaphragm, pleura, pericardium, and stomach has been reported to cause cough.[28–33] Whereas laryngeal and tracheobronchial

receptors appear to be irritated by both chemical and mechanical stimuli,[21] receptors in other sites most probably respond only to mechanical triggers.[21,28]

## Afferents

After stimulation of a cough receptor, impulses are conducted by the vagus and perhaps trigeminal, glossopharyngeal, and phrenic nerves to the central nervous system.

Irritation of tracheobronchial receptors initiates impulses in the pulmonary branches of the vagus nerve.[21] It appears that these impulses run through the ipsilateral nerve. This was demonstrated in patients with advanced bronchogenic carcinoma in whom transection of one vagus nerve between the origin of the pulmonary plexus and recurrent laryngeal nerves was found to reduce cough.[34] When a bronchoscope was subsequently introduced into the mainstem bronchus on the side of the vagotomy, cough was not induced. The same procedure performed on the other side resulted in violent coughing. Other branches of the vagus nerve may also carry impulses and produce cough.[29] These include the auricular branch (Arnold's nerve) conducting impulses from the external acoustic canal and eardrum; pharyngeal branches from the pharynx; superior laryngeal branch from the larynx; gastric branches from the stomach; pulmonary branches from the pleura; and cardiac and esophageal branches from the diaphragm. Impulses may also be carried in the glossopharyngeal nerve from the pharynx; the phrenic nerve from the pericardium[29]; and the trigeminal nerve from the nose and paranasal sinuses.[35]

Since cough may be voluntarily initiated, postponed, or suppressed, there may be afferent input from higher centers. Of all the complex defensive reflex mechanisms, cough appears to be unique in that it is the only one that can be voluntarily reduplicated in its entirety.

In addition to traveling to the "cough center," afferent impulses may stimulate secretion of mucus from airway submucosal glands.[36,37] This would serve as a physicochemical protective barrier against irritant chemicals as well as enhance the clearance of substances from the airways (see Pathophysiology section of this chapter).

## Central Pathway

The existence of a discrete central "cough center" is controversial. Evidence from experimental and animal studies suggests that afferent impulses are integrated into a coordinated cough response in the medulla oblongata of the brain stem, probably separate from the medullary centers that control breathing.[38] When neural structures above the medulla are ablated, cough can still be produced; but when the medulla is ablated also, cough cannot be produced.[39] Electrical stimulation studies of different areas in the medulla suggest that the "cough center" is diffusely located. However, even though electrical microstimulation of multiple areas of the medulla evokes a cough response,[40–43] a discrete "cough center" may still exist since these studies may have simultaneously stimulated the afferent limb of the cough reflex.[43] Identification of a discrete "cough center," if it exists, must await a better experimental approach.

Afferent fibers for coughing first relay in or near the nucleus of the tractus solitarius and the motor outputs are in the ventral respiratory group. The nucleus retroambigualis sends motorneurons to the respiratory muscles; and nucleus ambiguus, to the larynx and bronchial tree.[26]

## Efferents

The efferent impulses of the cough reflex are transmitted to the expiratory musculature including the diaphragm through the phrenic and other spinal motor nerves and to the larynx through the recurrent laryngeal branches of the vagi.[44] Vagal efferents also supply the tracheobronchial tree and mediate bronchial smooth muscle constriction which is believed to assist the cough effort by increasing the velocity of air flow.[21,45] Teleologically, bronchoconstriction may also serve another function; it may lessen the inflow of tussigenic material to deeper parts of the tracheobronchial tree.

Experiments in decerebrate cats have shown that these efferent pathways are anatomically distinct from those involved in normal spontaneous ventilation.[46] The clinical correlate to this was seen in a patient who underwent bilateral high cervical cordotomy and in whom spontaneous ventilation was severely impaired. Although his maximum vital capacity was only 200 mL, he coughed vigorously in response to tracheal stimulation and exhaled volumes up to 1500 mL.[46]

## Physiology

While the typical cough that originates in the tracheobronchial tree will be described in detail in this section, it is important to appreciate that the pattern of cough can vary depending on the site of initiation.[47] When cough is triggered from the tracheobronchial tree, it begins with a pronounced inspiration. When triggered from the larynx, cough may proceed without the inspiration. Since greater intrathoracic pressures (due to longer expiratory muscles) and expiratory flow rates can be achieved at high lung volumes, cough effectiveness is enhanced when cough begins with an inspiratory phase.

It is believed that there are usually four phases involved in the cough mechanism[47] (Figure 3). The first is an inspiratory phase which ends before closure of the glottis; the second is a compressive phase that is characterized by contraction of thoracic and abdominal musculature against a fixed diaphragm; the third is an expiratory phase which consists of the rapid expulsion of air when the glottis opens; and the fourth phase is the cessation of cough. The result of these actions is the production of sufficiently high expiratory velocity to dislodge and expel secretions or foreign bodies. The first three phases have been likened by Coryllos[48] to the three phases in the firing of a gun: "the inspiratory phase to the loading of the gun, the compressive phase to the deflagration of powder and production of gases under pressure, and the expiratory phase to the ejection of the bullet from the barrel of the gun."

## Inspiratory Phase

Cough is usually preceded by a deep inspiration. This initial inspiration is im-

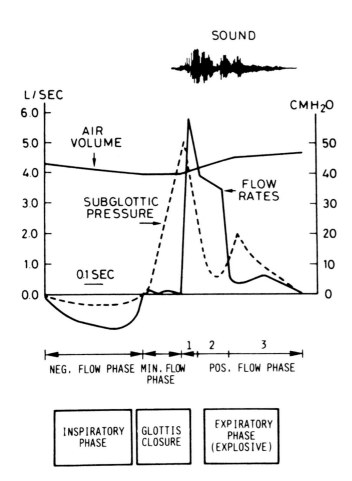

**Figure 3.** Schematic representation of changes in flow rate, intrathoracic volume, subglottic pressure, and sound during inspiratory, compressive, and expiratory phases of a typical cough. (Reproduced with permission from Bianco S, Robuschi M. Mechanics of cough. In: *Cough,* Braga PC, Allegra L, eds. Raven Press, New York, NY: Raven Press; 1989: 29–36.)

portant in producing an effective cough by permitting both expiratory pressure and flow to be maximal during the ensuing expiration.[49] This high–lung volume allows maximum expiratory flow rates by increasing static elastic recoil, the driving pressure, and by decreasing frictional resistance.[50,51]

During this phase of cough, the glottis opens widely as a result of contraction of the abductor muscles of the arytenoid cartilages.[52] This widens the airway opening between the vocal cords and permits the rapid entry of large amounts of air into the lungs. As the lower ribs become fixed by contraction of the thoracic and abdominal muscles as well as the diaphragm, the vertical and lateral dimensions of the chest increase with concomitant increase in lung volume.[53,54] Bronchographic studies have demonstrated that this change in lung volume is accompanied by an increase in caliber and an apparent lengthening of the bronchi caused by the unrolling of the spiral arrangement of the bronchial tree.[55–58]

## Compressive Phase

The compressive phase of cough begins with the closure of the glottis, continues with the active contraction of the expiratory muscles, and ends with the sudden opening of the glottis. It is during this phase that intrathoracic pressure is raised sufficiently to produce flow rates necessary for effective cough.

After a deep inspiration, the glottis rapidly and firmly closes through the actions of the adductor muscles of the arytenoid cartilages.[14,52,59] This completely occludes the larynx for approximately 0.2 seconds, trapping the previously inspired air within the thorax.[60] Although glottic closure is an integral part of the compressive phase, it is not essential for the production of an effective cough.[61] This is because the muscles of expiration are the most important determinant in producing elevated intrathoracic pressures and are capable of doing so even with an open glottis. For example, humans and animals

with tracheostomy or endotracheal tubes in place and patients with laryngeal infection or inflammation have been observed to cough effectively with an open glottis.

After closure of the glottis, the diaphragm contracts, rendering the base of the chest cavity rigid.[48] The action of the contracting thoracic and abdominal muscles is to pull the chest wall down and compress the trapped air in the chest against the fixed diaphragm.

## Expiratory Phase

It is during this phase that the function of cough is carried out; that is, the removal of undesired material from the respiratory tract. The coordinated movements of the glottis, respiratory muscles and tracheobronchial tree all contribute to this most important phase of the cough mechanism.

The expiratory phase of cough is initiated by the opening of the glottis, with the explosive release of the trapped intrathoracic air. As the vocal cords gradually separate, the width of the larynx diminishes at the level of the aryepiglottic folds.[62] Because of these dynamic changes, the vocal cords and the mucosal lining of the posterior laryngeal wall vibrate, shaking secretions loose from the larynx.[62]

While dynamic changes are taking place in the larynx, the same thoracic and abdominal muscles that were active during the compressive phase of cough contract further. The continued shortening of these muscles after the opening of the glottis serves to maintain the rapid flow of air by ensuring a high-pressure gradient between the intrathoracic airways and the mouth. Numerous studies have noted that maximum intrathoracic pressures during a cough occur after the opening of the glottis, attesting to the contribution of the expiratory muscles in maintaining high pressures, and therefore, high flow.[63–65] In fact, these muscles produce pleural pressures far in excess of those required to produce maximum flow.[66] These data lend further support to the observation that cough can be effective in patients who are unable to close their glottis.

The diaphragm also plays an important role in regulating the expiratory phase of cough. With the opening of the glottis, the diaphragm relaxes allowing the increased intra-abdominal pressure to be transmitted to the lung.[54] The degree to which the diaphragm relaxes determines the extent of the transmission of these pressures to the chest. Consequently, it does not directly assist in the expulsion of air from the lungs, but rather, regulates the forces brought to bear upon the chest.[48]

Along with the larynx and expiratory musculature, the tracheobronchial tree also undergoes dynamic changes that ensure an effective cough. The single most important parameter in the production of an effective cough is the linear velocity of the moving column of air.[60,66,67] The determinants of linear velocity are described by the following formula:

$$\text{Velocity} = \frac{\text{Flow}}{\text{Cross-sectional area}}$$

Since the velocity of the air stream (distance per unit time) increases directly with flow (volume per unit time), and inversely with the cross-sectional area of the airway in question, an effective cough depends primarily on a small cross-sectional area and high flow rates.[66]

Since cross-sectional area of the tracheobronchial tree becomes progressively larger with each generation of bronchi, the linear velocity of the air stream will be greatest in the trachea and large bronchi and progressively diminish in smaller airways. Consequently, this anatomic consideration indicates that cough will be most effective in clearing secretions in the larger airways where the total cross-sectional area is least. Probably more important in maintaining the small cross-sectional area is the dynamic compression that the tracheobronchial tree undergoes during the forced expiration.[66] It is the high–pleural or intrathoracic pressures produced by the contraction of the expiratory muscles that cause this compression. While studies in animals, as well as in normal man, have shown that this compres-

sion occurs most often in larger airways not located beyond segmental or third-generation bronchi, the site of dynamic compression can be influenced by lung volume.[68,69] Coughing at high–lung volumes will cause dynamic compression of larger airways while coughing at lower lung volumes should cause dynamic compression of smaller airways. In light of this, Macklem[66] has postulated the following series of events. During a series of coughs beginning with full inspiration, secretions are first cleared from the larger airways; as lung volume decreases with successive coughs, the secretions are moved from the smaller bronchi into successively larger ones. Following another deep breath and series of coughs, the secretions from all the airways are eventually eliminated. It is interesting to note that those airways in which cough is most effective in clearing secretions are the same airways that have the largest population of cough receptors sensitive to mechanical stimuli. Thus, the locations where cough is most likely to be evoked are the same areas that are most likely to be effectively cleared.

In addition to a small cross-sectional area, high flow is also an important determinant in producing an effective cough.[60] Since flow decreases as lung volume diminishes[66] and since maximum flows are achieved with only moderate muscular effort for any given lung volume,[70] it is clear that the most important factor necessary for achieving high flow rates is the initial deep breath of a cough. In addition to affecting the cross-sectional area of the airways, dynamic compression limits flow rates through these areas by increasing airway resistance.[69] Although this does not interfere with the cough mechanism in normal subjects, it may assume clinical significance in certain disease states that will be discussed.

## Cessation Phase

The cessation of cough begins with relaxation of the expiratory muscles. Expiratory flow rates become submaximal as abdominal, pleural, and alveolar pressures drop toward ambient pressure. "The glottis may close as the final event; there may be, instead, a voiced "huh" sound or simply quiet cessation of flow as antagonistic activity of inspiratory and expiratory muscles and elastic recoil of the respiratory system come into balance and alveolar pressure falls to ambient pressure."[47]

## Pathophysiology

Cough is an important defense mechanism that helps (1) clear excessive secretions and foreign material from the airways and (2) prevent foreign material from entering the lower respiratory tract. It is a reserve clearance mechanism to mucociliary transport and becomes operative when mucociliary clearance is overwhelmed or made inadequate due to an underlying disease such as chronic bronchitis.[71,72] When cough does not adequately serve its protective roles, adverse consequences can occur such as gas exchange abnormalities, atelectasis, pneumonia, lung abscess (Figure 4), bronchiectasis, and pulmonary fibrosis.

Cough effectiveness in clearing an airway theoretically depends on having secretions of sufficient thickness to be affected by two-phase gas-liquid flow[73] (Figure 5) and the linear velocity of air passing through its lumen.[66,73] In healthy people, voluntary coughing has been shown to be ineffective in clearing tagged particles from the lower respiratory tract. This is probably due to the moving stream

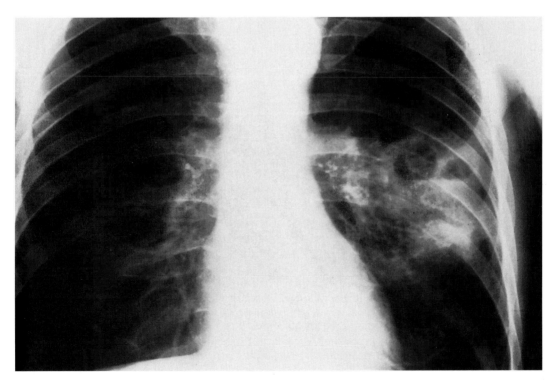

**Figure 4.** Lung abscess secondary to aspiration of a piece of fingernail. The chest roentgenograms (A and B) show a *Staphylococcus aureus* infected lung abscess in the superior segment of the left lower lobe. It developed there following aspiration of a fingernail (C), discovered at bronchoscopy, in a 55-year-old alcoholic, inveterate nail biter while he was lying supine in bed. It was likely that an alcoholic stupor depressed the patient's cough reflex, making it ineffective in preventing the fingernail from entering the lower respiratory tract and clearing it before it became lodged in the superior segmental bronchus.

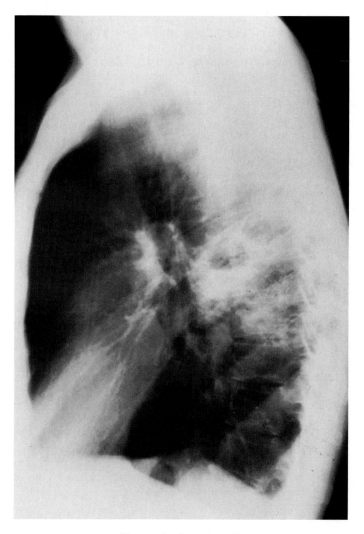

**Figure 4.** *(continued)*

of air being unable to interact adequately with the normally thin layer of mucus on which the particles were deposited.[74,75] However, once there is sufficiently thick mucus and/or material to be expelled from the airways, as occurs in patients with lung disease in which mucus is either overproduced and/or undercleared (eg, chronic obstructive pulmonary disease, asthma, bronchiectasis, pneumonia), cough effectiveness depends on a high expiratory flow rate of air and a small cross-sectional area of the airway to achieve a high linear velocity (distance traveled by gas molecules per unit of time). The relationship of these variables are described on page 8.

All clinically significant disorders that mitigate a cough's effectiveness interfere with the inspiratory or expiratory phases of cough, with most conditions adversely affecting both (Table II).[26] Disorders or interventions that might predominantly affect the compressive phase in a negative way are probably not clinically important.[25] For instance, although vocal cord closure is an important component of the compressive phase, it is not essential

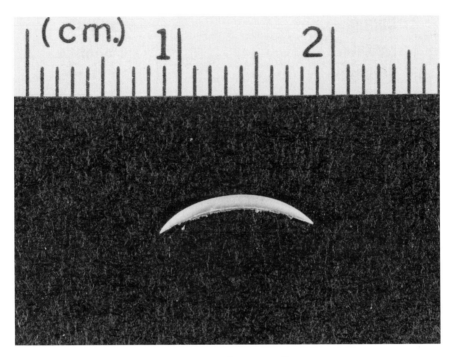

**Figure 4.** *(continued)*

for the production of an effective cough pressure.[76] The muscles of expiration appear to be the most important determinant in producing elevated intrathoracic pressures,[77] and they are capable of doing so even when an endotracheal tube is in place.[78]

### Ineffective Cough Due To Extrapulmonary Conditions

Numerous central and peripheral nervous system disorders, chest wall and respiratory muscle diseases, and upper airway conditions may cause cough to be ineffective as a clearance mechanism (Table II).[26] Because expiratory flow rates are directly related to lung volume and because greater expiratory muscle pressures are produced at high lung volumes as a result of enhancement of respiratory muscle length-tension relationships,[66,73] the inability or reluctance to take an initial deep breath and/or to give a forceful expiratory effort will place a patient at risk of producing an inadequate cough velocity. Without the initial breath and the strong expiratory effort, expiratory flow rates and dynamic compression of airways will be inadequate.

Patients with costochondritis, multiple rib fractures, acute surgical abdomens, and postoperative thoracic or upper abdominal incisions may have an ineffective cough because inspiratory and expiratory efforts are often limited to avoid pain.[79–83]

Diseases that lead to paralysis or weakness of the respiratory muscles theoretically can compromise cough effectiveness for the same pathophysiological reasons.[26] Compromised coughing has been seen in a variety of neuromuscular diseases, such as transection of the spinal cord,[84,85] Guillain Barré syndrome,[86,87] amyotrophic lateral sclerosis,[88,89] muscular dystrophy,[90] poliomyelitis,[85] and myasthenia gravis.[91,92] Based upon studies performed in healthy curarized subjects,[77] it appears that expiratory muscle weakness will most likely decrease cough effectiveness by reducing cough-induced

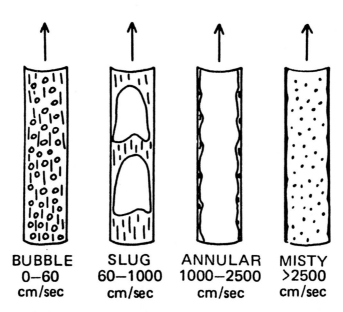

**Figure 5.** Main types of two-phase gas-liquid flow, with corresponding surface velocity of air. The range of velocities taken from the engineering literature applies to large rigid tubes and ordinary Newtonian fluids.[26] Although mucus is a non-Newtonian fluid, these examples help explain how airflow during coughing may move liquid in the form of excessive secretions. When flow rates are low, air will move through secretions as small bubbles; this is likely to occur at air velocities less than 60 cm/sec. As flow rates increase, bubbles increase in size and form plugs or slugs of air in the secretions; this is likely to occur at air velocities between 60 and 1000 cm/sec. Annular flow is a term that describes air passing through the secretions as a central wavelike core; this is likely to occur at air velocities between 1000 and 2500 cm/sec. Misty flow describes liquid carried as fine droplets in air; it occurs at air velocities greater than 2500 cm/sec. Because there is little interaction between air and liquid during bubble and annular flow, these types of flow are not likely to be effective in clearing secretions during coughing. Because air velocities usually easily exceed 2500 cm/sec in the central airways during dynamic compression, secretions in these airways are cleared by cough as mist or aerosols. (Reproduced with permission from Reference 73, p. 566. Courtesy of Marcel Dekkar, Inc.)

dynamic compression of the airways rather than decreasing expiratory flow rates.

Patients rendered unconscious by central nervous system disease, drug overdose, or general anesthesia will have central depression of the cough reflex,[26,93] thereby interfering with the inspiratory as well as expiratory phases of cough. Although there will not be any limitation to expiratory flow in a patient with a variable extrathoracic upper-airway obstructing lesion, cough effectiveness may theoretically become impaired if inspiratory flow limitation mitigates the patient's ability to take a sufficiently large initial breath.[94]

## Ineffective Cough Due to Pulmonary Conditions

Intrinsic pulmonary diseases can also impair a cough's clearance function (Table II).[26] These disorders are associated with decreased expiratory flow rates or excessive amounts of secretions. Both factors may be operative in asthmatic patients.[66,95] For instance, inflammation, edema, and smooth muscle contraction can cause narrowing of the airways, increasing resistance during inspiration and expiration. Thick, sticky secretions may obstruct the lumens of airways and completely occlude them. This combination,

## Table II
### Conditions Associated With an Ineffective Cough

*Extrapulmonary Disorders*
Pain
  Costochondritis
  Rib fractures
  Acute surgical abdomen
  Postoperative thoracic/abdomen incisions
Paralysis/weakness of respiratory muscles
  Transection of spinal cord
  Guillain-Barré syndrome
  Amyotrophic lateral sclerosis
  Muscular dystrophy
  Poliomyelitis
  Myasthenia gravis
Depression of cough center
  CNS disease
  Drug overdose
  Sedation
  General anesthesia
Extrathoracic upper airway obstruction

*Pulmonary Disorders*
Asthma
Cystic fibrosis
Chronic bronchitis and emphysema
Bronchiectasis
Tracheobronchomegaly
Intrathoracic upper airway obstruction
  Extrinsic compression lesion
  Endoluminal mass
  Airway stricture
  Small tracheostomy/endotracheal tube

All of these disorders either have been shown to interfere with cough effectiveness or may theoretically do so. While this listing is comprehensive, it is not meant to be exhaustive and all inclusive. CNS = central nervous system.

perhaps superimposed on respiratory muscle fatigue, can severely diminish expiratory flow rates. Due to tenacious secretions and debilitation preventing vigorous respiratory efforts, cough in cystic fibrosis patients may be similarly compromised.[61] In some patients with chronic bronchitis and emphysema, bronchiectasis, and the rare disorder of tracheobronchomegaly, expiratory flow rates may be further decreased due to a disproportionately greater dynamic compression of the larger, more central airways (eg, trachea, main-stem, and lobar bronchi).[56,64,65,96–102] These more central airways may undergo a much greater reduction in lumen size for a given change in transmural pressure than do the same airways in an asthmatic subject or a healthy subject due to an inherent increase in their compliance or compressibility.[66,97,99]

Theoretically, patients with saccular and varicose bronchiectasis may not be able to effectively clear secretions by coughing without postural drainage because there is no airflow through the blind sacs of the bronchiectatic segments and these sacs are distal to the more central airways undergoing dynamic compression.[26,101] It has also been postulated[66] that coughing in patients with saccular bronchiectasis may be more effective if it occurs at low lung volumes, because coughing at low lung volumes should cause dynamic compression of smaller airways.

Lastly, central obstructing intrathoracic lesions, such as an extrinsic compressing mass, endobronchial lesion, bronchial stricture, foreign body, or even a small tracheostomy tube may cause cough to be ineffective by reducing expiratory flow rates.[26,61]

## Determining the Effectiveness of Cough

From a physician's standpoint, it would be useful to be able to reliably predict when an individual patient has an ineffective cough, thereby placing the patient at risk of developing substantial gas exchange abnormalities, atelectasis, pneumonia, lung abscess, bronchiectasis, and pulmonary fibrosis. Unfortunately, there are no studies that have been published to predict cough effectiveness.[26] Data are few and have been generated in patients with muscular dystrophy[90] and myasthenia gravis[92]; they have suggested that maximal expiratory mouth pressure (MEP) measurements may be useful for assessing cough strength. Unfortunately, these measurements were not correlated with any clinical outcomes. In patients with muscular dystrophy,[90] using the absence of peak flow transients (Figure 6) during cough flow-volume curves to indicate inadequate expiratory muscle strength to dynamically compress the airways during coughing, the investigators found that the MEP was the most sensitive predictor of flow transient production during coughing. Patients who produced transients had MEP values greater than 60 cm $H_2O$ and all patients who could not produce transients had MEP values equal to or less than 45 cm $H_2O$. This latter value is consistent with clinical observations in patients with myasthenia gravis[92] in whom values less than 40 cm $H_2O$ were frequently associated with a difficulty in raising secretions without endotracheal suctioning.

## Complications of Coughing

During vigorous coughing, intrathoracic pressures up to 300 mmHg[103] and expiratory velocities up to 28,000 cm/sec or 500 miles per hour[104] (ie, 85% of the speed of sound) may be generated. While pressures and velocities of these magnitudes allow coughing to be an effective means of providing cardiopulmonary resuscitation (see last section of this chapter), they also can cause a variety of cardiovascular, central nervous system, gastrointestinal, musculoskeletal, respiratory, and miscellaneous complications (Table III).

## Cardiovascular Complications

Cough may be considered a modified Valsalva maneuver.[73,105] During the compressive and expiratory phases of cough, high intrathoracic pressures are generated and may impede systemic venous return and cause decreased cardiac output, arterial hypotension, and systemic venous hypertension. Arterial hypotension may cause loss of consciousness.[103,105–110] The increase in systemic venous pressure may cause rupture of subconjunctival, nasal, and anal veins [54,103]; it may also lead to dislodgment or malfunction of intravascular catheters.[111,112] Since cough may also

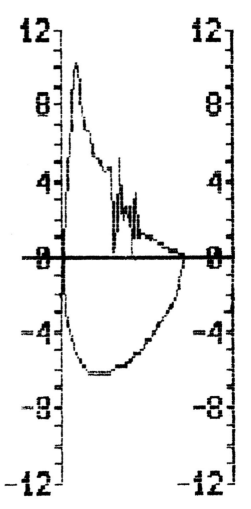

**Figure 6.** Cough flow-volume curve. The spikes seen in the cough flow-volume curve are called peak flow transients. They are thought to represent air that is rapidly displaced from the intrathoracic airways during dynamic compression. It follows that the dynamic compression briefly adds a spike of flow to the otherwise sustained maximal expiratory flow of air leaving the lungs. These transients are considered essential for achieving linear velocities of sufficient magnitude to clear secretions from the airways. Their absence implies a weak and probably ineffective cough. (Adapted from Irwin RS, Widdicombe RG. Cough. In: *Textbook of Respiratory Medicine*, Volume 1, 2nd edition. Murray JR, Nadel JA, eds. Philadelphia, Pa: WB Saunders Company; 1994:534.)

## Table III
### Complications of Cough

*Cardiovascular*
- Arterial hypotension
- Loss of consciousness
- Rupture of subconjunctival, nasal, and anal veins
- Dislodgement/malfunctioning of intravascular catheters
- Brady/Tachy-arrhythmias

*Neurological*
- Cough syncope
- Headache
- Cerebral air embolism
- Cerebrospinal fluid rhinorrhea
- Acute cervical radiculopathy
- Malfunctioning ventriculoatrial shunts
- Seizures
- Stroke due to vertebral artery dissection

*Gastrointestinal*
- Cough-induced gastroesophageal reflux events
- Hydrothorax in peritoneal dialysis
- Malfunction of gastrostomy button
- Splenic rupture
- Inguinal herniation

*Gastrourinary*
- Urinary incontinence
- Inversion of bladder through urethra

*Musculoskeletal*
- Ranges from asymptomatic elevations of serum creatine phosphokinase to rupture of rectus abdominis muscles
- Rib fractures

*Respiratory*
- Pulmonary interstitial emphysema, with potential risk of
  pneumatosis intestinalis
  pneumomediastinum
  pneumoperitoneum
  pneumoretroperitoneum
  pneumothorax
  subcutaneous emphysema
- Laryngeal trauma
- Tracheobronchial trauma (eg, bronchitis, bronchial rupture)
- Exacerbation of asthma
- Lung herniation

*Miscellaeneous*
- Petechiae and purpura
- Disruption of surgical wounds
- Constitutional symptoms
- Lifestyle changes
- Self-consciousness, hoarseness, dizziness
- Fear of serious disease
- Decrease in quality of life

be accompanied by a reflex increase in vagal tone, reflex bradycardia and second- or third-degree heart block may occur.[113] This increase in vagal tone may also abolish aberrant conduction in patients with supraventricular tachycardia by delaying conduction across the atrioventricular node.[114] Although the mechanism is unclear, cough has also been reported to induce nonsustained ventricular tachycardia[115] and a supraventricular tachycardia.[115a]

## Neurological Complications

Neurological complications may be expressed centrally and peripherally. Cough syncope was first described by Charcot in 1876 and has been the subject of numerous clinical reviews.[108–110, 116–118] While a number of mechanisms have been proposed to explain cough syncope, it is likely that cough syncope results from a combination of cardiovascular and neurological processes. Although a decrease in cardiac output during cough may lead to cerebral anoxia and loss of consciousness, this hemodynamic mechanism by itself does not explain the sudden syncope sometimes seen with cough. A more plausible explanation is that sudden rises in cerebrospinal fluid pressure, transmitted from intrathoracic and intra-abdominal pressures, may have the same effect as a cerebral concussion.[108,110,117] Or, if syncope is less sudden, it may be explained by a decrease in cerebral blood flow from the transmission of high intrathoracic pressures to the subarachnoid space. While syncope or near syncope due to coughing may occur with a frequency of approximately 5% in patients with persistently troublesome cough referred to a cough clinic (Table I), cough as a cause of syncope in general is much less common.[119] Cough syncope has been most commonly reported in middle-aged, cigarette-smoking men.[110] The typical patient is obese, large-chested and strong, and usually suffers from a mild, chronic-obstructive pulmonary disorder. Attacks may begin with a bout of coughing or be initiated by eating, drinking, or laughing.[109] While these patients have usually not had other comorbid conditions, scattered case reports have suggested that patients with cough syncope may also have other conditions that place them at risk of syncope. These conditions have included marked stenosis of both common carotid arteries,[118] idiopathic hypertrophic subaortic stenosis,[120] and congenital herniated cerebral tonsils.[121] The entire episode, from the initial paroxysm of cough to return of consciousness, usually lasts less than 1 minute.[108] Even though patients may have as many as 30 attacks per day, this condition is usually benign, with only a few fatalities reported in patients with severe cardiovascular disease.[110]

Headache induced by cough is also known as benign cough headache, a variant of benign exertional headache.[122–124] It presents as an intermittent, usually bilateral, severe bursting or explosive pain brought on by coughing. It can be located in the area of the vertex, frontal, or temporal regions. This headache comes on a few seconds after coughing and lasts approximately 1 minute. Before considering this headache to be benign, structural lesions, such as posterior fossa tumors, must be excluded. The pathogenesis of this headache is unknown.

Other neurological complications include cerebral air embolism as a consequence of barotrauma,[125] cerebrospinal fluid rhinorrhea,[126] acute cervical radiculopathy due to cervical disc herniation,[127] malfunctioning ventriculoatrial shunts caused by the circulatory dynamics of coughing,[111] stroke due to vertebral artery dissection,[127a] and seizures.[128] In patients with cough-induced seizures, it is important to exclude abnormalities of the brain and cerebral blood vessels as comorbid conditions that may be at the root of this complication.

## Gastrointestinal Complications

Cough and gastroesophageal reflux have been linked in a cause and effect relationship. Gastroesophageal reflux disease (GERD) is one of the most common causes of chronic cough, and cough can induce GER events[129] most likely by altering gastroesophageal transmural pressure changes that favor reflux. Cough has also been reported to facilitate hydrothorax in peritoneal dialysis,[130] and to cause malfunction of gastrostomy button,[130a] spontaneous splenic rupture,[130b] and inguinal herniation.[130c]

## Genitourinary Complications

Clinical observations have suggested why coughing can lead to urinary incontinence[130d] in women and inversion of the bladder through the urethra in children.[130e]

## Musculoskeletal Complications

Musculoskeletal pain is a common symptom of patients complaining of cough for at least a 3-week duration. It occurs with a frequency of about 44% (Table I). Muscle damage may be caused by severe paroxysms of coughing. It may range from the asymptomatic elevation of serum creatinine phosphokinase to the actual rupture of the rectus abdominis muscles.[54,131–137]

The clinical presentation of hemorrhage into the rectus sheath can mimic an intra-abdominal emergency. Typically, there is the sudden onset of abdominal pain, nausea, vomiting, and the sudden appearance of an abdominal mass that is often tender. The mass remains fixed and easily palpable during voluntary contraction of the rectus muscle. This last sign distinguishes a process involving the rectus abdominis muscle from an intraperitoneal condition. The drop in hematocrit signifies the hemorrhagic nature of the process. The pathogenesis of rectus sheath hematoma involves rupture of the rectus abdominis muscle itself or the arterial supply to the muscle. The arterial supply includes the superior epigastric artery, a branch of the internal mammary, and the inferior epigastric artery, a branch of the external iliac. In addition to trauma from the vigorous muscle contractions of coughing, rectus sheath hematoma has also been associated with anticoagulation therapy, collagen vascular diseases, blood dyscrasias, previous surgical procedures, degenerating disorders of muscles, and other forms of trauma associated with vigorous muscle contractions such as exercise, straining, delivery, and sexual intercourse. The diagnosis can be easily confirmed by real-time ultrasonography or an abdominal computed tomography scan.

Patients with cough are also susceptible to the development of spontaneous rib fractures.[138–142] While the true incidence is unknown, fractures due to chronic coughing have been estimated in patients with pulmonary tuberculosis to range from 0.73% to 6.5%.[142] In patients without pulmonary tuberculosis, cough has been found to be the cause of chest pain 7.6% of the time.[142] Most fractures occur at the lateral portion of the rib, where the serratus anterior and latissimus dorsi interdigitate with the external oblique muscles. Presumably, repeated stresses of cough may produce a small, undetectable rib fracture that my extend as cough continues. This observation may explain the chest wall discomfort experienced by many patients for several days prior to the detection of the rib fracture. Cough fractures have been reported in every rib with the uppermost and lowermost ribs being least commonly involved.[142] Underlying metabolic bone diseases have not been found to be a significant predisposing factor in the development of these fractures in adults even though they have been implicated in infants.[140] Since cough fractures are not usually displaced, serious complications are unusual. However, when these fractures become displaced, pneumothorax, hemothorax, major subcutaneous hemorrhage requiring blood transfusion, lung contusion, and flail chest may occur and may place the patient in a potentially life-threatening situation.[142,143]

## Respiratory Complications

Severe or prolonged coughing may lead to pulmonary interstitial emphysema.[145,146] After the rupture of alveolar walls, air escapes into interstitial tissue where it may dissect along perivascular and peribronchial tissue planes and lead to pneumatosis intestinalis, pneumomediastinum, pneumoperitoneum, pneumoretroperitoneum, pneumothorax, and subcutaneous emphysema. In adults, pneumomediastinum usually leads to subcutaneous emphysema and is almost always of no serious consequence. However, when it leads to pneumoperitoneum and pneumoretroperitoneum and simulates the presentation of a ruptured viscus, it assumes clinical significance.[147] In neonates, on the other hand, pneumomediastinum may not lead to subcutaneous emphysema and may cause circulatory collapse and death.[144]

Trauma from the high pressures and expiratory velocities of cough can cause an extrathoracic, variable upper airway obstruction due to vocal edema[5,148,149] as well as erythema and edema of the tracheobronchial tree.[54] Moreover, rupture of the bronchus has been reported from bronchoscopy during a paroxysm of coughing.[150] The effect of coughing on asthma is variable. Results of a recent questionnaire given to 187 asthmatics[151] indicated that while coughing appeared to cause an exacerbation of symptoms in approximately 42%, it may have brought relief, probably related to clearing the airways of excessive phlegm, in approximately 30% of the 187 asthmatics. Coughing appeared to have no effect in approximately 10% of the 187 asthmatics, and it inconsistently either brought relief or exacerbated asthma in approximately 18%. Coughing can also cause spontaneous lung herniation beyond the confines of the thoracic cavity.[151a,151b]

While protracted coughing has been implicated as a potential factor in the pathogenesis of pulmonary emphysema in the past,[152–154] support for this theory in recent years has not been forthcoming.[155] Advocates of this theory believe that the disruption of alveolar walls and elastic elements of the lung is caused by air trapped behind obstructed airways.

## Miscellaneous Complications

Adverse occurrences in this group of complications include the following: petechiae and purpura[156]; disruption of surgical wounds[54]; constitutional symptoms such as insomnia, exhaustion, anorexia, vomiting, sweating, and rise in body temperature due to the heat generated during vigorous muscle contractions associated with frequent coughing[54]; lifestyle changes[148]; exhaustion, self-consciousness, hoarseness, and dizziness (Table I); and fear of serious disease.[9]

The impact of the complications of cough on patients is to significantly decrease their quality of life.[9] Consequently, it behooves all physicians to be as knowledgeable as possible about how to diagnose and treat cough that is persistently troublesome.

## Diagnostic Evaluation of Cough

### Historical Perspective

A systematic manner of evaluating patients with cough was first proposed in 1977.[149] It was based upon evaluating the locations of the afferent limb of the cough reflex and was called an anatomic, diagnostic approach. At its core was the evaluation by history, physical examination, and laboratory testing of the anatomy of the afferent limb of the cough reflex (Figure 7). The inception of this approach to evaluating cough came from a review of animal histologic data, case reports of clinical observations in man, and a few prospective epidemiological studies. From this review, it was reasoned that cough could be caused by a multiplicity of diseases located in a variety of anatomic locations and that extrapulmonary as well as pulmonary diseases needed to be routinely considered as potential causes. This approach has led to the recognition that extrapulmonary conditions, such as postnasal drip syndrome (PNDS) and GERD, commonly cause persistent cough.

The duration of cough was first proposed in 1981 as the criterion for prospectively evaluating the usefulness of the anatomic, diagnostic protocol.[6] A duration of 3 weeks or more was chosen as the definition of chronic cough as a way of separating out most patients who had the transient cough of the common cold (Figure 1), the most common condition afflicting

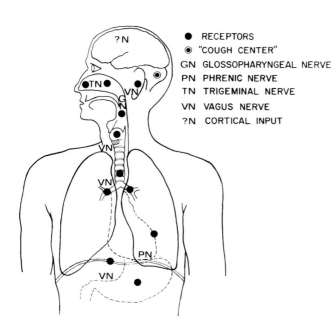

RECEPTORS
"COUGH CENTER"
GN GLOSSOPHARYNGEAL NERVE
PN PHRENIC NERVE
TN TRIGEMINAL NERVE
VN VAGUS NERVE
?N CORTICAL INPUT

**Figure 7.** Schematic representation of the anatomy of the cough reflex. This schematic representation comes from an amalgamation of clinical observations in man, and histological and physiological results in experimental animal studies. While it may not be anatomically exact, it has been found to be clinically useful. See the previous section "Anatomy of the Cough Reflex" for further discussion. (Reproduced with permission from Irwin RS, Rosen MJ, Braman SS. Arch Intern Med 1977; 137: 1186–1191. Copyright 1977, American Medical Association)

## Table IV
## Classification of Cough as a Symptom

ACUTE
- Lasting less than 3 weeks
- Most commonly transient and of minor consequence (eg, common cold)
- Occasionally potentially life-threatening (eg, pulmonary embolism, congestive heart failure, pneumonia)

CHRONIC
- Lasting 3 weeks or more

Based upon its duration, cough has been divided into two categories. Since an acute cough may become chronic, the categories are not mutually exclusive.

mankind, from patients with other more persistently troublesome conditions. From this study, a classification of cough as a symptom according to its duration was validated (Table IV). From a symptom standpoint, cough can be divided into two categories that are not mutually exclusive. It can be acute, lasting less than 3 weeks, or chronic, lasting 3 weeks or more. Acute cough is most commonly transient and of minor consequence as in the common cold; however, it could occasionally be potentially associated with life-threatening conditions, such as in pulmonary embolism, congestive heart failure, and pneumonia. Or acute cough can persist and become a chronic problem. Because there are patients with respiratory infections (eg, pertussis) more severe than the common cold who complain of cough for longer than 3 weeks and have it spontaneously disappear by 8 weeks, some authors have chosen to withhold a diagnostic workup for 4 or 8 weeks.[157]

Since 1977, a great deal has been learned about managing patients complaining of cough. This knowledge has primarily come from studies that have been faithful to the anatomic, diagnostic approach and studies that have been performed in North America in **immunocompetent** adults in university and community hospital settings and in children in tertiary care settings.

## Expected Results Utilizing the Anatomic, Diagnostic Protocol

Utilizing the anatomic diagnostic protocol and treatment guidelines initially established in 1981[6] and then modified in 1990,[7] the cause of chronic, persistent cough can be determined from 88% to 100% of the time with treatment success rates between 84% and 98%.[6,7,157–161] In the two studies with poorer rates of success, the authors appeared to have used treatment protocols other than those that have been consistently shown by others to be successful.[162,163]

While cough is most commonly due to a single cause (73% to 82%), it can be due to multiple causes in about one-fourth of cases (Figure 8).[6,7] Moreover, multiply-caused cough has been reported to have three explanations up to 8% of the time.[7]

Most smokers have a cough, but they have not been the group of patients who most commonly seek medical attention complaining of cough.[6,7]

In children older than 1 year old,[159] adults of all ages,[6,7] and the elderly,[164] PNDS, asthma, and GERD are the three most common causes of chronic cough (Figure 9).

In prospective studies,[6,7] chronic cough in adults has been due most commonly (91% to 94%) to four disorders (Figure 8): PNDS, asthma, GERD, and chronic bronchitis.

In prospective studies,[6,7,165] chronic cough has been uniformly due to three disorders—PNDS, asthma, and/or GERD—in adults with the following profile: (1) nonsmoker; (2) not taking an angiotensin-converting enzyme inhibitor (ACEI) drug; and 3) normal chest roentgenogram or one that shows nothing more than inconsequential, stable scarring.

Chronic cough can be the sole clinical manifestation of asthma and GERD up to 57%[6] and 75%[165] of the time, respectively. Nonspecific pharmacologic bronchoprovocation challenge testing and prolonged (24-hour) esophageal pH monitoring have been shown to be singularly useful in diagnosing these conditions.

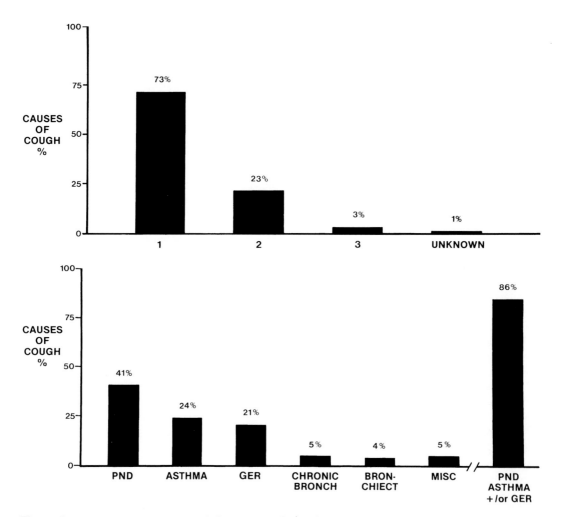

**Figure 8.** Representative causes of chronic cough in adults. (A) The cause of chronic cough was prospectively determined in 99% of patients; it was due to a single cause in 73% and multiple causes in 26%. (B) The spectrum and frequency of the 131 causes. (PND = postnasal drip syndrome; GERD = gastroesophageal reflux disease; bronch = bronchitis; bronchiect = bronchiectasis; misc = miscellaneous). The miscellaneous conditions included bronchogenic carcinoma in two patients; left ventricular failure in one patient, stage 3 pulmonary sarcoidosis in one patient, ACEI in one patient, and aspiration from a Zenker's diverticulum in one patient. (Reproduced with permission from Irwin RS, Curley FJ, French CL. Am Rev Respir Dis 1990; 141: 640–647.)

Fiberoptic bronchoscopy in adults will have a very low diagnostic utility (approximately 4%)[6,7] unless the chest roentgenogram is abnormal. However, this is an uncommon occurrence (approximately 5%).

The principal strength of the anatomic, diagnostic protocol is in ruling out suspected possibilities (Table V).[7] The principal limitation is that a positive test cannot necessarily be relied upon to establish the diagnosis[7]; a positive test has not been able to consistently predict a favorable response to "specific therapy." For example, the negative and positive predictive values of a methacholine inhalation challenge (MIC) have been prospectively reported to be 100% and 60%, respec-

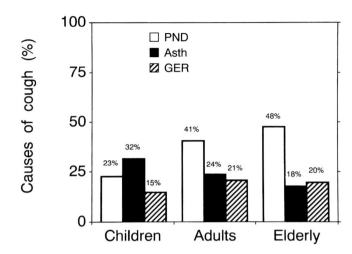

**Figure 9.** Spectrum and frequency of the three most common causes of chronic cough in three age groups. (Asth = Asthma; PND = postnasal drip syndrome; GER = gastro-esophageal reflux disease.)

tively.[7] In other words, when MIC is negative, asthma is essentially ruled out as a cause of cough, except for the patient who may have occupational asthma in its earliest stage.[166,167] However, in the occupational setting, the literature has shown that the test should become positive as the exposure continues. On the other hand, MIC can be falsely positive for predicting that asthma is causing the patient's cough (ie, the cough does not respond to asthma therapy but it does respond to specific therapy for another condition). This has been reported to occur in 22% of patients being evaluated for chronic persistent cough.[7] Therefore, it must be appreciated that a positive test, by itself, without witnessing a favorable response to therapy, is not diagnostic of asthma as the cause of cough.

## Guidelines for Evaluating Chronic Cough in Immunocompetent Patients

The following systematic, diagnostic approach has been validated in chronic cough in immunocompetent patients (Figure 10).

First, review the patient's history and perform a physical examination, concentrating on the anatomy of the afferent limb of the cough reflex and specifically the most common causes of chronic cough (eg, PNDS, asthma, GERD, chronic bronchitis, bronchiectasis, ACEI drug). The character (eg, paroxysmal, loose and self-propagating, productive or dry), sound quality (eg, barking, honking, brassy), or timing (eg, nocturnal, with meals) have not been shown in a prospective study to be of diagnostic help.[168]

Second, order a chest roentgenogram in nearly all patients. It is extremely useful for initially ranking differential diagnostic possibilities and directing laboratory testing. A normal roentgenogram or one which

**Table V**
Testing Characteristics of Anatomic Diagnostic Protocol

| Tests | n | Sens | Spec | PPV | NPV |
|---|---|---|---|---|---|
| Chest x-ray | 100 | 100 | 76 | 36 | 100 |
| Sinus x-ray | 98 | 100 | 79 | 57 | 100 |
| MIC | 86 | 100 | 67 | 60 | 100 |
| BaE | 54 | 48 | 76 | 63 | 63 |
| EPM | 25 | 100 | 100 | 100 | 100 |
| Bronchoscopy | 23 | 100 | 92 | 89 | 100 |

Sens = sensitivity; spec = specificity; PPV = positive predictive value; NPV = negative predictive value; MIC = methacholine inhalational challenge; BaE = barium esophagography; EPM = esophageal pH monitoring for 24-hours. (Adapted from Irwin RS, Curley FJ, French CL. Chronic cough: the spectrum and frequency of causes, key components of the diagnostic evaluation, and outcome of specific therapy. Am Rev Respir Dis 1990; 141:640–647.)

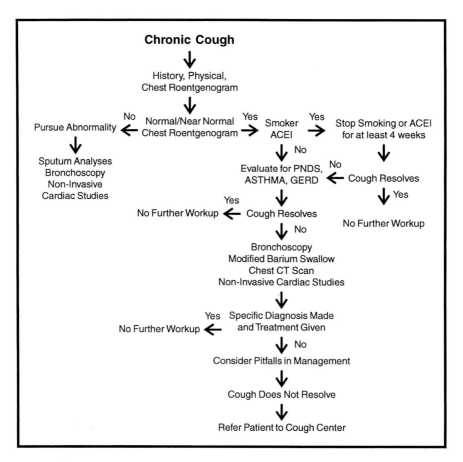

**Figure 10.** Diagnostic algorithm for managing chronic cough. ACEI = angiotensin-converting enzyme inhibitor; PNDS = postnasal drip syndrome; GERD = gastroesophageal reflux disease.

only shows an abnormality consistent with an old and unrelated process (eg, pleural scarring from prior pneumonia) makes PNDS, asthma, and/or GERD likely and makes bronchogenic carcinoma, sarcoidosis, and bronchiectasis unlikely. Chest roentgenograms do not have to be routinely ordered before beginning therapy for presumed PNDS in young nonsmokers or in pregnant women.

Third, do not order additional laboratory tests in present smokers or patients taking an ACEI until the response to cessation of smoking or discontinuation of the drug for 4 weeks can be assessed. Cough due to these causes should substantially improve or disappear during this period of abstinence.[169,170]

Fourth, depending on the results of the initial evaluation, smoking cessation, or discontinuation of the ACEI, the following may be obtained:

1) Sinus roentgenograms and allergy evaluation;
2) Spirometry prebronchodilator and postbronchodilator (BD) or MIC;
3) Barium esophagography (BaE) and/or 24-hour esophageal pH monitoring (EPM);
4) Sputum for microbiology and/or cytology;
5) Fiberoptic bronchoscopy;
6) Chest computed tomography scan;
7) Modified barium swallow;
8) Noninvasive cardiac studies.

Sinus roentgenograms and allergy evaluation are utilized to determine the possible causes of a PNDS; spirometry pre- and post-BD or MIC, asthma; and BaE or 24-hour EPM, "silent" GERD. While BaE is a much less sensitive and specific test than 24-hour EPM in diagnosing GERD as the cause of cough, it may occasionally be singularly helpful in this regard.[165] For instance, BaE can reveal reflux to the thoracic inlet at a time when refluxate from the stomach has a pH value similar to that of the normal esophagus, thus preventing its detection in the esophageal pH tracing. It is important to emphasize that diagnostic testing with BaE or 24–hour EPM for GERD is only recommended in patients who do not have upper gastrointestinal symptoms of GERD (ie, "silent" GERD). It is not indicated for those patients with cough who complain of weekly sour taste in the mouth, regurgitation, or heartburn since the frequency of these complaints is, by itself, indicative of GERD. If the chest roentgenogram is normal or shows nothing more than inconsequential, stable scarring in the immunocompetent patient, the order of tests is as listed above. On the other hand, if the chest roentgenogram is abnormal (eg, shows a mass, or localized/diffuse infiltrate), sputum studies and bronchoscopy should be ordered first. In patients with risk factors for aspiration due to pharyngeal dysfunction, modified barium swallow can be helpful. Unless history, physical examination, or chest roentgenograms suggest a cardiac cause of cough, noninvasive cardiac studies are ordered last. In this latter setting, consider ordering a high-resolution chest computed tomography scan to assess for bronchiectasis not suggested by routine chest roentgenograms before ordering cardiac studies.

Fifth, determine the cause(s) of cough by observing which specific therapy eliminates cough as a complaint. If the evaluation suggests more than one possible cause of cough, therapies should be initiated in the same sequence that the abnormalities were discovered. Since cough can be simultaneously caused by more than one condition, do not stop therapy that ap- pears to be partially successful; rather, sequentially add to it.

The role of empiric therapy in diagnosing the cause of chronic cough has not been rigorously studied. Nevertheless, it is reasonable to consider when PNDS, asthma, and/or GERD are likely possibilities and MIC and prolonged EPM studies are not available or cannot be performed. The setting in which these three conditions are extremely likely is as follows[165]: a patient has a chronic cough, is a non-smoker, is not taking an ACEI, and has a normal or near-normal chest roentgenogram. The success or failure of empiric therapy for these three common conditions will depend on which empiric treatment is chosen (eg, all $H_1$ antagonists are not equal); this will be discussed below.

## Guidelines for Evaluating Chronic Cough in Immunoincompetent Patients

While a systematic diagnostic approach has not been validated in these patients, guidelines similar to immunocompetent patients are likely to be helpful. The major modification to the algorithm in Figure 10 that is recommended is the active assessment by oximetry and blood $CD_4$ counts for the possibility of pulmonary parenchymal disease in the setting of a normal chest roentgenogram. For example, if oxygen saturation with exercise does not fall to 90% or less[165a,165b] or if blood $CD_4$ lymphocyte counts are greater than 200/cumm (.200 $\times$ $10^9$/L),[165c] it is unlikely that a clinically significant opportunistic lung infection in HIV positive patients is present and evaluation for such can be initially withheld.

## Guidelines for Evaluating Acute Cough

A clinical approach is recommended for evaluating acute cough; it consists of history, physical examination, and the estimated frequency of conditions. The most prevalent causes are the common cold, acute bacterial sinusitis, pertussis, exacerbation of chronic obstructive pulmonary disease, allergic rhinitis, and environmental irritant rhinitis. Less common causes include asthma, congestive heart failure, infectious pneumonia, aspiration syndromes, and pulmonary embolism.

## Differential Diagnosis and Pathogenesis of Cough

Cough can be caused by a multiplicity of disorders located in a variety of locations (Table VI).[171-257] Table VI has been constructed to highlight the fact that the causes of cough can be anatomically categorized. It is not meant to be exhaustive since literally hundreds of diseases can cause cough. Rather, the common and the most unusual and rare conditions have been selected as representatives of the spectrum of reported causes of cough. Because virtually any condition that stimulates cough receptors or afferent nervous pathways is capable of producing cough, only the most common will be discussed below in detail.

With respect to pathogenicity of cough, there are limited data which do not appear, at this time, to support one common unifying mechanism. For example, while excessive mucus production may lead to cough by mechanically stimulating the afferent limb of the cough reflex and extraluminal masses by compressing/distorting submucosal airway receptors, an increased sensitivity of the afferent limb of the cough reflex appears to be an important pathogenetic mechanism common to patients who have a nonproductive cough due to a variety of diseases (eg, asthma, upper respiratory infection, GERD, and ACEIs).[163] In this latter group, when there is improvement in cough with specific therapy, cough sensitivity assessed by capsaicin cough challenge has returned to normal.[163]

### Acute Cough

As previously defined, acute cough is less than 3 weeks in duration. While there are no published studies on the spectrum and frequency of causes of acute cough, clinical experience supports in overwhelming terms that upper respiratory tract infections are the most common causes of the acute, transient cough. Almost every person in the world has experi-

---

**Table VI**
Anatomic Categorization of the Causes of Cough

| Location | Disorder |
| --- | --- |
| CNS | Giles de la Tourette's disease[171-173] |
| | Psychogenic cough tic[174-177] |
| Head and Neck | Common cold[5] |
| | ACEI[170,178] |
| | Rhinitis/Sinusitis[6,7,148] |
| | Rhinolith[179] |
| | Nasal polyps[28,180] |
| | Elongated uvula[181] |
| | Enlarged, infected tonsils[181] |
| | Ear conditions[182-185] |
| | Neurilemmoma of vagus nerve[186] |
| | Neuroma internal laryngeal nerve[187] |
| | Aneurysm of ascending palatine artery[188] |
| | Osteophytes of cervical spine[188] |
| | Laryngeal disorders[189] |
| | *Syngamus laryngeus* infection[190,191] |
| | Thyroiditis[192] |

**Table VI**
**(*continued*)**

| Location | Disorder |
|---|---|
| Intrathoracic Airway Diseases | Asthma[6,7,157–161,193–195] |
| | Chronic bronchitis[6,7,169] |
| | Bronchiectasis[7] |
| | Bronchiolitis[196–200] |
| | Bronchogenic carcinoma[7,201,202] |
| | Foreign bodies[203,204] |
| | Inhaled medications[205,206*] |
| | Broncholith[207,208] |
| | Bronchial carcinoid[209–211] |
| | Sjogren's syndrome with xerotrachea[212,213] |
| | Endobronchial suture[214–216] |
| | Bacterial tracheitis[217] |
| | Herpetic tracheobronchitis[218,219] |
| | Influenza[220] |
| | *Klebsiella rhinoscleromatis* infection[221] |
| | Pertussis[222] |
| | Mycoplasma tracheobronchitis[223,224] |
| | Endobronchial tuberculosis[225,226] |
| | Aspergillus tracheobronchitis[227,228] |
| | Wegener's granulomatosis[229] |
| | Ulcerative colitis[230–232] |
| | Aspiration[233,234] |
| | Endobronchial sarcoidosis[235] |
| | Relapsing polychondritis[236,237] |
| Parenchymal Diseases | Metastatic carcinoma[6] |
| | Chronic interstitial pneumonia[238,239] |
| | Infectious pneumonia[240,241] |
| Mediastinal Masses | Neural tumors[242] |
| | Thymoma[243] |
| | Teratoma[244] |
| | Intrathoracic goiter[245] |
| | Bronchogenic cyst[159] |
| | Hodgkin's disease[246] |
| Cardiovascular Disease | Mitral stenosis[188,247] |
| | Left ventricular failure[188,247] |
| | Pulmonary embolism[248] |
| | Enlarged left atrium[249] |
| | Vascular ring[159,188] |
| | Aberrant innominate artery[159] |
| | Aortic aneurysm[28,247] |
| | Pericardial stimulation by transverse pacemaker[250] |
| Upper Gastrointestinal | Gastroesophageal reflux[6,7,165,251–253] |
| | Esophageal cyst[254] |
| | Tracheoesophageal fistula[28,159] |
| Pleural Conditions | Pneumothorax[54] |
| | Effusion[54] |
| | Thoracentesis[255–257] |
| Diaphragm | Stimulation by Transvenous Pacemaker[250] |

* Inhaled medications appear to provoke cough by irritating the larynx and/or tracheobronchial tree. CNS = central nervous system; ACEI = angiotensin-converting enzyme inhibitor.

enced such a cough at one time or another. The prevalence of cough without any treatment ranges from 83% within the first 48 hours to 26% on day 14. During a 14-day period, the prevalence is similar to that of postnasal drip, throat-clearing, nasal obstruction, and nasal discharge. Cough is significantly correlated with the presence of a reversible, extrathoracic, upper airway obstruction. Cough appears to arise from stimulation of the cough reflex in the upper respiratory tract by postnasal drip, throat-clearing, or both.

The diagnosis of the common cold is usually certain when patients present in the following manner: they develop an acute upper respiratory illness characterized by symptoms and signs referable predominantly to the nasal passages (eg, rhinorrhea, sneezing, nasal obstruction, and postnasal drip) with or without fever, lacrimation, and irritation of the throat, and they will have a normal physical examination of the chest. In this setting, diagnostic testing is not indicated because it is of such low yield. For instance, in immunocompetent patients in this setting, chest roentgenograms will be normal greater than 97% of the time.[257a] On the other hand, when immunocompromised patients, especially those with acquired immunodeficiency syndrome (AIDS) or at risk of AIDS, present with acute cough, pneumonia with a variety of organisms such as *Pneumocystis carinii* and *Mycobacterium tuberculosis* should be suspected early in the work-up, even when the physical examination and chest roentgenogram are normal. If oxygen saturation falls with exercise, pneumonia with these organisms, as well as other disorders involving the lower respiratory tract, should be vigorously pursued with other studies, such as induced sputa and bronchoscopy with bronchoalveolar lavage and transbronchoscopic lung biopsy.

Acute cough can also be the presenting manifestation of a disease that can be potentially life-threatening, such as pneumonia,[240,241] congestive heart failure,[188,247] pulmonary embolism,[248] or conditions that predispose to aspiration.[233,234] It is especially important to have a high index of suspicion for these disorders in the elderly patient with acute cough because the classic signs and symptoms of these diseases may be nonexistent or minimal. For example, because fever is frequently absent in the elderly with pneumonia,[258] a new onset of cough, especially when accompanied by either tachypnea or altered mental status and an abnormal physical examination of the chest, should raise the suspicion of pneumonia and warrant ordering a chest roentgenogram. It is often not appreciated that approximately 50% of patients with documented pulmonary embolism will complain of cough,[248] and that cough can occasionally be the predominant complaint. Consequently, when patients present with acute cough in association with risk factors for thromboembolic disease, pulmonary embolism must be entertained as a diagnostic possibility and evaluated as such. Because aspirated material can stimulate the afferent limb of the cough reflex in the large intrathoracic airways, acute cough may be due to any condition that interferes with normal pharyngeal- or esophageal-swallowing mechanisms or how the respiratory tract defends itself against inhalational assault.[234]

## Chronic Cough

When acute cough persists and becomes a persistently troublesome complaint, it qualifies as a chronic cough. As previously defined, a chronic cough is of more than 3 weeks' duration.

### Postnasal Drip Syndrome

Postnasal drip syndrome is a term that is used when respiratory complaints such as cough, dyspnea, or wheeze are due to postnasal drip.

Postnasal drip syndrome should be suspected as the cause of cough[7] when (1) patients describe the sensation of having something drip down into their throats, nasal discharge, and/or the need to frequently clear their throats; (2) friends/relatives notice that patients frequently clear their throats; or (3) physical examination of the nasopharynges and oropharynges reveal mucoid or mucopurulent secretions and/or a cobblestone appearance of the mucosa. Unfortunately, none of these criteria, by themselves, is very sensitive or specific. In a prospective study,[7] 100% of patients subsequently shown to have a chronic cough due to PNDS either complained of the sensation of postnasal drip, throat-clearing, or nasal discharge and/or had mucus or a cobblestone appearance observed in their oropharynges. However, only when all of these complaints and findings were absent was another cause found. Since postnasal drip and throat clearing are common complaints in the general population and in patients with chronic cough due to other conditions,[7] PNDS is diagnosed when cough responds favorably to specific therapy directed at eliminating the drip.[6,7]

Postnasal drip syndrome is a common cause of chronic cough in all age groups (Figure 9). It is second to asthma as the most common cause in children of all ages,[159] and the most common cause in adults[6,7] and the elderly.[164]

While the pathogenesis of chronic cough due to PNDS is not known for certain, all available data suggest that it arises from stimuli irritating the afferent limb of the cough reflex located in the pharynx and/or larynx.[5,148] The extrathoracic, variable upper airway obstruction that has been consistently observed with chronic cough due to PNDS[148] is most likely due to the act of coughing rather than to the postnasal drip.[5] Our group has speculated that chronic cough from any condition is liable to cause upper airway obstruction, since the act of coughing causes violent undulations of the laryngeal structures at a time when intrathoracic air, under pressures of as much as 300 mm Hg, traverses the vocal cords at velocities approaching 500 mph.[5]

Why only some individuals in the population that have postnasal drip sensation and/or clear their throats have chronic cough while most others do not is not known. Perhaps individuals in the group

### Table VII
### Spectrum and Frequency of PNDS Conditions Causing Cough

| Disorder | Frequency (%)* |
|---|---|
| Sinusitis | 39 |
| Perennial nonallergic rhinitis | 37 |
| Allergic rhinitis | 23 |
| Postinfectious rhinitis | 6 |
| Vasomotor rhinitis | 2 |
| Drug-induced rhinitis | 2 |
| Environmental irritant rhinitis | 2 |

* The combined frequencies of causes is more than 100% because many patients had more than one upper respiratory tract condition simultaneously contributing to the postnasal drip. The drug-induced rhinitis was angiotensin-converting enzyme-induced; the environmental irritant rhinitis was chlorine gas-induced. While gastroesophageal reflux disease (GERD) can irritate the upper respiratory tract and mimic the PNDS, cough in this setting will only resolve with treatment for GERD, not with therapy directed at other causes of PNDS such as those listed above. (Adapted from Irwin RS, Curley FJ, French CL. Chronic cough: the spectrum and frequency of causes, key components of the diagnostic evaluation, and outcome of specific therapy. Am Rev Respir Dis 1990; 141:640–647.)

that coughs also have inflammatory lesions that have sensitized the afferent limb of the cough reflex.

Any condition with the potential of irritating the upper respiratory tract may cause the PNDS. A spectrum of conditions has been reported in a contemporary, prospective study[7] and is tabulated (Table VII).

### Asthma

Asthma should be suspected as the cause of cough[7] when (1) patients complain of episodic wheezing, shortness of breath plus cough, and are heard wheezing; (2) reversible airflow obstruction is demonstrated by pulmonary function testing ($FEV_1$ increases at least 15% from baseline and approaches normal after inhaled beta$_2$-agonist) even in the absence of wheeze; (3) MIC is positive in the presence of normal or near-normal routine spirometry[166] even in the absence of wheeze. Since all that wheezes is not asthma,[259] and the presence of bronchial hyperresponsiveness can falsely predict asthma is the cause of cough,[7,166] the diagnosis of asthma as the cause of cough requires that (1) cough disappear with specific asthma medications, and (2) the patient's clinical course during follow-up observation be consistent with asthma. In this regard, the diagnosis of asthma is not made in any patient who experiences an obvious respiratory tract infection within 2 months prior to examination and testing, and in whom cough and bronchial hyperresponsiveness are transient and self-limited. Nonspecific, pharmacologic bronchoprovocation challenge testing with methacholine chloride or histamine phosphate is extremely helpful in ruling out asthma as a possible cause of cough. While it only has a positive predictive value of 60%,[7] it has a negative predictive value that approaches 100%.[7,166]

While cough can be associated with other respiratory complaints in the symptomatic asthmatic, it commonly is the sole presenting manifestation (ie, cough-variant asthma). In two prospectively evaluated series of patients with chronic cough, cough was the sole symptom in 28%[7] and 57%[6] of the asthmatic groups.

Asthma is a common cause of chronic cough in all age groups (Figure 9). It is the most common cause in children of all ages,[159] the second most common in adults of all ages,[6,7] and the third most common in the elderly.[164]

While the pathogenesis of cough due to asthma is thought to involve stimulation of sensitized afferent nerves in the airways of the lower respiratory tract, the stimuli for coughing are not known. What is known is that the stimuli for cough appear to be different from those for bronchoconstriction[260] and that cough is not necessarily dependent on bronchoconstriction[261] or degree of bronchial hyperresponsiveness (R.S.I., unpublished data, 1992). It is likely that the increased inflammatory process that is an integral part of symptomatic asthma sensitizes multiple types of afferent nerves[262] that subserve the cough reflex.

## Gastroesophageal Reflux Disease

Gastroesophageal reflux disease should be suspected as the cause of chronic cough[7] when (1) patients frequently complain (ie, daily to weekly) of heartburn or a sour taste in their mouths, or (2) upper gastrointestinal contrast roentgenograms demonstrate reflux of barium to the midesophagus or higher, and/or prolonged 24-hour EPM is abnormal in the absence of upper gastrointestinal complaints. The diagnosis of GERD as the cause of cough requires that cough disappears after antireflux therapy. While cough can be associated with upper gastrointestinal symptoms, it commonly is the sole presenting manifestation. In prospectively evaluated patients with chronic cough, cough has been the only symptom in 43%[7] and 75%[165] of the GERD groups. Contrary to common medical dogma, failure to obtain a history of nocturnal coughing should not dissuade one from considering GERD as a potential cause of cough. Cough due to GERD most commonly occurs while the patient is awake and upright, and it usually does not occur or is not noted at all during the night.[251]

Prolonged, 24-hour EPM is extremely helpful in linking "silent" GERD and cough in a potential cause and effect relationship.[7,165,251] Correlation of cough and reflux events is made possible by patients keeping a symptom diary during the monitoring session. The monitoring session can be considered consistent with GERD as the cause of chronic cough when reflux events (acid or alkaline) appear to induce a cough and/or any GERD parameter (eg, percentage of time that pH is less than 4) falls out of the normal physiologic range.[165] It has recently been reported that conventionally utilized diagnostic indices of GERD (eg, percentage of time that pH is less than 4) can be misleadingly normal and that observing GERD-induced coughs can be more frequently helpful.[165]

In all age groups, GERD is a common cause of chronic cough (Figure 9). It is the third most common cause in children of all ages,[159] and the third most common cause in adults of all ages,[6,7] and the second most common cause in the elderly.[164] As with PNDS and asthma, the precise mechanism by which GERD causes cough is not known. While GERD can stimulate cough by irritating the upper respiratory tract without aspiration (eg, larynx/hypopharynx) and by irritating the lower respiratory tract with microaspiration or macroaspiration, GERD appears to most commonly cause chronic cough by stimulating the distal esophagus, perhaps by an esophageal-bronchial reflex.[165,251,253]

Although GER most likely causes chronic cough by stimulating the distal esophagus, the weight of the available data suggests that the acid in gastric juice is not likely to be the sole mediator or trigger of cough in the majority of patients.[165]

### Chronic Bronchitis

Chronic bronchitis, especially from cigarette smoking, is one of the more common causes of chronic cough[6,7] (Figure 8). Dust, fumes, and smoke can theoretically stimulate the afferent limb of the cough reflex as well as nonspecific irritants by inducing inflammatory changes in the mucosa of the respiratory tract, by causing hypersecretion of mucus, and by slowing mucociliary clearance. Chronic bronchitis[263] should be considered when (1) the patient expectorates phlegm on most days during periods spanning at least 3 consecutive months, and such periods have occurred for more than 2 successive years; (2) alternative cough-phlegm syndromes, such as PNDS, asthma, and bronchiectasis, have been ruled out; and/or (3) the patient is known to be exposed to irritating dust, fumes, or smoke. The diagnosis is confirmed when cough goes away after elimination of the respiratory irritant. In cases caused by cigarette smoking, cough has gone away or markedly decreased in 94% of cases after abstinence for at least 4 weeks.[169]

### Bronchiectasis

Although bronchiectasis was not reported as a cause of chronic cough in the first prospective study on chronic cough,[6] it was the fifth most common cause in a second prospective study[7] (Figure 8) . The cough in this condition is likely due to the accumulation of excessive secretions from overproduction or underclearance, or both. While bronchiectasis should be suspected when cough is associated with expectoration of greater than 30 mL of purulent sputum in 24 hours (ie, bronchorrhea) with or without fever, hemoptysis, weight loss, and malaise, it is important to point out that bronchorrhea is not specific for bronchiectasis. In a prospective study, it was due to one cause 38% of the time; two causes 36% of the time; and three causes 26% of the time.[264] Moreover, PNDS was the most common cause of chronic cough with bronchorrhea 40% of the time, asthma 24% of the time, GERD 15% of the time, bronchitis 11% of the time, bronchiectasis 4% of the time, left ventricular failure 3% of the time, and miscellaneous conditions 3% of the time.[264] The plain chest roentgenogram should suggest the diagnosis in greater than 90% of cases.[265] Occasionally, high-resolution, thin-cut computed axial tomography of the chest may be necessary to reveal the bronchiectatic changes.[265]

### Angiotensin-Converting Enzyme Inhibitor-Induced Cough

Chronic cough has been reported to occur with the administration of ACEIs[178]; it has been typically described as being nonproductive and associated with an irritating, tickling, or scratching sensation in the throat. Cough appears to be a class effect of these drugs and not dose-related.[170,178] Although this association was originally reported with captopril, it has since been seen with all the ACEIs in clinical use.[266,267] When cough is experienced by a patient with use of one ACEI, it usually develops when another ACEI is tried.[268]

Although the frequency of cough associated with ACEIs has been reported to vary widely, from 0.2% to 33%,[269] chronic cough was prospectively reported to be due to ACEIs 2% of the time.[7] Cough has been reported to appear within a few hours of taking a first dose in many patients, but it may not become apparent for weeks or even months.[269]

The time course for recurrence and resolution of cough has been prospectively studied in a randomized, double-blind, placebo-controlled study[170] in patients who had previously experienced an ACEI-induced cough. During the lisinopril rechallenge period, the median time for patients to redevelop cough was 19 days (range 17 to 20 days). The median time to resolution during the placebo washout period was 26 days (range 24 to 27 days).[5]

The pathogenesis of ACEI induced-cough is unknown. It is likely that the cough is related to an accumulation of the inflammatory or proinflammatory mediators bradykinin, substance P, and/or prostaglandins,[170,269,270] and that these mediators in turn increase the sensitivity of the cough reflex.[269,270] Bradykinin and possibly substance P can be inactivated by angiotensin-converting enzyme. Because there is no laboratory test that will predict who will get the ACEI-induced cough, the diagnosis should be considered in any patient who develops a cough after initiation of an ACEI. The diagnosis is confirmed when cough disappears after the drug is discontinued.

## Postinfectious Cough

When patients complain of cough for more than 3 weeks after an acute upper and/or lower respiratory tract infection and have normal chest roentgenograms, some authors have referred to these coughs as postinfectious in causation.[157,158,161] In these studies, the frequency of postinfectious cough has ranged from 11% to 25%. While this cough has been reported to usually resolve on its own in approximately 4 weeks, the authors have occasionally felt the need to prescribe large doses of corticosteroids and antitussive medications and have been impressed that these medications helped in the recovery. Our group

has chosen not to use the terminology of the postinfectious cough because other diagnostic labels, such as PNDS and asthma, seem more appropriate from pathogenetic and treatment standpoints by the time we see such patients. An exception to this is when cough is due to **pertussis**,[222] an ancient disease, that has become more common again and that should be considered in adults as well as children.

The cough due to **pertussis** usually lasts 4 to 6 weeks. As the upper respiratory tract symptoms wane, cough worsens. While adult patients may not display the characteristic inspiratory whoop at the end of a coughing paroxysm, they often vomit with coughing and usually have the typical, initial catarrhal stage followed by paroxysmal and convalescent stages. In addition to this history, additional clues to the diagnosis include leukocytosis and lymphocytosis with mature lymphocytes in an afebrile patient with a normal chest roentgenogram. A nasopharyngeal smear for a direct fluorescent antibody test and culture for *Bordetella pertussis* will confirm the clinical diagnosis if the smear is taken early on in the illness.[222]

## Miscellaneous Diseases

Miscellaneous conditions have comprised no more than 6% of the causes of chronic cough in two prospective studies.[6,7] While they can include virtually any disease (Table VI) that may come in contact with the afferent limb of the cough reflex (Figure 7), the more common causes in the miscellaneous category have included metastatic carcinoma, sarcoidosis, left ventricular failure, aspiration from a Zenker's diverticulum, and bronchogenic carcinoma.

Although the frequency of cough in **bronchogenic carcinoma** varies on initial presentation from 21% to 87%, it occurs in 70% to 90% of these patients during the course of the disease.[271] Those patients with bronchogenic carcinoma who never complain of cough likely have more peripheral tumors arising from smaller bronchi and bronchioles where cough receptors are few in number or even absent. In this regard, it has been observed that peripheral tumors arising from small bronchi and bronchioles may attain large size without producing cough.[271] While cough is generally regarded as a common symptom associated with bronchogenic carcinoma, bronchogenic carcinoma is not a common cause of chronic cough (Figure 8).[6,7157, 158160,161] While it is very unlikely to be the cause of cough in patients with normal chest roentgenograms,[6,7,157,158,160,161,272] one should be suspicious that bronchogenic carcinoma is a potential cause when chest roentgenograms are abnormal and demonstrate centrally located lesions. In addition, in chronic cigarette smokers, coughs that develop for the first time and last for months or that change in character should also be considered suggestive of bronchogenic carcinoma.[272,273]

**Chronic Interstitial Pneumonia:** (eg, idiopathic pulmonary fibrosis) has not been reported as a common cause of chronic cough. Cough, however, has been reported along with breathlessness as a frequent presenting symptom in this disease.[238,239] Since the cause of cough in patients with chronic interstitial pneumonias has not been rigorously evaluated, it is not clear whether or not the chronic interstitial pneumonia is responsible for all or part of these coughs. Should these diseases be shown to cause chronic cough all by themselves, the mechanism may be related to the following: (1) stimulation of cough receptors in smaller airways by the concomitant, intrinsic, small airways disease that has been shown to be frequently present[238,274]; and/or (2) increased pressure and tension on the airways during breathing in the presence of decreased lung compliance.

**Psychogenic** or habit cough is reported to be relatively common,[157,158,160, 161,174–177] particularly in the pediatric population, but in our experience[6,7] it is a rare condition, even in patients with bizarre personalities. While the literature has suggested in the past that patients with psychogenic cough typically do not cough at night and they will have a barking or honking character to their coughs,[174–177] it is evident that the presence or absence of these characteristics is not diagnostically helpful. For instance, cough due to a variety of diseases (eg, chronic bronchitis, GERD) is unlikely to occur once patients fall asleep[3,251] and barking or honking coughs can be due to a variety of diseases (eg, bronchiectasis, GERD, PNDS).[168] Consequently, since there are no distinguishing clinical features and diagnostic tests of a psychogenic cough, it should be considered only after all other possibilities have been excluded. A referral to a specialty cough clinic has been shown to be successful in diagnosing and eliminating cough in all of patients who had been previously told that they would have to live with their cough because the cause could not be determined.[7] Many of these patients had been told that their cough was psychogenic in nature. Since patients with chronic cough seek medical attention because the cough adversely effects their quality of life,[9] every effort should be expended to come up with a specific, treatable cause of cough. It is inappropriate to minimize their complaint and/or advise them to "live with it."

For those interested in reading more about other specific diseases listed in Table VI, references have been provided.

## Treatment

### Overview

The treatment of cough can be divided into two main categories[275,276]: (1) therapy that controls, prevents or eliminates cough (**ie, antitussive therapy**); and (2) therapy that makes cough more effective (**ie, protussive therapy**).

Antitussive therapy can be either **specific** or **nonspecific**.[275,276] It is indicated when cough performs no useful function, such as clearing the airways in an infectious pneumonia. **Specific antitussive therapy** is directed at the causes (eg, smoking cessation in chronic bronchitis) or presumed operant pathophysiological mechanism responsible for cough (eg, eliminating the postnasal drip in allergic rhinitis); by its nature, it has the best chance of being definitive. **Nonspecific antitussive therapy** is directed at the symptom rather than the underlying causes or pathophysiology and aims to control rather than eliminate cough. It is indicated when definitive therapy cannot be given either because the cause of cough is unknown or because definitive therapy has not had a chance to work or will not work (eg, inoperable lung cancer).

Following utilization of an anatomical diagnostic protocol, **specific antitussive therapy** for chronic cough has been reported to have a success rate of between 84% and 98% (Figure 11).[6,7,157–161]. Because of the high probabilities of being able to determine the cause of cough and prescribe specific treatment that can be successful, there is a limited role for **nonspecific antitussive therapy**.[275,276]

**Protussive therapy** is indicated when cough performs a useful function and needs to be encouraged (eg, bronchiectasis, cystic fibrosis, pneumonia, postoperative atelectasis). However, there are no data that have convincingly demonstrated that any protussive agent is clinically useful.

## Specific Antitussive Therapy

Specific treatment for cough depends upon the cause; only the most common conditions will be discussed below in detail.

### Postnasal Drip Syndrome

Specific therapy for PNDS depends on the cause of the postnasal drip.[6,7] For instance, allergic, perennial nonallergic, postinfectious, environmental irritant, and vasomotor rhinitis can be treated with intranasal corticosteroids, or an antihistamine-decongestant (eg, dexbrompheniramine maleate plus d-isoephedrine) or antihistamine alone, and when feasible, avoidance of environmental precipitating factor(s). For perennial nonallergic rhini-

tis, my preference is to begin treatment with the antihistamine-decongestant medication for 3 to 4 weeks and, if there is a favorable response (eg, it usually begins within days to 1 week with this form of therapy), switch to intranasal corticosteroids for 3 months. Vasomotor rhinitis that fails to respond to the above measures can be treated with intranasal ipratropium bromide. Chronic sinusitis should be initially treated with antibiotics directed against *Hemophilus influenzae, Streptococcus pneumoniae,* and upper respiratory tract anaerobes and an antihistamine-decongestant oral medication for at least 3 weeks; and decongestant nasal spray (eg, oxymetazoline hydrochloride) for a maximum of 5 days. It appears that the newer, relatively nonsedating $H_1$-antagonists are only helpful in treating cough due to those conditions known to be mediated by histamine, such as allergic rhinitis. It is quite likely that these newer agents have failed in non-histamine-mediated conditions, such as the common cold, when the older, potentially more sedating $H_1$-antagonists have succeeded because the newer drugs possess relatively little if any anticholinergic activity.[276]

### Asthma

Uncomplicated, cough-variant asthma is easily treated. For example, in a recently completed double-blind, randomized, placebo-controlled, cross-over study,[277] patients with asthma had a significant decrease in cough severity after 1 week of therapy with inhaled beta-agonist (eg, two puffs of metaproterenol by metered dose inhaler with spacer device four times a day). Treatment with inhaled corticosteroid was added, and with combined therapy, cough disappeared. It is likely that all bronchodilator and anti-inflammatory asthma medications will be shown to be effective for the cough due to asthma. Such is already the case with nedocromil sodium[278] and cromolyn sodium.[279] Since cough due to uncomplicated asthma is almost always responsive to relatively safe and easy to deliver medications, broncho-

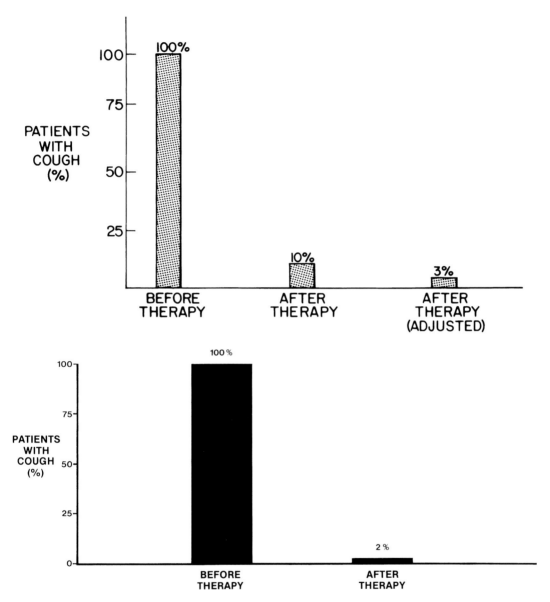

**Figure 11.** Outcome of specific therapy for chronic cough from two prospective studies carried out approximately 10 years apart. (A) An average of 18.9 months after therapy had been given in a study published in 1981, only 10% of patients continued to complain of cough. When success rate was adjusted for those patients who took the prescribed medicines, only 3% of patients complained of cough. (Reproduced with permission from Irwin RS, Corrao WM, Pratter MR. Am Rev Respir Dis 1981; 123: 413–417.) (B) An average of 3.2 months after therapy had been given in a study published in 1990, only 2% of patients continued to complain of cough. It took an average of 3.4 visits per patient, with a range of 1 to 14 visits, to diagnose and successfully treat these patients.

dilators and inhaled corticosteroids for initial treatment and for empiric, therapeutic trials should be tried first. Diagnostic-therapeutic trials with large doses of prednisone[280] are not necessary because systemic corticosteroids are not specific therapy for asthma since they will improve cough, at least transiently, from any inflammatory disease; and if bronchodilators and inhaled corticosteroids do not easily control cough, cough is either not due to asthma or it is due to asthma plus a condition making asthma difficult to control (eg, GERD).[251] A systematic protocol for managing difficult-to-control asthma can be found elsewhere.[281]

Occasionally, inhaled medications (eg, bronchodilators and corticosteroids) will provoke patients to cough.[205,206] If the use of spacer devices and switching brands is to no avail, begin treatment with oral bronchodilators. If the patient has uncomplicated cough-variant asthma, cough should subside[193] and allow the reinstitution of inhaled medications.

## Gastroesophageal Reflux Disease

Therapeutic recommendations are not clear-cut since therapy for cough due to GERD has not been systematically or rigorously studied and treatment with $H_2$-antagonists alone can fail.[251] Moreover, a number of the components of the treatment regimen can potentially be associated with morbidity (eg, side effects associated with drugs and/or surgery). And, successful therapy may have to be prolonged and requires perseverance on the part of patient and physician alike. Two prospective studies have shown that successful therapy for chronic cough due to GERD is usually relatively prolonged, taking, on average, 161 days[251] to 179 days.[97] This compares to the lengths of time of 70 and 67 days that have been reported for the successful treatment of coughs due to PNDS and asthma.[7]

While some investigators have occasionally found it necessary to resort to antireflux surgery[252] when medical therapy has failed, most investigators have found an intensive antireflux medical regimen to be highly efficacious. The regimen has multiple components: (1) a high-protein, low-fat (45 g) antireflux diet consisting of 3 daily meals, abstinence from foods and beverages (and medications)[282] that have the potential of lowering the lower esophageal sphincter pressure and are of low acidity, and nothing to eat or drink (except for taking medications) between meals or for 2 hours prior to reclining; (2) approximately 10–cm (4-in) head-of-bed elevation; and (3) medications[283] that include antacids, metoclopramide, cisapride, $H_2$-antagonists, proton pump inhibitors, and/or sucralfate. Since it has been our bias that the diet is the most important component of the regimen, most of our patients see a nutritionist in consultation and receive detailed verbal and written instructions on the diet each time they are seen in clinic. Adherence to the diet (and the antireflux regimen) is assessed by weighing patients when they return to clinic. It is reasonable to anticipate that most patients who adhere to the low-fat, antireflux diet should lose weight. Until recently, metoclopramide was usually included as part of our initial drug regimen. It was usually started at a low dose (eg, 5 mg, one-half hour before the evening meal and at bedtime) and gradually increased if needed and tolerated to 10 mg, one-half hour before 3 meals and at bedtime. Instead of metoclopramide, I now use cisapride and gradually increase the dose to 20 mg one-half hour before 3 meals and at bedtime. Compared to metoclopramide, cisapride is devoid of central or peripheral antidopaminergic effects (eg, drowsiness, restlessness, akathisia, dystonia, parkinsonism) and it is capable of maintaining a gastrokinetic effect under chronic administration.[284,285] When sucralfate is used, it is given as a slurry.

It has been our practice to continue therapy for an additional 3 months after cough has disappeared as a complaint and then to gradually discontinue it.

If medical therapy appears to have failed, consider that a comorbid disease (eg, obstructive sleep apnea[285a]) or treatment for a comorbid condition[282] (eg, progesterone, nitrates, or calcium channel blockers) may be making GERD difficult to control and make adjustments to treatment before referring the patient for antireflux surgery. If it is determined that obstructive sleep apnea is present, nasal continuous positive airway pressure (nasal CPAP) should be added to the patient's treatment regimen; it appears to be an effective way to treat GERD in such patients.[285a]

Failure of intensive medical therapy and consideration for surgery can be determined by performing 24-hour EPM while the patient is continuing the most intensive medical therapy.

## Chronic Bronchitis

The specific therapy of cough due to chronic bronchitis is removal of the environmental irritant, such as cigarette smoke. For those patients who seek medical attention complaining of cough, smoking cessation has been very successful.[6,7] Cough has been shown to disappear or markedly decrease in 94% of cases with smoking cessation; when it disappeared, 54% of the time, it did so within 4 weeks.[169]

## Bronchiectasis

The cough due to exacerbations of bronchiectasis has been successfully treated[7] with theophylline and/or a beta₂-agonist for their stimulatory affect on mucociliary clearance,[286,287] chest physiotherapy and postural drainage, and intermittent courses of antibiotics directed initially at *H influenzae*, *S pneumoniae*, and upper respiratory tract anaerobes.[288] If initial therapy is unsuccessful, the coverage may need to be expanded to include antibiotics that are effective against facultative gram-negative enteric rods and *Staphylococcus aureus*.[288] In our experience, it sometimes becomes necessary to extend antibiotic treatment for a duration of 3 weeks or longer. When exacerbations of bronchiectasis become chronic or recur-

rent, a reversible underlying cause for the bronchiectasis should be sought (eg, immunodeficiency state, endobronchial obstructing lesion, GERD with aspiration, alcoholism) and accurate cultures of the lower respiratory tract (eg, bronchoscopy with protected specimen brush quantitative cultures) should be performed while the patient is off of antibiotics to guide the next course of antibiotics.

## Angiotensin-Converting Enzyme Inhibitor-Induced Cough

Recent studies suggest that the mechanism for this cough in some way involves prostaglandins, mainly through the accumulation of bradykinin in the tissue of the tracheobronchial tree. Evidence supporting this comes from studies showing that sulindac, nifedipine, and indomethacin attenuated cough associated with ACEI.[289,290] Nifedipine is a dihydropyridine calcium antagonist which may inhibit prostaglandin synthesis. While reducing the severity of cough, it also acts to further lower blood pressure. Therefore, combining nifedipine and an ACEI can be attempted as a possible alternative to withdrawing the ACEI in those patients with troublesome ACEI-related cough.[289] Switching from one ACEI to another or decreasing the dose will usually not be beneficial.[170,178,268] Losartan, an angiotensin II receptor antagonist that has recently become available, can be used as an alternative drug to ACEIs. While losartan appears to effectively block the renin-angiotensin-aldosterone system by a mechanism other than ACE inhibition, its incidence of cough is significantly lower than that with the ACEI lisinopril and similar to that observed with hydrochlorothiazide.[170]

## Postinfectious Cough

Based upon the speculation that the postinfectious cough is due to inflammation of the upper/lower respiratory tract, some authors, based upon their personal experience, have advocated prescribing a brief course of corticosteroids, starting with 30 to 40 mg of prednisone (or equivalent) in the morning, tapering to zero over 2 to 3 weeks[291] for those patients whose coughs come on after a respiratory infection and become persistently troublesome. Since the majority of patients with chronic cough from a variety of causes, when asked, frequently provide a history that suggests that their chronic cough began after a respiratory infection, I believe that the diagnosis of postinfectious cough should be one of exclusion and only when other causes such as PNDS, asthma, and GERD have been ruled out. It follows that I would only recommend corticosteroids when these other conditions are deemed not present. A randomized, double-blind, placebo-controlled study suggests that inhaled ipratropium bromide may provide relief to some patients with postinfectious cough.[291a]

In the case of presumed **pertussis**, treatment with erythromycin for the sick individual and prophylaxis for exposed persons has been found to be effective in decreasing the severity and transmission of the disease to others if therapy is begun early (ie, within the first 8 days of the infection[222]).[292] It is reasonable to consider adding corticosteroids to the patient's drug regimen. In a pediatric study,[222] when adding a corticosteroid to erythromycin, there was a significant reduction in coughing paroxysms and episodes of vomiting, particularly in infants. Early results of experimental trials in adults and children using acellular pertussis vaccines suggest that pertussis may be safely and effectively prevented in the near future in all age groups.[293]

### Miscellaneous Diseases

Specific therapy for this category of conditions depends on the cause (Table VI). For instance, in a randomized, double-blind, placebo-controlled study,[5] the cough due to the common cold disappeared sooner in patients treated with an antihistamine-decongestant medication (eg, dexbrompheniramine maleate plus d-isoephedrine). Similar results have not occurred with the newer, relatively nonsedating $H_1$-antagonists loratadine and terfenadine probably because the common cold is not histamine-mediated and these newer agents are lacking in anticholinergic properties[276] that the older $H_1$-antagonists possess.

When cough has been due to irritation of the eardrum by a hair, it will go away when the hair is removed.[182] When it is due to an exposed endobronchial suture, it will disappear when the suture is removed.[214–216] The cough due to pneumonia will respond to an appropriate antibiotic; pulmonary embolism, to intravenous anticoagulation; resectable bronchogenic carcinoma, to surgery[7]; sarcoidosis, to corticosteroids[7]; and left ventricular failure associated with atrial fibrillation, to digitalis and diuretics.[6,7]

For those interested in reading more about specific therapy for other disease listed in Table VI, references are provided.

### Nonspecific Antitussive Therapy

Studies on artificially induced cough in animals and healthy human subjects were important in order to determine which drugs should be selected for clinical trials. However, these studies by themselves cannot be used to determine effectiveness since their efficacy has not always been reproducible in patients with pathologic cough.[275] In evaluating antitussive action, it is important not only to assess a change in the frequency of cough, but also a change in intensity or severity. Since objective cough counting can only evaluate cough frequency, while the patient's subjective assessment probably integrates both cough frequency and severity, it is possible for a drug to be considered effective when subjective and objective results deviate. Therefore, nonspecific antitussive agents can only be considered clinically useful if they have been shown to significantly decrease cough frequency or severity or both by objective cough counting or standardized questionnaires in randomized, double-blind, placebo-controlled studies in patients with pathologic cough.[275,276] With few exceptions, only those drugs that have been adequately evaluated according to these guidelines will be mentioned here.

To provide a framework for discussing nonspecific antitussive therapy, agents may be classified according to how and where they might theoretically control the cough reflex. Therefore, the following possibilities are considered:

1) drugs that change mucociliary factors irritating cough receptors;
2) drugs that increase the threshold and/or latency of the afferent limb;
3) drugs that increase the threshold and/or latency of the cough center;
4) drugs that increase the threshold and/or latency of the efferent limb;
5) drugs that decrease the strength of contraction of the respiratory muscles.

Because the site(s) of action of some drugs is not known for certain, and since it may be determined in the future that some agents may exert their effects on additional sites, this categorization, while not necessarily precise, is meant to facilitate this discussion of nonspecific antitussive medications.

Since nonspecific antitussive therapy has recently been extensively reviewed by us,[276] this form of therapy will be briefly reviewed here.

## Drugs Which Alter Mucociliary Factors

Drugs might theoretically alter lower respiratory tract secretions by: (1) increasing the volume of the secretions (ie, expectorants); (2) decreasing the production of mucus; (3) changing the consistency or regulation of mucus (ie, mucolytics); or (4) increasing mucociliary clearance.

Although a number of drugs have been shown to affect mucociliary factors in either **in vivo** or **in vitro** experimental preparations, there are few data published to date that convincingly demonstrate that drugs developed to alter mucociliary factors function as antitussives. Drugs that have been adequately evaluated in well-designed clinical studies and have been shown to be effective as nonspecific antitussive agents are listed in Table VIII.[276,294] Since ipratropium bromide may theoretically exert its antitussive effect by either altering mucociliary factors or increasing the latency or threshold of the efferent limb of the cough reflex, it is listed in both categories (Tables VIII and

## Table VIII
### Effective Drugs Acting on Mucociliary Factors

| Drug | Dosing | Disease |
|---|---|---|
| Ipratropium bromide | 40 $\mu$g qid aerosol | Chronic bronchitis |
| | 80 $\mu$g qid aerosol | Postinfectious |
| Iodopropylidne glycerol* | 60 mg qid po | Chronic bronchitis |
| | 60 mg qid po | Asthma |
| Dexbrompheniramine maleate plus | | Common cold |
| d-isoephedrine | 6 mg + 120 mg bid po | |
| Guaimesal | 500 mg tid po | Acute/chronic bronchitis |
| Dornase alfa | 2.5 mg qd-bid aerosol | Cystic fibrosis |

* Iodopropylidene has been removed from the market in the U.S. because of safety concerns; see text for additional information. Guaimesal is a synthetic agent whose chemical structure includes salicylate and guaiacol rings. Qid = 4 times a day; bid = 2 times a day; po = by mouth. The disease refers to the diagnosis of the study subjects in which the drug was shown to be effective. (Adapted from Irwin RS, Curley FJ, Bennett FM. Appropriate use of antitussives and protussives: a practical review. Drugs 1993; 46:80–91.

**Table IX**
Effective Drugs Acting on the Efferent Limb

| Drug | Dosing | Disease |
|------|--------|---------|
| Ipratropium bromide | 40 μg qid aerosol 80 μg qid aerosol | Chronic bronchitis Postinfectious |

Qid = four times a day.

IX). While iodopropylidene glycerol has been shown to be an effective antitussive agent, it has been removed from the market in the United States because of potential safety concerns (eg, carcinogenesis). It is important to be aware that Wallace Laboratories, Cranbury, NJ in the United States has reformulated their Organidin family of antitussive drugs by replacing iodopropylidene glycerol with guaifenesin and that guaifenesin has not been shown to be efficacious.

Because of conflicting results, data on the efficacy of bromhexine and carbocysteine (S-carboxy-methyl-cysteine) are inconclusive.[276] Moreover, studies suggesting efficacy of inhaled fenoterol and sodium cromoglycate as nonspecific antitussives must also be regarded as inconclusive since the patient groups that served as study subjects were not well-characterized and may have included patients with asthma.[276] Often recommended nonspecific antitussive therapies, such as ammonium chloride, hydration by the oral and intravenous routes, theophylline, and aromatic chest rubs[276] have not been adequately evaluated.

## Drugs That Increase the Threshold and/or Latency of the Afferent Limb

Drugs included in this section may work by altering the sensitivity of either the cough receptors or afferent neural pathways (Table X). Every bronchoscopist can attest to the transient antitussive effect of topically administered lidocaine. Intravenous lidocaine has been convincingly shown to suppress the persistent, almost uninterrupted cough in patients after they awaken from general anesthesia following bronchoscopy.[276] Despite these observations, lidocaine by either route has not been evaluated in appropriately designed clinical trials in patients with chronic cough. When given topically, the maximum recommended dose of lidocaine applied to the respiratory tract at any one time is 4 mg/kg of lean body weight[295]; once this dose is reached, additional lidocaine should not be given for a substantial period of time because of the increased risk of potentially life-threatening central nervous system and cardiovascular complications. The half-life of lidocaine is approximately 90 minutes. Conceivably, intravenous lidocaine may also work by having an effect on the cough center.

Levodropropizine, a nonnarcotic antitussive, has been shown to decrease cough in patients with bronchitis and asthma[296] and thought to do so through a peripheral

**Table X**
Effective Drugs Acting on the Afferent Limb

| Drug | Dosing | Disease |
|------|--------|---------|
| Lidocaine | ≤4 mg/kg* topical | Bronchoscopy |
| Levodropropizine | 60 mg tid po | Acute/chronic bronchitis, asthma |
| Naproxen | 400–500 mg loading dose, then 200—500 mg tid po | Rhinovirus colds |

* This maximum dose is of lean body weight; half-life of lidocaine is approximately 90 minutes. tid = 3 times a day; po = by mouth.

**Table XI**
Effective Drugs Acting on the Cough Center

| Drug | Dosing | Disease |
|---|---|---|
| Narcotics | | |
| Codeine* | 30–60 mg sd po | Bronchitis |
| | 20 mg bid po | Tuberculosis, cancer, bronchitis, pulmonary fibrosis |
| Nonnarcotics | | |
| Dextromethorphan | 60 mg sd po | Bronchitis |
| | 10–20 mg qid po | Bronchitis |
| | 20 mg bid po | Tuberculosis, cancer, pulmonary fibrosis, bronchitis |
| Glaucine | 30 mg sd po | Bronchitis |
| | 30 mg tid po | Upper respiratory tract infection |
| | 30 mg sd po | Bronchitis, cancer, pneumonia, asthma |
| Caramiphen | 10 mg qid po | Bronchitis |
| | 20 mg tid po | Bronchitis, tuberculosis |
| Diphenhydramine | 25–50 mg q4h po | Bronchitis, sarcoidosis |
| Viminol | 70–140 mg sd po | Bronchitis |
| | 60 mg sd po | Bronchitis |

* Since it is reasonable to assume that all narcotics of the phenanthrene alkaloid group are effective, only codeine, the prototypical agent is listed. sd = single dose; bid = twice a day; po = by mouth; qid = four times a day; tid = three times a day; q4h = every 4 hours. (Adapted from Irwin RS, Curley FJ, Bennett FM. Appropriate use of antitussive and protussives: a practical review. Drugs 1993; 46:80–91.

nervous system mechanism, primarily at the rapidly-adapting irritant receptors.[276]

Naproxen, an inhibitor of prostaglandin synthesis and anti-inflammatory drug, reduced cough in experimental rhinovirus colds.[297]

*Drugs That Increase the Threshold and/ or Latency of the Cough Center*

An extensive number of narcotic and nonnarcotic agents have been adequately evaluated in clinic trials. Narcotics of the phenanthrene alkaloid group (eg, morphine and codeine) are effective antitussives.[298] Codeine and the nonnarcotic agents that have been adequately evaluated and shown to be efficacious appear in Table XI.

Codeine is the standard to which other central antitussives are compared. While codeine has been shown to be effective in a variety of conditions, it has not been uniformly efficacious in all diseases. In a recent double-blind, randomized, placebo-controlled study,[299] codeine was no more effective than syrup vehicle in controlling coughs in patients with acute viral infection of the upper respiratory tract. The decrease in cough following vehicle or codeine may have been due to the demulcent action of the syrup vehicle. It has been suggested that the efficacy of cough mixtures containing opiates may be a result of the sugar-based vehicle.[300] However, the demulcent action of syrup cannot explain the many reports of efficacy of codeine, since the drug also has substantial antitussive effects when administered as a capsule formulation.[301] Rather, it is more probable that the essential mechanism of cough and/or the importance of the central component in the cough reflex is not the same in induced cough, chronic cough, or cough caused by upper respiratory tract infection.

While dextromethorphan hydrobromide, glaucine, diphenhydramine, caramiphen, viminol, and levodropropizine have been shown to be effective nonnarcotic antitussive agents, ethyl dibunate, pholcodine, and brospamin have not.[276] The efficacy of levopropoxyphene is currently unclear.[276] While it was found to be effective in a subjective study, an objective study utilizing cough counting found it to be ineffective. Racemic glaucine has been shown to be an effective, centrally-acting, nonnarcotic antitussive, but it is only available, to our knowledge, in some Eastern European countries.[276] Readers should be cautioned that the drug marketed in Europe by the trade name, Glaucine, is not the same drug, and it should not be prescribed as an antitussive; it is a beta-adrenergic blocker, metipranolol.

### Drugs That Increase the Threshold and/ or Latency of the Efferent Limb

Ipratropium bromide, an atropine-like anticholinergic drug, has been shown to be effective when given as an aerosol, in patients with chronic bronchitis[302] and postinfectious cough (Table IX).[303] It may exert its antitussive effect either on the efferent limb or on the cough receptor by altering mucociliary factors.

### Drugs That Decrease the Strength of Contraction of the Respiratory Skeletal Muscles

Although not normally classified as antitussive drugs, neuromuscular blocking agents may be considered as such in those patients who can not be mechanically ventilated because of uncontrollable spasms of coughing (ie, "bucking the ventilator"). The nondepolarizing neuromuscular blockers (eg, pancuronium bromide, vecuronium bromide, atracurium besylate)[304] are typically used in this situation. A study on artificially induced cough in normal volunteers has suggested that narcotics may exert some of their antitussive effect by decreasing the intensity of contraction of the abdominal muscles.[305]

### Protussive Therapy

Protussive therapy is treatment that increases cough effectiveness with or without increasing cough frequency.[275] The results of subjective studies alone are impossible to evaluate since patients may sense that mucus has been changed by agents that may alter mucociliary factor(s) when there has actually been no improvement in clearance. Since it is theoretically possible to change the consistency of mucus and the volume of expectorated sputum without improving cough clearance, objective studies that measure only these parameters are impossible to evaluate. For instance, the volume of sputum may increase without improving cough effectiveness because (a) the patient swallowed less mucus during the study period, (b) the drug stimulated the production of saliva, or (c) the drug actually increased the volume of airway secretions without improving cough effectiveness. Therefore, protussive therapy can only be considered clinically useful if it has been shown to

### Table XII
Protussive Agents that Increase Cough Clearance

| Drug | Dosing | Disease |
|---|---|---|
| Hypertonic saline | aerosol bid | Bronchitis |
| | aerosol sd | Bronchitis |
| Amiloride* | 10 mmol/L sd aerosol | Cystic fibrosis |
| | 10 mmol/L bid aerosol | Cystic fibrosis |
| Terbutaline | 5 mg sd aerosol following CPT and PD | Bronchiectasis |

* Amiloride improved a calculated cough clearability measure that is not a direct measure of cough clearance. sd = single dose; bid = twice a day; CPT = chest physiotherapy; PD = postural drainage.

significantly increase the clearance of particles from the lower airways during coughing in randomized, double-blind, placebo-controlled studies in patients with pathologic cough.[275,276]

## Cough Clearance

Drugs that have been adequately evaluated in well-designed clinical studies and shown to be effective are listed in Table XII. While hypertonic saline aerosol improved cough clearance in patients with bronchitis, there was no improvement in either pulmonary function or subjective assessment.[306,307] In one prospective, open-label, placebo-controlled, parallel-group trial of patients with cystic fibrosis, ultrasonically nebulized hypertonic saline significantly improved $FEV_1$ (15% versus 2.8%) after 2 weeks; however, cough clearance was not measured. Moreover, 6 of 58 patients had to withdraw from the study, one due to severe coughing and one due to hemoptysis associated with the hypertonic saline.[307a] Amiloride aerosol in patients with cystic fibrosis has been shown to improve a calculated cough clearability measure (not a direct measure of cough clearance) without improving pulmonary function.[308] While aerosolized ipratropium bromide diminished the effectiveness of cough for clearing radiolabeled particles from the airways in chronic obstructive pulmonary disease,[309] aerosolized terbutaline following chest physiotherapy significantly increased cough clearance in patients with bronchiectasis.[310]

The divergent results with these two different types of bronchodilators suggest that terbutaline sulfate achieved its favorable effect by increasing hydration of mucus or by enhancing ciliary beating and these overcame any negative effects that bronchodilation had on cough clearance. If bronchodilators result in too much smooth muscle relaxation of large airways, flow rates can actually decrease even in healthy individuals[311] when more compliant large airways narrow too much because they cannot withstand dynamic compression during forced expirations.

Although hypertonic saline, amiloride, and terbutaline, by aerosol following chest physiotherapy, have been shown to increase cough clearance, their clinical utility remains to be determined in future studies that assess short- and long-term effects of these agents on the patient's condition.

It has been proposed that cough effectiveness could be improved by mechanical therapies. For example, positive insufflation followed by manual compression of the lower thorax and abdomen may be helpful in quadriparetic patients.[312] Similarly, an abdominal push maneuver that assists expiratory efforts in patients with spinal cord injuries[313] or combining abdominal binding and muscle training of the clavicular portion of the pectoralis major may aid tetraplegic patients.[314] A combination involving positive expiratory pressure and chest physiotherapy may assist patients with chronic bronchitis.[315] The utility of the first three measures in improving clinical outcomes has yet to be studied. While combining short bouts of positive expiratory pressure breathing, forced expirations and chest physiotherapy resulted in reduced coughing, less mucus production, and fewer acute exacerbations in patients with chronic bronchitis compared with chest physiotherapy alone,[315] the effect of these combined maneuvers on cough clearance was not assessed. At this time, there does not appear to be a clear benefit of combining any form of chest physiotherapy with coughing over vigorous coughing alone to increase cough clearance.[316,317]

## Cough Frequency

A number of agents can increase cough frequency with varying success. While these effects have been primarily used to induce cough in animals and human volunteers to evaluate the effectiveness of antitussive drugs and better understand the pathogenesis of cough, none of the following have been studied as potentially clinically useful protussive agents[275]: (1) drugs that inhibit angiotensin-converting enzyme; (2) inhalations of a variety of agents that include solutions of low osmolarity and low ion concentration (eg, distilled water) or high osmolarity and high ion concentration (eg, hypertonic sodium chloride), capsaicin, citric acid, acetic acid, ethyl ether, acrolein, ammonia, sulfuric acid, sulfur dioxide, and acetylcholine; and (3) intravenous injections of lobeline and paraldehyde.

## Common Pitfalls in Managing Patients with Chronic Cough

If patients continue to complain of persistently troublesome cough even after an extensive evaluation, reconsider the following pitfalls in management previously mentioned throughout this chapter as possible contributing factors:

1) assuming that a positive MIC, all by itself, is diagnostic of asthma as the cause of cough;

2) not considering that inhaled medications prescribed for cough due to asthma may be making the cough worse;

3) assuming that all $H_1$-antagonists are equal and that the newer, relatively nonsedating $H_1$-antagonists will effectively treat the postnasal drip of non-histamine-mediated conditions;

4) not considering that more than one condition is simultaneously contributing to the cough;

5) failing to consider the commonest causes of cough in the presence of other seemingly "obvious" diagnostic culprits (eg, solitary pulmonary nodule);

6) not appreciating that "silent" GERD can be the cause of cough and that it may take up to 2 to 3 months of treatment before the cough starts to improve and, on average, 5 to 6 months before the cough disappears;

7) not appreciating the possibility that $H_2$-antagonist therapy alone may be inadequate in treating cough due to GERD;

8) not appreciating the importance of prolonged EPM in diagnosing GERD as the cause of cough and how to interpret the study (eg, conventional indices of reflux may be misleadingly normal);

9) not appreciating that patients with cough due to GERD may fail to improve with the most intensive medical therapy and that the adequacy of the treatment regimen (and/or need for surgery) can be assessed by performing 24-hour EPM while the patient continues to take medical therapy.

## Cough Cardiopulmonary Resuscitation

In the 1960s and 1970s, coronary angiographers initially observed that by coughing a patient could maintain consciousness during potentially lethal arrhythmias and/or convert these arrhythmias to more viable and normal cardiac rhythms.[318,319] Since those initial observations, cough cardiopulmonary resuscitation has assumed an established place in clinical practice[320] and has been found to be beneficial in the electrocardiographically monitored, conscious patient with (1) asystole, (2) profound bradycardia with hypotension, and (3) ventricular tachycardia. While voluntary coughing is unlikely to convert ventricular fibrillation to a more viable rhythm,[321] it can maintain blood pressure and oxygenation while the defibrillator is being readied. It has been shown that patients with ventricular fibrillation, asystole, or heart block can maintain consciousness in catheterization laboratories or coronary care units with forceful, abrupt coughing at 1- to 3-second intervals for 39 to 92 seconds.[322,323]

Data exist that allow us to understand why cough cardiopulmonary resuscitation is effective in the situations mentioned above. Coughing produces hemodynamic changes that compare favorably to chest compressions. During the expiratory phase of a vigorous cough, systolic pressures approach 140 mm Hg compared to 75 mm Hg during chest compressions.[320] It has been estimated that a vigorous cough can generate from 1 to 25 J of energy.[324] Adequate ventilation should be maintained during coughing since, following the inspiratory phase of cough, 1 to 3 L of air can normally be measured during the expiratory phase.[53,325] While it is not known why the heart rate in a patient with profound bradycardia can increase with coughing, the most plausible explanation is that it is due to enhanced oxygenation of the myocardium afforded by an increase in blood pressure.

While cough cardiopulmonary resuscitation can be successful, it has two major limitations. It must be initiated before loss of consciousness occurs, and because the act of coughing expends more than a modest amount of energy, it cannot be continued indefinitely.

## References

1. Rabiner LR, Schafer RW. *Digital Processing of Speech Signals.* Englewood Cliffs, NJ: Prentice Hall, 1978.
2. Loudon RG. Cough in health and disease. Current research in chronic obstructive lung disease. In: *Proceedings of the Tenth Emphysema Conference.* U.S. Department of Health, Education, and Welfare; 1967:41–53.
3. Power JT, Stewart IC, Connaughton JJ, Brash HM, et al. Nocturnal cough in patients with chronic bronchitis and emphysema. Am Rev Respir Dis 1984; 130: 999–1001.
4. Schappert SM. National ambulatory medical care survey: 1991: Summary. In: *Vital and Health Statistics.* U.S. Department of Health and Human Services; 1993. Publication No. 230: 1–20.
5. Curley FJ, Irwin RS, Pratter MR, et al. Cough and the common cold. Am Rev Respir Dis 1988; 138: 305–311.
6. Irwin RS, Corrao WM, Pratter MR. Chronic persistent cough in the adult: the spectrum and frequency of causes and successful outcome of specific therapy. Am Rev Respir Dis 1981; 123: 413–417.
7. Irwin RS, Curley FJ, French CL. Chronic cough: the spectrum and frequency of causes, key components of the diagnostic evaluation, and outcome of specific therapy. Am Rev Respir Dis 1990; 141: 640–647.
8. Cough Remedies: Which ones work best? Consumer Reports. 1983; February: 59–61.
8a. Couch RB. The common cold: Control? J Infect Dis 1984; 150: 167–173.
9. French CL, Irwin RS, Curley FJ, et al. The impact of chronic cough on quality of life. Am J Respir Crit Care Med. 1995; 151, Part: A450.
10. Das RM, Jeffery PK, Widdicombe JG. The epithelial innervation of the lower respiratory tract of the cat. J Anat 1978; 126: 123–131.
11. Elftman AG. The afferent and parasympathetic innervation of the lungs and trachea of the dog. Am J Anat 1943; 72: 1–27.
12. Honjin R. On the nerve supply of the lung of the mouse, with special reference to the structure of the peripheral vegetative nervous system. J Comp Neurol 1956; 105: 587–625.
13. Gaylor JB. The intrinsic nervous mechanism of the human lung. Brain 1934; 57: 143–160.
14. Pressman JJ, Kelemen G. Physiology of the larynx. Physiol Rev 1955; 35: 506–554.
15. Bucher K. Pathophysiology and pharmacology of cough. Pharmacol Rev 1958; 10: 43–58.
16. Larsell O, Burget GE. The effects of mechanical and chemical stimulation of the tracheobronchial mucous membrane. Am J Physiol 1924; 70: 311–321.
17. Widdicombe JG. Rapidly adapting mechano-receptors in the trachea of the cat. J Physiol 1952; 118: 46P-47P.
18. Widdicombe JG. Receptors in the trachea and bronchi of the cat. J Physiol 1954; 123: 71–104.
19. Widdicombe JG. Respiratory reflexes from the trachea and bronchi of the cat. J Physiol 1954; 123: 55–70.
20. Tedeschi RE, Tedeschi DH, Hitchens JT, et al. A new antitussive method involving mechanical stimulation in unanesthetized dogs. J Pharmacol Exp Ther 1959; 126: 338–344.
21. Widdicombe JG. Respiratory reflexes. In: *Handbook of Physiology, Respiration.* Vol I. In: Fenn WO and Rahn H, ed. Baltimore, Md: Williams & Wilkens; 1964: 585–630.
22. Boyd EM. Expectorants and respiratory tract fluid. Pharmacol Rev 1954; 6: 521–542.
23. Karlsson J-A, Sant'Ambrogio G, Widdicombe JG. Afferent neural pathways in cough and reflex bronchoconstriction. J Appl Physiol 1988; 65: 1007–1023.
24. Sant'Ambrogio G. Afferent pathways for

the cough reflex. Clin Resp Physiol 1987; 23 (Suppl 10): 19S-23S.

25. Widdicombe JG. Reflexes from the upper respiratory tract. In: *Handbook of Physiology, (Section 3: The Respiratory System: Volume II, Control of Breathing, Part 1,* . Cherniack NS and Widdicombe JG, eds. Bethesda, Md: American Physiological Societyσ86:363–394.

26. Irwin RS, Widdicombe JG. Cough. In: *Textbook of Respiratory Medicine* (Volume 1). 2nd edition. Murray JF and Nadel JA, eds. Philadelphia, Pa; WB Saunders Company, 1994: 529–544.

27. Tatar M, Webber SE, Widdicombe JG. Lung C-fibre receptor activation and defensive reflexes in anaesthetized cats. J Physiol 1988; 22: 411–420.

28. Clerf LJ. Cough as a symptom. Med Clin North Am 1947; 31: 1393–1399.

29. Bickerman HA. Bronchial drainage and the phenomena of cough. In: *Clinical Cardiopulmonary Physiology.* 3rd edition. Gordon BL et al., eds. New York, NY: Grune and Stratton Inc; 1960:494–506.

30. Ishrat-Husain S. Rhinolith—-A rare cause of chronic cough. Can Med Assoc J 1967; 97: 540–541.

31. Lillie HI, Thornell WC. Arnold's nerve reflex cough syndrome. Ann Otol Rhinol Laryngol 1944; 53: 770–773.

32. Wolff AP, May M. The tympanic membrane: a source of the cough reflex. JAMA 1973; 223: 1269.

33. Banyai AL. Fifteen years' experience with carbon dioxide in the management of cough. Chest 1947; 13: 1–19.

34. Klass KP, Morton DR, Curtis GM. The clinical physiology of the human bronchi. III. The effect of vagus section on the cough reflex, bronchial caliber, and clearance of bronchial secretions. Surgery 1951; 29: 483–490.

35. Gray H. *Anatomy of the Human Body.* 27th edition.CM Goss, ed. Philadelphia, Pa; Lea & Febigerσ64:960.

36. Coleridge HM, Coleridge JCG. Reflexes evoked from tracheobronchial tree and lungs. In: *Handbook of Physiology, Section 3: The Respiratory System,* vol II Control of Breathing, Part 1. Cherniack NS and Widdicombe JG, eds. Bethesda, Md: American Physiological Society; 1986: 395–429.

37. Davis B, Roberts AM, Coleridge HM, Coleridge JCG. Reflex tracheal gland secretion evoked by stimulation of bronchial C-fibers in dogs. J Appl Physiol 1982; 53: 985–991.

38. Friebel H, Kuhn HF. Uber husten-und atemdepressorische wirkung. Arch Exp Path 1962; 243: 162–173.

39. Lumsden T. Observations on the respiratory centres. J Physiol 1923; 57: 354–367.

40. Borison JL. Electrical stimulation of the neural mechanism regulating spasmodic respiratory acts in the cat. Am J Physiol 1948; 154: 55–62.

41. Chakravarty NK, Matallana A, Jensen R, et al. Central effects of antitussive drugs on cough and respiration. J Pharmacol Exp Ther 1956; 117: 127–135.

42. Kase Y, Wakita Y, Kito G, et al. Centrally-induced coughs in the cat. Life Sci 1970; 9: 49–59.

43. Mori M, Sakai Y. Re-examination of centrally-induced cough in cats using a micro-stimulation technique. Jap J Pharmacol 1972; 22: 635–643.

44. Furstenberg AC, Crosby E. Neuron arcs of clinical significance in laryngology. Ann Otol Rhinol Laryngol 1948; 57: 298–310.

45. Simonsson BG, Jacobs FM, Nadel JA. Role of autonomic nervous system and the cough reflex in the increased responsiveness of airways in patients with obstructive airway disease. J Clin Invest 1967; 46: 1812–1818.

46. Davis JM, Plum F. Separation of descending spinal pathways to respiratory motoneurons. Exp Neurol 1972; 34: 78–94.

47. Leith DE, Butler JP, Sneddon SL, Brain JD. Cough. In *Handbook of Physiology, Section 3: The Respiratory System, vol III, Mechanics of Breathing, Part 1.* Macklem PT, Mead J, eds. Bethesda, Md: American Physiological Society; 1986:315–336.

48. Coryllos PN. Action of the diaphragm in cough. Experimental and clinical study on the human. Am J Med Sci 1937; 194: 523–535.

49. Yanagihara N, von Leden H, Werner-Kukuk E. The physical parameters of cough: the larynx in a normal single cough. Acta Otolaryngol 1966; 61: 495–510.

50. Hyatt RE, Schilder DP, Fry DL. Relationship between maximum expiratory flow and degree of lung inflation. J Appl Physiol 1958; 13: 331–336.

51. Mead J, Turner JM, Macklem PT, Little JB. Significance of the relationship between lung recoil and maximum expiratory flow. J Appl Physiol 1967; 22: 95–108.

52. Green JH, Neil E. The respiratory function

of the laryngeal muscles. J Physiol 1955; 129: 134–141.

53. Franklin KJ, Janker R. Coughing studied by means of x-ray cinematography. J Physiol 1938; 92: 467–472.

54. Banyai AL, Joannides M. Cough hazard. Chest 1956; 29: 52–61.

55. DiRienzo S. Bronchial dynamism. Radiology 1949; 53: 168–186.

56. Fraser RG. Measurements of the calibre of human bronchi in three phases of respiration by cinebronchography. J Can Assoc Radiol 1961; 12: 102–112.

57. Huizinga E. On the changes of the lumen of the bronchi during respiration and cough. Acta Otolaryngol 1967; 63: 273–279.

58. Huizinga E. The "tussive squeeze" and the "bechic blast" of the Jacksons. Ann Otol Rhinol Laryngol 1967; 76: 923–934.

59. Faaborg-Andersen K. Electromyographic investigation of intrinsic laryngeal muscles in humans. IV. Closure of the laryngeal aperture with cough, glottal click and swallow. Acta Physiol Scand 1957; 41(Suppl 140): 77–83.

60. Ross BB, Gramiak R, Rahn H. Physical dynamics of the cough mechanism. J Appl Physiol 1955; 8: 264–268.

61. Leith DE. Cough. Phys Ther 1968; 48: 439–447.

62. von Leden H, Isshiki N. An analysis of cough at the level of the larynx. Arch Otolaryngol 1965; 81: 616–625.

63. Whittenberger JL, Mead J. Research in tuberculosis and related subjects: respiratory dynamics during cough. Trans Nat Tuberc Assoc 1952; 48: 414–418.

64. Langlands J. The dynamics of cough in health and in chronic bronchitis. Thorax 1967; 22: 88–96.

65. Loudon RG, Shaw GB. Mechanics of cough in normal subjects and in patients with obstructive respiratory disease. Am Rev Respir Dis 1967; 96: 666–677.

66. Macklem PT. Physiology of cough. *Ann Otol* 1974; 83: 761–768.

67. Harris RS, Lawson TV. The relative mechanical effectiveness and efficiency of successive voluntary coughs in healthy young adults. Clin Sci 1968; 34: 569–577.

68. Macklem PT, Mead J. Factors determining maximum expiratory flow in dogs. J Appl Physiol 1968; 25: 159–169.

69. Macklem PT, Wilson NJ. Measurement of intrabronchial pressure in man. J Appl Physiol 1965; 20: 653–663.

70. Fry DL, Hyatt RE. Pulmonary mechanics: a unified analysis of the relationship between pressure, volume and gasflow in the lungs of normal and diseased human subjects. Am J Med 1960; 29: 672–689.

71. Hasani A, Pavia D. Cough as a clearance mechanism. In: *Cough.* Braga P, Allegra L, eds. New York, NY: Raven Press; 89: 39–52.

72. Puchelle E, Zahm JM, Girard F, et al. Mucociliary transport in vivo and in vitro. Relations to sputum properties in chronic bronchitis. Eur J Respir Dis 1980; 61 (Suppl): 254–264.

73. Leith DE. Cough. In: *Respiratory Defense Mechanisms. Part II. Lung Biology in Health and Disease.* Brain JD, Proctor DF, Reid LM, eds. New York, NY: Marcel Dekker; 1977: 545–592.

74. Camner P. Studies on the removal of inhaled particles from the lungs by voluntary coughing. *Chest* 1981; 80 (Suppl): 824–826.

75. Kim CS, Sackner MA, Gebhart J, et al. Studies of cough efficacy by aerosol photometric technique (Abstract). Am Rev Respir Dis 1981; 123: 215A.

76. McCool FD, Leith DE. Pathophysiology of cough. Clin Chest Med 1987; 8: 189–195.

77. Arora NS, Gal TJ. Cough dynamics during progressive expiratory muscle weakness in healthy curarized subjects. J Appl Physiol 1981; 51: 494–498.

78. Gal TJ. Effects of endotracheal intubation on normal cough performance. Anesthesiology 1980; 52: 324–329.

79. Greene BA, Berkowitz S. The preanesthetic induced cough as a method of diagnosis of preoperative bronchitis. Ann Intern Med 1952; 37: 723–732.

80. Greene BA, Berkowitz S. The prevention of atelectasis or pneumonia following abdominal operations. Anesthesiology 1953; 14: 160–179.

81. Egbert LD, Laver MB, Bendixen JJ. The effect of site of operation and type of anesthesia upon the ability to cough in the postoperative period. Surg Gynecol Obstet 1962; 115: 295–298.

82. Greene BA, Berkowitz S. Atelectasis and pneumonia as preoperative complications of the "acute surgical abdomen." NY State J Med 1953; 53: 1976–1982.

83. Yamazaki S, Ogawa J, Shohzu A, et al. Intrapleural cough pressure in patients after thoracotomy. J Thorac Cardiovasc Surg 1980; 80: 600–604.

84. Siebens AA, Kirby NA, Poulos DA. Cough following transection of spinal cord at C-

6. Arch Phys Med Rehabil 1966; 47: 705–710.

85. Kirby NA, Barnerias MJ, Siebens AA. An evaluation of assisted cough in quadriparetic patients. Arch Phys Med Rehabil 1966; 47: 705–710.

86. Moore P, James O. Guillain-Barré syndrome: incidence, management and outcome of major complications. Crit Care Med 1981; 9: 549–555.

87. Chevrolet J-C, Deleamont P. Repeated vital capacity measurements as predictive parameters for mechanical ventilation need and weaning success in the Guillain-Barré syndrome. Am Rev Respir Dis 1991; 144: 814–818.

88. Fromm GB, Wisdom PJ, Block AJ. Amyotrophic lateral sclerosis presenting with respiratory failure: diaphragmatic paralysis and dependence on mechanical ventilation in two patients. Chest 1977; 71: 612–614.

89. Schiffman PL, Belsh JM. Effect of inspiratory resistance and theophylline on respiratory muscle strength in patients with amyotrophic lateral sclerosis. Am Rev Respir Dis 1989; 139: 1418–1423.

90. Szienberg A, Tabachnik E, Rashed N, et al. Cough capacity in patients with muscular dystrophy. Chest 1988; 94: 1232–1235.

91. Stuart WD. The otolaryngologic aspects of myasthenia gravis. Laryngoscope 1965; 75: 112–121.

92. Gracey DR, Divertie MB, Howard FM, Jr. Mechanical ventilation for respiratory failure in myasthenia gravis: two-year experience with 22 patients. Mayo Clin Proc 1983; 58: 597–602.

93. Calvert JR, Steinhaus JE, Lange SJ. Halothane as a depressant of cough reflex. Anesth Analg 1966; 45: 76–81.

94. Kryger M, Bode F, Antic R, Anthonisen N. Diagnosis of obstruction of the upper and central airways. Am J Med 1976; 61: 85–93.

95. Bickerman HA, Itkin SE. The effect of a new bronchodilator aerosol on the aMw flow dynamics of the maximum voluntary cough of patients with bronchial asthma and pulmonary emphysema. J Chronic Dis 1958; 8: 629–636.

96. Macklem PT, Fraser RG, Brown WG. Bronchial pressure measurements in emphysema and bronchitis. J Clin Invest 1965; 44: 897–905.

97. Macklem PT, Fraser RG, Bates DV. Bronchial pressures and dimensions in health and obstructive airway disease. J Appl Physiol 1963; 18: 699–706.

98. Rayl JE. Tracheobronchial collapse during cough. Radiology 1965; 85: 87–92.

99. Wright RR. Bronchial atrophy and collapse in chronic obstructive pulmonary emphysema. Am J Pathol 1960; 37: 63–75.

100. Johnston RF, Green RA. Tracheobronchomegaly. Am Rev Respir Dis 1965; 91: 35–50.

101. Fraser RG, Macklem PT, Brown WG. Airway dynamics in bronchiectasis: a combined cinefluorographic-manometric study. Am J Roentgenol Radium Ther Nucl Med 1965; 93: 821–835.

102. Williams J, Campbell P. Generalized bronchiectasis associated with deficiency of cartilage in the bronchial tree. Arch Dis Child 1960; 35: 182–191.

103. Sharpey-Schafer EP. The mechanism of syncope after coughing. Br Med J 1953; 2: 860–863.

104. Comroe JH, Jr. Special acts involving breathing. In: *Physiology of Respiration: An Introductory Text.* 2nd edition. Chicago, Ill: Year Book Medical Publishers; 1974: 230–231.

105. Sharpey-Schafer EP. Effects of coughing on intrathoracic pressure, arterial pressure and peripheral blood flow. J Physiol (Lond.) 1953; 122: 351–357.

106. Wilkins RW, Friedland CK. Laryngeal epilepsy due to increased intrathoracic pressure (Abstract). J Clin Invest 1944; 23: 939.

107. McCann WS, Bruce RA, Lovejoy FW Jr, et al. Tussive syncope. Arch Intern Med 1949; 84: 845–856.

108. McIntosh HD, Estes EH, Warren JV. The mechanism of cough syncope. Am Heart J 1956; 52: 70–82.

109. Skolnick JL, Dines DE. Tussive syncope. Minn Med 1969; 52: 1609–1613.

110. Kerr A, Jr, Derbes VJ. The syndrome of cough syncope. Ann Intern Med 1953; 39: 1240–1253.

111. Cogbill TH, Keimowitz RM. Injection port silastic catheter dislodgement caused by tussive (cough) paroxysm. Wisc Med J 1987; 86: 21–22.

112. Natelson SE, Molnar W. Malfunction of ventriculoatrial shunts caused by the circulatory dynamics of coughing. J Neurosurg 1972; 36: 283–286.

113. Irani F, Sanchis J. Inspiration- and cough-induced atrioventricular block. Can Med Assoc J 1971; 105: 735–736.

114. Francis CK, Singh JB, Polansky BJ. Inter-

ruption of aberrant conduction of atrioventricular junctional tachycardia by cough. N Engl J Med 1972; 286: 357–358.

115. Reisin L, Blaer Y, Jafari J, et al. Cough-induced nonsustained ventricular tachycardia. Chest 1994; 105: 1583–1584.

115a. Omori I, Yamada C, Inoue D, et al. Tachyarrhythmia provoked by coughing and other stimuli. Chest 1984; 86: 797–799.

116. Hamilton WF, Woodburn RA, Harper HT, Jr. Arterial, cerebrospinal and venous pressures in man during cough and strain. Am J Physiol 1944; 141: 42–50.

117. Kerr A, Eich RH. Cerebral concussion as a cause of cough syncope. Arch Intern Med 1961; 108: 138–142.

118. Strauss MJ, Longstreth WT, Thiele BL. Atypical cough syncope. JAMA 1984; 251: 1731.

119. Kapoor WN, Karpf M, Wieand S, et al. A prospective evaluation and follow-up of patients with syncope. N Engl J Med 1983; 309: 197–204.

120. White CW, Zimmerman TJ, Ahmad M. Idiopathic hypertrophic subaortic stenosis presenting as cough syncope. Chest 1975; 68: 250–253.

121. Larson SJ, Sances A, Jr, Baker JB, et al. Herniated cerebellar tonsils. J Neurosurg 1974; 40: 524–528.

122. Williams B. Cough headache due to craniospinal pressure dissociation. Arch Neurol 1980; 37: 226–230.

123. Sands GH, Newman L, Lipton R. Cough, exertional, and other miscellaneous headaches. Med Clin North Am 1991; 75: 733–747.

124. Moncada E, Graff-Radford SB. Cough headache presenting as a toothache: a case report. Headache 1993; 33: 240–243.

125. Ulyatt DG, Judson JA, Trubuhovich RV, et al. Cerebral arterial air embolism associated with coughing on a continuous positive airway pressure circuit. Crit Care Med 1991; 19: 985–987.

126. Shugar JMA, Som PM, Eisman W, et al. Non-traumatic cerebrospinal fluid rhinorrhea. Laryngoscope 1981; 91: 114–120.

127. Torrington KG, Adornato BT. Cough radiculopathy—another cause of pain in the neck. West J Med 1984; 141: 379–380.

127a. Herr RD, Call G, Banks D. Vertebral artery dissection from neck flexion during paroxysmal coughing. Ann Emerg Med 1992; 21: 88–91.

128. Morgan-Hughes JA. Cough seizures in patients with cerebral lesions. Br J Med 1966; 2: 494–496.

129. Patterson WG, Murat BW. Combined ambulatory esophageal manometry and dual-probe pH-metry in evaluation of patients with chronic unexplained cough. Dig Dis Sci 1994; 39: 1117–1125.

130. Bundy JT, Pontier PJ. Cough-induced hydrothorax in peritoneal dialysis. Peritoneal Dialysis International 1994; 14: 293.

130a. Sanyal A, Jefferson PA, Kirby DF. Percutaneous endoscopic gastrostomy button malfunction with severe cough. Gastrointestinal Endoscopy 1989; 35: 118–119.

130b. Wergowske GL, Carmody TH. Splenic rupture from coughing. Arch Surg 1983; 118: 1227.

130c. Lord R. Factors predisposing to inguinal hernia: an analysis of 1,100 cases. NZ J Surg 1968; 37: 377–381. 130d. Warrell DW. Incontinence in women. *The Practitioner* 1980; 224:885.

130d. Warrell DW. Incontinence in women. *The Practitioner* 1980; 224: 885.

130e. El-Hammady S, Ghoneim M. Acute complete inversion of the bladder. Br Med J 1971; 3: 306–307.

131. Schen RJ, Zurkowski S. Increased serum creatine phosphokinase activity with violent coughing. N Engl J Med 1973; 289: 328–329.

132. Horsburgh AG. Medical memoranda. Rupture of the rectus abdominis muscle. Br J Med 1962; 2: 898.

133. Love W. Rupture of rectus abdominis muscle. Br J Med 1962; 2: 1130.

134. McCarthy D, Durkin TE. Rupture of the rectus abdominis muscle. Br J Med 1963; 2: 58–59.

135. Anderton RL. Rectus abdominal muscle pulled by coughing. JAMA 1972; 222: 486.

136. Ducatman BS, Ludwig J, Hurt RD. Fatal rectus sheath hematoma. JAMA 1983; 249: 924–925.

137. Lee TM, Greenberger PA, Hahrwold DL, et al. Rectus sheath hematoma complicating an exacerbation of asthma. J Allergy Clin Immunol 1986; 78: 290–292.

138. Derbes VJ, Haran T. Rib fractures from muscular effort with particular reference to cough. Surgery 1954; 35: 294–321.

139. Long AE. Stress fracture of the ribs associated with pregnancy. Surg Clin North Am 1962; 42: 909–919.

140. Kopscanyi I, Laczay A, Nagy L. Cough fracture of ribs in infants with dyspnoea.

Acta Paediatr Acad Sci Hung 1969; 10: 93–98.

141. Lorin MI, Slovis TL, Haller JO. Fracture of ribs in psychogenic cough. NY State J Med 1978; 78: 2078–2079.

142. Roberge RJ, Morgenstern MJ, Osborn J. Cough fracture of the ribs. Am J Emerg Med 1984; 2: 513–517.

143. Hjalmarsson S, Asmundsson T, Sigurdsson J, et al. Major hemorrhage as a complication of cough fracture. Chest 1993; 104: 1310.

144. Macklin MT, Macklin CC. Malignant interstitial emphysema of the lungs and mediastinum as an important occult complication in many respiratory diseases and other conditions: an interpretation of the clinical literature in the light of laboratory experiment. Medicine 1944; 23: 281–358.

145. Naggar CZ. Pneumatosis intestinalis following common upper-respiratory-tract infection. JAMA 1976; 235: 2221–2222.

146. Roe PF, Kulkarni BN. Pneumomediastinum in children with cough. Br J Med 1967; 61: 147–150.

147. Glauser FL, Bartlett RH. Pneumoperitoneum in association with pneumothorax. Chest 1974; 66: 536–540.

148. Irwin RS, Pratter MR, Holland PS, et al. Postnasal drip causes cough and is associated with reversible upper airway obstruction. Chest 1984; 85: 346–352.

149. Irwin RS, Rosen MJ, Braman SS. Cough: a comprehensive review. Arch Intern Med 1977; 137: 1186–1191.

150. Benedict EB. Rupture of the bronchus from bronchoscopy during a paroxysm of coughing. JAMA 1961; 178: 509–510.

151. Young S, Bitsakou H, Caric' D, et al. Coughing can relieve or exacerbate symptoms in asthmatic patients. Respir Med 1991; 85, Suppl. A: 7–12.

151a. Prasud R, Mukerji PK, Gupta H. Herniation of the lung. Ind J Chest Dis All Sci 1990; 32: 129–132.

151b. Sheka KP, Williams LG. Spontaneous intercostal lung hernia. J National Med Assoc 1984; 76: 1210–1213.

152. Abbott OA, Hopkins WA, VanFleit WE, et al. A new approach to pulmonary emphysema. Thorax 1953; 8: 116–132.

153. McClean KH. The pathogenesis of pulmonary emphysema. Am J Med 1958; 25: 62–74.

154. Fisher CM. The possible role of coughing in the pathogenesis of pulmonary emphysema. Can Med Assoc J 1964; 91: 351–352.

155. Snider GL. Emphysema: the first two centuries—-and beyond. A historical overview, with suggestions for future research: Part 2. Am Rev Respir Dis 1992; 146: 1615–1622.

156. Kravitz P. The clinical picture of "cough purpura," benign and non-thrombocytopenic eruption. VA Med 1979; 106: 373–374.

157. Poe RH, Harder RV, Israel RH, et al. Chronic persistent cough: experience in diagnosis and outcome using an anatomic diagnostic protocol. Chest 1989; 95: 723–728.

158. Poe RH, Israel RH, Utell MJ, et al. Chronic cough: bronchoscopy or pulmonary function testing? Am Rev Respir Dis 1982; 126: 160–162.

159. Holinger LD, Sanders AD. Chronic cough in infants and children: an update. Laryngoscope 1991; 101: 596–605.

160. Pratter MR, Bartter T, Akers S, et al. An algorithmic approach to chronic cough. Ann Intern Med 1993; 119: 977–983.

161. Hoffstein V. Persistent cough in nonsmokers. Can Respir J 1994; 1: 40–47.

162. Puolijoki H, Lahdensuo A. Causes of prolonged cough in patients referred to a chest clinic. Ann Med 1989; 21: 425–427.

163. O'Connell F, Thomas VE, Pride NB, et al. Capsaicin cough sensitivity decreases with successful treatment of chronic cough. Am J Respir Crit Care Med 1994; 150: 374–380.

164. Smyrnios NA, Curley FJ, French CL, et al. Chronic cough in the elderly: causes and outcome of diagnostic evaluation and specific therapy. Am Rev Respir Dis 1993; 147 (Part 2): A381.

165. Irwin RS, French CL, Curley FJ, et al. Chronic cough due to gastroesophageal reflux: clinical, diagnostic, and pathogenetic aspects. Chest 1993; 104: 1511–1517.

165a. Smith DE, Wyatt J, McLuckie A, et al. Severe exercise hypoxaemia with normal or near normal x-rays: a feature of Pneumocystis carinii infection. Lancet 1988; 2: 1049–1051.

165b. Stover DE, Greeno RA, Gagliardi AJ. The use of a simple exercise test for the diagnosis of Pneumocystis carinii pneumonia in patients with AIDS. Am Rev Respir Dis 1989; 139: 1343–1346.

165c. Masur H, Ognibene FP, Yarchoan R, et al. CD$_4$ counts as predictors of opportunistic pneumonias in human immunodeficiency virus (HIV) infection. Ann Intern Med 1989; 111: 223–231.

166. Irwin RS, Pratter MR. The clinical value of pharmacologic bronchoprovocation challenge. Med Clin North Am 1990; 74: 767–778.

167. Hargreave FE, Ramsdale EH, Pugsley SO. Occupational asthma without bronchial hyperresponsiveness. Am Rev Respir Dis 1984; 130: 513–515.

168. Mello CJ, Irwin RS, Curley FJ. The predictive values of the character, timing, and complications of chronic cough in diagnosing its cause. Arch Intern Med 1996; 156: 997–1003.

169. Wynder EL, Kaufman PL, Lesser RL. A short-term follow-up study on ex-cigarette smokers: with special emphasis on persistent cough and weight gain. Am Rev Respir Dis 1967; 96: 645–655.

170. Lacourciere Y, Brunner H, Irwin R, et al. and the Losartan Cough Study Group. J Hypertension 1994; 12: 1387–1393.

171. Moldofsky J, Tullis C, Lamon R. Multiple tic syndrome (Gilles de la Tourette's syndrome): clinical, biological, and psychosocial variables and their influence with haloperidol. J Nerv Ment Dis 1974; 159: 282–292.

172. Golden GS. Tics and Tourette syndrome. Hosp Prac 1979; Nov: 91–100.

173. Van Woert MH, Yip LC, Balis ME. Purine phosphoribosyl-transferase in Gilles de la Tourette syndrome. N Engl J Med 1977; 296: 210–212.

174. Bernstein L. A respiratory tic: "the barking cough of puberty." Report of a case treated successfully. Laryngoscope 1963; 73: 315–319.

175. Cohlan SQ, Stone SM. The cough and the bedsheet. Pediatrics 1984; 74: 11–15.

176. Blager FB, Gay ML, Wood RP. Voice therapy techniques adapted to treatment of habit cough: a pilot study. J Commun Disord 1988; 21: 393–400.

177. Gay M, Blager F, Bartsch K II, et al. Psychogenic habit cough: review and case reports. J Clin Psychiatry 1987; 48: 483–486.

178. Israili ZH, Hall WD. Cough and angioneurotic edema associated with angiotensin-converting enzyme inhibitor therapy: a review of the literature and pathophysiology. Ann Intern Med 1992; 117: 234–242.

179. Ishrat-Husain S. Rhinolith—-a rare cause of chronic cough. Can Med Assoc J 1967; 97: 540–541.

180. Sokoloff MJ. Mechanisms and management of cough. Med Clin North Am 1961; 45: 1437–1442.

181. Ghosh S. Cough in children. J Ind Med Assoc 1966; 47: 325–328.

182. Paulose KO, Shenoy PK, Sharma RK. Otogenic reflex cough: implanted hair in the bony external auditory canal. Arch Otolaryngol Head Neck Surg 1988; 114: 1334.

183. Bloustine S, Langston L, Miller T. Earcough (Arnold's) reflex. Ann Otol 1976; 85: 406–407.

184. Sheehy JL, Lee S. chronic cough due to cholesteatoma: a case report. Am J Otol 1988; 9: 392.

185. Wolff AP, May M, Nuelle D. The tympanic membrane: a source of the cough reflex. JAMA 1973; 223: 1269.

186. Leichtling JJ, Lesnick GJ, Garlock JH. Neurilemmomas of vagus nerve in the neck: a significant diagnostic sign. JAMA 1963; 183: 143–145.

187. To SS, Gupta ARD. Traumatic neuroma of the internal laryngeal nerve as a cause of severe cough. J Laryngol Otol 1986; 100: 843–845.

188. Banyai AL. A symptom connoting many causes and sequels. Chest 1971; 60: 355.

189. Fitzpatrick TM, Whitlock WL. Chronic cough: sometimes you have to look at a tree to see the forest. Chest 1991; 100: 1180.

190. de Lara TDAC, Barbosa MA, de Oliveira MR, de Godoy I, Queluz TT. Human syngamosis:; two cases of chronic cough caused by Mammomonogamus laryngeus. Chest 1993; 103: 264–265.

191. Weinstein L, Molavi A. Syngamus laryngeus infection (syngamosis) with chronic cough. Ann Intern Med 1971; 74: 577–580.

192. Irwin RS, Pratter MR, Hamolsky MW. Chronic persistent cough: an uncommon presenting complaint of thyroiditis. Chest 1982; 81: 386–388.

193. Corrao WM, Braman SS, Irwin RS. Chronic cough as the sole presenting manifestation of bronchial asthma. N Engl J Med 1979; 300: 633–637.

194. Glauser FL. Variant asthma. Ann Allergy 1972; 30: 457–459.

195. McFadden ER Jr. Exertional dyspnea and cough as preludes to acute attacks of bronchial asthma. N Engl J Med 1975; 292: 555–559.

196. Kinney WW, Angelillo VA. Bronchiolitis in systemic lupus erythematosus. Chest 1982; 82: 646–649.

197. Lahdensuo A, Mattila J, Vilppula A. Bron-

chiolitis in rheumatoid arthritis. Chest 1984; 85: 705–708.

198. Kraft M, Mortenson RL, Colby TV, et al. Cryptogenic constrictive bronchiolitis: a clinico-pathologic study. Am Rev Respir Dis 1993; 148: 1093–1101.

199. Kindt GC, Weiland JE, Davis WB, et al. Bronchiolitis in adults: a reversible cause of airway obstruction associated with airway neutrophils and neutrophil products. Am Rev Respir Dis 1989; 140: 483–492.

200. Wright JL, Cagle P, Churg A, et al. Diseases of the small airways. Am Rev Respir Dis 1992; 146: 240–262.

201. Hyde L, Hyde CI. Clinical manifestations of lung cancer. Chest 1974; 65: 299–306.

202. Weiss W, Seidman J, Boucot KR. The Philadelphia pulmonary neoplasm research project: symptoms in occult lung cancer. Chest 1978; 73: 57–61.

203. Abdulmajid O, Ebeid AM, Motaweh MM, et al. Aspirated foreign bodies in the tracheobronchial tree: report of 250 cases. Thorax 1976; 31: 635–640.

204. Limper AH, Prakash UBS. Tracheobronchial foreign bodies in adults. Ann Intern Med 1990; 112: 604–609.

205. Shim C, Williams MH Jr. Cough and wheezing from beclomethasone aerosol. Chest 1987; 91: 207–209.

206. Shim CS, Williams MH Jr. Cough and wheezing from beclomethasone dipropionate aerosol are absent after triamcinolone acetonide. Ann Intern Med 1987; 106: 700–703.

207. Aust MR, Prakash UBS, McDougall JC, et al. Bronchoscopic broncholithotripsy. J Bronchology 1994; 1: 37–41.

208. Starkey GWB. Case records of the Massachusetts General Hospital. Weekly clinicopathological exercises. N Engl J Med 1978; 298: 1353–1357.

209. Lawson RM, Ramanathan L, Hurley G, et al. Bronchial adenoma: review of an 18-year experience at the Brompton Hospital. Thorax 1976; 31: 245–253.

210. Blondal T, Grimelius L, Nou E, et al. Argyrophil carcinoid tumors of the lung: incidence, clinical study, and follow-up of 46 patients. Chest 1980; 78: 840–844.

211. Grote TH, Macon WR, Davis B, et al. Atypical carcinoid of the lung: a distinct clinicopathologic entity. Chest 1988; 93: 370–375.

212. Constantopoulos SH, Drosos AA, Maddison PJ, et al. Xerotrachea and interstitial lung disease in primary Sjogren's syndrome. Respiration 1984; 46: 310–314.

213. Constantopoulos SH, Papadimitriou CS, Moutsopoulos HM. Respiratory manifestations in primary Sjogren's syndrome: a clinical, functional, and histologic study. Chest 1985; 88: 226–229.

214. Baumgartner WA, Mark JBD. Bronchoscopic diagnosis and treatment of bronchial stump suture granulomas. J Thorac Cardiovasc Surg 1981; 81: 553–555.

215. Albertini RE. Cough caused by exposed endobronchial sutures. Ann Intern Med 1981; 94: 205–206.

216. Shure D. Endobronchial suture: a foreign body causing chronic cough. Chest 1991; 100: 1193–1196.

217. Valor RR, Polnitsky CA, Tanis DJ, Sherter CB. Bacterial tracheitis with upper airway obstruction in a patient with the acquired immunodeficiency syndrome. Am Rev Respir Dis 1992; 146: 1598–1599.

218. Jordan SW, McLaren LC, Crosby JH. Herpetic tracheobronchitis. Arch Intern Med 1975; 135: 784–788.

219. Sherry MK, Klainer AS, Wolff M, et al. Herpetic tracheobronchitis. Ann Intern Med 1988; 109: 229–233.

220. Louria DB, Blumenfeld HL, Ellis JT, et al. Studies on influenza in the pandemic of 1957–1958. II. Pulmonary complications of influenza. J Clin Invest 1959; 38: 213–265.

221. Colt HG, Gumpert BC, Harrell JH. Tracheobronchial obstruction caused by Klebsiella rhinoscleromatis: diagnosis, pathologic features, and treatment. J Bronchology 1994; 1: 31–36.

222. Olson LC. Pertussis. Medicine 1975; 54: 427–469.

223. Murray HW, Masur H, Senterfit LB, et al. The protean manifestations of Mycoplasma pneumoniae infection in adults. Am J Med 1975; 58: 229–242.

224. Mansel JK, Rosenow EC III, Smith TF, et al. Mycoplasma pneumoniae pneumonia. Chest 1989; 95: 639–646.

225. Albert RK, Petty TL. Endobronchial tuberculosis progressing to bronchial stenosis. Chest 1976; 70: 537–539.

226. Smith JL, Elliott CG, Schmidt CD, et al. Bronchial stenosis: a complication of healed endobronchial tuberculosis. West J Med 1986; 144: 361–362.

227. Kramer MR, Denning DW, Marshall SE, et al. Ulcerative tracheobronchitis after lung transplantation: a new form of invasive

aspergillosis. Am Rev Respir Dis 1991; 144: 552–556.

228. Pervez NK, Kleinerman J, Kattan M, et al. Pseudomembranous necrotizing bronchial aspergillosis: a variant of invasive aspergillosis in a patient with hemophilia and acquired immune deficiency syndrome. Am Rev Respir Dis 1985; 131: 961–963.

229. Cordier J-F, Valeyre D, Guillevin L, et al. Pulmonary Wegener's granulomatosis: a clinical and imaging study of 77 cases. Chest 1990; 97: 906–912.

230. Vasishta S, Wood JB, McGinty F. Ulcerative tracheobronchitis years after colectomy for ulcerative colitis. Chest 1994; 106: 1279–1281.

231. Wilcox P, Miller R, Miller G, et al. Airway involvement in ulcerative colitis. Chest 1987;92: 18–22.

232. Butland RJA, Cole P, Citron KM, et al. Chronic bronchial suppuration and inflammatory bowel disease. Q J Med 1981; New Series L, 197: 63–75.

233. Buckler RA, Pratter MR, Chad DA, et al. Chronic cough as the presenting symptom of oculopharyngeal muscular dystrophy. Chest 1989; 95: 921–922.

234. Irwin RS. Aspiration. In: *Intensive Care Medicine*, 2nd Edition. Edited by Rippe JM, Irwin RS, Alpert JS, Fink MP, eds. Boston, Ma: Little, Brown and Company; 1991: 525–532.

235. Fouty BW, Pomeranz M, Thigpen TP, et al. Dilatation of bronchial stenosis due to sarcoidosis using a flexible fiberoptic bronchoscope. Chest 1994; 106: 677–680.

236. Arkin CR, Masi AT. Relapsing polychondritis: review of current status and case report. Semin Arthrit Rheum 1975; 5: 41–62.

237. Center C. Case records of the Massachusetts General Hospital. Weekly clinicopathological exercises. N Engl J Med 1985; 313: 1530–1537.

238. Guerry-Force ML, Muller NL, Wright JL, et al. A comparison of bronchiolitis obliterans with organizing pneumonia, usual interstitial pneumonia, and small airways disease. Am Rev Respir Dis 1987; 135: 705–712.

239. Crystal RG, Fulmer JD, Roberts WC, et al. Idiopathic pulmonary fibrosis: clinical, histologic, radiographic, physiologic, scintigraphic, cytologic, and biochemical aspects. Ann Intern Med 1976; 85: 769–788.

240. Research Committee of the British Thoracic Society and the Public Health Laboratory Service. Community-acquired pneumonia in adults in British hospitals in 1982–1983: a survey of aetiology, mortality, prognostic factors and outcome. Q J Med 1987; 239 (New Series 62): 195–220.

241. Fang G-D, Fine M, Orloss J, et al. New and emerging etiologies for community-acquired pneumonia with implications for therapy: a prospective multicenter study of 359 cases. Medicine 1990; 69: 307–316.

242. Davidson KG, Walbaum PR, McCormack RJM. Intrathoracic neural tumours. Thorax 1978; 33: 359–367.

243. Hodge J, Aponte G, McLaughlin E. Primary mediastinal tumors. J Thoracic Surg 1959; 37: 730–744.

244. Ferrucci JT Jr. Case records of the Massachusetts General Hospital. Weekly clinicopathological exercises. N Engl J Med 1977; 296: 1467–1473.

245. Ellis FH Jr, Good CA. Intrathoracic goiter. Ann Surg 1952; 135: 79–90.

246. Akers SM, Bartter TC, Pratter MR. Chronic cough as the sole manifestation of Hodgkin's disease. Chest 1992; 101: 853–854.

247. Currens JH, White PD. Cough as a symptom of cardiovascular disease. Ann Intern Med 1949; 30: 528–543.

248. Moser KM. Pulmonary embolism. Am Rev Respir Dis 1977; 115: 829–852.

249. Kleiber EE. Long standing productive cough as chief clinical manifestation in mitral stenosis: a case complicated by thrombosis of left auricle. Ann Intern Med 1941; 15: 899–910.

250. Kang J, Gupta M, Catangay PA, et al. Paroxysmal cough induced by transvenous pacemaker. Am Heart J 1971; 81: 719–720.

251. Irwin RS, Zawacki JK, Curley FJ, et al. Chronic cough as the sole presenting manifestation of gastroesophageal reflux. Am Rev Respir Dis 1989; 140: 1294–1300.

252. Fitzgerald JM, Allen CJ, Craven MA, et al. Chronic cough and gastroesophageal reflux. Can Med Assoc J 1989; 140: 520–524.

253. Ing AJ, Ngu MC, Breslin ABX. Pathogenesis of chronic persistent cough associated with gastroesophageal reflux. Am J Respir Crit Care Med 1994; 149: 160–167.

254. Bowton DL, Katz PO. Esophageal cyst as a cause of chronic cough. Chest 1984; 86: 150–152.

255. Collins TR, Sahn SA. Thoracocentesis: clinical value, complications, technical

problems, and patient experience. Chest 1987; 91: 817–822.

256. Seneff MG, Corwin RW, Gold LH, et al. Complications associated with thoracocentesis. Chest 1986; 89: 97–100.

257. Light RW, Stanbury DW, Brown SE. The relationship between pleural pressures and changes in pulmonary function after therapeutic thoracocentesis. Am Rev Respir Dis 1986; 133: 658–661.

257a. Diehr P, Wood RW, Bushyhead JB, et al. Prediction of pneumonia in outpatients with acute cough. J Chronic Dis 1984; 37: 215–225.

258. Niederman MS, Fein AM. Pneumonia in the elderly. Geriatr Clin North Am 1986; 2: 241–268.

259. Pratter M, Hingston DM, Irwin RS. Diagnosis of bronchial asthma by clinical evaluation: an unreliable method. Chest 1983; 84: 42–47.

260. Eschenbacher WL, Boushey HA, Sheppard D. Alteration in osmolarity of inhaled aerosols cause bronchoconstriction and cough, but absence of a permeant anion causes cough alone. Am Rev Respir Dis 1984; 129: 211–215.

261. Sheppard D, Rizk NW, Boushey HA, et al. Mechanism of cough and bronchoconstriction induced by distilled water aerosol. Am Rev Respir Dis 1983; 127: 691–694.

262. Fuller RW, Jackson DM. Physiology and treatment of cough. Thorax 1990; 45: 425–430.

263. Medical Research Council. Committee report on the aetiology of chronic bronchitis. Definition and classification of chronic bronchitis for clinical and epidemiologic purposes. Lancet 1965; 1: 775–778.

264. Smyrnios NA, Irwin RS, Curley FJ. Chronic cough with a history of excessive mucus production: the spectrum and frequency of causes, key components of the diagnostic evaluation, and outcome of specific therapy. Chest 1995; 108: 991–997.

265. Fraser RG, Pare' JAP, Pare' PD, et al. Diseases of the airways. In: *Diagnosis of Diseases of the Chest.* 3rd edition. Volume 3. Philadelphia, Pa: WB Saunders Company; 1990: 2092–2201.

266. Sesko S, Kaneko Y. Cough associated with the use of captopril. Arch Intern Med 1985; 145: 1524.

267. Sebastian JL, McKinney WP, Kaufman J, et al. Angiotensin-converting enzyme inhibitors and cough. Chest 1991; 99: 36–39.

268. Faison EP, Nelson EB, Irvin JD. Profile of angiotensin-converting enzyme inhibitor (ACEI) associated cough: incidence and clinical characteristics. Am J Hypertension 1991; 4 (Part 2): 28A.

269. Berkin KE. Respiratory effects of angiotensin-converting enzyme inhibition. Eur Respir J 1989; 2: 198–201.

270. Morice AH, Lowry R, Brown MJ, et al. Angiotensin-converting enzyme and the cough reflex. Lancet 1987; 2: 1116–1118.

271. Hyde L, Hyde CI. Clinical manifestations of lung cancer. Chest 1974; 65: 299–306.

272. Weiss W, Seidman H, Boucot KR. The Philadelphia pulmonary neoplasm research project: symptoms of occult lung cancer. Chest 1978; 73: 57–61.

273. Boucot KR, Cooper DA, Weiss W, et al. Cigarettes, cough, and cancer of the lung. JAMA 1966; 196: 167–172.

274. Fulmer JC, Roberts WC. Small airways and interstitial pulmonary disease. Chest 1980; 77: 470–477.

275. Irwin RS, Curley FJ. The treatment of cough: a comprehensive review. Chest 1991; 99: 1477–1484.

276. Irwin RS, Curley FJ, Bennett FM. Appropriate use of antitussives and protussives: a practical review. Drugs 1993; 46: 80–91.

277. Irwin RS, French CL, Smyrnios NA et al. The effect of inhaled metaproterenol on cough-variant asthma. Am Rev Respir Dis 1992; 145 (Part 2): A12.

278. Barnes PJ. Effect of nedocromil sodium on airway sensory nerves. J Allergy Clin Immunol 1993; 92: 182–186.

279. Petty TL, Rollins DR, Christopher K, et al. Cromolyn sodium is effective in adult chronic asthmatics. Am Rev Respir Dis 1989; 139: 694–701.

280. Doan T, Patterson R, Greenberger PA. Cough variant asthma: usefulness of a diagnostic-therapeutic trial with prednisone. Ann Allergy 1992; 69: 505–509.

281. Irwin RS, Curley FJ, French CL. Difficult to control asthma: contributing factors and outcome of a systematic management protocol. Chest 1993; 103: 1662–1669.

282. Richter JE, Castell DO. Drugs, foods, and other substances in the cause and treatment of reflux esophagitis. Med Clin North Am 1981; 65: 1223–1234.

283. Sontag SJ. The medical management of reflux esophagitis. Gastroenterol Clin North Am 1990; 19: 683–712.

284. Schapira M, Henrion J, Heller FR. The

current status of gastric prokinetic drugs. Acta Gastro-enterologica Belgica 1990; LIII: 446–457.

285. Barone JA, Jessen LM, Colaizzi JL, et al. Cisapride: a gastrointestinal prokinetic drug. Ann Pharmacotherapy 1994; 28: 488–500.

285a. Kerr P, Shoenut JP, Millar T, et al. Nasal CPAP reduces gastroesophageal reflux in obstructive sleep apnea syndrome. Chest 1992: 101: 1539–1544.

286. Sackner MA. Effect of respiratory drugs on mucociliary clearance. Chest 1978: 73 (Suppl).: 958–966.

287. Sutton PP, Pavia D, Bateman JRM, et al. The effect of oral aminophylline on lung mucociliary clearance in man. Chest 1981; 80 (Suppl).: 899–892.

288. Bjerkestrand G, Digranes A, Schreiner A. Bacteriological findings in transtracheal aspirates from patients with chronic bronchitis and bronchiectasis: a preliminary report. Scand J Resp Dis 1975; 56: 201–207.

289. Fogari R, Zoppi A, Tettamanti F, et al. Effects of nifedipine and indomethacin on cough induced by angiotensin-converting enzyme inhibitors: a double-blind, randomised, cross-over study. J Cardiovasc Pharmacol 1992; 19: 670–673.

290. McEwan JR, Choudy NB, Fuller RW. The effect of sulindac on the abnormal cough reflex associated with dry cough. J Pharmacol Exp Ther 1990; 255: 161–164.

291. Poe RH, Israel RH. Evaluating and managing that nagging chronic cough. J Respir Dis 1990; 11: 297–313.

291a. Holmes PW, Barter CE, Pierce RJ. Chronic persistent cough: use of ipratropium bromide in undiagnosed cases following upper respiratory tract infection. Respir Med 1992; 86: 425–429.

292. Herwaldt LA. Pertussis in adults: what physicians need to know. Arch Intern Med 1991; 151: 1510–1512.

293. Herwaldt LA. Pertussis and pertussis vaccines in adults. JAMA 1993; 269: 93–94.

294. Fuchs HJ, Borowitz DS, Christiansen DH, et al, for the Pulmozyme Study Group. Effect of aerosolized recombinant human DNase on exacerbations of respiratory symptoms and on pulmonary function in patients with cystic fibrosis. N Engl J Med 1994; 331: 637–642.

295. Reed AP. Preparation of the patient for awake flexible fiberoptic bronchoscopy. Chest 1992; 101: 244–253.

296. Allegra L, Bossi R. Clinical trials with the new antitussive levodropropizine in adult bronchitic patients. Arzneimittel-Forschung 1988; 38: 1163–1166.

297. Sperber SJ, Hendley JO, Hayden FG, et al. Effects of naproxen on experimental rhinovirus colds: a randomized, double-blind, controlled trial. Ann Intern Med 1992; 117: 37–41.

298. Eddy NB, Friebel H, Hahn K-J, et al. Codeine and its alternates for pain and cough relief: 4. Potential alternatives for cough relief. Bull WHO 1969; 40: 639–719.

299. Eccles R, Morris S, Jawad M. Lack of effect of codeine in the treatment of cough associated with acute upper respiratory infection. J Clin Pharm Ther 1992; 17: 175–180.

300. Fuller RW, Jackson DM. Physiology and treatment of cough. Thorax 1991; 45: 425–430.

301. Mathys H, Bleicher B, Bleicher U. Dextromethorphan and codeine: objective assessment of antitussive activity in patients with chronic cough. J Intern Med Res 1983; 11: 92–100.

302. Ghafouri MA, Patil KD, Kass I. Sputum changes associated with the use of ipratropium bromide. Chest 1984; 86: 387–393.

303. Holmes PW, Barter CE, Pierce RJ. Chronic persistent cough: use of ipratropium bromide in undiagnosed cases following upper respiratory tract infection. Respir Med 1992; 86: 425–429.

304. Wheeler AP. Sedation, analgesia, and paralysis in the intensive care unit. Chest 1993; 104: 566–577.

305. Cox ID, Wallis PJW, Hughes DTD, et al. An electromyographic method of objectively assessing cough intensity and use of the method to assess effects of codeine on the dose-response curve to citric acid. Br J Clin Pharmacol 1984; 18: 377–382.

306. Clarke SW, Lopez-Vidriero MT, Pavia D, et al. The effect of sodium 2-mercaptoethane sulphonate and hypertonic saline aerosols on bronchial clearance in chronic bronchitis. Br J Clin Pharmacol 1979; 7: 39–44.

307. Pavia D, Thomson ML, Clarke SW. Enhanced clearance of secretions from the human lung after the administration of hypertonic saline aerosol. Am Rev Respir Dis 1978; 117: 199–203.

307a. Eng PA, Morton J, Douglas JA, et al. Short-term efficacy of ultrasonically nebulized hypertonic saline in cystic fibrosis. Pediatr Pulmonol 1996; 21: 77–83,

308. App EM, King M, Helfesrieder R, et al. Acute and long-term amiloride inhalation in cystic fibrosis therapy. Am Rev Respir Dis 1990; 141: 605–612.

309. Bennett WD, Chapman WF, Mascarella JM. The acute effect of ipratropium bromide bronchodilator therapy on cough clearance in COPD. Chest 1993; 103: 488–495.

310. Sutton PP, Gemmell JG, Innes N, et al. Use of nebulized saline and nebulized terbutaline as an adjunct to chest physiotherapy. Thorax 1988; 43: 57–60.

311. Bouhuys A, Van de Woestijne KP. Mechanical consequences of airway smooth muscle relaxation. J Appl Physiol 1971; 30: 670–676.

312. Kirby NA, Barnerias MJ, Siebens AA. An evaluation of assisted cough in quadriparetic patients. Arch Phys Med Rehab 1966; 47: 705–710.

313. Braun SR, Giovannoni R, O'Connor M. Improving the cough in patients with spinal cord injury. Am J Phys Med 1984; 63: 1–10.

314. Estenne M, De Troyer A. Cough in tetraplegic subjects: an active process. Ann Intern Med 1990; 112: 22–28.

315. Christensen EF, Nedergaard T, Dahl R. Long-term treatment of chronic bronchitis with positive expiratory pressure mask and chest physiotherapy. Chest 1990; 97: 645–650.

316. de Boeck C, Zinman R. Cough versus chest physiotherapy. Am Rev Respir Dis 1984; 129: 182–184.

317. Rossman CM, Waldes R, Sampson D, et al. Effect of chest physiotherapy on the removal of mucus in patients with cystic fibrosis. Am Rev Respir Dis 1982; 126: 131–135.

318. Sones FM Jr. Cine coronary arteriography. In: *The Heart*. Hurst JW, Logue RD, eds. New York, NY: McGraw-Hill; 1970: 377–385.

319. Conti CR. Coronary arteriography. Circulation 1977; 55: 227–241.

320. Schultz DD, Olivas GS. The use of cough cardiopulmonary resuscitation in clinical practice. Heart Lung 1986; 15: 273–280.

321. Caldwell G, Millar G, Quinn E, et al. Simple mechanical methods for cardioversion: defence of the precordial thump and cough version. Br Med J 1985; 291: 627–630.

322. Criley JM, Blaufuss AH, Kissel GL. Cough induced cardiac compression: self-administered form of cardiopulmonary resuscitation. JAMA 1976; 236: 1246–1250.

323. Niemann JT, Rosborough J, Hausknecht M, et al. Cough CPR: documentation of systemic perfusion in man and in an experimental model: a window to the mechanism of blood flow in external CPR. Crit Care Med 1980; 8: 141–146.

324. Wei JY, Greene HL, Weisfeldt ML. Cough-facilitated conversion of ventricular tachycardia. Am J Cardiol 1980; 45: 174–176.

325. Evans JM, Jaeger MJ. Mechanical aspects of coughing. Pneumonologie 1975; 152: 253–257.

# 2

# Dyspnea

Frederick J. Curley, M.D.

## Introduction

Dyspnea is a common symptom occurring in up to 20% of the general population and it is associated with a marked increase in mortality.[1] This risk of death in a dyspneic population followed for 6 years was 1.7 to 2.0 times above the risk predicted in a general population.[1] Since physicians encounter dyspnea in all medical practice settings, in all age groups, and in association with innumerable diseases, all physicians should have a fundamental understanding of how to systematically evaluate and manage the dyspneic patient. When a systematic evaluation of dyspnea was not used, the cause of dyspnea was not determined in 73% of cases and 61% of dyspneic patients were unimproved.[2] On the other hand, a systematic evaluation and treatment of dyspnea performed in a pulmonary clinic has been shown to almost always identify the causes of dyspnea and result in a decrease of symptoms.[3]

This chapter aims to review the physiology of dyspnea, the relationship of specific diseases to the sensation of dyspnea, and how this information can be used to guide the cost-effective evaluation and management of the dyspneic patient. Although dyspnea in children and acute dyspnea will be discussed, this chapter will focus more on the adult patient presenting with chronic dyspnea.

## Definition

Dyspnea comes from the Greek roots "dys" and "pnoia" and literally could be translated as "bad breathing." The medical definition of dyspnea has varied among authors, but generally reflects the following broad working definition: dyspnea is a distressing sensation of difficult, labored, or unpleasant breathing. Each word in the above definition is carefully chosen.

This chapter deals with dyspnea as a symptom—indicating that the patient identifies that his or her breathing is *distressing*. Although labored or difficult breathing may be encountered by healthy individuals while exercising, it may not qualify as dyspnea because it may not be perceived as distressing. Individuals may perceive similar physiologic challenges differently and may describe a different intensity or quality to the sensation. The fact that the sensation of dyspnea is often poorly or vaguely described may, in part, reflect that dyspnea may actually be several sensations that we group as one. Of the five major senses, touch is the most used to describe dyspnea. In common

From Irwin RS, Curley FJ, Grossman RF (eds): Diagnosis and Treatment of Symptoms of the Respiratory Tract. Armonk, New York, Futura Publishing Company, Inc., © 1997.

usage, we include in the sensation of touch our ability to judge the weight, firmness, smoothness, and temperature of an object. Physiologically, we know that these perceptions utilize different neuroreceptors that share neural pathways and are probably processed in several areas of the central nervous system (CNS). Similarly, when patients describe their breathing as gasping, tight, or short, these perceptions may involve different receptors, neural pathways, or areas of the CNS, yet we speak of them all as a part of dyspnea. Until our understanding of the physiology of dyspnea is advanced enough to explain how differences in perception arise or in many cases whether the difference in perception is due to a difference in the pathophysiology of dyspnea, we must accept a broad working definition of dyspnea.

In order to have a common understanding of the definition of dyspnea, we must broaden our discussion of definition by expanding on attempts to better characterize the quality and intensity of the dyspneic sensation.

## Describing the Quality of Dyspnea

Failure to appreciate the varied ways that patients describe dyspnea or the imprecise definition can contribute to a clinician's failure to appreciate its presence as a problem. Any description of the quality of dyspnea must be affective. Patients may perceive their breathing to be difficult with regard to its (1) timing—"I cannot breathe fast enough"; (2) depth—"I feel I need more air" or "I cannot take a deep enough breath"; (3) effort—"I am struggling to breathe"; or (4) taste or feel—"My air is bad" or "My chest is raw when I breathe."

Moreover, several descriptors may apply to the same problem in a single patient. These varied qualities of breathing lead to a wide range of descriptors of the dyspneic sensation. In the broadest definition of dyspnea, one would consider all of these as a type of difficult breathing.

Due to the affective nature of dyspnea some patients may have a difficult time describing their dyspnea and some may select unusual descriptions for the sensation of dyspnea. When dyspneic patients are administered a questionnaire asking them to describe how their breathing feels, most can relate to common descriptors: short of breath, hard to breathe, feel like I need air, rapid breathing, shallow breathing, panting, or hard to get breath out.[4] Eliott et al.[5] offered a choice of 45 different descriptors to 208 dyspneic patients with cardiopulmonary disease. Table I indicates the most and least common descriptors selected by this group. Once it is clear that the patient is describing dyspnea, he or she may also select descriptors not typically associated with breathing. When I asked 89 dyspneic patients to choose appropriate descriptors for their breathing discomfort from a list of pain descriptors in the McGill Melzack Pain Rating Questionnaire,[6] 23% of the patients described their dyspnea as pricking, 21% as cool, and 5% as flickering. This heterogeneity of description may easily confound the clinician attempting to elicit a history of dyspnea or an investigator attempting to ensure that dyspneic patients actually have the sensation they wish to study. The clinician must listen closely to the patient and not dismiss unusual statements or the complaint may be missed.

## Describing the Intensity of Dyspnea

To determine the severity of the patient's complaint and assess the impact of therapy on the progression of the disease causing dyspnea, the clinician should attempt to quantify dyspnea. Clinicians have typically assessed the intensity of dyspnea by measuring the patient's ability to perform exertion. Scales have been developed that simply quantify the magnitude of exertion the patient can perform before stopped by breathlessness. The most widely used scale to quantify dyspnea was developed by Fletcher under funding of the British Medical Research Council (BMRC) in the 1950s.[7] This scale (see Appendix A), referred to as the British Medical Research Council (BMRC) scale, grades dyspnea from 1 to 5, with 5 indicating that the patient has dyspnea on the

**Table I**
Frequency of Descriptors of Dyspnea in Cardiopulmonary Patients

*12 Most Frequent Descriptors—selected by more than 60%*

| | |
|---|---|
| I feel short of breath | I want to take in more air |
| I am aware of my breathing | I feel a need to take a deeper breath |
| I feel out of breath | It is difficult to breathe |
| I feel breathless | I can't get enough air into my chest |
| I feel puffed | I feel a need to breathe |
| I feel I cannot breathe deeply enough | I feel I am gasping for breath |

*12 Least Frequent Descriptors—selected by less than 30%*

| | |
|---|---|
| I feel that air does not taste right | I feel that I am breathing bad air |
| My breathing is too deep | I feel that my breathing stops |
| I feel a raw sensation in my chest | I feel winded in my chest |
| My breath does not go out enough | I feel I am smothering |
| I cannot breathe out fast enough | I feel I am suffocating |
| I feel a raw sensation deep in my throat | I cannot breathe fast enough |

Adapted from reference 5 Eliott MW et al. Am Rev Respir Dis 1991;144:826–832.

slightest exertion. The American Thoracic Society[8] modified this scale (see Appendix B) to range from 0 to 4 instead of 1 to 5, leaving the descriptors of the amount of exertion needed to cause dyspnea essentially unchanged. Both of these scales have the advantage of simplicity and ease of use. Both are, however, unidimensional and not applicable to all patients. Neither scale quantifies the amount of effort used by the patient to perform a task and neither quantifies a degree of impairment. Patients may have dyspnea on minor exertion but remain gainfully employed. They may compensate for their dyspnea by eliminating the most strenuous tasks in their daily life or performing tasks very slowly.

In order to address these limitations, Mahler et al.[9] published a more elaborate index (see Appendix C) that corrects these deficiencies by using three subscales to assess the severity of dyspnea: (1) the magnitude of effort needed to produce dyspnea, (2) the magnitude of task needed to produce dyspnea, and (3) the degree of functional impairment due to dyspnea. Each subscale ranges from 0 to 4, where the higher the number the less the severity of the dyspnea and the lower the number the greater the severity of the dyspnea. Each subscale score is added to provide a total score of 0 to 12.

Mahler and colleagues made an additional modification that uses three similar subscales to measure an improvement or deterioration in dyspnea from baseline (see Appendix D).[9] This permits quantification of fine gradations of change (transitional index) in the level of dyspnea. Using the BMRC dyspnea index, a patient with dyspnea on dressing (Grade 5) needs to improve to be able to walk 100 yards or walk a few minutes (Grade 4) to have a measurable improvement. Using the transitional index, improvement may be seen due to fewer pauses or less of a sense of effort while performing the same task.

Visual analog scales (VAS) (Figure 1) or modified Borg scales (Table II) can also be used to assess the severity of dyspnea. The most frequently used visual analog scales employ a fixed-length vertical or horizontal line with anchoring statements at each end. A patient may then be asked to mark on the line the point that best corresponds to the severity of their dyspnea between anchoring statements such as none and maximal. If a 10-cm line is used, the scores are easily graded by measuring from 0 to 100 mm. Modified Borg scales

Please mark on the line below the point that best describes the amount of difficulty you have with your breathing.

None                                                                    Maximal

**Figure 1.** Visual analog scale of dyspnea severity. If a line is drawn to be 100 mm long, the result may be easily calculated.

typically present the patient with a scale ranging from 0 to 10 with each integer between corresponding to an anchoring descriptor. The Borg scale quantifies sensation in a nonlinear fashion—mild dyspnea starts at 1 and severe dyspnea starts at 5. This asymmetric distribution of descriptors recognizes the psychometric principle that the perceived intensity of sensation is exponentially related to physiologic intensity. Construction of a scale in this fashion permits more valid comparisons among different subjects.[10,11]

Visual analog scales and modified Borg scales categorize the patient's perception of dyspnea in relation to a particular task or challenge well. However, they lack the global descriptor quality of the BMRC or Mahler's index. Clinically, they have been most useful in quantifying changes in dyspnea during a brief time period in response to measurable physiologic changes. For example, these scales are excellent to describe the increase in dyspnea during an incremental exercise test, during a 12-minute walk test, or as the patient walks on a treadmill at fixed settings over the course of a rehabilitation program. In daily clinical practice, the scales can also be used to record the patient's estimate of the dyspnea that results from standard tasks—climbing stairs, making a bed, or bathing. Improvement or deterioration could be judged by comparisons between recorded levels of dyspnea at different visits.

### Table II
#### Modified Borg Scale

| | |
|---|---|
| 0 | Nothing at all |
| 0.5 | Very, very slight (just noticeable) |
| 1 | Very slight |
| 2 | Slight |
| 3 | Moderate |
| 4 | Somewhat severe |
| 5 | Severe |
| 6 | |
| 7 | Very severe |
| 8 | |
| 9 | Very, very severe (almost maximal) |
| 10 | Maximal |

Modified from Borg GAV. Psychophysical bases of perceived exertion. Med Sci Sports Exerc 1982;14: 377–381.

## Prevalence of Dyspnea

The lack of a precise definition of dyspnea has confounded attempts to provide an accurate estimate of the prevalence and incidence of dyspnea. Estimates of the prevalence of dyspnea come primarily from large, well-designed, epidemiologic surveys and smaller, uncontrolled studies conducted in office practices.

### General Population

Several well-done epidemiologic studies have provided enough similar data

**Table III**
Prevalence of Dyspnea

| Country | N | Age | Sex | Frequency |
|---|---|---|---|---|
| Sweden[12] | 855 | 50 years | men | 2.8% |
|  |  | 67 years | men | 10% |
| France[13] | 3777 | >65 years | men | 15% |
|  |  |  | women | 19% |
| Italy[14] | 2322 | >20 years | men | 14% |
|  |  |  | women | 21% |
| USA[15] | 3948 | >25 years | men | 3.3% |
|  |  |  | women | 6.2% |

that we can conclude that the prevalence of dyspnea in the general population increases with age, increases rapidly after age 50, and is higher in women. Table III[12–15] summarizes the results of several large studies and suggests that the prevalence of dyspnea of BMRC severity grade 2 or higher is approximately 3% to 5% in a younger population, exceeds 10% in older men, and approaches 20% in older women. When one looks for the prevalence of any grade of dyspnea, the numbers are much higher. Dyspnea of any grade may occur in 16% to 22% of the general USA population younger than 50 years and in 19% to 34% of those older than 50 years.[1] The prevalence of any degree of dyspnea in an older French population was 60% in men and 64% in women.[13] In all studies, dyspnea appeared to be more common with older age and in women.

Several studies have also shown that dyspnea is directly related to smoking, occupation, and obesity (Table IV). When a

**Table IV**
Risk Factors for Developing Dyspnea

Older Age
Female Sex
Tobacco Smoking
Occupation
Rural Residence
Obesity: BMI >30 kg/m$^2$

BMI, body mass index.

cohort of 1722 adult smokers and ex-smokers in Poland and the USA were followed over 13 years,[16] the prevalence of dyspnea in smokers was 7.3% and ex-smokers was 8.2%, while the incidence of dyspnea was 15.9% and 17.4%, respectively. The incidence rates for attacks of breathlessness were significantly reduced in ex-smokers. The prevalence rates probably appear lower than those studies discussed above because 90% of the subjects included in this study were younger than 56 years of age and 59% were 40 years old or less. The incidence rates, despite the younger age, appear much higher in smokers and ex-smokers than in the general population.

Studies from Italy and France support a significant influence of occupation on the prevalence of dyspnea. In a study of more than 1600 subjects in Italy,[17] the odds ratio for having BMRC grade 2 or higher dyspnea was 2.76 for men and 3.74 for women in those exposed to occupational dusts, chemicals, or gases, as compared with unexposed subjects. In France, a survey examining dyspnea in relationship to occupation[13] showed that dyspnea was common in all occupations (Figures 2 and 3), but appeared highest in farm workers, unskilled blue collar workers, and domestic service employees. An urban place of residence had a significantly protective effect (odds ratio 0.7).

In a study of 1006 obese Swedish subjects with a body mass index greater than 30 kg/m$^{2,18}$ the prevalence of dyspnea was 70.4% for men and 82.6% for women aged

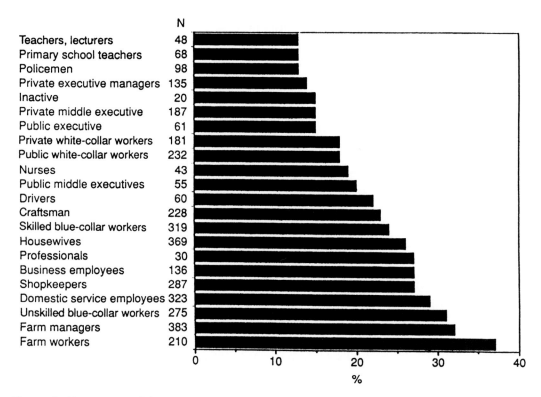

**Figure 2.** Percentage of dyspneic subjects according to their principal occupational category. (Adapted from reference 13: Nejjari C, et al. Int J Epidemiol 1993; 22: 848–854.

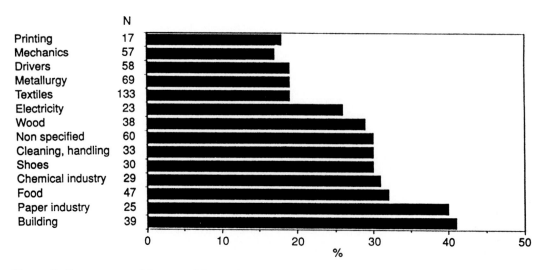

**Figure 3.** Percentages of dyspneic blue-collar workers according to the type of industry. (Adapted from reference 13: Nejjari C, et al. Int J Epidemiol 1993; 22: 848–854.

37 to 42 and 75.9 % for men and 92.3% for women aged 53 to 57. At age 50, the odds ratio for dyspnea in obese subjects compared to controls was 4.3 for men and 4.7 for women. A 5-ft tall person exceeds a body mass index of 30 kg/m$^2$ at 146 pounds, a 5 ft 6 in person at 182 pounds, and a 6 ft person at 212 pounds. This suggests that obesity may be an extremely common cause of dyspnea.

## Physician Practice

The prevalence of dyspnea in the population of patients seen by a physician differs from the prevalence in the general population. Although exact figures are difficult to obtain because few studies have been performed, dyspnea is most common in the inpatient setting and less common in the outpatient setting. The highest prevalence of dyspnea has been found among psychiatric patients. On an inpatient psychiatry service, 40% to 47% of patients may complain of dyspnea.[19] Primarily due to the high prevalence of patients with cardiopulmonary diseases admitted to the hospital, the prevalence of dyspnea among nonpsychiatric inpatients may approach 15% to 25%.[20–23] In the emergency department, 2.7% of patient have been reported to be dyspneic.[21]

Although there are no reliable data estimating the prevalence of dyspnea in the outpatient internal medicine or family practice office, one would expect that at least 5% of patients in a busy practice would be dyspneic. In one study that retrospectively reviewed the charts of 1000 outpatients seen in the outpatient clinic of an internal medicine training program, dyspnea was the seventh most common symptom prompting evaluation and occurred in 3.7% of patients.[2] In fact, 12% to 17% of adults report attacks of shortness of breath each year.[24] Studies have estimated that 10% of visits to an internist are due to a hyperventilation syndrome and that 90% of these patients complain of dyspnea.[25] By extrapolation, it is easy to estimate that most busy outpatient physicians should expect to see on average at least one to two patients with significant dyspnea each day.

## Physiology

### Overview

The physiology of dyspnea remains unclear despite more than 40 years of active investigation. A simplistic single neural pathway has been superseded by a complex, multiple neural pathway paradigm.

For years, investigators have attempted to construct a physiologic model for dyspnea that describes a single neural pathway between a respiratory stimulus and the sensation of dyspnea (Figure 4). This pathway requires that a stimulus activates a receptor, generating a signal that is carried by a nerve to the brain stem and higher cortical centers. The higher centers then receive, acknowledge, and evaluate the signal, creating the sensation of dyspnea. The difficulty with such models lies in the fact that no one model has been able to account for all types of dyspnea. Each new revelation regarding dyspnea has been refuted by others who can show that the latest model does not apply to a given problem.

Since the respiratory system itself is extremely complex and redundant in its control mechanisms, it is quite likely that there are multiple stimuli, receptors, nerves, and neural pathways that mediate the sensation of dyspnea. Logic supports this view. Clinical practice has proven that patients can severely injure components of the respiratory system and continue to perform adequately. In a teleological sense, if one views dyspnea as a defense mechanism against respiratory failure and subsequent death, it is unlikely that an organism that possessed a single pathway-mediating respiratory distress would have survived. If one accepts this perspective, then the conflicting physiologic models seeking a unitary explanation can easily be reconciled—multiple respiratory signals reaching the brain stem are probably gated in a complex control mechanism that passes a

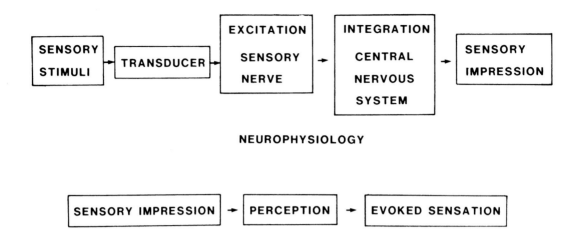

**Figure 4.** Schematic diagram of the steps required for conscious sensation of a physiologic stimulus (Adapted from reference 260: Killian KJ. Chest 1985; 88:85S). The top panel indicates the neurophysiologic model and the bottom panel indicates the behavioral psychologic model for the sensation of dyspnea. Both models are correct but developed from different theoretical assumptions.

diversity of signals at different times to higher centers and alters central processing and perception. Signals relating to a sense of effort, $Paco_2$, $Pao_2$, work, and fatigue arise with each breath and are probably integrated and balanced centrally and differently under a variety of physiologic conditions.

This multiple neural pathway model of dyspnea suggests that the sensation of dyspnea may arise due to abnormalities in the afferent pathways, the efferent pathways, or the central control centers of the respiratory system (Figure 5). A fundamental understanding of the anatomy of each of these major areas will be beneficial in developing a clinical approach for evaluating and treating dyspnea. Consequently, the remainder of this section will aim to review the basic anatomy and physiology of the efferent, afferent, and control systems that pertain to dyspnea.

cles. They extend from the brain stem and exit at all levels between cranial nerves IX and L1 (Figure 5). These pathways are activated when the act of breathing involves a signal that is generated either voluntarily by higher centers or reflexly by the brain stem and is passed to the spinal cord, the anterior horn cells, the peripheral nerves, and the neuromuscular junction. The respiratory muscles are anchored to the thoracic cage and, when stimulated, generate a pressure gradient that deforms the thoracic cage and lung to create inspiration and expiration. The resultant gas flow through the upper and lower airways permits exchange of air with the alveolar capillaries. The vasculature then permits carried gases to exchange with the tissues. Any defect in the above schema may impair the efficacy of respiration and lead to dyspnea.

## Efferent Respiratory Pathways

The efferent pathways are the motor nerves that innervate the respiratory mus-

## Afferent Respiratory Pathways

Afferent pathways feed back to the CNS from virtually all levels of the efferent

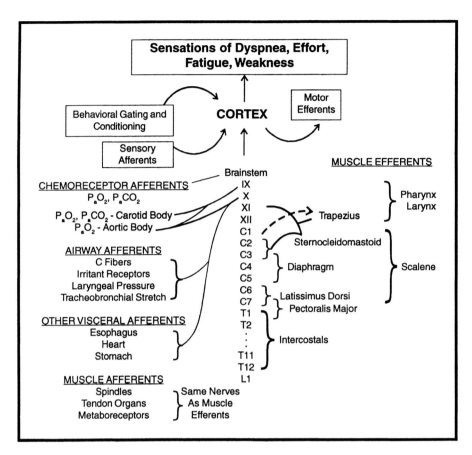

**Figure 5.** Schematic diagram of the afferent and efferent motor nerves serving the respiratory system. The cortex integrates sensory afferent (left) and efferent data (right) with experience and produces sensations of dyspnea, effort, fatigue, and weakness.

pathway. Afferent information likely to be generated with each breath now is thought to include measures of muscle force, rate of change of muscle length, muscle metabolic state, airway pressure and stretch, $Pao_2$, $Paco_2$, lung edema, and temperature. Nerve activity is phasic with respiration. Muscle afferents are thought to mediate respiratory responses to changes in load and posture. Thin fiber muscle afferents known as metaboreceptors end in free-nerve endings and respond to ischemia, hypoxemia, and acidosis.

Muscles generate afferent information regarding mechanics from spindle and tendon organs and metabolic conditions from metaboreceptors.[26] Muscles then pass this information to the spinal cord via

the dorsal root of the same nerve as the efferent signal. Tendon organs provide a measure of the force of muscle contraction. Spindles are involved in detecting the magnitude and velocity of the change in muscle length and provide a measure of load or tension. Information regarding intercostal muscles is also transmitted via costovertebral joint receptors.

Afferent information from virtually all thoracic and upper abdominal organs, including the pharynx, larynx,[27] airways, lung parenchyma, esophagus, heart, and stomach travel via their respective branches of the vagus nerve (X) to the medulla. This information arises from a variety of receptor sources. Irritant receptors, located within the airways, respond to inhaled noxious stimuli. C fibers are lung and airway afferent fibers that respond to large volume-lung inflation and deflation, changes in pulmonary circulation, lung edema, and an increase in temperature. Activation increases vagal traffic to the brain stem and may result in vasodilation, apnea, airway constriction, and mucus production.[28] Tracheobronchial stretch receptors and laryngeal pressure receptors respond to changes in laryngeal and lung volume and may result in airway constriction or dilation. All of these receptors are probably involved in coordinating complex respiratory behaviors, such as speech, cough, and vomiting. Numerous other receptors in the gastrointestinal tract and heart, mostly vagally mediated receptors, help coordinate complex activities, such as swallowing and respiratory sinus arrhythmia.

The dyspnogenic stimuli of $Paco_2$ and $Pao_2$ are sensed differently. $Pao_2$ is sensed by the carotid body, the aortic body, and central receptors. The predominant location for the detection of changes in $Paco_2$ is the carotid body. Signals from the carotid body reach the medulla via the carotid sinus nerve to the glossopharyngeal nerve (IX). Although chemoreceptor discharge persists in the carotid body at arterial $Pao_2$ values above 500 mmHg, discharge increases abruptly near an arterial $Pao_2$ of 75 mmHg and reaches a maximum near a $Pao_2$ of 10 to 20 mmHg.[29] While neurotransmission is primarily adrenergic- and dopaminergic-mediated, acetycholine, serotonin, opioids, substance P, vasoactive intestinal peptide, neuropeptide Y, and adenosine are also involved in neurotransmission and control of carotid body vascular flow.[29] The aortic body is stimulated by reductions in $O_2$ content and primarily induces changes in the phase timing of respiration rather than the hyperventilation produced by the carotid body. Central nervous system hypoxia decreases neural excitation and leads to hypoventilation. Apnea may occur with reductions in $O_2$ content of 50% and gasping with reductions of 80%.[30]

$CO_2$ receptors exist centrally and peripherally in the carotid body. Central $CO_2$ receptors appear to be clustered at the ventrolateral medullary surface. Deeper receptors also exist within the medulla. Any local increase in acid or $CO_2$ in these areas results in hyperventilation.[31] Control by central chemoreceptors predominates over input of $CO_2$ receptors in the carotid body. The mediators of this action have not been identified as well as those for changes in $Po_2$.

## Central Integration of the Afferent and Efferent Systems and the Sensation of Dyspnea

The perception of dyspnea must involve some type of thalamic, limbic, and/or cortical process. The challenge is to determine which physiologic stimuli create this sensation. Afferent information may result in sensation by creating a sensory impression of the specific afferent receptor stimulus. Efferent information may create a sensory impression by evoked motor commands, an assumption by the brain that an action resulted from an efferent command. Higher centers influence these sensory impressions through experience, learning, and emotion. Since the final common pathway for the perception of dyspnea is above the brain stem, multiple stimuli may play a role in eliciting dyspnea. Hypercapnia, hypoxemia, and muscle afferent data appear to be the major dyspnogenic stimuli.

Several experiments attempting to explain the origin of dyspnea have altered sensory afferent data from the vagus nerve, muscles, afferents, and chemoreceptors and then evaluated the resultant effects on the sensation of dyspnea.

### Vagus Nerve Experiments

Attempts to remove the input from C, stretch, and irritant fibers have included the inhalation of topical anesthetics and sectioning the vagus. Pharyngeal lidocaine has decreased the sensation of dyspnea associated with breathing through a mouthpiece.[32] Blocking the cervical vagus has resulted in the ability to prolong a breath hold at a higher $P_{CO_2}$ with less dyspnea[33-35] and has lessened dyspnea in interstitial fibrosis.[36] In evaluating deafferented patients after heart-lung transplant, Kimoff found no difference in the sensation of dyspnea for a given level of inspiratory drive, $P_{0.1}$. Taguchi reported that inhaled prostaglandin E2 increased dyspnea by stimulating C fibers. These experiments suggest that vagal afferents are not necessary for the sensation of dyspnea but probably in some circumstances contribute significantly to it. However, one would suspect by the nature of the receptors that these might be more important in dyspnea due to lung edema states, irritant stimuli (eg, smoke inhalation) airway burns due to thermal injury or acid inhalation, or pneumothorax. Dyspnea due to upper airway inflammation, such as during the common cold, may also be more mediated by vagal and laryngeal pharyngeal afferents.

## Muscle Afferent Experiments

The role of muscle afferents in evoking dyspnea has been extensively studied. A group of investigators led by Campbell in the early 1960s formulated the theory that dyspnea related to a sense of muscle length-tension imbalance or inappropriateness. Paralyzed volunteers were able to sustain longer apnea without a sensation of dyspnea than when awake and asked to hold their breath. Dyspnea remained absent in some paralyzed subjects despite a rise in $Pa_{CO_2}$ to 70 mmHg.[37,38] The sensation of dyspnea at the breaking point of breath holding could be decreased by breathing a gas similar in composition to exhaled gas[39] or even by performing an isovolume maneuver (ie, moving the thorax and abdomen but not moving air at the mouth).[40] This work strongly suggested that the dyspnea of breath-holding was primarily sensed by muscle afferents and not chemoreceptors. Block of intercostal muscles[41] or study of C5 quadriplegics[42] indicated that breath-holding time and dyspnea scaling were unchanged, sug-

gesting that the diaphragm was the primary source of dyspnogenic muscle afferents.

In studying patients undergoing large volume thoracentesis for relief of dyspnea from pleural effusion, Estenne et al.[43] concluded that the relief of dyspnea was associated with improved muscle function secondary to a change in the inspiratory pressure-volume curve due to a reduction in the size of the thorax. These experiments and others also suggested that these muscle afferents were responsible for the sensations of internal and external load and effort[44] and that these muscle afferents combine to generate sensations of effort, load, impedance, and possibly of length-tension inappropriateness and weakness. The work of Sibuya et al.[45] supports the role of muscle afferents in causing dyspnea. When vibration at 100 Hz was delivered to inspiratory intercostal muscles during inspiration and expiratory intercostals during expiration (ie, when in-phase vibration was delivered, dyspnea decreased, and when out-of-phase vibration was delivered, dyspnea increased). Because changes in gas exchange were minimal during vibration, these authors speculated that the change in dyspnea was mediated by muscle or, less likely, by vagal afferents. The integration of these sensations by the CNS was felt to provide a common pathway for dyspnea in diseases that severely altered lung and muscle mechanics, such as asthma, chronic obstructive pulmonary disease (COPD), muscle weakness, and interstitial fibrosis.

## Chemoreceptor Experiments

Evidence gathered over the past decade has contradicted the above work and suggested a more primary role for the chemoreceptor afferents in dyspnea. Banzett and colleagues[34,46] and Gandevia et al.[47] repeated the paralysis/breath-holding experiments of Campbell in an elegantly controlled fashion and examined breath-holding and breathing sensation in quadriplegics. They were able to demonstrate that dyspnea could occur without muscle contraction and with an approximately 10 mmHg rise in $Pa_{CO_2}$. Transcranial stimulation of the motor cortex resulted in the perception of illusory movements of the limbs but without a sense of effort, suggesting that dyspnea was unlikely to arise from cortical projections of outgoing motor command (ie, evoked respiratory muscle activity). Mathematical models of control during breath-holding have demonstrated that chemoreceptor control is likely more important than nonchemical factors.[48] Although normal subjects can not voluntarily regulate $CO_2$ to precise levels, normals can detect changes in $CO_2$.[49] These studies now firmly establish that $CO_2$ levels can be sensed and, at times, produce dyspnea.

Several studies have compared the dyspnea resulting from voluntary hyperventilation with that resulting from exercise, hypercapnia, and hypoxemia. When the severity of dyspnea is compared at the same level of minute ventilation, hypercapnia (due to $CO_2$ rebreathing) appears to be the greatest dyspnogenic stimulus, exercise and hypoxemia are intermediate dyspnogenic stimuli, and voluntary hyperventilation is the least dyspnogenic stimulus.[50-54] Ward and Whipp[55] examined the combination of stimuli by combining exercise with hypoxemia or hypercapnia. When these subjects were compared at equal levels of minute ventilation, the intensity of dyspnea was greater during isocapnic hypoxemia than during hypercapnic hyperoxia. This suggests that during exercise hypoxemia may be a stronger dyspnogenic stimulus than hypercapnia.

Emotion, learning, experience, and psychiatric state also clearly alter the sensation of dyspnea, and there is evidence that these associations are related to changes in $CO_2$ responsiveness. Dudley et al.,[56] in studying psychiatrically impaired patients, were able to demonstrate dyspnea brought on by anger and anxiety during hyperventilation and hyperpnea, and by depression during hypoventilation. Studies have found a blunted $CO_2$ response in depression[57] and an elevated $CO_2$ response in extroverts.[58] Studies in identical twins[59,60] have demonstrated that although there is a genetic control of respiratory chemosensitivity, especially with regard to change in tidal volume in relation to $P_{CO_2}$ and minute ventilation in response to hypoxia, nongenetic or personality factors contribute to the dyspnea sensation and rate response to $CO_2$. Improved understanding of the central neurotransmitters in psychiatric diseases may provide a better understanding in the future of how emotion and psychiatric condition alter dyspnea perception.

## Perspective

Investigators have struggled to redefine dyspnea in more physiologic terms. Wasserman[61,62] states that dyspnea is an "unsatisfied ventilatory drive." Killian[11,63] indicates that dyspnea arises from a sense of "inappropriateness," a deviation of the respiratory system from its learned expectations. Such statements elegantly indicate that dyspnea results from the higher brain centers' viewing of efferent and afferent data in a uncomfortable fashion. As will be seen in the next section, the precise physiologic pathways that are activated for diseases producing dyspnea remain unknown.

The general concept that dyspnea may result from inappropriate, unsatisfied, or uncomfortable effort, tension, weakness, or gas tensions appears to have at least descriptive validity. Several indices of effort or work relate well to dyspnea. Wilson et al.[64] found a strong relationship between exertional dyspnea measured on the Borg scale and minute ventilation. Minute ventilation divided by the maximum voluntary ventilation can be used as a reliable dyspnea index. Any index of control system efficiency such as $P_{0.1}/\dot{V}e$, $P_{0.1}/P_{CO_2}$, $P_{di}/\dot{V}e$ is also likely to relate to dyspnea.[65] These general conclusions are useful in considering the physiology of dyspneic states when the specific physiology is unknown.

There are several important conclusions regarding the physiology of dyspnea that have significant clinical importance:

(1) because dyspnea may frequently arise by several mechanisms, no one treatment is likely to be universally effective; (2) hypoxemia and hypercapnia appear to be important dyspnogenic stimuli; (3) information regarding load, effort, and impedance from muscle afferents appears to contribute to dyspnea; (4) the importance of vagal afferents appears limited to specific types of dyspnea, and vagal afferants that are unlikely to contribute to most exertional dyspnea; and (5) as dyspnea intensity is modulated by learning, experience, and emotional/psychiatric state, behavioral therapies and psychoactive drug therapy may be helpful.

## Differential Diagnosis and Pathophysiology of Dyspnea

### Prevalence of Causes of Dyspnea

Although numerous diseases have been reported to cause dyspnea (Table V),[66–111] most cases of dyspnea are due to cardiac, pulmonary, or gastrointestinal dysfunction or the hyperventilation anxiety syndrome. The frequency of these and the less common causes of dyspnea would be expected to vary depending on whether the dyspnea was acute or chronic, the age of the patient group studied, and whether the setting for evaluation of dyspnea was outpatient or inpatient. This section will briefly summarize the limited data available regarding the prevalences of the causes of dyspnea.

### Acute Dyspnea

Acute dyspnea might be characterized as dyspnea present for only a few days that is severe enough to prompt an urgent evaluation in an emergency department or a hospital admission. In the emergency department, Fedullo et al.[21] demonstrated that of 162 patients with a chief complaint of dyspnea, 26% had heart failure, 25% asthma, 19% COPD, 5% arrhythmias, 4% psychogenic causes, 3% infection, and 18% unknown or miscellaneous causes. In patients admitted to the hospital with a chief complaint of dyspnea, 79% to 92% will have common cardiopulmonary causes of dyspnea[22,23]: asthma in 20% to 33% of patients; congestive heart failure (CHF) 30% to 31%; arrhythmia 0 to 7%; COPD 9% to 17%; or infection 5% to 12%. In a larger series, one would expect to see epiglottitis, spontaneous pneumothorax, and other less frequent causes of acute, severe dyspnea.

### Chronic Dyspnea

In the outpatient setting, studies have focused mostly on the population of patients with difficult-to-explain dyspnea evaluated by a consulting pulmonologist. Most of these patients have chronic, moderate-to-severe dyspnea. DePaso et al.[112] evaluated 58 such patients and found that the cause of dyspnea could be clearly identified in 76%: 17% cardiac causes (coronary artery disease, cardiomyopathy, arrhythmia, intracardiac shunt, constrictive pericarditis); 41% pulmonary causes, with 38% intrapulmonary causes (asthma, interstitial fibrosis, intrathoracic airway obstruction, bullae, thromboembolic disease, and primary pulmonary hypertension) and 3% extrapulmonary causes (extrathoracic airways obstruction, pectus excavatum); 24% hyperventilation syndrome; 5% gastroesophageal reflux disease (GERD); 3.4% thyroid disorders; 3.4% neuromuscular disorders; and 3.4% deconditioning. Pratter et al.[3] found 75% of the cases due to pulmonary causes, 10% cardiac causes, 5% hyperventilation, 5% deconditioning, and 5% GERD. Martinez et al.[113] found 32% of cases due to pulmonary causes, 28% deconditioning/obesity, 18% hyperventilation, 14% cardiac, and 2% GERD. If the data from these studies is combined one might conclude that cardiopulmonary diseases cause 75% to 92% of dyspnea cases in emergency department patients and inpatients and 46% to 85% of dyspnea cases in outpatients. More importantly, 94% of dyspnea cases appear to result from one of the five major causes

**Table V**
Differential Diagnosis of Dyspnea by Organ/Disease System

*Cardiac*
  Arrhythmia
  Coronary Artery Ischemia
  Cardiomyopathy
  Hypotension
  Left-to-right Shunt
  Myxoma
  Pacemaker syndrome
  Valvular Disease with Pulmonary Edema
  Pericarditis
  Tamponade
*Deconditioning/Obesity*
*Dermatologic*
  Herpes Zoster[66,67]
*Endocrine*
  Acromegaly[68]
  Ectopic Thyroid
  Goiter
  Hypoparathyroidism[68]
  Hyperthyroidism[69–72]
  Thyroiditis[73]
*Gastrointestinal*
  Gastroesophageal Reflux Disease
  Aspiration
*Hematologic*
  Anemia
  Polycythemia
*Infectious*
  Common Cold[74]
  Epiglottitis
  HIV
  HSV
  Laryngitis
  Mononucleosis[75]
  Pneumonia
  Sinusitis
*Larynx and Upper Airway*
  Arytenoid dysfunction
  Dyskinesia
  Foreign body
  Meige syndrome
  Recurrent layngeal nerve injury
  Spastic Dysphonia
  Shy-Drager syndrome
  Trauma
*Neuromuscular*
  Acid Maltase Deficiency[76]
  Amyotrophic Lateral Sclerosis
  Multiple Sclerosis[77,78]
  Muscular Dystrophy[79]
  Myasthenia gravis
  Neuralgic Amyotrophy[80]
  Parkinson's Disease[81–83]
  Postcardioplegia Phrenic Nerve Paralysis[84]
  Postpolio Syndrome[85,86]
  Quadri- or Paraplegia[87]
  Shy-Drager Syndrome

*Nutritional*
  Excess Carbohydrate Intake
  Malnutrition
*Oncologic*
  Lung Cancer
  Tumor Emboli
*Pharmacologic*
  Angiotensin Converting Enzyme Inhibitors[88]
  L-tryptophan[89]
  Neuroleptics[82,83]
  Nitrofurantoin[90]
  Nonsteroidal Anti-inflammatories[91]
*Pregnancy[92–94]*
*Pulmonary*
  Airway tumors
  Asthma
  Bronchiectasis
  Chest Wall Deformities
  Compressive Lesions of the Airways
  COPD
  Cystic Fibrosis
  Interstitial Fibrosis
  Mechanical Ventilation
  Pleural effusion
  Pneumoconiosis
  Pneumothorax
  Pneumomediastinum[95]
  Postpneumonectomy
  Tracheobronchial Malacia
  Vocal Cord Dysfunction
*Psychiatric*
  Anxiety
  Depression
  Panic
*Renal*
  Dialysis
  Metabolic acidosis
  Renal failure[96–99]
*Rheumatologic*
  Amyloidosis[100]
  Ankylosing Spondylitis[101]
  Fibromyalgia[102,103]
  Polymyositis[104]
  Rheumatoid Arthritis[105–108]
  Scleroderma[109]
  Systemic Lupus Eythematosis[110]
  Vasculitis[111]
*Vascular*
  Left-to-right Shunt
  Pulmonary Artery Compression
  Pulmonary Embolism
  Pulmonary Hypertension
  Right-to-left Shunt

HIV, human immunodeficiency virus; HSV, herpes simplex virus; COPD, chronic obstructive pulmonary disease.

of dyspnea: (1) cardiac, (2) pulmonary, (3) psychogenic/hyperventilation, (4) GERD, and (5) deconditioning.

## Pathophysiology of Diseases Causing Dyspnea

The mechanism by which diseases produce dyspnea varies with the disease. Some diseases affect afferent pathways, others efferent pathways, and others integrative sensations. The causes of dyspnea might therefore be categorized by grouping them according to putative physiologic mechanisms, the anatomic site of the primary causative defect, or by a traditional organ/disease systems of classification (Table V). Since the precise physiologic defects associated with many diseases which give rise to dyspnea are not clearly known, a physiologic classification is not extremely useful to the clinician. Therefore, the discussion of disease-specific mechanisms of dyspnea in this section will be organized according to the traditional organ/disease systems classification approach. This approach has the advantage of reflecting clinical practice and overlapping with the anatomic categorization. An understanding of the mechanisms by which the common diseases result in dyspnea remains fundamental for the later discussion of rationales for therapy.

In many diseases, the precise mechanism by which dyspnea occurs is unknown or unstudied. For the sake of brevity, this discussion will review only the data that help clarify the effect of disease on the afferent, efferent, and integrative sensory pathways and will focus only on the most common diseases.

## Pulmonary

Although dyspnea may arise from diseases involving the upper airway, intrinsic or extrinsic compression of the lower airways, parenchymal diseases, or pleural diseases, virtually all studies regarding the mechanism of dyspnea in lung disease have been performed on patients with the two common obstructive airways diseases – COPD or asthma. The mechanism by which airways obstruction produces dyspnea remains controversial. In asthma and COPD, inflammation and bronchoconstriction may activate vagal, muscle, and chemoreceptor afferents. Even though obstruction is common to both diseases and may stimulate the sensation of dyspnea, the intensity of dyspnea does not correlate well to the degree of obstruction. Therefore, most studies have attempted to define other mechanical or neurochemical factors that would account for dyspnea.

### Asthma

Studies on the genesis of dyspnea in asthmatic patients reveal that mechanical, blood-gas, and psychological factors probably all play a role. Brand et al.[114] studied the variability in the perception of airway obstruction in 412 middle-aged subjects. An increase in Borg dyspnea score in response to histamine bronchoprovocation challenge was associated with younger age, more airway responsiveness, atopy, and female sex, but not in forced expiratory volume in 1 second ($FEV_1$) or change in $FEV_1$. Bellofiore et al.[115] demonstrated that pretreatment with naloxone prior to methacholine challenge increased post-challenge dyspnea, respiratory rate, and inspiratory flow. This would suggest that individual variations in the secretion of endogenous opioids may account for some of the variability in the sensation of asthmatic dyspnea. Dyspnea in responders to bronchoprovocation challenge appeared to relate to reactivity not degree of obstruction. Turcotte and Boulet[116] evaluated the relationship of fall in $FEV_1$ to Borg scale dyspnea in 28 asthmatic patients during early and late asthmatic responses to antigen challenge. The rate of fall of the $FEV_1$ best correlated with the perception of dyspnea. As the late phase fall tended to be slower the bronchoconstriction was less perceived as dyspnea. Although acute dyspnea in individuals may relate to the speed and degree of change in obstruction, the average daily Borg dyspnea score does not appear to correlate with lability in daily peak flow values.[117] Lougheed et al.[118] performed a careful study of Borg scale dyspnea in 21 asthmatic patients to determine what factors accounted for the difference in the perceived intensity of dyspnea at equal levels of obstruction. Reduced inspiratory capacity, increase in esophageal pressure to tidal volume ratio, and an increase in end-expiratory lung volume highly correlated with the sensation of dyspnea. The application of 5 to 7.5 cm $H_2O$ of continuous positive airway pressure to asthmatic patients in acute exacerbation has been shown to decrease dyspnea without affecting gas exchange or $FEV_1$.[119] This would presumably work by improving resting muscle lengths, reducing air trapping, decreasing functional residual capacity, and reducing the work of breathing. During exercise dyspnea in asthmatic patients has been shown to relate to higher inspiratory flows, tidal volumes, respiratory rates, and inspiratory mouth pressures.[120] Killian et al.[121] were able to demonstrate that asthmatic patients with a high level of dyspnea during bronchoprovocation challenge also had a high level of dyspnea during exercise. Few studies have carefully reported the relationship between $Po_2$ and $Pco_2$ and dyspnea in asthma. In a small study of exacerbated asthmatic patients in an emergency department, Kunitoh et al.[122] were able to demonstrate a significant relationship between Borg scale dyspnea and $Pco_2$. Kikuchi et al.[123] demonstrated that asthmatic patients with a history of near fatal attacks had a reduced response to hypoxia and a reduced sensation of dyspnea.

## Chronic Obstructive Pulmonary Disease (COPD)

Chronic obstructive pulmonary disease differs from asthma in its chronicity, type of parenchymal lung damage, and baseline gas exchange balance. Studies on the mechanism of dyspnea in COPD suggest that mechanical factors and gas exchange variables interact to produce the sensation. Compared with asthma, $Paco_2$ and $Pao_2$ appear to play a greater role while the effects on mechanics are similar. When COPD patients with severe breathlessness were compared with those with mild breathlessness, the greatest predictors of breathlessness were a reduction in the diffusing capacity and elevation in the $\dot{V}e/\dot{V}co_2$ ratio.[124] On exercise, the more breathless group desaturated more and developed a higher ventilatory response. An increase in dyspnea on exertion in COPD patients appears to relate to an increased motor output of the inspiratory muscles. Several studies have demonstrated a relationship between exertional breathlessness and increased minute ventilation, tidal volume, respiratory rate, and inspiratory flow,[120,125–127] a reduction in inspiratory reserve volume, end-expiratory lung volume, and respiratory rate.[128] Dyspnea increased with increasing inspiratory muscle activity with the greatest breathlessness experienced by those approaching their ventilatory maximum or with an acute change in end-expiratory lung volume.

Reduction in dyspnea due to inhaled bronchodilator appears to relate to an improvement in the inspiratory lung capacity.[129] As in asthma, the reduction in dyspnea seen with the application of continuous positive airway pressure is presumably mediated by reducing functional residual capacity, improving resting muscle length, and decreasing inspiratory work. The relief of dyspnea by sitting forward in the leaning position has occurred more in hyperinflated, air-trapped patients,[130] has been correlated with postural improvements in the inspiratory and expiratory maximal pressures,[131] and has been associated with a greater portion of the inspiratory work being assumed by the intercostal and accessory muscles than the diaphragm.[130] No study has examined the effect of posture change on gas exchange.

Little data are available regarding the role of vagal afferents in COPD. Some patients do appear to have a reduction in dyspnea with vagotomy.[132] Hypercapnia and hypoxemia occur frequently in moderate-to-severe COPD and are potent mediators of dyspnea.

## Interstitial Lung Disease

The dyspnea resulting from interstitial lung disease has been much less well-studied. Interstitial diseases include more than 100 distinct causes that share a common pathophysiological mechanism. Alveolitis results in interstitial fibrosis with consequent gas-exchange impairment, reduced pulmonary compliance, abnormal resting respiratory muscle lengths, and an increased work of breathing. Similar to the obstructive diseases, dyspnea in interstitial diseases is probably affected by abnormal gas exchange, impaired muscle function due to changes in length-tension relationships, and activation of parenchymal stretch and C receptors. Vagotomy has been reported to reduce dyspnea in interstitial disease.[133] Vagal block and inhalation of an anesthetic aerosol, however, did not reduce exertional dyspnea.[36]

Multiple physiologic mechanisms probably interact over the course of the disease to cause dyspnea. Patients with early interstitial disease may complain of dyspnea when spirometry and lung volumes remain normal, but there is a mild decrease in diffusing capacity. In more advanced stages of disease, the addition of supplemental oxygen may improve dyspnea but does not eliminate the sensation.

## Compression of the Tracheobronchial Tree and Laryngeal Dysfunction

Compression of the tracheobronchial tree and laryngeal dysfunction presumably result in dyspnea by creating airways obstruction similar to COPD and perhaps by triggering local irritant and stretch receptors. The following diseases in this category have been reported to cause dyspnea: intrinsic airway obstruction by tumor[134,135] or tracheal stenosis; extrinsic obstruction by an aortic aneurysm[136]; herniated lung after pneumonectomy[137]; thymoma[138]; liposarcoma[139]; and goiter. Arytenoid tremble[140]; dyskinesia; laryngeal closure[141] or laryngospasm due to hypocalcemia, tetanus, or neurologic dysfunction; vocal cord paresis or paralysis due to recurrent laryngeal nerve section, Shy-Drager syndrome,[142] or compression by surrounding structures or ectopic calcification[143]; and vocal cord trauma[144] may all present with dyspnea. Meige syndrome[145,146] is a spastic cranial dystonia characterized by intermittent spasm of facial, oral, and laryngeal muscles. Women appear more commonly affected than men. Onset is typically in the sixth decade of life. Other causes of airway compression probably have been underreported as causes of dyspnea since the causal relationship to compression appears to be self-evident. Adductor spastic dysphonia may also be seen in Tourette's syndrome, torsion dysphonia, and torticollis.[147] Laryngeal dyspnea may be severe and acute, suggesting that mechanoreceptors in the larynx, pharynx, and muscles may mediate the sensation.

## Compression of Lung Tissue and Distortion of the Thoracic Cage

Compression of lung tissue and distortion of the thoracic cage size and shape by pneumothorax, tumor, or pleural effusion produces dyspnea. These lesions would likely trigger C and stretch receptors and alter gas exchange. When patients undergo thoracentesis and drainage of large volume pleural effusions, relief of dyspnea is associated with improved muscle function due to a reduction in the size of the thorax and a resultant change in the inspiratory pressure-volume curve.[43]

Kyphoscoliosis and similar chest wall deformities may alter gas exchange and clearly alter resting muscle length-tension relationships. Mechanical ventilation may severely alter lung mechanics, change resting muscle lengths, alter gas exchange, and produce patient anxiety. Interestingly, the mode of ventilation does not appear to alter the sensation of dyspnea.[148]

## Cardiovascular

Dyspnea from cardiac disease probably occurs due to activation of vagal afferents, muscle afferents, and in pulmonary edema due to gas exchange abnormalities. The best evidence that vagal afferents are involved in producing dyspnea from mild pulmonary venous congestion comes from a well-studied case of a 43-year-old woman who had severe dyspnea from a unilateral pulmonary venous obstruction.[149] Her right pulmonary vein had thrombosed after an unsuccessful attempt at repair of an anomalous venous connection. Dyspnea at rest and on exertion resolved after right vagotomy. In this patient with no known airway or cardiac disease, dyspnea occurred without significant pulmonary hypertension, was faster in onset and departure during exercise than would be expected to result from airway edema, and was not accompanied by abnormal oxygen or $CO_2$ tensions. Vagotomy also resulted in the resolution of an inappropriate respiratory alkalosis during exercise. Although the right lung remained underperfused, ventilation at each workload was reduced after vagotomy. This evidence would strongly support that C and stretch receptors mediate the sense of dyspnea due to mild pulmonary venous congestion.

Conversely, the improvement in dyspnea seen after relief of more severe pulmonary congestion appears to be related to changes in gas exchange. In patients undergoing percutaneous mitral commissurotomy, dyspnea during exercise was significantly reduced.[150] A decrease in $\dot{V}e$/$\dot{V}CO_2$ was correlated with a decrease in dead space. There was no improvement in exercise capacity. Although this did not rule out improvement in muscle function, it suggested that improved gas exchange may be a significant factor in reducing dyspnea. In patients with chronic heart failure, McParland et al.[151] found that inspiratory and expiratory muscle strength was less than in controls, and the degree of reduced strength correlated with dyspnea on daily activities. Nishimura et al.[152] were able to demonstrate that inspiratory muscle strength declined with increasing heart failure. Although Mancini et al.[153] were unable to demonstrate diaphragmatic fatigue in patients with chronic CHF during exercise, they did show that diaphragmatic work had significantly increased in these patients and approached levels associated with fatigue in normals. Increased work resulted from the need to maintain gas exchange in the face of reduced compliance and increased dead space. Metaboreceptors may mediate some of the sensation of muscle fatigue. Caidahl et al.[154] performed a multivariate analysis to relate cardiac parameters to the sensation of dyspnea in 42 67-year-old Swedish men. Angina, pulmonary congestion, and Q waves on electrocardiogram explained 47% of the variability in dyspnea severity. Left atrial size and a left atrial emptying index accounted for 16% of the variability. Diastolic left ventricular dysfunction appeared more important than systolic dysfunction on multivariate analysis.

Dyspnea during tamponade probably also relates to elevated atrial pressure and altered gas exchange (eg, blood flow to the lungs is reduced). The prompt relief of symptoms with pericardiocentesis would argue against muscle fatigue or weakness due to hypoperfusion as the underlying cause.

Several studies have documented that dyspnea on exertion is common in patients with fixed rate ventricular pacing (VVI).[155–157] Up to 65% of these patients may experience moderate-to-severe dyspnea on exertion. The mean severity of dyspnea has decreased from 3.3/10 to 0.8/10 when pacemakers have been reprogrammed to a dual-chamber mode. Tani et al.[157] demonstrated that dual-chamber pacing (DDD) or rate-responsive ventricular pacing (VVIR) reduced $\dot{V}e$ and $\dot{V}e$/$\dot{V}CO_2$ when measured just prior to the anaerobic threshold. Tidal volume and minute ventilation did not change but respiratory rate was increased with VVI pacing. As some patients in this study had normal left ventricular function, the rise in pulmonary capillary wedge pressure seen during VVI pacing appears to be due to superimposition of atrioventricular contraction.[155]

These patients were hypocapnic on exertion, suggesting that the increased minute ventilation was not carotid body-mediated but perhaps due to vagal afferents. Arrhythmias presumably may create dyspnea via similar mechanisms.

There do not appear to be any studies on dyspnea due to hypotension, low cardiac output with a normal wedge pressure, or valvular disease associated with normal wedge pressures such as aortic stenosis without mitral insufficiency. Either muscle metaboreceptors or cardiac baroreceptors with stretch receptors could mediate this sensation. Right atrial myxoma can produce ventilation-perfusion inequalities through myxomatous embolism or transient interruption of blood flow.

Vascular malformations probably mediate the sensation of dyspnea primarily through their effect on ventilation-perfusion mismatch and gas exchange and by excitation of vagally mediated C receptors. Right-to-left shunts in the pulmonary parenchyma, great vessels, or heart probably produce dyspnea primarily due to hypoxemia. Large volume shunts may activate C fibers or cardiac stretch receptors and baroreceptors; dyspnea resolves on closure of the shunt.[158,159] Terry et al.[158] reported 10 patients with pulmonary AV malformations. Patients had hypoxemia and hyperventilation at rest with a mean ventilation of 12 L/min and $P_{CO_2}$ of 28 mmHg. $\dot{V}_E/\dot{V}_{CO_2}$ was increased on exercise compared to normals. They speculated that patients were similar to those acclimatized to altitude and that dyspnea resulted from inappropriately high levels of minute ventilation for a given workload magnified by hypoxemia.

Pulmonary hypertension and pulmonary embolism produce dyspnea by yet unexplained mechanisms. Both would likely stimulate C fibers and vagally mediated atrioventricular stretch receptors. Both alter $P_{CO_2}$ and $P_{O_2}$. Compression of the pulmonary artery by a bronchogenic cyst may present with a normal chest roentgenogram, decreased perfusion on lung scan, and dyspnea.[160] Dyspnea may also occur with unilateral pulmonary venous obstruction as discussed above.[149]

## Gastroesophageal Reflux Disease

Gastroesophageal reflux disease has been reported to cause dyspnea and has appeared in some series to be a common cause.[3] Since reflux may occur in more than 25% of the asymptomatic population[161] with some regularity, it would appear that only a small percentage of reflux patients perceive their reflux as dyspnea. The mechanism by which reflux disease results in dyspnea remains unclear. Since patients may have normal lungs, exercise capacity, muscle strength, and gas exchange, dyspnea may be due to stimulation of gastroesophageal vagal afferents mediating the perception of dyspnea. In patients with regurgitation of food or acid to the vocal cords, dyspnea may be due to intense laryngospasm.[162]

## Hyperventilation Syndrome, Anxiety, Panic, and Psychologic Dyspnea

Anxiety, panic, depression, and other psychologic diseases cause dyspnea. Because these patients typically have normal cardiopulmonary function, normal efferent pathways, and no obvious afferent pathway defects, it is tempting to explain the sensation of dyspnea as a "nonbiologic" perceptual CNS problem. However, in many patients, symptoms of anxiety, panic, fear, dyspnea, chest pain, and/or lightheadedness arise during periods of hyperventilation. This suggests that an increased minute ventilation with a reduction in $P_{CO_2}$ may also be associated with dyspnea.

Behavioral models (Figure 6) of this "hyperventilation syndrome" suggest that symptoms such as dyspnea, chest pain, or panic result from the patient's misattribution of the sensation of hyperventilating. This is supported by recognition that hyperventilation, not organic disease or danger, is the problem, and adherence to different breathing strategies prevents hyperventilation and relieves the symptoms.[163,164]

Physiologic data describing patients

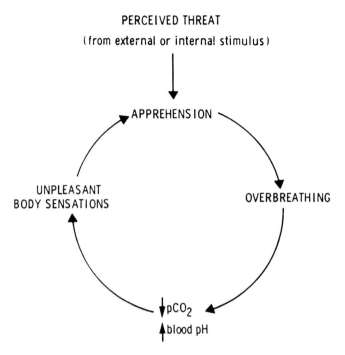

**Figure 6.** Schematic diagram of the development of a hyperventilation or panic attack. (Adapted from Clark DM et al.[163] J Behav Ther Exp Psychiat 1985;16:24.)

with the hyperventilation syndrome and dyspnea remain scarce. Tiller et al.[165] contrasted the responses of normal controls to patients with chronic anxiety disorders during inspiratory resistive loading. In the control group dyspnea was clearly related to the muscular effort of countering the inspiratory load, whereas in the anxiety group there was no relationship between dyspnea and muscular effort. He concluded that anxious patients depended on other stimuli for their perception of breathlessness. Several investigators have commented that the pattern of breathing in these patients appeared abnormal with frequent sighing and increased variability in both respiratory rate and tidal volume. This suggests that patients may have a defect in respiratory control. Garsson[166] compared changes in respiratory pattern in normals and hyperventilation patients exposed to mild stress and demonstrated an exaggerated response in the hyperventilation patients.

Since many patients with hyperventilation syndrome have chronic hypocapnia, other investigators have specifically focused on the relationship of $CO_2$ and its control to the production of symptoms. Saltzman et al.[167] performed $CO_2$ stimulation challenges before and after 20 minutes of voluntary hypocapnia in healthy subjects. Since subjects had either a decreased or increased ventilatory response to $CO_2$ following hypocapnia, he suggested that those normals with an increased responsiveness to hypocapnia may be prone to the hyperventilation syndrome. Okel and Hurst[168] found that a few deep breaths were enough to trigger carpopedal spasm and tetany during voluntary prolonged hyperventilation, suggesting that in chronic hyperventilation, small changes in breathing pattern may produce profound physiologic effects. Margarian[25] suggests that many of the symptoms associated with hyperventilation are related to the changes in cellular phosphate concentrations due to alkalosis. Hormbrey et al.[169] discriminated between the chronic hyperventilation syndrome in which patients have chronic hypocapnia and the eucapneic patients who develop atypical symptoms during hyperventilation. In this latter group, he demonstrated abnormal control of breathing as seen in an increased variability in breathing but not related to an increased chemoreceptor responsiveness. Since psychiatric diagnoses occur in hyperventilators 2.5 times more frequently than in controls and since psychiatric diseases are increasingly found to relate to neurotransmitter imbalance, it is interesting to speculate that the defects in psychiatric control affect respiratory control via shared pathways or neurotransmitters. Chronic hypocapnia as seen in hyperventilation, cirrhosis, and pregnancy may also destabilize control mechanisms. Much more basic investigation will be required to adequately reconcile the conflicting information cited above.

The diagnosis of a hyperventilation/anxiety syndrome remains troublesome. Hyperventilation and anxiety may occur with common diseases that cause dyspnea. Therefore, the clinician needs to make sure that common diseases that may be triggered by anxiety, such as asthma, are not misdiagnosed as hyperventilation and that patients with the hyperventilation syndrome are evaluated for other common causes of dyspnea. Bass and Garner[170] evaluated 21 patients with chronic hyperventilation and $P_{CO_2}$ <30 mmHg who had functional complaints. Chest pain was a more common complaint, but dyspnea was near universal. Of the 21 patients, 2 had asthma, 1 had COPD, 2 had probable pulmonary embolism, 9 had panic, 3 had phobia, and 6 displayed no psychiatric or organic cause.

Magarian's[25] summary of the signs and symptoms of hyperventilation syndromes are the most frequently used to screen for the diagnosis (Table VI). The majority of these symptoms are very nonspecific. The most common symptoms are dyspnea, chest pain, and lightheadedness. Historical items that may have a higher specificity for a hyperventilation syndrome would include dyspnea that begins after rather than during exercise, parasthesias accompanying dyspnea, carpopedal spasm with dyspnea, and overt psychosis. Psychiatric diagnoses, especially anxiety neurosis, occur in 65% of the patients with unexplained breathlessness, 2.5 times

---

**Table VI**
Signs and Symptoms of the Hyperventilation Syndrome

| | |
|---|---|
| General: | Chronic and easy fatigability, weakness, sleep disturbances, headache, excessive sweating, sensation of feeling cold, poor concentration, and performance of tasks. |
| Neurologic: | Numbness and tingling especially of distal extremities, giddiness, syncope, blurring or tunneling of vision, and impaired thinking. |
| Respiratory: | Sensation of breathlessness or inability to take a deep enough breath with sighing, yawning, and excessive use of upper chest and accessory muscles of respiration, nocturnal dyspnea superficially mimicking paroxysmal nocturnal dyspnea of cardiovascular origin, and nonproductive cough with frequent clearing of throat. |
| Cardiovascular: | Chest pains often mimicking angina, palpitations, and tachycardia. |
| Gastrointestinal: | Aerophagia resulting in full/bloated sensation, belching, flatus, esophageal reflux and heartburn, sharp lower chest pain, dry mouth, and sensation of lump in throat. |
| Musculoskeletal: | Myalgias, increased muscle tone with muscle tightness (stiffness), cramps with occasional carpopedal spasms and rarely a more generalized tetany. |
| Psychiatric: | Anxious, irritable, and tense though may superficially appear calm (suppression of emotional release), depersonalization or a feeling of being far away, phobias, and panic attacks. |

## Table VII
### Provocative Test for the Hyperventilation Syndrome

1. Instruct patients that you are going to have them do a breathing test and that they are only to pay complete attention to how they feel during the test. The test should be done before you discuss hyperventilation with the patient so that they may more spontaneously recognize the association of their symptoms with hyperventilation. Others inform patients in advance that the test is being performed to provoke their symptoms.
2. Tell the patient to expect a very dry mouth and that it may be somewhat tiring, otherwise offer no suggestions of what they may experience during the trial.
3. It is often of value to breathe with them initially to demonstrate the rate and depth you wish for them to breathe and show them using arm motions to increase the speed or depth of respirations if they slow down during the trial. A rate of 30 to 40 deep breaths per minute is usually used.
4. Patients should be encouraged to tell you whatever sensations they may feel as they hyperventilate. The test should be continued until 4 to 5 minutes of vigorous hyperventilation has occurred or until the patient complains of dizziness. If replication of at least some of the symptoms have not occurred by this time, an arterial blood gas should be obtained to document the absence of the patient's symptoms despite a respiratory alkalotic state. If respiratory alkalosis is not present, the test is inadequate.
5. For those with chest pain as a primary complaint, the test should be performed with electrocardiographic monitoring. If ischemic appearing changes occur, other diagnostic maneuvers will be necessary to distinguish whether this represents the "pseudoischemia" of hyperventilation or is reflective of true myocardial ischemia.
6. If symptoms are reproduced, it is desirable for the patient to make the connection spontaneously before asking them if they are feeling any of the symptoms they have been previously experiencing.
7. After the patient's recognition of the symptoms, bag rebreathing is used to demonstrate its ability to quickly relieve the symptoms and how they can thereby regain control.

more frequently than in controls.[25] Burns[171] notes that hyperventilation attacks are common in patients with depressive psychosis. He felt that breathlessness at rest, rapidly fluctuating severity of breathlessness, sighing, and delusions of imminent death were helpful in separating this group from controls with COPD. Bass et al.[172] studied 37 patients with unexplained breathlessness who had undergone cardiac catheterization and compared them with controls. Patients with the unexplained breathing disorder had frequent sighing or gasping at rest, inability to take a deep satisfying breath, dyspnea after trivial exertion, and dyspnea associated with faintness or giddiness. This cluster of symptoms significantly discriminated between patients with and without coronary obstruction.

A provocation test[25] (Table VII) may be performed in suspected patients by having the patients perform voluntary hyperventilation. The sensitivity of this test may be as high as 94%.[173] Some authors recommend that a blood gas be drawn if hyperventilation fails to produce symptoms in order to demonstrate that a provocative level of alkalosis was developed.[174] The test, however, lacks specificity. Most patients with cardiopulmonary disease would experience dyspnea on hyperventilating for 4 to 5 minutes. Because the provocative test will be nonspecific and potentially harmful to patients with suspected cardiopulmonary disease, it should not be performed prior to further diagnostic evaluation in this group of patients.

### Deconditioning

Deconditioning implies a less-than-healthy level of fitness of the cardiovascular system and skeletal muscles. Deconditioning presumably increases the sensation of dyspnea by requiring an abnormally high minute ventilation to perform a task. This increased effort of breathing is perceived as inappropriate to the level of difficulty of the task performed and is sensed as dyspnea. As little experimental data are available regarding the pathophysiology of dyspnea in deconditioning, one can only hypothesize regarding the underlying mechanism. The cause of dyspnea in these patients is likely to be multifactorial and involve minor abnormalities in afferent, efferent, and integrative pathways as well as an alteration in sensory perception. Relative respiratory muscle weakness may result in abnormal activation of afferent pathways via spindle or metaboreceptors. Impaired left ventricular response to abrupt increases in demand may activate vagal afferents via localized, transient passive pulmonary congestion or intracardiac receptors. A lowered anaerobic threshold results in the early onset of increased minute ventilation with exercise. The dyspnea seen in obese individuals, weak and malnourished individuals, and people debilitated by systemic illnesses probably share these general mechanisms.

## Other Diseases

Most other diseases that result in dyspnea do so by the direct involvement of the heart or lungs or secondary deconditioning. Muscle weakness in neurologic disease, interstitial lung involvement in the collagen vascular diseases, or compression of the trachea by an enlarged thyroid produce dyspnea similarly to the mechanisms described above. These diseases will not be reviewed in detail and the reader is referred to the references cited in Table V for further information. Controversy in the literature and/or the frequency of some diseases in clinical practice merit a brief discussion of dyspnea due to anemia, overfeeding, and cancer.

Anemia can be a common problem in patients with hematologic diseases, during menstruation in young women, during pregnancy, after chemotherapy, with parasitic infection, and with chronic malnutrition. Although virtually all review articles cite anemia as a cause of dyspnea, data regarding the prevalence of dyspnea due to anemia or the degree of anemia necessary to induce dyspnea remain scarce. Porter and James[175] published clinical observations on patients with anemia due to hookworm infection and concluded that dyspnea at rest was uncommon, "the most frequent symptom is dyspnea on effort," and that "pulmonary ventilation consistently increased on exercise in anemic patients with hemoglobin of 7 g/dL or less." Anemia to this degree is infrequent in clinical practice and is usually easily recognized. Given these data, it is likely that anemia alone is a rare cause of dyspnea. It is possible, however, that lesser degrees of anemia amplify the sensation of dyspnea when another cause of dyspnea is already present. Anemia lowers oxygen content in the blood and may trigger receptors in the aortic body. The carotid body responds to $PaO_2$ not oxygen content. Reduced oxygen carrying capacity could produce a more rapid desaturation of hemoglobin as it passes through a capillary from systemic artery to vein. In exercising muscle, this may exhaust the local oxygen supply creating an earlier dependence on anaerobic metabolism. This local ischemia may trigger muscle metaboreceptors. Wasserman et al.[176] report that anemia, as compared with the nonanemic state, lowers the anaerobic threshold, increasing the acidosis associated with a given workload. By triggering the chemoreceptors, anemia also increases the ventilation necessary for that workload. This produces a higher minute ventilation at a lower maximum workload compared to normals.

High levels of carbohydrate ingestion or overfeeding have been reported to cause an increased level of dyspnea in patients with COPD.[177] Since the respiratory quotient ($\dot{V}CO_2/\dot{V}O_2$) for carbohydrate is higher than that for fat, eating a high-fat diet should result in a lower postprandial resting minute ventilation. The increase in minute ventilation with high levels of carbohydrate results in dyspnea, presumably similarly to exercise-induced dyspnea. Angelillo confirmed that $\dot{V}CO_2$ was lower in COPD patients eating a reduced-carbohydrate, high-fat diet, and Brown showed that high carbohydrate loads reduced exercise performance in COPD. Since the severity of dyspnea increases as minute ventilation approaches maximum voluntary ventilation, it would be expected that changes induced by diet would be significant mainly in those with reductions in maximum voluntary ventilation to levels approximating rest ventilation. If one were able to achieve a maximal reduction in the respiratory quotient from 1.0 to 0.7, the minute ventilation of a patient with a resting ventilation of 10.0 L/min would fall to 7.0 L/min and minute ventilation of a patient with a resting ventilation of 6.0 L/min would fall to 4.2 L/min. Since even minimal exertion may increase ventilation 1.8 to 3.0 L/min, the phenomenon of carbohydrate-induced dyspnea would likely be observed predominantly in patients with rest dyspnea.

Dyspnea may be the initial complaint in 15% of patients with lung cancer and occur in 65% of lung cancer patients at some point during their course.[178] Dyspnea may be severe in that in one survey 52% to 56% of late-stage cancer patients experienced dyspnea on talking, eating, or getting dressed and 95% experienced dyspnea on stair climbing.[179] When Reuben and Mor[178] surveyed 1754 terminally ill patients with cancer, they found a 70% prevalence of dyspnea in the last 6 weeks of life. More than 14 primary sites of cancer were included in this study, and 24% of these dyspneic cancer patients had no known lung or pulmonary involvement by cancer. Dyspnea in cancer thus appears to be multifactorial in etiology. It also occurs so frequently in this population that exhaustive diagnostic evaluations for occult causes of dyspnea would be unnecessary. Dyspnea in many of these patients might have occurred as a complication of radiation, chemotherapy, or resectional lung surgery. Microscopic tumor emboli may also result in pulmonary hypertension and dyspnea and may present without obvious radiographic abnormality.[105] Debility and muscle weakness from cancer or its treatment must affect the respiratory muscles and result in dyspnea due to an increased sense of respiratory effort.

## Clinical Evaluation

### Overview

While there is a large number of diseases that can result in dyspnea and the mechanisms by which they can cause dyspnea are complex, the knowledgeable clinician can usually document the cause or causes of dyspnea. Although some suggest that it is not possible, our group was able to identify the cause of chronic outpatient dyspnea in virtually all patients who agreed to a complete evaluation.[3] A review of the literature suggests that three algorithms will suffice for the evaluation of most dyspneic patients. Figure 7 presents an algorithm for evaluating dyspnea in the pediatric population. Figure 8 depicts a strategy for the evaluation of acute dyspnea in adults. Figure 9 outlines a diagnostic strategy for adult patients with outpatient, chronic dyspnea.

The key conclusions that influenced the development of these strategies include: (1) since five disease groups (cardiac, pulmonary, psychogenic, deconditioning, gastroesophageal reflux) account for 75% to 90% of the causes of dyspnea, these diseases should always be screened for first; (2) most causes of pulmonary dyspnea involve the pulmonary parenchyma, not the upper airway or chest wall; (3) because dyspnea experts overdiagnose the common causes of dyspnea at the time of initial evaluation, confirmatory tests are required even when common causes are suspected; (4) tests with higher predictive values, such as chest roentgenogram, methacholine challenge, spirometry, and diffusing capacity, should act as diagnostic branch points; (5) the exercise test is the only test to offer confirmatory evidence of the absence of cardiopulmonary disease and presence of psychogenic disease or deconditioning; (6) patients with upper airway symptoms and unexplained dyspnea should undergo laryngotracheoscopy; and (7) GERD may be a clinically silent but frequent cause of dyspnea and may require ambulatory esophageal pH monitoring to confirm the diagnosis. Schmitt et al.[20] em-

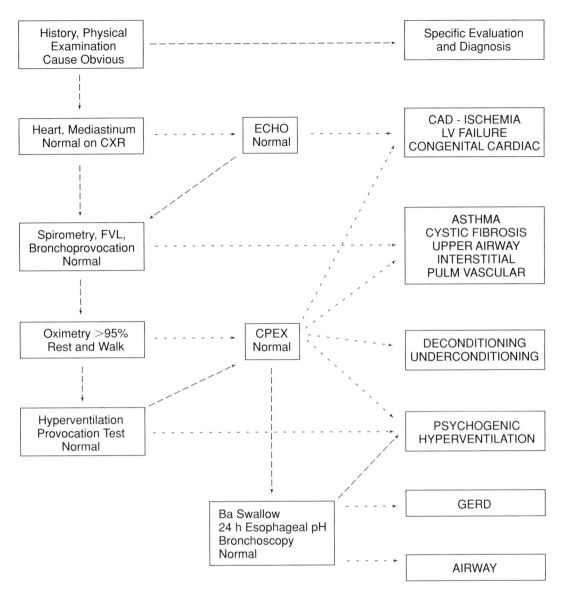

**Figure 7.** Schematic algorithm for the evaluation of moderate-to-severe dyspnea in a child. Ba = Barium, CAD = coronary artery disease, CPEX = cardiopulmonary exercise test, CXR = Chest roentgenogram, ECHO = cardiac echocardiography, FVL = flow-volume loop, GERD = gastroesophageal reflux disease, LV = left ventricle, PULM = pulmonary.

phasize that up to 34% of inpatients with dyspnea in their series had multiple causes of dyspnea. In all patients who fail to improve appropriately with specific therapy for the problem identified, further evaluation must be performed.

In devising a cost-effective strategy for evaluating the dyspneic patient, it will be helpful to recall that 94% of dyspnea cases can usually be explained by the five categories of disease reviewed above: pulmonary disease, cardiovascular disease, GERD, deconditioning, and the anxiety hyperventilation syndrome. Since the

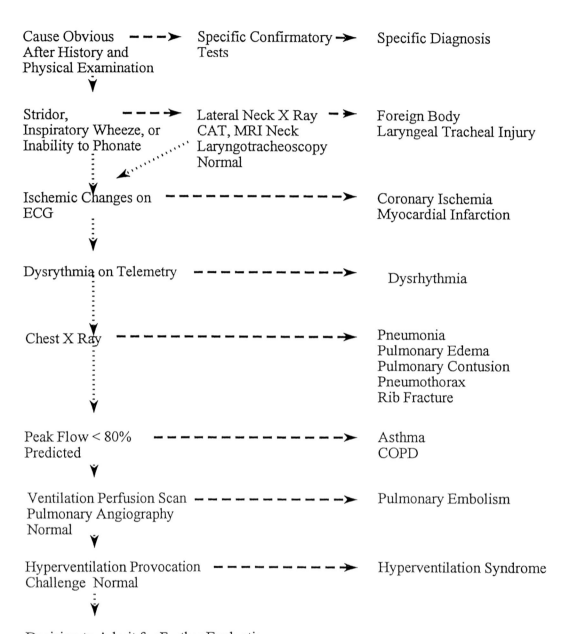

Decision to Admit for Further Evaluation

**Figure 8.** Schematic algorithm for the evaluation of acute moderate-to-severe dyspnea in adults in the urgent care setting. . . . . . . . = a false answer to the statement, ——— = a true answer to the statement; CAT = computer-assisted tomography, COPD = chronic obstruction pulmonary disease, ECG = electrocardiogram, MRI = magnetic resonance imaging.

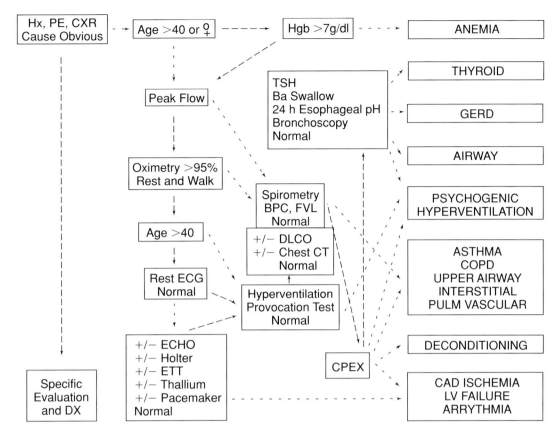

**Figure 9.** Schematic algorithm for the evaluation of chronic dyspnea in adults in the ambulatory setting. . . . . = a false answer to the statement in the box, ——— = True answer to the statement in the box; Ba = barium, BPC = bronchoprovocation challenge, CAD = coronary artery disease, Chest CT = computer-assisted tomography of the chest, COPD = chronic obstructive pulmonary disease, CPEX = cardiopulmonary exercise testing, CXR = chest roentgenogram, DLCO = diffusing capacity of carbon monoxide, DX = diagnosis, ECG = electrocardiogram, ECHO = cardiac echocardiography, Holter = 24-hour ambulatory arrhythmia monitoring, ETT = cardiac exercise tolerance test, FVL = flow-volume loop, GERD = gastroesophageal reflux disease, Hx = history, LV = left ventricular, pacemaker = check of pacemaker integrity or programming mode, PE = physical examination, psychogenic = anxiety, depression, hyperventilation syndrome and psychoses, pulm vascular = pulmonary hypertension syndrome, Thallium = cardiac nuclear perfusion exercise test, TSH = thyroid stimulating hormone, 24 h Esophageal pH = ambulatory esophageal pH monitoring.

prevalence of causative diseases will vary depending on the population studied, the strategy employed for diagnosing the cause of the dyspnea must vary with the population. Age, severity of symptoms, and chronicity are probably all useful discriminators in narrowing the differential diagnosis. In a pediatric population, tests evaluating for COPD and CHF are unlikely to be helpful, whereas tests evaluating for asthma would be expected to have a high yield. Acute dyspnea (Table VIII) is likely to have different causes than chronic dyspnea (Table IX). Mild dyspnea (Table X) may occur frequently under certain conditions and may require no special evaluation. With the prevalence of these causes in mind, it would be useful to review the value of the traditional evaluation for dyspnea—history, physical examination, and

## Table VIII
### Common Causes of Acute, Moderate-to-Severe Dyspnea

Anxiety/Hyperventilation Syndrome
Cardiac
  Angina
  Arrhythmia
  Pulmonary Edema
  Pericarditis
Pulmonary
  Asthma
  COPD
  Spontaneous Pneumothorax
  Pulmonary Embolism
  Noncardiogenic Pulmonary Edema
Gastroesphageal Reflux Disease
Trauma
  Pulmonary Contusion
  Rib Fracture
  Pneumothorax
  Shock
  Laryngeal/Tracheobronchial Injury
Upper Airway Conditions
  Laryngospasm
  Epiglottitis
  Foreign Body
Pneumonia

COPD, chronic obstructive pulmonary disease.

## Table IX
### Common Causes of Chronic, Moderate-to-Severe Dyspnea

Cardiac
  Arrhythmia
  Cardiomyopathy
  Ischemia
  Pacemaker syndrome
  Valvular Disease
Pulmonary
  Asthma
  COPD
  Interstitial Lung Disease
Gastroesophageal Reflux Disease
Anxiety/Hyperventilation
Deconditioning
Obesity

COPD, chronic obstructive pulmonary disease.

## Table X
### Common Causes of Mild Dyspnea

Anxiety/Hyperventilation
Deconditioning
Common Cold
Obesity
Postnasal Drip Syndrome
Pregnancy

chest roentgenogram. The potential value of more specific diagnostic tests, for example cardiopulmonary exercise testing and methacholine challenge, will also be discussed.

### History, Physical Examination, and Chest Roentgenogram

The clinical evaluation of the dyspneic patient should always document the severity and character of dyspnea and then include a history, physical examination, and objective tests aimed at identifying the diseases or conditions responsible for producing the dyspnea.

A proper history of the chief complaint is necessary in order to establish that the patient is indeed complaining of dyspnea. As noted earlier, the terms patients select to describe their breathing may not immediately cause the physician to identify the problem as dyspnea. The physician must question the patient carefully in that a patient who does not exert himself will not have exertional symptoms. Enough questions should be asked so that the interviewer can easily classify the patient's dyspnea on both the BMRC index and Mahler's baseline dyspnea index. Specific markers of severity need to be identified for each patient in order to later assess improvement with treatment. Severity and chronicity help narrow the differential diagnosis as noted above.

Although a thorough history, including a complete review of systems (Table XI) and physical examination (Table XII) directed to dyspnea are always recommended and traditionally felt to be help-

**Table XI**
Review of Systems for Dyspneic Patients

| | | |
|---|---|---|
| *Cardiac* | *Infectious* | *Pharmacologic* |
| History of Infarct, Angina, Arrhythmia | Cough | Street Drugs |
| | Fever | Chemotherapy |
| History of CABG | Pleurisy | Methotrexate |
| Pacemaker | Periorbital Pain | Amiodarone |
| Hypertension | Epistaxis | ACE |
| Tobacco History | Postnasal Drip | NSAIDS |
| Family History | Nasal Polyps | Nitrofurantoin |
| Diabetes | *Larynx—Upper Airway* | Neuroleptics |
| Heart Murmur | Trauma | *Pregnancy* |
| Chest Pain | Aspiration | Most Recent Menses |
| Cardiac Radiation | Hoarseness | *Pulmonary* |
| Cardiotoxic Chemotherapy | Speech Difficulty | Cough |
| *Deconditioning/Obesity* | Facial Spasms | Wheeze |
| Exercise Habits | Neck Surgery | Hemoptysis |
| Weight change in past 1 to 5 years | *Neuromuscular* | Sputum Production |
| | Weakness | Tobacco Use |
| *Dermatologic* | Easy Fatiguability | Occupational History |
| Painful Rash | Shoulder Pain | Intubation |
| *Endocrine* | Trauma | Pleurisy |
| Thyroid Surgery | *Nutritional* | *Psychiatric* |
| Thyroid Hormone Use | Dietary Habits | Anxiety |
| *Gastrointestinal* | Change in Weight | Panic |
| Heartburn | *Oncologic* | Depression |
| Indigestion | Prior Cancer | *Renal Failure* |
| Dysphagia | Prior Radiation | Dialysis |
| Coffee Consumption | Prior Chemotherapy | *Rheumatologic* |
| Antacid Use | Recent Mammogram | Known Diagnosis |
| *Hematologic* | Recent Cervical PAP | Rheumatoid Arthritis |
| Recent Pregnancy | Recent Rectal Exam, Hemoccults, or Endoscopy | Dysphagia |
| Menses | | Skin Rash |
| | Recent CXR | *Vascular* |
| | | Pleurisy |
| | | Platypnea |

CABG, coronary artery bypass grafting; ACE, angiotensin-converting enzyme; NSAIDS, nonsteroidal anti-inflammatory drugs; CXR, chest x-ray.

ful, several studies dispute the value of the traditional evaluation of the dyspneic patient with a history, physical examination, and chest roentgenogram. The predictive value of this traditional evaluation appears highest in acute dyspnea and in patients with the more common causes of dyspnea. In evaluating inpatients with acute dyspnea, Schmitt et al.[20] reported that a senior physician could accurately determine the causative diagnosis in 74% of cases after history alone. In this series of inpatients, dyspnea was caused by asthma, left ventricular failure, COPD, ar-rhythmia, pneumonia, or interstitial lung disease in 89% of patients. Mustchin and Tiwari[23] evaluated 77 patients referred for admission to the hospital for dyspnea by general practitioners in Great Britain. In 66%, the general practitioner was able to indicate the correct diagnosis in his office prior to emergency evaluation and, in 92% of the cases, the correct diagnosis was established in the emergency department prior to any further inpatient evaluation. Pratter et al.[3] reported that in only 66% of cases, the initial clinical impression of a pulmonary consultant evaluating outpa-

**Table XII**
Pertinent Items for Evaluation on Physical Examination

| *Cardiac* | *Gastrointestinal* | *Pulmonary* |
|---|---|---|
| Pulse | Tenderness | Stridor |
| Blood Pressure | Tympany | Expiratory wheeze |
| Arrhythmia | *Hematologic* | Cough |
| Gallop | Orthostasis | Inspiratory crackles |
| Murmur | Splenomegaly | Kyphoscoliosis |
| Rub | Pallor | Thoracic dullness |
| Hepatojugular Reflex | *Infection* | Decreased Breath Sounds |
| Response to Valsalva | Wheeze | *Rheumatologic* |
| Pulsus Paradoxicus | Thoracic Dullness | Subcutaneous Nodules |
| *Deconditioning* | Periorbital Tenderness | Deforming Arthritis |
| Weight | Purulent Rhinorrhea | Rash |
| Height | *Larynx and Upper Airway* | Sclerodactyly |
| Body Mass Index | Nasal Polyp | *Vascular* |
| *Dermatologic* | Hoarseness | Telangiectasia |
| Herpetic Rash | Stridor | Rub |
| Dermatomyositis | *Neuromuscular* | Hepatomegaly |
| *Endocrine* | Fasiculations | Murmur |
| Goiter | Power | |
| Exophthalmos | *Pregnancy* | |
| Stridor | Uterine size | |
| Hoarseness | | |
| Acromegalic Facies | | |

tients following history, physical examination, and chest roentgenogram was correct. Clinical impression was most accurate, at 81% accuracy, when the cause was asthma, COPD, interstitial lung disease, or cardiomyopathy. This suggests the initial evaluation of the dyspneic patient is frequently either pathognomonic or unhelpful. Certain other diagnoses become obvious on history—for example, trauma, lung resection, or prior psychiatric hospitalization. However, there are no studies to support a belief that history and physical examination alone can separate those patients with cardiac dyspnea from pulmonary dyspnea, discriminate between the five major causes of dyspnea listed above, or reliably identify the less frequent causes of dyspnea. The studies by Pratter et al.,[3] DePaso[112] and Martinez[113] all suggest that "historical features were unlikely to yield a specific diagnosis without further testing."

The study by Pratter et al.[3] indicates that the major role of the history and physical examination appears to be in ruling out

a diagnosis. Table XIII lists the positive and negative predictive values of major items from the history and physical examination. Most items have a high-negative predictive value and a low-positive predictive value. For example, a prior diagnosis of asthma or a history of wheezing had a positive predictive value of a diagnosis of asthma of less than 50%, a history of smoking had a positive predictive value for a diagnosis of COPD of only 20%, and the presence of crackles on auscultation had a positive predictive value of a diagnosis of heart failure of only 21%. Conversely, negative predictive values tended to be high. If crackles were absent on examination, the likelihood of not having interstitial lung disease as the cause of dyspnea was 98% and the likelihood of not having a cardiomyopathy as the cause of dyspnea was 92%.

Other studies have specifically attempted to separate patients with cardiac conditions from patients with pulmonary conditions on the basis of history and

**Table XIII**
Positive and Negative Predictive Value of History and Physical
Examination in 85 Dyspneic Patients[3]

| Parameter | Dx | Predictive Value | |
|---|---|---|---|
| | | *Positive* | *Negative* |
| History | | | |
| Previous diagnosis of COPD | COPD | .45 | .95 |
| Cigarette smoking | COPD | .29 | 1.00 |
| History of cough | COPD | .42 | .81 |
| Previous diagnosis of asthma | Asthma | .48 | .76 |
| History of wheezing | Asthma | .42 | .83 |
| History of throat clearing | UA | .12 | .97 |
| History of postnasal drip | UA | .12 | .94 |
| History of wheezing | UA | .05 | .88 |
| Physical Examination | | | |
| Wheeze | COPD | .42 | .89 |
| Wheeze | Asthma | .33 | .72 |
| Crackles | ILD | .79 | .98 |
| Crackles | Cardiac | .21 | .89 |

UA, upper airway; ILD, interstitial lung disease; Cardiac, cardiomyopathy; COPD, chronic
obstructive pulmonary disease.

physical examination. Unfortunately, no bedside test appears to be both accurate and convenient. Surprisingly, the findings of orthopnea, paroxysmal nocturnal dyspnea, leg edema, jugular venous distention, heart murmur, an S3 gallop, response to a Valsalva maneuver or a hepatojugular reflux test, or pattern of speech have not been shown to be sensitive or specific in separating these two groups. Eriksson and colleagues[12,180] attempted to develop a scoring system, based on history, physical examination, and chest roentgenogram, that would discriminate cardiac from pulmonary causes of dyspnea. In 644 men with a mean age of 67 years old, they could find no significant difference between the frequency of pitting leg edema, jugular venous distention, a third heart sound, or heart murmur grade III or louder between the groups without dyspnea or those with cardiac or pulmonary dyspnea. Zema et al.[181] studied 37 subjects with COPD, attempting to differentiate those with left ventricular failure from those without. Although orthopnea and dyspnea on exertion had a higher prevalence in those with left ventricular failure (71% versus 35%

and 100% versus 80%, respectively) they concluded that "the low specificity of both resulted in an unacceptably low predictive value when applied to an individual patient." While there was no difference in prevalence of paroxysmal nocturnal dyspnea and ankle edema between these groups, Zema et al. documented a high sensitivity (88%) and accuracy (88%) of a bedside Valsalva maneuver in detecting dyspnea due to left ventricular dysfunction. In this study, a blood pressure cuff was inflated 15 mmHg higher than diastolic pressure and the patient was asked to perform a Valsalva maneuver for 10 seconds. The pattern of Korotkoff sounds was recorded by auscultation over the brachial artery compressed by the sphygmomanometer. Patients with left ventricular dysfunction had an abnormal systolic arterial pressure response characterized by an absent overshoot or a square-wave response (Figure 10). In normals, Korotkoff sounds are heard during most of the Valsalva maneuver and reappear 3 to 5 seconds after cessation of Valsalva. Absence of this return of sounds corresponds to lack of the pressure overshoot or a square-

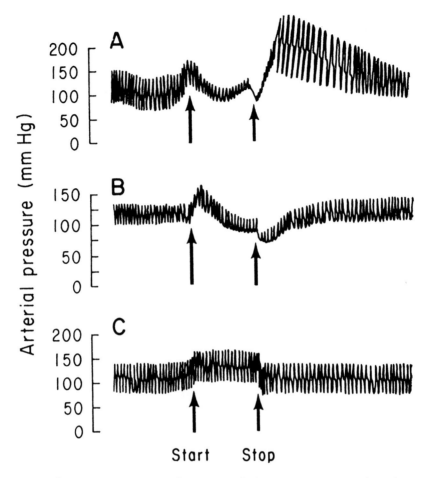

**Figure 10.** Arterial pressure responses during a Valsalva maneuver. Panel A shows a normal sinusoidal response, B shows the absent overshoot response, and C shows the square-wave response. (Adapted from reference 181: Zema et al. Br Heart J, 1980, 44:562.)

wave response. The specificity of this response was comparable to the chest roentgenogram for detecting left ventricular failure but far more sensitive (88% versus 59%). Left ventricular ejection fraction in the normal sinusoidal response group was 64%, in the absent overshoot group 42%, and in the square-wave response group 19%. In a similar study Marantz et al.[182] found a sensitivity of 78% and specificity of 65% for the Valsalva maneuver in detecting left ventricular failure in dyspneic patients. Patients with arrhythmias or on beta blockers would be ineligible for this test. Some authors have advocated using the hepatojugular reflux to discriminate cardiac from pulmonary dyspnea. However, this may be abnormal in patients with emphysema and has a low sensitivity (24%) for detecting heart failure.[183]

Dyspneic patients may complain about breathing difficulty during speech, and speech patterns in these patients have been found to be different.[184] During speech most dyspneic patients have a higher respiratory rate and spend more time in inspiration than controls (Ti/Ttot). Different strategies of balancing metabolic and communication needs occur in different diseases. While the speech pattern can be used to separate asthma, emphysema, sarcoid, and healthy patients from each

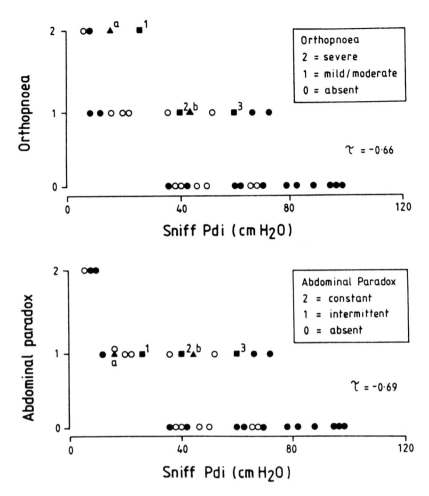

**Figure 11.** Relationship between inspiratory muscle strength as measured by transdiaphragmatic pressure during a sniff maneuver (Sniff $P_{di}$) and the severity of orthopnea (upper panel) and abdominal paradox (lower panel). Men are indicated by closed circles and women by open circles. Closed squares (1 to 3) and closed triangles (a and b) represent two men patients studied as their clinical condition improved (Adapted from reference 185: Mier-Jedrzejowicz A et al. Am Rev Respir Dis 1988; 137:877)

other, only 54% of patients can be correctly classified by this method.

One might suspect that diseases that involve respiratory muscles might be detected on examination. However studies reveal that it is difficult to detect moderate respiratory muscle weakness by history or physical examination. In one study of 30 breathless patients,[185] patients with the weakest diaphragms had more severe orthopnea and abdominal paradox (Figure 11). No patient with a sniff transdiaphrag-

matic pressure above 80 cm $H_2O$ had orthopnea or paradox. All patients with a transdiaphragmatic pressure less than 30 cm $H_2O$ had both symptoms. Patients with sniff pressures between 30 cm and 80 cm $H_2O$ only sometimes had orthopnea or paradox. Thus, orthopnea and inspiratory abdominal paradox appear specific for muscle severe weakness but insensitive for moderate or mild weakness.

Several studies suggest that the chest roentgenogram has excellent testing characteristics and is clearly helpful. Thirty-four percent of patients presenting to a walk-in clinic with new pulmonary complaints had a chest roentgenogram abnormal enough to prompt urgent intervention or follow-up.[186] In Pratter's population of patients referred for dyspnea,[3] a chest roentgenogram was a high yield test with a positive predictive value of 75% and negative predictive value of 91% when all diagnoses were considered. One would expect the chest roentgenogram to be most helpful, or at least have a high-negative predictive value, in establishing a diagnosis of pneumothorax, foreign body or airway obstruction, cardiomyopathy, pleural effusion, and interstitial fibrosis. Roetgenographic abnormalities in the lung fields predicted pulmonary causes of dyspnea and roentgenographic abnormalities of the heart predicted cardiac dyspnea.

## Positional and Nocturnal Dyspnea

Some would suggest that a history of positional dyspnea (Table XIV) may be helpful in narrowing the differential diagnosis. Trepopnea, dyspnea that increases when one side is dependent, is extremely nonspecific in that it might occur with any

---

**Table XIV**
Causes of Positional Dyspnea

Platypnea
  Right-to-left shunts
    Intracardiac
      Postpneumonectomy[258]
    Lung Parenchyma
      Congenital
      Cirrhotic[259]
    Ileus[188]
    Pericarditis[187]
Orthopnea
  Cardiomyopathy
  COPD
  Respiratory Muscle Weakness or Paralysis
Trepopnea
  Any lung disease affecting one lung more than the other

---

COPD, chronic obstructive pulmonary disease.

---

**Table XV**
Causes of Nocturnal Dyspnea

Asthma
Gastroesophageal Reflux Disease
Cardiomyopathy
COPD
Trepopnea*

---

* See Table 10.

---

asymmetric lung disease. Since trepopnea may occur with common diseases such as COPD or CHF, any given patient is more likely to have one of the common causes of dyspnea such as COPD or CHF causing trepopnea than the infrequent causes of trepopnea such as a paralyzed hemidiaphragm (Table XV). Orthopnea, an increase in dyspnea on recumbency, occurs with COPD, CHF, and respiratory muscle weakness. As noted above, it lacks the sensitivity and specificity to separate cardiac from pulmonary causes of dyspnea. Platypnea, an increase in dyspnea in the upright position, may result from pericarditis, ventilation-perfusion ratio mismatch, ileus, or right-to-left shunts. The presence of orthodeoxia, a decrease in $Po_2$ on sitting upright, suggests shunts more than the other causes. One patient with no demonstrable shunt developed platypnea due to a post pneumonectomy constrictive pericarditis that resolved postpericardiectomy.[187] Ileus with presumed impaired abdominal muscle contraction has caused platypnea in a patient with COPD.[188] Right-to-left shunts may be congenital, such as in the hereditary hemorrhagic telangiectasia syndrome, or acquired such as postinfection, tumor, or with cirrhosis. There are little data on the sensitivity or specificity of platypnea with regard to predicting the cause of dyspnea. As all of the above syndromes may also occur without platypnea or orthodeoxia, the sensitivity of these descriptors is likely low.

Nocturnal dyspnea (Table XV) may be useful to help limit the differential diagnosis, but the predictive value of this symptom has not been prospectively evaluated. Nocturnal dyspnea has been associated with COPD, GERD, asthma, and CHF. In patients with COPD, Zema et al.[181] found that 25% had nocturnal dyspnea, but that this increased to 47% if left ventricular failure was also present. In the absence of cardiopulmonary disease, a history of nocturnal dyspnea may suggest GERD.

## Age and Chronicity of Dyspnea

Age and chronicity probably are helpful diagnostic considerations. Diagnoses such as coronary ischemia, interstitial fibrosis, and cancer would clearly be more likely in the adults. While there are no studies describing the spectrum of causes of dyspnea in the pediatric population, it could be expected that in the pediatric age group a greater proportion of dyspnea might result from asthma, congenital cardiac abnormalities, and cystic fibrosis. The prevalence of the postnasal drip syndrome and the common cold in children should be the same or perhaps higher than in adults.

Several problems may be encountered in the pediatric age group not seen in adults: children may select different or unusual descriptors of their breathing, diagnostic tests may be less easily performed on children, and the presenting symptoms may be influenced by parental perceptions. Although the differential diagnosis may be more limited in children, the evaluation may be more challenging. Bronchoprovocation challenge can usually be reliably performed in children older than 8 years old. Peak flows, exercise challenge, electrocardiogram, echocardiography, and oximetry may greatly help guide diagnosis. A cardiopulmonary exercise test has the advantage of attempting to reproduce the symptoms while measuring all the pertinent physiology. Exercise testing may also demonstrate that the physically fit, normal individual who cannot compete with the best peer athletes has no significant cardiopulmonary disease and exercises to a normal capacity. See Figure 7 for the evaluation of chronic moderate-to-severe dyspnea in children.

The chronicity of dyspnea is probably helpful in that the differential diagnosis is smaller when the dyspnea is chronic (contrast tables 8 and 9). Clinical experience would suggest that many of the diagnoses that present with acute dyspnea would be apparent after initial clinical evaluation and limited confirmatory testing.[20] Most of these diagnoses are established by history, physical examination, chest roentgenogram, electrocardiogram, peak flow or spirometry, and response to therapy. Figure 8 displays an algorithm for evaluating acute dyspnea with an emphasis on common causes and ruling out the more lethal diseases, such as pulmonary embolism and myocardial infarction. Patients with persistent severe dyspnea despite this evaluation would require admission for further study.

## Role of Diagnostic Testing and Identification of Specific Causes

In patients with chronic dyspnea, objective testing appears necessary to confirm clinical impression. Board certified pulmonologists were able to correctly identify asthma, COPD, interstitial fibrosis, and cardiomyopathy 81% of the time when these diseases caused the patient's dyspnea. When these diseases were not the cause of dyspnea, initial clinical impression was accurate only 33% of the time.[3]

Several diagnostic tests have been helpful in diagnosing the cause of dyspnea. (Table XVI) Most were best at ruling out diagnoses. Tests with a high-negative predictive value included: methacholine bronchoprovocation challenge which was 100% predictive for ruling out asthma; spirometry which was 100% predictive for ruling out COPD; diffusing capacity which was 95% predictive for ruling out interstitial disease; and a barium swallow which was 83% predictive for ruling out GERD. Few tests had a high-positive predictive value: methacholine bronchoprovocation challenge was 95% predictive for asthma; diffusing capacity was 79% predictive of interstitial disease, and radionuclide ventriculography was 66% predictive of left ventricular failure.

**Table XVI**
Predictive Value of Diagnostic Tests in the Evaluation of Dyspnea[3]

| Objective Test | Dx | # | Predictive Value Positive | Predictive Value Negative |
|---|---|---|---|---|
| Spirometry | COPD | 84 | .32 | 1.00 |
| Spirometry | Asthma | 84 | .18 | .72 |
| Bonchoprovocation | Asthma | 62 | .95 | 1.00 |
| Diffusion Capacity | ILD | 32 | .79 | .95 |
| Echocardiogram | Cardiac | 11 | .44 | 0.00 |
| RVG | Cardiac | 9 | .66 | 0.00 |
| Barium swallow | GERD | 15 | .33 | 0.83 |
| Comprehensive ETT | All Dx | 15 | .93 | 0.00 |
| Chest roentgenogram | All Dx | 84 | .75 | 0.91 |
| Spirometry | All Dx | 84 | .80 | 0.56 |

#, number of cases; Dx, diagnosis; COPD, chronic obstructive pulmonary disease; UA, upper airway disorder; ILD, interstitial lung disease; Cardiac, cardiomyopathy; ETT, exercise test; RVG, radionuclide ventriculogram; GERD, gastroesophageal reflux disease; Bronchoprovocation, methacholine inhalation bronchoprovocation challenge.

Buehler and Gracey[189] have suggested that lung volumes may be helpful in discriminating between COPD and CHF. Congestive heart failure has a normal or restricted pattern (reduced lung volumes) and COPD has an air-trapped (increased residual volume, functional residual capacity, and/or residual volume-to-total lung capacity ratio) or hyperinflated pattern (increased total lung capacity). A diffusing capacity appears to be an adequate screening test for dyspnea due to interstitial lung disease. Prior to change on chest roentgenogram, an interstitial impairment may be diagnosed at rest by a reduction in the diffusing capacity or on exertion by desaturation. A study by Mohensifar et al.[190] indicates that exertional tests are unnecessary in this setting since 97% of patients with a diffusing capacity above 70% of predicted will not have exertional desaturation. Studies by Andersen et al.[191] would also support this approach. If a diffusing capacity is not conveniently available, tests for exertional desaturation should be at least as sensitive.

All of the above series of studies do confirm that the diagnosis of the major cardiopulmonary disease causing dyspnea can be confirmed by traditional methods.

## Asthma, COPD, Interstitial Lung Disease

A diagnosis of asthma as the cause of dyspnea may be confirmed by an appropriate history, evidence of reversible airways obstruction on pulmonary function testing, positive bronchoprovocation challenge, and response to antiasthmatic therapy. Interstitial lung disease can be diagnosed[192,193] when there is an interstitial pattern on the chest roentgenogram, a reduction in diffusing capacity or desaturation on exertion, biopsy or chest computed-assisted tomography evidence of alveolitis or fibrosis, and/or pulmonary function tests indicating restriction. A diagnosis of COPD[194] can be established by demonstrating obstruction on spirometry that fails to respond to steroids and bronchodilator. Left ventricular dysfunction can be confirmed by echocardiography or radionuclide scans.

## Gastroesophageal Reflux Disease

Dyspnea due to GERD may be difficult to evaluate. As noted above, gastroesophageal reflux occurs frequently in the general population and only in a small percentage of patients does it produce dyspnea. Thus, even if gastrointestinal symptoms are clearly present or the reflux is confirmed by diagnostic testing, a causal relationship cannot be established unless the patient responds to specific therapy. Patients with suspected reflux disease should still be screened for the other common cardiopulmonary causes of dyspnea. Dyspnea that occurs nocturnally may suggest GERD triggered dyspnea. All dyspneic patients should be questioned regarding dysphagia, choking, heartburn, indigestion, regurgitation of food, antacid use, caffeine consumption, and fat content of their diets. The prevalence of dyspnea as the sole symptom of GERD is unknown. Good medical practice calls for treatment of symptomatic reflux whether dyspneic or not. A trial of antireflux therapy can be advocated in all patients with dyspnea and gastrointestinal symptoms of reflux. Patients with a high-risk profile for GERD, no symptoms of GERD apart from dyspnea, and no obvious cardiopulmonary cause of dyspnea may require a barium swallow or ambulatory 24-hour esophageal pH monitoring to help establish the diagnosis.

## Hyperventilation Syndromes

The diagnosis of the hyperventilation syndrome in a young individual with no risk factors for cardiopulmonary disease can probably be safely established with an appropriate history, a positive provocative test, and response to specific therapy. Specific therapy for the hyperventilation syndrome (discussed below) is available, is highly effective, and may work within weeks of institution.

In the older population, where the prevalence of cardiopulmonary disease is higher, the diagnosis might be suspected but other common causes of dyspnea need to be ruled out first. For instance, in individuals older than 40 years of age with no cardiopulmonary risks, simple office tests (eg, peak flow or spirometry, resting and walking oximetry, electrocardiogram, and history evaluating possible angina) may be used to screen for the common cardiopulmonary causes of chronic dyspnea. In patients with moderate risks of cardiopulmonary disease, negative screening tests, and a positive provocative challenge, an empiric trial of therapy should delay further evaluation only by a few weeks. When hyperventilation syndrome is suspected in a patient with a greater risk of cardiopulmonary disease or one who fails appropriate therapy, the most cost-effective evaluation strategy is likely to involve cardiopulmonary exercise testing.

## Pregnancy

The dyspneic pregnant patient poses a complex diagnostic challenge. Because dyspnea is so common during pregnancy, it is difficult to know which patients require further evaluation. Although dyspnea is common, it rarely interferes enough with daily activity[195] to prompt patient complaint and physician evaluation.

Rest dyspnea or dyspnea hindering exercise is rare and requires further evaluation.[196,197] Moreover, dyspnea accompanied by clubbing, cyanosis, hemoptysis, a systolic murmur louder than grade III, syncope, chest pain, or cough also should prompt further evaluation. Due to the large number of physiologic changes that occur during pregnancy, diagnostic tests must be carefully evaluated in that results that are clearly abnormal in nonpregnant women may be quite normal during pregnancy. Echocardiography may be helpful in evaluating possible pulmonary hypertension, cardiomyopathy, congenital heart diseases, and rheumatic heart disease. Pulmonary function tests can help evaluate a question of asthma. Methacholine challenge is not contraindicated in pregnancy. Pregnant patients may develop acute dyspnea due to embolism of air, amniotic fluid, or thrombus. Noninvasive evaluation of the legs with impedance plethysmography or duplex scanning poses no risk to the fetus. Transesophageal echocardiography, when feasible, may suggest embolism by the presence of acute right ventricular overload or confirm embolism by detecting proximal pulmonary artery clots. Although the dose of radioactivity delivered to a fetus with a ventilation/perfusion scan is only 300 Gy and less than that of a pulmonary arteriogram, it is advisable to reserve these tests only for life-threatening situations.[198]

## Occupational Dyspnea

Occupational dyspnea is an increasingly common problem that may require a special evaluation. Individuals with normal or mildly impaired cardiopulmonary fitness may experience dyspnea in unusual work environments. Jobs which place individuals at altitude, at high atmospheric pressure, or with higher levels of ambient $Pco_2$ may precipitate dyspnea which otherwise would not occur. Normal individuals may perceive mild dyspnea in the "tight building syndrome." Individuals forced to exert themselves while wearing pressure demand respirators may experience dyspnea related to a reduced ventilatory capacity. Scuba divers, firefighters, and others performing exhaustive endurance work with pressure demand respirators have a reduced work capacity and increased breathing discomfort when the respirator is worn.[199] In studies of healthy individuals performing sustained exercise at 70% maximum $\dot{V}o_2$, the maximum minute ventilation increased 22% when the patient wore a pressure demand ventilator[199] and the sensation of dyspnea increased.[200] Standards for respirators are currently determined to satisfy the ventilatory needs of the average individual performing sustained exertion at 50% maximum oxygen consumption. Differences in body size, degree of fitness, and degree of expected exertion render these standards inadequate for some individuals. In order to better accommodate 99% of the population ,it has been recommended that respirators be redesigned to permit minute ventilations of 199 L/min, inspiratory peak flows of 400 L/min, expiratory peak flows of 496 L/min, and pressure swings of 30 cm $H_2O$ across the mask. The maximum

voluntary ventilation appears to be the best screening test for evaluating individuals for respirator use.

## Cardiopulmonary Exercise Testing

Several authors advocate the use of cardiopulmonary exercise testing in dyspneic patients.[61,113,201–204] In this test, a patient typically undergoes a test with incrementally increasing workloads on a treadmill or stationary cycle ergometer. The electrocardiogram is performed continuously, gas exchange is measured by a metabolic cart, oximeter, and/or arterial cannula, and dyspnea is recorded on a visual analog or Borg scale. Testing continues until the patient can no longer sustain maximum effort. The main strength of the test lies in its ability to quantify cardiac and pulmonary function while the patient experiences dyspnea.

A healthy individual will exercise until maximum predicted heart rate is attained. At this point, the individual usually has a large breathing reserve, reaching a minute ventilation of only 60% to 80% of his or her predicted maximum.

Patients with cardiovascular disease demonstrate this type of pattern, but typically at a reduced work rate, and may show evidence of poor left ventricular function [eg, a low oxygen pulse (oxygen consumption/heart rate) at maximum exercise or a low anaerobic threshold, the oxygen consumption at which anaerobic metabolism starts as oxygen demand exceeds supply], electrocardiogram changes suggestive of ischemia, exercise-induced arrhythmia, or exercise-induced hypertension or hypotension.

Patients with a pulmonary limitation to exercise typically have a low breathing reserve and may not reach maximum predicted heart rate, may desaturate, have evidence of gas exchange inequality as seen by $\dot{V}e/\dot{V}co_2$ and $\dot{V}e/\dot{V}o_2$, or develop obstruction on postexercise spirometry indicative of asthma.

Cardiopulmonary exercise testing also provides measures of overall fitness. In normal subjects, the maximum oxygen consumption and anaerobic threshold provide objective evidence of the degree of physical conditioning. Patients with an anxiety/hyperventilation syndrome may hyperventilate at rest and show a rise in $CO_2$ as exercise starts.

The test has been reported to be helpful in identifying almost all diseases that cause dyspnea except GERD. Since physicians generally do well identifying patients with asthma, COPD, interstitial lung disease or cardiomyopathy, the test would be most cost-effective when these diagnoses are not suspected or if confirmed when dyspnea fails to respond to specific treatment. The test would then be useful in directing further evaluation toward other possible causes of dyspnea. Cardiopulmonary exercise testing is the only objective test to provide evidence that suspected deconditioning, psychogenic factors, anemia, metabolic acidosis, or muscle weakness are causally related to dyspnea. Martinez et al.[113] suggest that further evaluation may be needed to distinguish deconditioning from cardiac disease. There is some suggestion that the test may be less sensitive in patients with mild pulmonary vascular disease.

### Flow-Volume Loop

Much has been written about how to use the flow-volume loop to diagnose upper airway disease. The literature suggests that it is not likely to be often helpful. Parkinson's disease and redundant pharyngeal tissue in patients with sleep apnea may create a fluttering in the expiratory loop.[205,206] Neither disease is typically subtle enough or a common enough cause of dyspnea that one would expect to establish the diagnosis with flow-volume loops rather than with more traditional tests, and this finding is not specific for these conditions. Reduced inspiratory flows may be due to poor patient effort, postnasal drip, laryngeal dyskinesia, and tracheal masses. Since postnasal drip and poor patient effort are by far more common than the other processes, the specificity of reduced inspiratory flows is poor. In patients without upper airway symptoms, upper airway causes of dyspnea are rare.[3] In patients with upper airway symptoms, a laryngotracheoscopy would be a more definitive and cost-effective procedure.[140,144]

## Treatment

Treatment for dyspnea may either be disease-specific or disease-nonspecific. Specific therapy treats the underlying disease. Nonspecific therapy treats the symptoms of dyspnea. This review will demonstrate that specific therapy when available is more effective than nonspecific therapy. Therefore, whenever possible, the underlying cause of dyspnea should be identified and specific treatment provided for the underlying disease.

### Specific Therapy

The study by Pratter et al.[3] indicates that 76% of patients improve with specific therapy. All patients with asthma, postnasal drip syndrome, psychogenic causes, deconditioning, or GERD improved. Only 33% of patients with COPD, 58% of patients with interstitial lung disease, and 78% of patients with cardiomyopathy improved. Patients with interstitial lung disease and cardiomyopathy all continued to have some dyspnea despite treatment. When one of the less common diseases (eg, laryngeal edema) was the cause of dyspnea, specific therapy was effective in only 12%.

### Asthma

The treatment of asthma is more completely discussed in the chapter on wheeze. Few studies have specifically focused on the relief of dyspnea in asthma. Conventional therapy for asthma appears to reduce dyspnea as well as other asthmatic symptoms. Recent NIH guidelines[207] indicate that asthma is best managed when: (1) a physician and an educated patient work together; (2) triggers are identified and reduced; (3) therapy is guided by daily use of peak flow meters; (4) inhaled anti-inflammatory drugs, such as inhaled steroids, cromolyn, or nedocromil are taken on a daily basis; (5) inhaled beta agonists are taken only as needed; and (6) a written asthma management plan is used to guide therapy and determine the need for adding drugs, including oral steroids, or increasing drug dosage. Acute asthmatic dyspnea has also been reported to decrease with 2.5 to 7.5 cm $H_2O$ continuous positive airway pressure therapy.[119]

### Interstitial Lung Disease

Interstitial lung diseases are a diverse group of diseases that share a similar pathophysiology.[192,193] If the cause of the interstitial lung disease is known, specific treatment protocols are frequently available for individual diseases. In the 35% of cases where the cause can be identified, the patient should be removed from sources of further exposure to that agent. Therapy in general is aimed at preventing progression of the alveolitis to a stage where irreversible interstitial damage occurs. Traditional therapy calls for high-dose oral steroids taken for at least 9 months to 1 year. For example, the traditional NIH protocol was prednisone 1 mg/kg daily for 6 weeks, then tapered 2.5 mg per week until a maintenance dose of 0.25 mg/kg was reached. Therapy is then tapered or increased based on tests of objective response to treatment. Although numerous other anti-inflammatory agents besides steroids have been studied, none has achieved popular acceptance.[208] Cyclophosphamide and azathioprine are the most common second-line drugs added when patients fail to improve with steroids. The most recent data suggest that first-line treatment for idiopathic interstitial fibrosis with azathioprine and prednisone may improve outcome and minimize toxicity.[209] This protocol recommends prednisone at 1.5 mg/kg daily for the first two weeks (not to exceed 100 mg/day), followed by a biweekly taper (20 mg decrease every 2 weeks to a dose of 40 mg/day, then 5 to 10 mg decrease every 2 weeks) to a maintenance dose of 20 mg/day. Azathioprine is administered at a daily dose of 3 mg/kg (not to exceed 200 mg/day).

### COPD

The treatment of COPD is more completely discussed in Chapter 3, Wheeze. It is in this chapter that the role of corticosteroids and antibiotics are discussed in detail. In brief, the treatment of COPD should always include smoking cessation. Patients may benefit from exercise rehabilitation programs,[210] oxygen therapy when indicated, [211] and upper body exercises designed to strengthen accessory muscles.[212,213] Use of inhaled ipratropium or inhaled beta agonists remains first line pharmacotherapy.[214] Teramoto et al.[214] were able to demonstrate a reduction in dyspnea during exercise in 19 COPD patients who received 300 $\mu$g of a newer anticholinergic drug, oxitropium bromide, pre-exercise, in a randomized, placebo-controlled fashion. Theophylline has been shown to reduce dyspnea in COPD,[215] but is no longer considered a first-line drug for the disease.

### Upper Airway Diseases

Epiglottitis is treated with stabilization of the airway with intubation or tracheostomy if necessary and antibiotics. In children and adults, the most common causative bacterial organism is *Hemophilus influenza*, and the treatment is cefuroxime, a third generation cephalosporin, or trimethoprim-sulfamethoxazole. Angioedema usually responds to H1 and H2 blockers and systemic steroids. A typical urgent treatment regimen might call for diphenhydramine, ranitidine, and prednisone. In severe cases, intubation or tracheostomy to preserve the airway may be necessary. Laryngeal dyskinesia improves with the treatment of Parkinson's disease and may improve with the withdrawal of neuroleptic agents. Speech therapy may be helpful in other laryngeal dysfunction syndromes.[216] Postnasal drip syndrome may result from acute or chronic sinusitis, allergic rhinitis, perennial nonallergic rhinitis, occupational rhinitis, vasomotor rhinitis, infectious pharyngitis, and GERD. Treatment is discussed in detail in the chapter on rhinitis.

## Cardiac Diseases

The treatment for ischemic coronary disease is fully outlined in Chapter 6, Chest Pain: Diagnostic Strategies and Treatment. Dyspnea due to arrhythmias may be treated empirically by adding a drug known to normalize the arrhythmia or on the basis of an electrophysiologic study. Pacing may be necessary for the control of some arrhythmias. In patients with a pacemaker syndrome, the pacemaker should be reprogrammed in a mode that best permits synchronized atrioventricular contraction and permits reflex increases in heart rate from the sinus node. In most patients, this would be DDD or VVIR pacing. Dyspnea may result from cardiomyopathies of diastolic or systolic dysfunction or both. Therapy differs depending on the type of left ventricular dysfunction.[217] Systolic dysfunction is characterized by a reduction in the left ventricular ejection fraction and typically becomes clinically significant when the ejection fraction falls below 40%. Symptomatic patients with clinically significant left ventricular systolic dysfunction benefit from inotropes, diuretics, angiotensin converting enzyme (ACE) inhibitors, and vasodilators. Diastolic dysfunction is typical of hypertrophic cardiomyopathies and stiff ventricles from coronary disease. Dysfunction is characterized by increased diastolic pressures and a normal ejection fraction. Symptomatic patients with diastolic dysfunction benefit from treatment with negative inotropes, such as beta blockers or calcium channel blockers.

Pulmonary shunts due to arteriovenous malformations close with emboliza-tion or, if too large for embolization, resection. Embolization is more fully described in Chapter 4, Hemoptysis.

## Obesity/Deconditioning

Both obesity and deconditioning respond to diet and exercise. In patients who are obese or deconditioned enough to complain of dyspnea, consultation with a dietician and starting a regular exercise regimen is recommended. Patients should be strongly encouraged to establish the habit of exercise. Exercise initially may need only be walking on level ground as much as comfortably tolerated for 30 minutes 3 to 5 days per week. If patients are unable to be active continuously for the full 30 minutes, they should rest until fatigue and dyspnea resolve and then resume exercise until the 30 minute time is over. Depending on the severity of the impairment, patients may take over a year to have dyspnea resolve, but most note improvement by 3 months. Reardon et al.[210] randomized deconditioned patients with COPD to a nonintervention group and a group that underwent 12 3-hour sessions over 6 weeks of an education and exercise program. Dyspnea at maximum treadmill workload significantly decreased and the transitional dyspnea index significantly increased.

## Psychogenic Causes

Many patients with a hyperventilation/anxiety syndrome respond simply to acknowledging the diagnosis and reassurance.[112] Many patients require treatment aimed at understanding the disorder and teaching a new breathing strategy. Such treatment typically includes (a) allowing the patient to identify that their symptoms result from hyperventilation by performing a period of voluntary brief hyperventilation, (b) counseling the patient to emphasize that symptoms result from hyperventilation and not other causes, and (c) training in a respiratory control technique. Authors recommend learning to

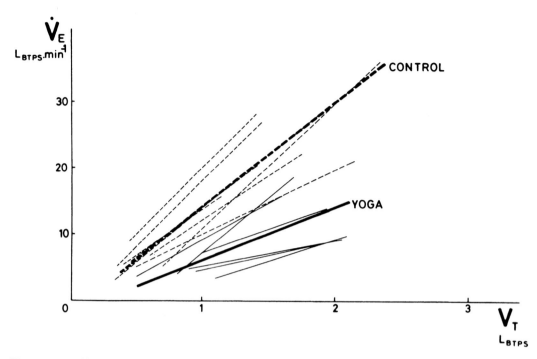

**Figure 12.** Effect of yoga on $CO_2$ response test. Yoga practitioners are less stimulated to increase ventilation as $CO_2$ increases. (Adapted from reference 219: Stanescu DC et al. J Appl Physiol 1981; 51:1625.)

breathe slowly with the aid of a pacing tape[163] or acoustic feedback device,[218] bag rebreathing into a 6X12-in bag,[25] and slow abdominal breathing.[164]

Controlled studies suggest that breathing retraining is effective.[218] Of 640 patients treated with the above general strategy, Lum[164] reported that 70% were rendered asymptomatic, 20% to 25% were improved, and 5% to 10% failed to respond. One-third were completely treated in two to three visits.[25]

The mechanism of improvement with specific breathing strategies remains speculative. Breathing control therapy appears to alter $CO_2$ responsivity.[218,219] Stanescu et al.[219] have demonstrated that practitioners of ujjai slow deep-breath yoga have a decreased response to $CO_2$ (Figure 12). They suggest that this behavioral strategy may alter control of breathing by modifying vagal traffic due to chronic overstimulation of stretch receptors, loss of response of the CNS to vagal afferents due to habi-

tuation, or decreased adrenergic tone. Tandon[220] has used yoga successfully also to reduce dyspnea in COPD. Panic disorder should be treated similarly with counseling, behavioral breathing strategies, and if refractory with pharmacotherapy. Beta blockade has been helpful in some patients, but studies overall have had conflicting results. Fluoxetine hydrochloride (Prozac®) and sertraline hydrochloride (Zoloft®) have been helpful in patients with panic attacks who have failed behavioral therapy. Acute situational anxiety may be treated with short-term anxiolytics. Major psychiatric disorders involving psychosis may require psychotherapy or pharmacotherapy with psychoactive drugs.

## Gastroesophageal Reflux Disease

The strategy for treating GERD is reviewed in more detail in Chapter 1, Cough.

The intensity of the regimen necessary to treat GERD-induced dyspnea remains unclear. In order to relieve GERD-induced cough patients require on average 5.5 months of multidrug therapy and extensive lifestyle modification.[221] Patients with mild or infrequent symptoms might be started on a minimal regimen involving: antacids when symptomatic either with dyspnea or heartburn, a low-fat diet, and simple avoidance techniques and mechanical measures. Patients without prompt relief to this regimen or with more severe or frequent symptoms should have an H2 blocker added and can be considered for a promotility agent, such as metoclopramide or cisapride. Patients with severe symptoms can be treated with omeprazole 20 to 40 mg daily and cisapride 10 mg 15 to 30 minutes before meals and at bedtime. Patients refractory to this regimen may require fundoplication. Tibbling and Gibellino[222] evaluated dyspnea in 113 patients undergoing fundoplication and reported a significant decrease in the prevalence of dyspnea from 32% preoperatively to 13% postoperatively.

### Neuromuscular diseases

Neuromuscular diseases, such as myasthenia gravis, respond to conventional therapy for the disease. As the overall disease improves, the dyspnea improves. In other cases, one should aim to exercise weak muscles, rest fatigued muscles, and pace denervated muscles. Quadriplegia may benefit from specific respiratory muscle exercise with an inspiratory muscle trainer.[223] The goal in this case is to develop hypertrophy and strength in the respiratory muscles that remain innervated. Diseases which involve possible muscle weakness, such as muscular dystrophy, or require compensatory hypertrophy of remaining muscles, such as amyotrophic lateral sclerosis, multiple sclerosis, or the postpolio syndrome, could theoretically benefit from such a strategy. Inspiratory muscle rest by use of nocturnal or intermittent positive or negative pressure ventilators may provide relief for some patients with amyotrophic lateral sclerosis or muscular dystrophy.[224] Speech therapy may be able to teach some patients a glossopharyngeal breathing technique that ameliorates dyspnea.[216] Diaphragmatic pacing may benefit patients having cervical spine injuries with intact phrenic nerves.

## Nonspecific Therapy

Nonspecific therapy is therapy that is directed at the symptom rather than at the disease. In this category, one would need to include: conditioning regimens, stress reduction and coping skills, oxygen, mechanical ventilation, respiratory muscle training, vagotomy, muscle vibration, and pharmacotherapy with narcotics, anxiolytics, and phenothiazines.

### Conditioning Regimens

Aerobic conditioning aims to reduce dyspnea by increasing cardiovascular efficiency and reducing the $CO_2$ production and minute ventilation associated with a given workload. Conditioning lowers the $\dot{V}e/\dot{V}o_2$ slope and raises the anaerobic threshold.[176] Aerobic conditioning is specific therapy for patients who are deconditioned. The value of aerobic conditioning for other patients, while unproven, appeals to common sense. Patients with COPD who are able to aerobically exercise show a reduction in dyspnea.[225–227] Given the lack of evidence supporting the role of aerobic conditioning in most diseases resulting in dyspnea, it is difficult to recommend a preferred training regimen. In general, one would recommend a gradual progression to 30 minutes of aerobic exercise at least 3 days per week. Once reconditioned, patients are advised to continue exercise for enhanced performance status at workloads and frequencies acceptable to their level of dyspnea and cardiovascular state.

## Nutrition

Nutritional state may affect dyspnea due to obesity, malnutrition, or carbohydrate loading. As dyspnea in general appears to increase with body mass index,[18] all patients above ideal body weight might benefit from weight reduction.

Since respiratory muscle function significantly affects dyspnea, it is also likely that patients with protein malnutrition will experience a decrease in dyspnea with nutritional repletion. Rogers et al.[228] performed a controlled, randomized study that supports this conclusion. They were able to demonstrate a reduction in dyspnea in malnourished COPD patients after a 3-month refeeding intervention. A low-carbohydrate diet has been shown to reduce $\dot{V}_{CO_2}$ in COPD patients by lowering the respiratory quotient. As discussed above, the strategy of reducing carbohydrates in the diet will be beneficial in a very small number of patients. Restricting carbohydrate-intake prior to exercise may be more generally recommended.

## Stress Reduction and Coping Skills

Stress reduction and coping skills presumably decrease dyspnea by altering cortical assessments of dyspnogenic stimuli and altering daily routines to minimize dyspnea. Carrieri-Kohlman and colleagues[229–232] provide extensive suggestions for decreasing dyspnea by activity modification and energy conservation. All patients with moderate dyspnea should receive instruction in modifying their activities to reduce dyspnea from a skilled healthcare provider. Detailed suggestions for decreasing dyspnea during grooming, bathing, dressing, meal preparation, cleaning, washing, and sex are available. Most of these strategies emphasize planning, rest breaks, recognition of physical limitations, advantageous postures, and work aids.

## Oxygen

Patients with reduced oxygen saturations at rest or on exertion may experience a reduction in dyspnea by oxygen therapy. Oxygen therapy may reduce dyspnea by several actions. In patients who are hypoxemic, oxygen will eliminate the dyspnogenic stimulus. In patients with $\dot{V}/\dot{Q}$ ratio mismatch, an increase in alveolar oxygen may increase perfusion to poorly ventilated alveoli thereby favorably altering gas exchange. In patients with COPD, supplemental oxygen increases exercise time[233] and reduces dyspnea.[234] Recent studies of patients with transtracheal oxygen have demonstrated an improvement in exercise tolerance but no improvement in dyspnea in COPD patients receiving transtracheal oxygen as opposed to nasal cannula.[235]

There are no data to support the use of continuous oxygen therapy in patients with oxygen saturations above 85%. However, in patients with mild desaturation on exertion supplemental oxygen during exercise may be beneficial. Dean et al.[211] report improved dyspnea and exercise duration in 12 patients with severe COPD during exercise receiving 40% oxygen, with a mean postexercise $P_{O_2}$ of 63 mmHg during the control room air trial.

## Vagotomy

Vagotomy decreases dyspnea by eliminating afferent vagal information and theoretically may help those with vagally mediated dyspnea. Vagotomy has been reported to reduce dyspnea in patients with COPD, interstitial disease, and pulmonary venous occlusion.[33,132,133,149] Although modern surgical techniques allow selective pulmonary vagotomy to be performed thoracoscopically at the level of the hilum with minimal expected complications, no large series of patients undergoing vagotomy for dyspnea exists. Therefore, vagotomy cannot be recommended as a general therapy. In end-stage patients, especially those with pulmonary vascular congestion, it is reasonable to attempt vagotomy if other nonspecific therapy fails.

## Muscle Vibration

Sibuya et al.[45] delivered 100 Hz vibrations to 15 patients with chronic dyspnea.

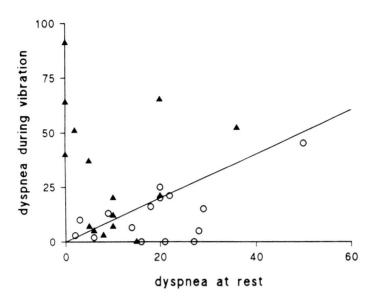

**Figure 13.** Effect of intercostal muscle vibration on dyspnea. Dyspnea was measured in 15 COPD patients and plotted as response on a 150 mm visual analog scale. Circles indicate in-phase vibration and triangles indicate out-of-phase vibration. The diagonal line is a line of identity. In-phase vibration decreases dyspnea and out-of-phase vibration increases dyspnea. (Adapted from Reference 45: Sibuya M et al. Am J Respir Crit Care Med 1994; 149: p 1237.)

Vibration to the inspiratory intercostals during inspiration and expiratory intercostals during expiration, called in-phase vibration, reduced dyspnea whereas out-of-phase vibration increased dyspnea. Of the 15 patients, 8 patients had a significant decrease in dyspnea with in-phase vibration (Figure 13). Patients with the greatest degree of rest dyspnea appeared to have the greatest benefit. The mechanism of action is unclear, but a decrease in dyspnea would presumably result from altering muscle afferent signals. This technique remains experimental and has not been adapted for ambulatory patient use. Should further studies prove confirmatory it offers an exciting possibility for alleviating dyspnea of many causes.

## Respiratory Muscle Training

Inspiratory resistive loading has been shown to increase both respiratory muscle strength and endurance. However, inspiratory muscle training has not been conclu-sively shown to reduce dyspnea. Virtually all studies have been performed in COPD patients. Most document an improvement or no change in exercise performance and a decrease in dyspnea. Because many studies are uncontrolled, the value of resistive training remains unclear. Kim et al.[236] report a 6-month randomized, controlled trial of 67 patients with COPD. In this study, 38% of the treatment group noticed a reduction in dyspnea as compared to 40% of the control group. Placebo effect appears to be significant with this intervention. One would expect the greatest benefit in patients with weak inspiratory muscles and those whose dyspnea is mediated by muscle weakness. Even if one limits this intervention to patients with known muscle weakness measured by maximal inspiratory mouth pressure, one cannot be assured that improving muscle strength will decrease dyspnea. I agree with Mahler[237] that inspiratory resistive training should be reserved for those patients with weak muscles who have failed all other conventional therapies. Patients with neuromuscular disorders could, however, use inspiratory resistive training as a specific therapy.

The easiest patient devices to prescribe are the PFLEX (Healthscan, Upper Montclair, NJ) and the Threshold (Healthscan Products Inc, Cedar Grove, N.J.). The PFLEX creates an increased inspiratory resistance by allowing the patient to breathe in through a small orifice. The appropriate resistance may be selected by varying the orifice size. Patients who breathe at slow inspiratory flows through this device do not achieve the desired inspiratory load and visual feedback may be necessary for success. The Threshold is a spring-loaded device that requires the patient to inspire to a given pressure to compress a spring and allow entry of air. If prescribed, the patient should exercise for at least 30 minutes per day, in one or two sessions, at least 4 to 5 days per week. Initial workloads should be in the range of 25% maximal inspiratory pressure and increased approximately every 2 weeks as symptoms permit to a maximum of 50% maximal inspiratory pressure. Because improvements may be seen as early as 1 month, the maximal inspiratory pressure should be remeasured at least every 2 months so that new targets may be set. As with other types of exercise, inspiratory resistive training may lead to desaturation. Each patient should be monitored with oximetry for a 10- to 15-minute observed training session before being sent home with the device. Both devices include adapters for supplemental oxygen if necessary.

Exercises that strengthen the upper chest and shoulder muscles may reduce dyspnea. Celli et al.[213] noted that muscles with both a rib cage and shoulder/humerus attachment could function to aid respiration or arm/shoulder movement. When the arms move, the serratus anterior, trapezius, latissimus dorsi, and pectoralis major and minor may be unable assist in ventilation. One would expect that when the arms are unsupported in an activity, their inability to assist ventilation would be even greater. Patients who rely on accessory muscles for ventilatory support may have difficulty performing unsupported arm activity and may complain of dyspnea during shampooing or tooth-brushing. The same patient may have little difficulty in scrubbing a floor if the arms are leaned upon during the activity.

Shoulder muscles may be strengthened and endurance increased by an exercise regimen emphasizing frequent repetitions with light weights.[212] Patients may easily perform the exercises at home with no special equipment. A simple regimen would be to have a patient lift a 1- to 4-lb broom handle with both arms until arms are horizontal, hold for 6 seconds, and repeat 10 times. This should be done three to five times per day.

Ries et al.[238] have shown a decrease in dyspnea with upper extremity exercise after 6 weeks of arm cycling. The use of arm cycling should be encouraged when a patient has access to a fitness center since it cannot be easily performed at home.

Although the studies that support the above exercises are few and have been performed only in COPD patients, they theoretically could reduce dyspnea associated with arm activity in any patient, are simple, can be performed at home, and have no reported morbidity. All patients with arm-use dyspnea should be prescribed this simple exercise program.

### Mechanical Ventilation

Mechanical ventilation can be adjusted to decrease inspiratory muscle work, provide muscle rest, reduce muscle fatigue and metaboreceptor stimulation, and thereby reduce dyspnea when ventilation is subsequently withdrawn. Continuous mechanical ventilation can be used to decrease dyspnea in patients willing to undergo this. In most cases where continuous mechanical ventilation could be considered for dyspnea relief, the underlying disease would be so advanced that issues regarding prolongation of life would also need to be addressed. Mechanical ventilation can normalize $PaCO_2$, $PaO_2$, decrease muscle work and decrease dead space.

Patients who should experience a decrease in dyspnea from intermittent muscle rest with intermittent mechanical ventilation would be expected to have a disease that mediates dyspnea via muscle fatigue. Although muscle rest may benefit some patients with COPD, CHF, thyroid disease, malnutrition, or neuromuscular diseases, it would be extremely unlikely to benefit the majority of the patients in any of these groups. Systematic studies have been performed only in COPD patients.[239–245] These report an increase in muscle strength and endurance and a reduction in $Pco_2$. Although some studies suggest a decrease in dyspnea, dyspnea has not been systematically evaluated. The largest, randomized, sham-controlled study of negative-pressure ventilation showed no improvement in quality of life or dyspnea.[246]

Although some patients with dyspnea may benefit from nocturnal ventilation, we do not know how to prospectively identify them. In patients with neuromuscular disease or kyphoscoliotic respiratory failure, a trial of nocturnal ventilation could be attempted when disabling levels of dyspnea are reached despite maximal conventional therapy. In other patients nocturnal ventilation cannot be routinely recommended. In most patients requiring only intermittent nocturnal ventilation, a nasal positive-pressure ventilator works well.[224] Although numerous other negative-pressure devices may be used effectively to provide nocturnal ventilation, most patients find them less convenient.

### Pharmacotherapy

Studies suggest that benzodiazepines, phenothiazines, and narcotics may all reduce dyspnea in some patients. These drugs are nonspecific therapy in that they probably function by altering CNS perception of the dyspnea signal. Al-Damluji[247] reported the only trial of a drug not in these classes. He notes that medroxyprogesterone acetate, 20 mg tid, administered to COPD patients lowered $Pco_2$ and increased $Po_2$ but did not alter dyspnea.

Benzodiazepines function as anxiolytics and may be specific therapy for patients with anxiety-exacerbated dyspnea. In other patients, these drugs may act through ventilatory depression. The few patient studies suggesting benefit[248,249] suffer from small sample sizes, populations limited primarily to COPD, and lack of controls. The only two controlled studies of benzodiazepines showed no reduction in dyspnea in COPD patients.[250,251] Based on these results, benzodiazepines cannot be recommended.

Phenothiazines may act as specific therapy in patients with psychiatric illnesses. In other patients, the mechanism of action is unclear. Results to date have been controversial. Studies are limited to COPD patients in small numbers participating in uncontrolled trials. Woodcock et al.[250] reported a reduction in dyspnea with promethazine hydrochloride, whereas Rice[252] did not. There are not enough data to support the generalized use of these drugs.

Opiates might reduce dyspnea by a blunting of perception and a respiratory depression. Several studies have evaluated different opiates for relief of dyspnea in COPD. Giron et al.[253] administered dextromethorphan hydrobromide, 60 mg, in a single-blind placebo-controlled trial and concluded that there were no differences in hypoxic or hypercapnic drive, exercise endurance, or rest or exercise dyspnea. Woodcock et al.,[250] in a different study, were able to demonstrate (a) a reduction in dyspnea during treadmill exercise after oral dihydrocodeine 1 mg/kg, (b) a reduction in exercise dyspnea after dihydrocodeine, 30 mg tid, but not after 60 mg tid or placebo, and (c) a decrease in dyspnea after dihydrocodeine, 15 mg tid. Rice found no improvement in dyspnea after codeine, 30 mg qid for 1 month. Light et al.[254] reported improved exercise performance and reduced dyspnea in 13 COPD patients after treatment with oral morphine sulfate 0.8 mg/kg. Robin[255] demonstrated a benefit of hydromorphone hydrochloride (Dilaudid), 3 mg, rectal suppositories in an individual patient. New drugs such as Duragesic, a transdermal fentanyl patch, and controlled-release morphine preparations, MS Contin and MSIR, have been used with success in individual patients but not studied in a controlled fashion. All drugs in this class have substantial side effects of mental depression, constipation, and addiction. Any decision to attempt reduction of dyspnea with these agents must be balanced with the side effects.[256] In the dying patient, morphine may allow death to occur with comfort and dignity. Efficacy can be titrated in this situation with naloxone, if desired.[257]

## References

1. Hammond EC. Some preliminary findings on physical complaints from a prospective study of 1,064,004 men and women. Am J Public Health 1964; 54: 11–23.
2. Kroenke K, Mangelsdorff D. Common symptoms in ambulatory care: incidence, evaluation, therapy, and outcome. Am J Med 1989; 86:262–266.
3. Pratter MR, Curley FJ, Dubois J, et al. Cause and evaluation of chronic dyspnea in a pulmonary disease clinic. Arch Intern Med 1989; 149:2277–2282.
4. Janson-Bjerklie S, Carrieri VK, Hudes M. The sensations of pulmonary dyspnea. Nurs Res 1986; 35:154–159.
5. Eliott MW, Adams L, Cockroft A, et al. The language of breathlessness: the use of verbal descriptors by patients with cardiopulmonary disease. Am Rev Respir Dis 1991; 144:826–832.
6. Melzack R. The McGill pain questionnaire: major properties and scoring methods. Pain 1975; 1:277–299.
7. Fletcher CM. The clinical diagnosis of pulmonary emphysema. An experimental study. Proceedings of the Royal Society of Medicine 1952; 45:577
8. Brooks SM. Task group on surveillance for respiratory hazards in the occupational setting: surveillance for respiratory hazards. ATS News 1982; 8:12–16.
9. Mahler DA, Weinberg DH, Wells CK, et al. The measurement of dyspnea: contents, interobserver agreement, and physiologic correlates of two new clinical indices. Chest 1984; 85:751–757.
10. Mahler DA, Harver A. Clinical measurement of dyspnea. In: Donald A, Mahler MD, eds. Dyspnea. Mount Kisco: Futura Pubishing Company; 1990:56–74.
11. Killian KJ, Jones NL. Respiratory muscles and dyspnea. Clin Chest Med 1988; 9: 237–248.
12. Eriksson H, Svardsudd K, Larsson B, et al. Dyspnoea in a cross-sectional and a longitudinal study of middle-aged men: the Study of Men Born in 1913 and 1923. Eur Heart J 1987; 8:1015–1023.
13. Nejjari C, Tessier JF, Dartigues JF, et al. The relationship between dyspnoea and main lifetime occupation in the elderly. Int J Epidemiol 1993; 22:848–854.
14. Viegi G, Paoletti P, Carrozzi L, et al. Effects of home environment on respiratory symptoms and lung function in a general population sample in North Italy. Eur Respir J 1991; 4:580–586.
15. Sherman CB, Xu X, Speizer FE, et al. Longitudinal lung function decline in subjects with respiratory symptoms. Am Rev Respir Dis 1992; 855–859.
16. Krzyzanowski M, Robbins DR, Lebowitz MD. Smoking cessation and changes in respiratory symptoms in two populations followed for 13 years. Int J Epidemiol 1993; 22:666–673.
17. Viegi G, Prediletto R, Paoletti P, et al. Respiratory effects of occupational exposure in a general population sample in North Italy. Am Rev Respir Dis 1991; 143: 510–515.
18. Sjostrom L, Larsson B, Backman L, et al. Swedish obese subjects (SOS). Recruitment for an intervention study and a selected description of the obese state. Int J Obesity 1992; 16:465–479.
19. Altose M, Cherniack N, Fishman AP. Respiratory sensations and dyspnea. J Appl Physiol 1985; 58:1051–1054.
20. Schmitt BP, Kushner MS, Wiener SL. The diagnostic usefulness of the history of the patient with dyspnea. J Gen Intern Med 1986; 1:386–393.
21. Fedullo AL, Swineburne AJ, McGuire-Dunn C. Complaints of breathlessness in the emergency department: the experience at a community hospital. NY State J Med 1986; 86:4–6.
22. Pearson SB, Pearson EM, Mitchel JRA. The diagnosis and management of patients admitted to hospital with acute breathlessness. Postgrad Med 1981; 57: 419–424.
23. Mustchin CP, Tiwari I. Diagnosing the breathless patient. Lancet 1982; 2: 907–908.

24. Dodge RR, Burrows B. The prevalence and incidence of asthma and asthma-like symptoms in a general population sample. Am Rev Respir Dis 1980; 122: 567–575.

25. Magarian GJ. Hyperventilation syndromes: infrequently recognized common expressions of anxiety and stress. Medicine 1982; 61:219–236.

26. Jammes Y, Speck DF. Respiratory control by diaphragmatic and respiratory muscle afferents. In: Dempsey JA, Pack AI, eds. *Regulation of Breathing.* 2nd ed. New York, NY: Marcel Dekker, Inc; 1995: 543–582.

27. Mathew OP, Ghosh TK. Role of airway afferents on upper airway muscle activity. In: Dempsey JA, Pack AI, eds. *Regulation of Breathing.* 2nd ed. New York, NY: Marcel Dekker Incα95:511–544.

28. Kubin L, Davies RO. Central pathways of pulmonary and airway vagal afferents. In: Dempsey JA, Pack AI, eds. *Regulation of Breathing.* 2nd ed. New York, NY: Marcel Dekker Inc;:219–284.

29. Gonzalez C, Dinger BG, Fiidone SJ. Mechanisms of carotid body chemoreception. In: Dempsey JA, Pack AI, eds. *Regulation of Breathing.* 2nd ed. New York, NY: Marcel Dekker Inc; 1995:391–472.

30. Bisgard GE, Neubauer JA. Peripheral and central effects of hypoxia. In: Dempsey JA, Pack AI, eds. *Regulation of Breathing.* 2nd ed. New York, NY: Marcel Dekker,-Inc. 1995:617–828.

31. Nattie EE. Central chemoreception. In: Dempsey JA, Pack AI, editors. *Regulation of Breathing.* 2nd ed. New York, NY: Marcel Dekker Inc; 1995:473–510.

32. Simon PM, Basner RC, Weinberger SE, et al. Oral mucosal stimulation modulates intensity of breathlessness induced in normal subjects. Am Rev Respir Dis 1991; 144:419–422.

33. Guz A, Noble MIM, Widdicombe JG, et al. The role of vagal and glossopharyngeal afferent nerves in respiratory sensation, control of breathing, and arterial pressure regulation in conscious man. Clin Sci 1966; 30:161–170.

34. Banzett RB, Lansing W, Brown R. High level quadriplegics perceive lung volume change. J Appl Physiol 1987; 62:567–573.

35. Guz A, Noble MIM, Eisele JH, et al. The effect of bilateral block of vagus and glossopharyngeal nerves on the ventilatory response to $CO_2$ of conscious man. Respir Physiol 1966; 1:206–210.

36. Winning AJ, Hamilton RD, Guz A. Ventilation and breathlessness on maximal exercise in patients with interstitial lung disease after local anaesthetic aerosol inhalation. Clin Sci 1988; 74:275–281.

37. Campbell EJM, Freedman S, Clark TJH, et al. The effect of muscular paralysis induced by tubocurarine on the duration and sensation of breathholding. Clin Sci 1967; 32:425–432.

38. Campbell EJM, Godfrey S, Clark TJH, et al. The effect of muscular paralysis induced by tubocurarine on the duration and sensation of breathholding during hypercapnia. Clin Sci 1969; 36:323–328.

39. Fowler WS. Breaking point in breathholding. J Appl Physiol 1954; 6:539–545.

40. Rigg JRA, Rebuck AS, Campbell EJM. A study of factors influencing relief of discomfort in breath-holding in normal subjects. Clin Sci Mol Med 1974; 47:193–199.

41. Eisele J, Trenchard D, Burki NK, et al. The effect of chest wall block on respiratory sensations and control in man. Clin Sci 1968; 35:23–33.

42. Gottfried SB, Leech I, DiMarco AF, et al. Sensation of respiratory force following low cervical spinal transection. J Appl Physiol 1984; 57:989–994.

43. Estenne M, Yernault JC, De Troyer A. Mechanism of relief of dyspnea after thoracocentesis in patients with large pleural effusions. Am J Med 1983; 74:813–819.

44. Killian KJ, Campbell EJM. Dyspnea. In: Roussos C, Macklem PT, eds. *The Thorax.* New York, NY: Marcel Dekker Inc; 1985: 787–828.

45. Sibuya M, Yamada M, Kanamaru A, et al. Effect of chest wall vibration on dyspnea in patients with chronic respiratory disease. Am J Respir Crit Care Med 1994; 149:1235–1240.

46. Banzett RB, Lansing RW, Brown R, et al. 'Air hunger' from increased $P_{CO_2}$ persists after complete neuromuscular block in humans. Respir Physiol 1990; 81:1–18.

47. Gandevia SC, Killian KJ, McKenzie DK, et al. Respiratory sensations, cardiovascular control, kinaesthesia, and transcranial stimulation during paralysis in humans. J Physiol 1993; 470:85–107.

48. Kimoff RJ, Cheong TH, Cosio MG, et al. Pulmonary denervation in humans: effects on dyspnea and ventilatory pattern during exercise. Am Rev Respir Dis 1990; 142:1034–1040.

49. Schwartzstein RM, LaHive K, Pope A, et

al. Detection of hypercapnea by normal subjects. Clin Sci 1987; 73:333–335.

50. Adams L, Lane R, Shea SA, et al. Breathlessness during different forms of ventilatory stimulation: a study of the mechanisms in normal subjects and in respiratory patients. Clin Sci 1985; 69: 663–672.

51. Chonan T, Mulholland MB, Leitner J, et al. J Appl Physiol 1990; 68:2100–2106.

52. Demediuk BH, Manning H, Lilly J, et al. Dissociation between dyspnea and respiratory effort. Am Rev Respir Dis 1992; 146:1222–1225.

53. Lane R, Cockroft A, Guz A. Voluntary isocapneic hyperventilation and breathlessness during exercise in normal subjects. Clin Sci 1987; 73:519–523.

54. Freedman S, Lane R, Guz A. Breathlessness and respiratory mechanics during reflex or voluntary hyperventilation in patients with chronic airflow obstruction. Clin Sci 1987; 73:311–318.

55. Ward SA, Whipp BJ. Effects of peripheral and central chemoreflex activation on the isopneic rating of breathing in humans. J Physiol 1989; 411:27–43.

56. Dudley DL, Martin CJ, Holmes TH. Dyspnea: psychologic and physiologic observations. J Psychosom Res 1968; 11: 325–339.

57. Shershow JC, Kanarek DH, Kazemi H. Ventilatory response to carbon dioxide inhalation in depression. Psychosom Med 1976; 38:282–287.

58. Saunders NA, Heilpern S, Rebuck AS. Relation between personality and ventilatory response to carbon dioxide in normal subjects: a role in asthma? Br Med J 1972; 1:719–721.

59. Arkinstall WW, Nirme K, Klissouras V, et al. Genetic differences in the ventilatory response to inhaled $CO_2$. J Appl Physiol 1974; 36:6–11.

60. Kobayashi S, Nishimura M, Yamamoto M, et al. Dyspnea sensation and chemical control of breathing in adult twins. Am Rev Respir Dis 1993; 147:1192–1198.

61. Wasserman K. Dyspnea on exertion. Is it the heart or the lungs? JAMA 1982; 248: 2039–2043.

62. Wasserman K. Physiology of gas exchange and exertional dyspnoea. Clin Sci 1981; 61:7–13.

63. Killian KJ, Campbell EJM. Mechanisms of dyspnea. In: Mahler DA, ed. *Dyspnea*. Mount Kisco: Futura Publishing Company; 1990:55–74.

64. Wilson RC, Oldfield WL, Jones PW. Effect of residence at altitude on the perception of breathlessness on return to sea level in normal subjects. Clin Sci 1993; 84: 159–167.

65. Burki NK. Dyspnea. Clin Chest Med 1980; 1:47–55.

66. Passerini L, Cosio MG, Newman SL. Respiratory muscle dysfunction after herpes zoster. Am Rev Respir Dis 1985; 132: 1366–1367.

67. Dornhurst AC. Respiratory insufficiency. Lancet 1955; 1:1185

68. Dujovny M, Osgood CP, Segal R. Acute acromegalic dyspnea. Laryngoscope 1976; 86:1397–1401.

69. Ayres J, Rees J, Clark TJ, et al. Thyrotoxicosis and dyspnea. Clin Endocrinol (Oxf) 1982; 16:65–71.

70. Mier A, Brophy C, Wass JAM, et al. Reversible respiratory muscle weakness in hyperthyroidism. Am Rev Respir Dis 1989; 139: 529–533.

71. Small D, Gibbons W, Levy RD, et al. Exertional dyspnea and ventilation in hyperthyroidism. Chest 1992; 101:1268–1273.

72. McElvaney GN, Wilcox PG, Fairbarn MS, et al. Respiratory muscle weakness and dyspnea in thyrotoxic patients. Am Rev Respir Dis 1990; 141:1221–1227.

73. Leigh M, Holman G, Rohn R. Dyspnea as the presenting symptom of thyroid disease.Two unusual cases. Clin Pediatr (Phila) 1980; 11:773–774.

74. Curley FJ, Irwin RS, Pratter MR, et al. Cough and the common cold. Am Rev Respir Dis 1988; 138:305–311.

75. Morgan EJ, Altmeyer R, Khakoo R, et al. Pulmonary function in infectious mononucleosis. Chest 1982; 81:699–700.

76. Lightman NI, Schooley RT. Adult-onset acid maltase deficiency. Case report of an adult with severe respiratory difficulty. Chest 1977; 72:250–252.

77. Howard RS, Wiles CM, Hirsch NP, et al. Respiratory involvement in multiple sclerosis. Brain 1992; 115:479–494.

78. Cooper CB, Trend PSJ, Wiles CM. Severe diaphragm weakness in multiple sclerosis. Thorax 1985; 40:633–634.

79. Begin R, Bureau MA, Lupien L, et al. Pathogenesis of respiratory insufficiency in myotonic dystrophy. The mechanical factors. Am Rev Respir Dis 1982; 125: 312–318.

80. Mulvey DA, Aquilina RJ, Elliott MW, et al. Diaphragmatic dysfunction in neuralgic amyotrophy: an electrophysiologic

evaluation of 16 patients presenting with dyspnea. Am Rev Respir Dis 1993; 147: 66–71.

81. Zupnick HM, Brown LK, Miller A, et al. Respiratory dysfunction due to L-dopa therapy for Parkinsonism: diagnosis using serial pulmonary function tests and respiratory inductive plethysmography. Am J Med 1990; 89:109–114.

82. DeBruin PFC, DeBruin VMS, Lees AJ, et al. Effects of treatment on airway dynamics and respiratory muscle strength in Parkinson's disease. Am Rev Respir Dis 1993; 148:1576–1580.

83. Weiner WJ, Goetz CG, Nausieda PA, et al. Respiratory dyskinesias: extrapyramidal dysfunction and dyspnea. Ann Intern Med 1978; 88:327–331.

84. Chandler KW, Rozas CJ, Kory RC, et al. Bilateral diaphragmatic paralysis complicating local cardiac hypothermia during open heart surgery. Am J Med 1984; 77: 243–249.

85. Knobil K, Becker FS, Harper P, et al. Dyspnea in a patient years after severe poliomyelitis. The role of cardiopulmonary exercise testing. Chest 1994; 105:777–781.

86. Cashman NR, Maselli R, Wollmann RL, et al. Late denervation in patients with antecedent paralytic poliomyelitis. N Engl J Med 1987; 317:7–12.

87. De Troyer A, Heilporn A. Respiratory mechanics in quadriplegia. The respiratory function of the intercostal muscles. Am Rev Respir Dis 1980; 122:591–600.

88. Lunde H, Hedner T, Samuelsson O, et al. Dyspnoea, asthma, and bronchospasm in relation to treatment with angiotensin converting enzyme inhibitors. Br Med J 1994; 308:18–21.

89. Read CA, Clauw D, Weir C, et al. Dyspnea and pulmonary function in the L-tryptophane-associated eosinophilia-myalgia syndrome. Chest 1992; 101:1280–1286.

90. Rosenow EC. Drug-induced pulmonary disease. In: Murray JF, Nadel JA, eds. *Textbook of Respiratory Medicine.* Philadelphia, Pa: W B Saunders Company; 1994:2117–2144.

91. Goodwin SD, Glenny RW. Nonsteroidal anti-inflammatory drug-associated pulmonary infiltrates with eosinophilia: Review of the literature and Food and Drug Administration adverse drug reaction reports. Arch Intern Med 1992; 152: 1521–1524.

92. Gilbert R, Auchincloss JHJ. Dyspnea of pregnancy. Clinical and physiological ob-

servations. Am J Med Sci 1966; 252: 270–276.

93. Zeldis SM. Dyspnea during pregnancy. Distinguishing cardiac from pulmonary causes [Review]. Clin Chest Med 1992; 13:567–585.

94. Milne J, Howie A, Pack A. Dyspnea during normal pregnancy. Br J Obstet Gynaecol 1978; 85:260–263.

95. Panacek EA, Singer AJ, Sherman BW, et al. Spontaneous pneumomediastinum: clinical and natural history. Ann Emerg Med 1992; 21:1222/67–1227/72.

96. Ahluwalia M, Ishikawa S, Gellman M, et al. Pulmonary functions during peritoneal dialysis. Clin Nephrol 1995; 18: 251–256.

97. Singh S, Dale A, Morgan B, et al. Serial studies of pulmonary function in continuous ambulatory peritoneal dialysis: A prospective study. Chest 1986; 6: 874–877.

98. Sebert P, Bellet M, Girin E, et al. Ventilatory and occlusion pressure responses to hypercapnia in patients with chronic renal failure. Respiration 1984; 45: 191–196.

99. Lee HY, Stretton TB. The lungs in renal failure. Thorax 1975; 30:46–53.

100. Santiago RM, Scharnhorst D, Ratkin G, et al. Respiratory muscle weakness and ventilatory failure in amyloidosis with muscular pseudohypertrophy. Am J Med 1987; 83:175–178.

101. Rosenow EC III, Strimlan CV, Muhm JR, et al. Pleuropulmonary manifestations of ankylosing spondylitis. Mayo Clin Proc 1977; 52:641–649.

102. Caidahl K, Lurie M, Bake B, et al. Dyspnoea in chronic primary fibromyalgia. J Intern Med 1989; 226:265–270.

103. Schmalstieg EJ, Peters BH, Schochet SS, et al. Neuropathy presenting as prolonged dyspnea. Arch Neurol 1977; 34:473–476.

104. Thomas MR, Lancaster R. Polymyositis presenting with dyspnoea, greatly raised muscle enzymes, but no apparent muscular weakness. BJCP 1990; 44:378–381.

105. Greene NB, Solinger AM, Baughman RP. Patients with collagen vascular disease and dyspnea. The value of gallium scanning and bronchoalveolar lavage in predicting response to steroid therapy and clinical outcome. Chest 1987; 91: 698–703.

106. Turner-Warwick M, Courtenay Evans R. Pulmonary manifestations of rheumatoid

disease. Clin Rheumatol Dis 1977; 3: 594–604.

107. Brannan HM, Good CA, Divertie MB, et al. Pulmonary disease associated with rheumatoid arthiritis. JAMA 1964; 189: 914

108. Patterson CD, Harville WE, Pierce JA. Rheumatoid lung disease. Ann Intern Med 1965; 685

109. Bettman MA, Kantrowitz F. Rapid onset of lung involvement in progressive systemic sclerosis. Chest 1979; 75:509–510.

110. Jacobelli S, Moreno R, Massardo L, et al. Inspiratory muscle dysfunction and unexplained dyspnea in systemic lupus erythematosus. Arthritis Rheum 1985; 28: 781–788.

111. Fauci AS, Haynes BF, Katz P, et al. Wegener's granulomatosis: prospective clinical and therapeutic experience with 85 patients for 21 years. Ann Intern Med 1983; 98:76–85.

112. DePaso WJ, Winterbauer RH, Lusk JA, et al. Chronic dyspnea unexplained by history, physical examination, chest roentgenogram, and spirometry. Chest 1991; 100:1293–1299.

113. Martinez FJ, Stanopoulos I, Acero R, et al. Graded comprehensive cardiopulmonary exercise testing in the evaluation of dyspnea unexplained by routine evaluation. Chest 1994; 105:168–174.

114. Brand PL, Rijcken B, Schouten JP, et al. Perception of airway obstruction in a random population sample. Relationship to airway hyperresponsiveness in the absence of respiratory symptoms. Am Rev Respir Dis 1992; 146:396–401.

115. Bellofiore S, DiMaria GU, Privitera S, et al. Endogenous opioids modulate the increase in ventilatory output and dyspnea during severe acute bronchoconstriction. Am Rev Respir Dis 1990; 142:812–816.

116. Turcotte H, Boulet LP. Perception of breathlessness during early and late asthmatic responses. Am Rev Respir Dis 1993; 148:514–518.

117. Peiffer C, Toumi M, Marsac J, et al. Relationship between spontaneous dyspnoea and lability of airway obstruction in asthma. Clin Sci 1992; 82:717–724.

118. Lougheed MD, Lam M, Forkert L, et al. Breathlessness during acute bronchoconstriction in asthma. Pathophysiologic mechanisms. Am Rev Respir Dis 1993; 148:1452–1459.

119. Shivaram U, Miro AM, Cash ME, et al. Cardiopulmonary responses to continu-ous positive airway pressure in acute asthma. J Crit Care 1993; 8:87–92.

120. Mahler DA, Faryniarz K, Lentine T, et al. Measurement of breathlessness during exercise in asthmatics: predictor variables, reliability, and responsiveness. Am Rev Respir Dis 1991;144:39–44.

121. Killian KJ, Summers E, Watson RM, et al. Factors contributing to dyspnoea during bronchoconstriction and exercise in asthmatic subjects. Eur Respir J 1993; 6: 1004–1010.

122. Kunitoh H, Watanabe K, Sajima Y. Dyspnea in acute bronchial asthma in an emergency room. Ann Allergy 1994; 72: 250–254.

123. Kikuchi Y, Okabe S, Tamura G, et al. Chemosensitivity and perception of dyspnea in patients with a history of near-fatal asthma. N Engl J Med 1994; 330: 1329–1334.

124. O'Donnell DE, Webb KA. Breathlessness in patients with severe chronic airflow limitations. Chest 1992; 102:824–831.

125. Silverman M, Barry J, Hellerstein HI, et al. Variability in perceived sense of effort in breathing during exercise in patients with chronic obstructive pulmonary disease. Am Rev Respir Dis 1988;137: 206–209.

126. O'Donnell DE, Sanii R, Giesbrecht G, et al. Effect of continuous positive airway pressure on respiratory sensation in patients with chronic obstructive pulmonary disease during submaximal exercise. Am Rev Respir Dis 1988; 138:1185–1191.

127. O'Donnell DE, Sanii R, Younes M. Improvement in exercise endurance in patients with chronic airflow limitation using continuous positive airway pressure. Am Rev Respir Dis 1988; 138: 1510–1514.

128. O'Donnell DE, Webb KA. Exertional breathlessness in patients with chronic airflow limitation: the role of lung hyperinflation. Am Rev Respir Dis 1993; 148: 1351–1357.

129. Noseda A, Schmerber J, Prigogine T, et al. How do patients with either asthma or COPD perceive acute bronchodilation? Eur Respir J 1993; 6:636–644.

130. Sharp JT, Druz S, Moisan T, et al. Postural relief of dyspnea in severe chronic obstructive pulmonary disease. Am Rev Respir Dis 1980; 122:201–211.

131. ONeill S, McCarthy DS. Postural relief of dyspnoea in severe chronic airflow limi-

tation: relationship to respiratory muscle strength. Thorax 1983; 38:595–600.

132. Bradley GW, Hale T, Pimble J, et al. Effect of vagotomy on the breathing pattern and exercise in emphysematous patients. Clin Sci 1982; 62:311–319.

133. Guz A, Noble NIM, Eisele JH, et al. Experimental results of vagal block in cardiopulmonary disease. In: Porter R, ed. *Breathing: Ciba Foundation Hering-Breuer Centenary Symposium.* New York, NY: Churchill Livingstone Inc; 1970:315–336.

134. Abdullah AK, Danial BH, Zeid A, et al. Solitary bronchial papilloma presenting with recurrent dyspnea attacks: case report with computed tomography findings. Respiration 1991; 58:62–64.

135. Leach KR, Martinez FJ, Morelock JW, et al. Dyspnea and tracheal mass in an elderly man. Chest 1994; 105:1555–1556.

136. Phillips GD, Smith EE, Millard FJ. Positional dyspnoea due to aneurysm of the thoracic aorta. Eur Respir J 1994;7: 412–414.

137. Whyte KF, McMahon G, Wightman AJA, et al. Bronchial compression as a result of lung herniation after pneumonectomy. Thorax 1991;46:855–857.

138. Tsubota N, Murotani A, Yoshimura M. A huge non-invasive thymoma causing acute dyspnea. Tohoku J Exp Med 1993; 171:229–233.

139. Carroll F, Kramer MD, Acinapura AJ, et al. Pleural liposarcoma presenting with respiratory distress and suspected diaphragmatic hernia. Ann Thorac Surg 1992; 54:1212–1213.

140. Nagai A, Matsumiya H, Hayashi M, et al. Lesions of the arytenoid region in a patient with exertional dyspnoea. Eur Respir J 1993; 6:1065–1066.

141. Campbell AH, Mestitz H, Pierce R. Brief upper airway (laryngeal) dysfunction. Aust NZ J Med 1990; 20:663–668.

142. Bawa R, Ramadan HH, Wetmore SJ. Bilateral vocal cord paralysis with Shy-Drager syndrome. Otolaryngol Head Neck Surg 1993;109:911–914.

143. Karlins NL, Yagan R. Dyspnea and hoarseness: a complication of diffuse idiopathic skeletal hyperostosis. Spine 1991;16:235–237.

144. Bollinger CT, Sopko J, Maurer P, et al. The flow volume loop in bilateral vocal cord paralysis. Chest 1993;104:1302–1304.

145. O'Hollaren MT. Masqueraders in clinical allergy: laryngeal dysfunction causing asthma. Ann Allergy 1990;65:351–356.

146. Tolosa E, Kulisevsky J, Fahn S. Meige syndrome: primary and secondary forms. Adv Neurol 1988;50:509–515.

147. Hartman DE, Abbs JH, Vishwnant B. Clinical investigations of adductor spastic dysphonia. Ann Otol Rhinol Laryngol 1989; 97:247–252.

148. Knebel AR, Janson-Bjerklie SL, Malley JD, et al. Comparison of breathing comfort during weaning with two ventilatory modes. Am J Resp Crit Care Med 1994; 149:14–18.

149. Davies SF, McQuaid KR, Iber C, et al. Extreme dyspnea from unilateral pulmonary venous obstruction: demonstration of a vagal mechanism and relief by right vagotomy. Am Rev Respir Dis 1987; 136: 184–188.

150. Tanabe Y, Suzuki M, Takahashi M, et al. Acute effect of percutaneous transvenous mitral commissurotomy on ventilatory and hemodynamic responses to exercise: pathophysiological basis for early symptomatic improvement. Circulation 1993; 88:1770–1778.

151. McParland C, Krishnan B, Wang Y, et al. Inspiratory muscle weakness and dyspnea in chronic heart failure. Am Rev Respir Dis 1992; 146:467–472.

152. Nishimura Y, Maeda H, Tanaka K, et al. Respiratory muscle strength and hemodynamics in chronic heart failure. Chest 1994; 105:355–359.

153. Mancini DM, Henson D, LaManca J, et al. Respiratory muscle function and dyspnea in patients with chronic congestive heart failure. Circulation 1992; 86:909–918.

154. Caidahl K, Eriksson H, Hartford M, et al. Dyspnoea of cardiac origin in 67-year-old men: (1) Relation to systolic left ventricular function and wall stress/The Study of Men Born in 1913. Br Heart 1988; 59: 319–328.

155. Fujiki A, Tani M, Mizumaki K, et al. Pacemaker syndrome evaluated by cardiopulmonary exercise testing. PACE 1990; 13: 1236–1241.

156. Heldman D, Mulvihill D, Nguyen H, et al. True incidence of pacemaker syndrome. PACE 1990; 13:1742–1750.

157. Tani M, Fujiki A, Asanoi H, et al. Effects of chronotropic responsive cardiac pacing on ventricular response to exercise in patients with complete AV block. PACE 1992; 15:1482–1491.

158. Terry PB, White RI, Barth KH, et al. Pulmonary arteriovenous malformations: physiologic observations and results of

therapeutic balloon embolization. N Engl J Med 1983; 308:1197–1200.

159. Brack MJ, Hubner PJB, Firmin RK. Successful operation on a coronary arteriovenous fistula in a 74-year-old woman. Br Heart J 1991; 65:107–108.

160. Worsnop CJ, Teichtahl H, Clarke CP. Bronchogenic cyst: a cause of pulmonary artery obstruction and breathlessness. Ann Thorac Surg 1993; 55:1254–1255.

161. Koufman JA, Wiener GJ, Wu WC, et al. Reflux laryngitis and its sequelae: the diagnostic role of ambulatory 24-hour pH monitoring. J Voice 1988; 2:78–89.

162. Orenstein SR, Orenstein DM, Whitington PF. Gastroesophageal reflux causing stridor. Chest 1983; 84:301–302.

163. Clark DM, Salkovskis PM, Chalkley AJ. Respiratory control as a treatment for panic attacks. J Behav Ther Exp Psychiat 1985; 16:23–30.

164. Lum LC. The syndrome of chronic habitual hyperventilation. In: Hill OW, ed. Modern Trends in Psychosomatic Medicine. London, England: Buttersworth; 1976:196

165. Tiller J, Pain M, Biddle N. Anxiety disorder and perception of inspiratory resistive loads. Chest 1987; 91:547–551.

166. Garssen B. Role of stress in the development of the hyperventilation syndrome. Psychother Psychosom 1980; 33: 214–225.

167. Saltzman HA, Heyman AH, Sieker HO. Correlation of clinical and physiologic manifestations of sustained hyperventilation. N Engl J Med 1963; 268:1431–1436.

168. Okel BB, Hurst JW. Prolonged hyperventilation in man: associated electrolyte changes and subjective symptoms. Arch Intern Med 1961;108:757–762.

169. Hormbrey J, Jacobi MS, Patil CP, et al. $CO_2$ response and pattern of breathing in patients with symptomatic hyperventilation, compared to asthmatic and normal subjects. Eur Respir J 1988; 1:846–852.

170. Bass C, Garner WN. Respiratory and psychiatric abnormalities in chronic symptomatic hyperventilation. Br Med J 1985; 290:1387–1390.

171. Burns BH. Breathlessness in depression. Brit J Psychiat 1971; 119:39–45.

172. Bass C, Wade C, Gardner WN, et al. Unexplained breathlessness and psychiatric morbidity in patients with normal and abnormal coronary arteries. Lancet 1983; 2: 605–609.

173. Folerging H, Colla P. Some anomalies in the control of $Paco_2$ in patients with a hyperventilation syndrome. Bull Eur Physiopath Resp 1978;14:503–512

174. Neill WA, Pantley GA, Nakornchai V. Respiratory alkalemia during exercise reduces angina threshold. Chest 1981; 80: 149–153.

175. Porter WB, James GW. The heart in anemia. Circulation 1953; 8:111–116.

176. Wasserman K, Hansen JE, Sue DY, et al. Principles of Exercise Testing and Interpretation. 2nd ed. Philadelphia, Pa: Lea & Febiger; 1994.

177. Talpers SS, Romberger DJ, Bunce SB, et al. Nutritionally associated increase in carbon dioxide production. Excess total calories vs high proportion of carbohydrate calories. Chest 1992; 102:551–555.

178. Reuben DB, Mor V. Dyspnea in terminally ill cancer patients. Chest 1986; 89: 234–236.

179. Roberts DK, Thorne SE, Pearson C. The experience of dyspnea in late-stage cancer. Patients' and nurses' perspectives. Cancer Nurs 1993; 16:310–320.

180. Eriksson H, Caidahl K, Larsson B, et al. Cardiac and pulmonary causes of dyspnoea—validation of a scoring test for clinical-epidemiological use: the Study of Men Born in 1913. Eur Heart J 1987; 8: 1007–1014.

181. Zema MJ, Masters AP, Margouleff D. Dyspnea: the heart or the lungs? Differentiation at bedside by use of the simple Valsalva maneuver. Chest 1984; 85:59–64.

182. Marantz PR, Kaplan MC, Alderman MH. Clinical diagnosis of heart failure in patients with acute dyspnea. Chest 1990; 97: 776–781.

183. Mulrow CD, Lucey CR, Farnett LE. Discriminating causes of dyspnea through clinical examination. J Gen Intern Med 1993; 8:383–392.

184. Lee L, Loudon RG, Jacobson BH, et al. Speech breathing in patients with lung disease. Am Rev Respir Dis 1993; 147: 1199–1206.

185. Mier-Jedrzejowicz A, Brophy C, Moxham J, et al. Assessment of diaphragm weakness. Am Rev Respir Dis 1988; 137: 877–883.

186. Butcher BL, Nichol KL, Parenti CM. High yield of chest radiography in walk-in clinic patients with chest symptoms. J Gen Intern Med 1993; 8:115–119.

187. Mashman WE, Silverman ME. Platypnea related to constrictive pericarditis. Chest 1994; 105:636–637.

188. Desjardin JA, Martin RJ. Platypnea in the intensive care unit: a newly described cause. Chest 1993; 104:1308–1309.

189. Buehler JH, Gracey DR. Laboratory differentiation of cardiac and primary pulmonary dyspnea. Mod Concept Cardiovasc Dis 1974; 43:113–118.

190. Mohensifar Z, Collier J, Belman MJ, et al. Isolated reduction in single-breath diffusing capacity in the evaluation of exertional dyspnea. Chest 1992; 101:965–969.

191. Andersen SJ, Arvidsson U, Fransson L, et al. The relationship between the transfer factor obtained at rest, and arterial oxygen tension during exercise, in patients with miscellaneous pulmonary diseases. J Intern Med 1992; 232:415–419.

192. Crystal RG, Bitterman PB, Rennard SJ, et al. Interstitial lung diseases of unknown cause: disorders characterized by chronic inflammation of the lower respiratory tract (part I). N Engl J Med 1984; 310:154–166.

193. Crystal RG, Bitterman PB, Rennard SI, et al. Interstitial lung diseases of unknown cause: disorders characterized by chronic inflammation of the lower respiratory tract (second of two parts). N Engl J Med 1984; 310:235–244.

194. Petty TL. Definitions in chronic obstructive pulmonary disease. In: Hodgkin JE, ed. *Chronic Obstructive Pulmonary Disease*. Philadelphia, Pa: W B Saunders; 1990:363–374.

195. Leontic E. Respiratory diseases in pregnancy. Med Clin North Am 1977; 61:111–128.

196. Huch R, Errkola R. Pregnancy and exercise-exercise and pregancy: a short review. Br J Obstet Gynaecol 1990; 97:208–214.

197. Gilbert R, Auchincloss J. Dyspnea of pregnancy: clinical and physiological observation. Am J Med Sci 1966; 252:270–276.

198. Markisz JA. Radiologic and nuclear medicine diagnosis. In: Goldhaber SZ, ed. *Pulmonary Embolism and Deep Venous Thrombosis*. Philadelphia, Pa: W B Saunders; 1985:41–75.

199. Wilson JR, Raven PB, Morgan WP, et al. Effects of pressure-demand respirator wear on physiological and perceptual variables during progressive exercise to maximal levels. Am Ind Hyg Assoc J 1989; 50:85–94.

200. Wilson JR, Raven PB, Zinkgraf SA, et al. Alterations in physiological and perceptual variables during exhaustive endurance work while wearing a pressure-demand respirator. Am Ind Hyg Assoc J 1989; 50:85–94.

201. Blackie SP, Pardy RL. Exercise testing in the assessment of pulmonary disease. Clinical Reviews in Allergy 1990; 8:215–227.

202. Palange P, Carlone S, Forte S, et al. Cardiopulmonary exercise testing in the evaluation of patients with ventilatory vs circulatory causes of reduced exercise tolerance. Chest 1994; 105:1122–1126.

203. Cockcroft A. Treadmill testing in the evaluation of breathlessness. Pract Cardiol 1986; 12:133–141.

204. Stark RD, Gambles SA, Chatterjee SS. An exercise test to assess clinical dyspnoea: estimation of reproducibility and sensitivity. Br J Dis Chest 1982; 76:269–278.

205. Vincken WG, Gauthier SG, Dolfuss RE. Involvement of upper airway muscles in extrapyramidal disorders: a cause of airflow limitation. N Engl J Med 1984; 311:438–442.

206. Tammelin BR, Wilson AF, de Berry Borowiecki B. Flow-volume curves reflect pharyngeal airway abnormalities in sleep apnea syndrome. Am Rev Respir Dis 1983; 128:712–715.

207. National Asthma Education Program: Expert Panel Report. Executive summary: Guidelines for the diagnosis and management of asthma. Office of prevention, education, and control. National Heart, Blood, and Lung Institute. Bethesda, MD: National Institutes of Health, Publication No. 94–3042A; July 1994.

208. Smith CM, Moser KM. Management of interstitial lung disease: state of the art. Chest 1989; 95:676–678.

209. Raghu G, DePaso WJ, Cain K, et al. Azathioprine combined with prednisone in the treatment of idiopathic pulmonary fibrosis: a prospective double-blind, randomized, placebo-controlled trial. Am Rev Respir Dis 1991; 144:291–296.

210. Reardon J, Awad E, Normandin E, et al. The effect of comprehensive outpatient pulmonary rehabilitation on dyspnea. Chest 1994; 105:1046–1052.

211. Dean NC, Brown JK, Himelman RB, et al. Oxygen may improve dyspnea and endurance in patients with chronic obstructive pulmonary disease and only mild hypoxemia. Am Rev Respir Dis 1992; 146:941–945.

212. Breslin EH. Dyspnea-limited response in chronic obstructive pulmonary disease:

reduced unsupported arm activities. Rehabil Nurs 1992; 17:12–20.

213. Celli B, Criner G, Rassulo J. Ventilatory muscle recruitment during unsupported arm exercise in normal subjects. J Appl Physiol 1988; 64:1936–1941.

214. Teramoto S, Fukuchi Y, Orimo H. Effects of inhaled anticholinergic drug on dyspnea and gas exchange during exercise in patients with chronic obstructive pulmonary disease. Chest 1993; 103:1774–1782.

215. Mahler DA, Matthay RA, Snyder PE, et al. Sustained-release theophylline reduces dyspnea in nonreversible obstructive airway disease. Am Rev Respir Dis 1985; 131:22–25.

216. Larsen GL. A role for the speech pathologist in neuromuscular dyspnea. Milit Med 1972; 137:20–21.

217. Gaasch WH. Diagnosis and treatment of heart failure based on left ventricular systolic or diastolic dysfunction [Review]. JAMA 1994; 271:1276–1280.

218. Grossman P, DeSwart CG, Defares PB. A controlled study of a breathing therapy for treatment of hyperventilation syndrome. J Psychosomatic Res 1985; 29:49–58.

219. Stanescu DC, Nemery B, Veriter C, et al. Pattern of breathing and ventilatory response to $CO_2$ in subjects practicing hatha-yoga. J Appl Physiol 1981; 51:1625–1629.

220. Tandon MK. Adjunct treatment with yoga in chronic severe airways obstruction. Thorax 1978; 33:514–517.

221. Irwin RS, Zawacki JK, Curley FJ, et al. Chronic cough as the sole presenting manifestation of gastroesophageal reflux. Am Rev Respir Dis 1989; 140:1294–1300.

222. Tibbling L, Gibellino F. Remission of angina pectoris and dyspnea by fundoplication in gastro-oesophageal reflux disease. Ann Med 1992; 24:457–459.

223. Gross D, Ladd HW, Riley EJ, et al. The effect of training on strength and endurance of the diaphragm in quadriplegia. Am J Med 1980; 68:27–35.

224. Meyer TJ, Hill NS. Noninvasive positive pressure ventilation to treat respiratory failure. Ann Intern Med 1994; 120:760–770.

225. Chester EH, Belman MJ, Bahler RC. Multidisciplinary treatment of chronic pulmonary insufficiency: The effect of physical training on cardiopulmonary performance in patients with chronic obstructive pulmonary disease. Chest 1977; 72:695–702.

226. Strijbos JH, Sluiter HJ, Postma DS. Objective and subjective performance indicators in COPD. Eur Respir J 1989; 2:666–669.

227. Pierce AK, Taylor HF, Archer RF. Response to exercise training in patients with emphysema. Arch Intern Med 1964; 113:28–36.

228. Rogers RM, Donahoe M, Costantino J. Physiologic effects of oral supplemental feeding in malnourished patients with chronic obstructive pulmonary disease. A randomized control study. Am Rev Respir Dis 1992; 146:1511–1517.

229. Carrieri VK, Janson Bjerklie S. Strategies patients use to manage the sensation of dyspnea. West J Nurs Res 1986; 8:284–305.

230. Carrieri VK, Janson Bjerklie S, Jacobs S. The sensation of dyspnea: a review. Heart Lung 1984; 13:436–447.

231. Carrieri-Kohlman V, Douglas MK, Gormley JM, et al. Desensitization and guided mastery: treatment approaches for the management of dyspnea [Review]. Heart Lung 1993; 22:226–234.

232. Kohlman-Carrieri V, Janson-Bjerklie S. Coping and self-care strategies. In: Mahler DA, ed. *Dypsnea*. Mount Kisco: Futura Publishing Company; 1990:201–230.

233. Woodcock AA, Gross ER, Geddes DM. Oxygen relieves breathlessness in "pink puffers." Lancet 1981; i:907–909.

234. Davidson AC, Leach R, George RJD. Supplemental oxygen and exercise ability in chronic obstructive airways disease. Thorax 1988; 43:965–971.

235. Dewan NA, Bell CW. Effect of low flow and high flow oxygen delivery on exercise tolerance and sensation of dyspnea. A study comparing the transtracheal catheter and nasal prongs. Chest 1994; 105:1061–1065.

236. Kim MJ, Larson JL, Covey MK, et al. Inspiratory muscle training in patients with chronic obstructive pulmonary disease. Nurs Res 1993; 42:356–363.

237. Mahler DA. Therapeutic strategies. In: Mahler DA, ed. *Dyspnea*. Mount Kisco: Futura Publishing Company; 1990:231

238. Ries AL, Ellis B, Hawkins RW. Upper extremity exercise training in chronic obstructive pulmonary disease. Chest 1988; 93:688–692.

239. Rochester DF, Braun NM. The diaphragm and dyspnea. Evidence from inhibiting

diaphragmatic activity with respirators. Am Rev Respir Dis 1979; 119:77–80.

240. Cropp A, DiMarco A. Effects of intermittent negative pressure ventilation on respiratory muscle function in patients with severe chronic obstructive pulmonary disease. Am Rev Respir Dis 1987; 135:1056–1061.

241. Braun NMT, Marino WD. Effects of daily intermittent rest of respiratory muscles in patients with severe chronic airflow limitation (CAL). Chest 1984; 85:59S-60S.

242. Zibrak JD, Hill NS, Federman EC, et al. Evaluation of intermittent long-term negative-pressure ventilation in patients with severe chronic obstructive pulmonary disease. Am Rev Respir Dis 1988; 138:1515–1518.

243. Rochester DF, Braun NMT, Laine S. Diaphragmatic energy expenditure in chronic respiratory failure; the effect of assisted ventilation with body respirators. Am J Med 1977; 63:223–232.

244. Celli B, Lee H, Criner G. Controlled trial of external negative pressure ventilation in patients with severe chronic airflow obstruction. Am Rev Respir Dis 1989; 140:1251–1256.

245. Gutierrez M, Beroiza T, Contreras G. Weekly cuirass ventilation improves blood gases and inspiratory muscle strength in patients with chronic airflow limitation and hypercapnia. Am Rev Respir Dis 1988; 138:617–623.

246. Martin JG. Clinical intervention in chronic respiratory failure. Chest 1990; 97:105S-109S.

247. Al Damluji S. The effect of ventilatory stimulation with medroxyprogesterone on exercise performance and the sensation of dyspnoea in hypercapnic chronic bronchitis. Br J Dis Chest 1986; 80: 273–279.

248. Mitchell-Heggs P, Murphy K, Minty K, et al. Diazepam in the treatment of dyspnea in the 'pink puffer' syndrome. Q J Med 1980; 49:9–20.

249. Man GC, Hsu K, Sproule BJ. Effect of alprazolam on exercise and dyspnea in patients with chronic obstructive pulmonary disease. Chest 1986; 90:832–836.

250. Woodcock AA, Gross ER, Geddes DM. Drug treatment of breathlessness: contrasting effects of diazepam and promethazine in pink puffers. Br Med J 1981; 283: 343–346.

251. Eimer M, Cable T, Gal P. Effects of clorazepate on breathlessness and exercise tolerance in patients with chronic airflow obstruction. J Fam Pract 1985; 21: 359–362.

252. Rice KL. Treatment of dyspnea with psychotropic agents [editorial]. Chest 1986; 90:789–790.

253. Giron AE, Stansbury DW, Fischer CE, et al. Lack of effect of dextromethorphan on breathlessness and exercise performance in patients with chonic obstructive pulmonary disease (COPD). Eur Respir J 1991; 4:532–535.

254. Light RW, Muro JR, Sato RI. Effects of oral morphine on brreathlessness and exercise tolerance in patients with chronic airflow obstruction. Am Rev Respir Dis 1989; 139:126–133.

255. Robin ED. Single-patient randomized clinical trial. Opiates for intractable dyspnea. Chest 1986; 90:832–836.

256. Cohen MH, Johnston-Anderson A, Krasnow SH, et al. Treatment of intractable dyspnea: clinical and ethical issues. Cancer Investigations 1992; 10:317–321.

257. Hsu DH. Dyspnea in dying patients [Review]. Canadian Family Physician 1993; 39:1635–1638.

258. Mercho N, Stoller JK, White RD, et al. Right-to-left interatrial shunt causing platypnea after pneumonectomy. A recent experience and diagnostic value of dynamic magnetic resonance imaging. Chest 1994; 105:931–933.

259. Lambrecht GL, Malbrain ML, Coremans P, et al. Orthodeoxia and platypnea in liver cirrhosis: effects of propranolol. Acta Clinica Belgica 1994; 49:26–30.

260. Killian KJ. The objective measurement of breathlessness. Chest 1985; 88:84S-90S.

## Appendix A. Initial Pneumoconiosis Research Unit Dyspnea Questionnaire

**Grade 1:** Is the patient's breath as good as that of other men of his own age and build at work, on walking, and on climbing hills or stairs?

**Grade 2:** Is the patient able to walk with normal men of own age and build on the level but unable to keep up on hills or stairs?

**Grade 3:** Is the patient unable to keep up with normal men on the level, but able to walk about a mile or more at his own speed?

**Grade 4:** Is the patient unable to walk more than about 100 yards on the level without a rest?

**Grade 5:** Is the patient breathless on talking or undressing, or unable to leave his house because of breathlessness?

From: Fletcher CM. The clinical diagnosis of pulmonary emphysema-an experimental study. Proc R Soc Med 1952; 45:577–584. Reprinted with permission.

## Appendix B. American Thoracic Society Dyspnea Scale

| Grade | Degree |
| --- | --- |
| 0 None | Not troubled with breathlessness except with strenuous exercise. |
| 1 Slight | Troubled by shortness of breath when hurrying on the level or walking up a slight hill. |
| 2 Moderate | Walks slower than people of the same age on the level because of breathlessness or has to stop for breath when walking at own pace on the level. |
| 3 Severe | Stops for breath after walking about 100 yards or after a few minutes on the level. |
| 4 Very Severe | Too breathless to leave the house or breathless when dressing or undressing. |

## Appendix C. Baseline Dyspnea Index

Functional Impairment

**Grade 4: No Impairment.** Able to carry out usual activities* and occupation without shortness of breath.

**Grade 3: Slight Impairment.** Distinct impairment in at least one activity but no activities completely abandoned. Reduction, in activity at work **or** in usual activities, that seems slight or not clearly caused by shortness of breath.

**Grade 2: Moderate Impairment.** Patient has changed jobs **and/or** has abandoned at least one usual activity due to shortness of breath.

**Grade 1: Severe Impairment.** Patient unable to work **or** has given up most or all usual activities due to shortness of breath.

**Grade 0: Very Severe Impairment.** Unable to work **and** has given up most or all usual activities due to shortness of breath.

**W: Amount Uncertain.** Patient is impaired due to shortness of breath, but amount cannot be specified. Details are not sufficient to allow impairment to be categorized.

**X: Unknown.** Information unavailable regarding impairment.

**Y: Impaired for Reasons Other than Shortness of Breath.** For example, musculoskeletal problem or chest pain.

Magnitude of Task

**Grade 4: Extraordinary.** Becomes short of breath only with extraordinary activity such as carrying very heavy loads on the level, lighter loads uphill, or running. No shortness of breath with ordinary tasks.

**Grade 3: Major.** Becomes short of breath only with such major activities as walking up a steep hill, climbing more than three flights of stairs, or carrying a moderate load on the level.

**Grade 2: Moderate.** Becomes short of breath with moderate or average tasks such as walking up a gradual hill, climbing less than three flights of stairs, or carrying a light load on the level.

**Grade 1: Light.** Becomes short of breath with light activities such as walking on the level, washing or standing.

**Grade 0: No Task.** Becomes short of breath at rest, while sitting, or lying down.

**W: Amount Uncertain.** Patient's ability to perform tasks is impaired due to shortness of breath, but amount cannot be specified. Details are not sufficient to allow impairment to be categorized.

**X: Unknown.** Information unavailable regarding limitation of magnitude of task.

**Y: Impaired for Reasons Other than Shortness of Breath.** For example, musculoskeletal problem or chest pain.

Magnitude of Effort

**Grade 4: Extraordinary.** Becomes short of breath only with the greatest imaginable effort. No shortness of breath with ordinary effort.

**Grade 3: Major.** Becomes short of breath with effort distinctly submaximal, but major proportion. Tasks performed with-

---

From Mahler DA, Weinberg DH, Wells CK, et al. The measurement of dyspnea: Contents, interobserver agreement, and physiologic correlates of two new clinical indexes. Chest 1984; 85:751–758. Reprinted with permission.
*Usual activities refer to requirements of daily living, maintenance, or upkeep of residence, yard work, gardening, shopping, etc.

out pause unless the task requires extraordinary effort that may be performed with pauses.

**Grade 2: Moderate.** Becomes short of breath with moderate effort. Tasks performed with occasional pauses and requiring longer to complete than the average person.

**Grade 1: Light.** Becomes short of breath with little effort. Tasks performed with little effort or more difficult tasks performed with frequent pauses and requiring 50% to 100% longer to complete than the average person might require.

**Grade 0: No Effort.** Becomes short of breath at rest, while sitting, or lying down.

**Grade W: Amount Uncertain.** Patient's exertional ability is impaired due to shortness of breath, but amount cannot be specified. Details are not sufficient to allow impairment to be categorized.

**Grade X: Unknown.** Information unavailable regarding limitation of effort.

**Grade Y: Impaired for Reasons Other than Shortness of Breath.** For example, musculoskeletal problems or chest pain.

## Appendix D. Transitional Dyspnea Index

Change in Functional Impairment

**−3: Major Deterioration.** Formerly working and has had to stop working **and** has completely abandoned some of usual activities due to shortness of breath.

**−2: Moderate Deterioration:** Formerly working and has had to stop working **or** has completely abandoned some of usual activities due to shortness of breath.

**−1: Minor Deterioration.** Has changed to a lighter job **and/or** has reduced activities in number or duration due to shortness of breath. Any deterioration less than preceding categories.

**−0: No Change.** No change in functional status due to shortness of breath.

**+1: Minor Improvement.** Able to return to work at reduced pace **or** has resumed some customary activities with more vigor than previously due to improvement in shortness of breath.

**+2: Moderate Improvement.** Able to return to work at nearly usual pace **and/or** able to return to most activities with moderate restriction only.

**+3: Major Improvement.** Able to return to work at former pace **and** able to return to full activities with only mild restriction due to improvement of shortness of breath.

**Further Impairment for Reasons Other than Shortness of Breath.** Patient has stopped working, reduced work, or has given up or reduced other activities for other reasons. For example, other medical problems, being "laid off" from work, etc.

Change in Magnitude of Task

**−3: Major Deterioration.** Has deteriorated two grades or greater from baseline status.

**−2: Moderate Deterioration.** Has deteriorated at least one grade but less than two grades from baseline status.

**−1: Minor Deterioration.** Has deteriorated less than one grade from baseline. Patient with distinct deterioration within grade, but has not changed grades.

**0: No Change.** No change from baseline.

**+1: Minor Improvement.** Has improved less than one grade from baseline. Patient with distinct improvement within grade, but has not changed grades.

**+2: Moderate Improvement.** Able to do things with fewer pauses and distinctly greater effort without shortness of breath. Improvement is greater than preceding category, but not of major proportion.

**+3: Major Improvement.** Able to do things with much greater effort than previously with few, if any, pauses. For example, activities may be performed 50% to 100% more rapidly than at baseline.

**Z: Further Impairment for Reasons Other than Shortness of Breath.** Patient has reduced exertional capacity, but not related to shortness of breath. For example, musculoskeletal problem or chest pain.

From Mahler DA, Weinberg DH, Wells CK, et al. The measurement of dyspnea: Contents, interobserver agreement, and physiologic correlates of two new clinical indexes. Chest 1984; 85:751–758. Reprinted with permission.

# 3

# Wheeze

Nicholas A. Smyrnios, M.D.
Richard S. Irwin, M.D.

## Introduction

Wheeze may be either a symptom or a sign. In some cases, a patient will hear a continuous noise produced when he or she breathes and this may prompt that person to seek medical attention. In other cases, wheezing may be discovered by the physician during a physical examination when a patient presents for another reason. In either situation, wheezing signifies the obstruction of an airway that may vary in significance from trivial to life-threatening.

Wheeze can be caused by hundreds of different diseases. Rather than discuss each disease individually, the intent of this chapter is to present an approach to evaluating and managing this very common complaint. Wheeze can be evaluated in a systematic and cost-efficient manner, and specific therapy can be provided in most cases.

## Defining Wheeze

Although the lungs are among the most commonly examined organs, often very little is done with the results of that examination. Studies that looked at the descriptions of lung sounds found considera-

ble variation among the ways different examiners describe the same sounds.[1-3] Different words were used to describe the same entity, and different observers interpreted the terms used in varying ways. Many adjectives that were used to further refine the descriptions of lung sounds were not found to be useful in distinguishing between major diseases, leading to confusion both in clinical decision making and in research efforts.[1]

It was because of this confusion that an American College of Chest Physicians-American Thoracic Society Joint Committee recommended that the terms used to describe lung sounds be simplified and standardized.[4] These terms should be the only terms used to describe the findings on auscultation of the lungs. Adventitious or abnormal breath sounds are divided into two major categories: (1) discontinuous sounds or crackles and (2) continuous sounds or wheezes. Crackles are interrupted explosive sounds lasting less than 20 milliseconds. They are heard in various diseases including pulmonary edema states, interstitial fibrosis, and pneumonia. Crackles are produced by more than one mechanism including: (1) the sudden opening of a series of small airways and (2) the bubbling of air through secretions.[5] The term "rale" has been used synony-

From Irwin RS, Curley FJ, Grossman RF (eds): Diagnosis and Treatment of Symptoms of the Respiratory Tract. Armonk, New York, Futura Publishing Company, Inc., © 1997.

mously with crackle, although this should be discouraged. Although they have not been found to be helpful in differentiating between diseases, the terms "fine" and "coarse" have been found by Holford to correlate with different acoustic characteristics and are occasionally used to distinguish between crackles.[5]

Wheezes are continuous, musical sounds that last longer than 250 milliseconds.[5] Wheezes can be inspiratory or expiratory, be high- or low-pitched, and consist of single or multiple notes. Stridor is another descriptor that is synonymous with inspiratory wheeze. Wheezing can originate from airways of any size, from the large extrathoracic upper airway down to the intrathoracic small airways. Large airways are defined as those that are 2 mm in diameter or greater; small airways are less than 2 mm in diameter.[6] This definition has as its basis the different physiological characteristics of flow through large and small airways. The pitch of a wheeze is determined by the mass and elastic properties of the structures that are oscillating and has nothing to do with the size of the airway from which the wheeze originates.[7]

While the pitch of a wheeze is not determined by the location of its origin, its timbre may help to determine its location. A polyphonic wheeze consists of multiple musical notes; it is typically produced by dynamic compression of the large, more central bronchi.[7] A monophonic wheeze consists of a single musical note that frequently reflects disease in small airways.[7] There will often be multiple monophonic wheezes in this situation. However, monophonic wheezes can also be detected in upper airway obstruction (UAO).[7] While recognizing that the polyphonic or monophonic nature of expiratory wheezes may theoretically be helpful in localizing the site of obstruction, there are no studies that have looked at their sensitivity or specificity.

Technology that should help analyze both the acoustic and clinical characteristics of breath sounds now exists. Techniques, such as digital respirosonography, time-expanded waveform analysis and Fast Fourier transform analysis, are used experimentally to describe the physical properties of what clinicians hear daily through their stethoscopes.[8,9] These techniques may permit the examination of the chest in a more consistent and effective manner.

## Epidemiology of Wheeze

Wheeze is a common symptom. The Normative Aging Study examined the frequency of wheezing and the risk factors for developing wheezing illness in men. Wheezing was defined as a positive response to one of the following four questions: (1) Do you wheeze occasionally, apart from colds? (2) Do you wheeze mostly on days or nights? (3) Have you ever had an attack of wheezing that made you feel short of breath? and (4) Have you ever received a diagnosis of asthma? The investigators detected a prevalence of wheezing in 13.3% of 1069 adult men.[10] Among those without wheezing at the time of initial evaluation, 28 (4.5%) developed wheezing over the subsequent 3 years. Active smoking, postural heart rate change, and level of responsiveness to inhaled methacholine (in nonsmokers only) were found to be independent predictors of the development of wheezing. Although the 28 men who developed wheezing during the follow-up period had lower forced expiratory volume in 1 second ($FEV_1$) and lower $FEV_1$/forced vital capacity (FVC) values than the other subjects, only seven of them had levels of pulmonary function that would be classified as abnormal. The specific causes of wheeze in these patients were not addressed in this study. Nevertheless, the study confirms that diseases other than chronic obstructive pulmonary disease (COPD) play a role in the development of wheezing in adult men. Similar rates of wheezing have been detected by questionnaire surveys in adults of both sexes in a farming community in Canada[11] and in a group of children in Leicestershire, UK.[12] While asthma and wheezing in childhood have been shown to increase absenteeism from school, these children achieved similar final levels of educational achievement, employment, economic status, and housing as compared to those in a group of initially healthy children.[13,14]

## Physiology of Wheeze

Wheezing is produced by oscillation of opposing walls of an airway that is narrowed almost to the point of closure.[7] This is akin to the noise produced by the detached mouthpiece of an oboe whose reeds are nearly touching. Earlier analogies suggested a similarity with the sounds produced by the pipes of an organ. However, in addition to the obvious physical dissimilarities (ie, the longest airway is approximately 1 ft, while organ pipes producing similar frequencies range from 4 to 8 ft, the pitch of a wheeze is unchanged when helium replaces nitrogen in the air, whereas the pitch produced by an organ pipe will rise. Therefore, the analogy to the organ pipe has been abandoned.[7]

Wheezes may be transmitted through the airways and heard by the patient who is therefore prompted to seek medical attention, or wheezes may be transmitted through the lung parenchyma and auscultated by the physician. Transmission through the airways seems to be more complete. Various investigators have compared wheezes detected at the chest wall to those recorded from either within or over the trachea.[5,15,16] In general, these studies have found that the highest frequency components of the wheeze are better transmitted through a patent airway than through normal lung parenchyma. High frequency sound transmission is much better when the lung tissue is consolidated.[7]

Wheezing can be categorized as inspiratory or expiratory. Inspiratory wheezes are typically associated with obstruction in the extrathoracic upper airway, although there are small airway causes also (eg, asthma). An inspiratory wheeze is likely to originate from the extrathoracic upper airway since this portion of the airway preferentially narrows during inspiration. This relates to the dynamic transmu-

ral pressure changes that normally occur with the respiratory cycle[17] (Figure 1).

Expiratory wheezes are typically associated with intrathoracic upper or lower airway obstructions. Obstruction in the intrathoracic, rather than the extrathoracic, component of the upper airway typically presents with expiratory wheezing since this portion of the airway preferentially narrows during expiration (Figure 1). While lower airway obstruction may produce either inspiratory or expiratory wheezes, multiple monophonic expiratory wheezes tend to predominate.

## Diagnosis

### History and Physical Examination

The physiologic evaluation of wheeze is discussed in the next section. Expiratory wheezing obtained by patient history or detected by physical examination is lacking in sensitivity and specificity in diagnosing asthma.[18,19] Symptomatic asthma can present without wheeze, and wheezing associated with other conditions may mimic asthma. In a prospective study of patients referred to a pulmonary clinic because of wheeze, a history of wheeze predicted asthma 35% of the time, the physical finding of expiratory monophonic wheeze predicted asthma 43% of the time, and a prior clinical diagnosis of asthma by a referring physician predicted asthma only 62% of the time.[18] While unforced expiratory wheezing heard on physical examination has been shown to be significantly correlated with the severity of obstruction in patients with asthma and COPD, the correlations were not strong enough to permit consistent prediction for clinical purposes.[20] Wheezing heard during forced expirations has not been shown to correlate with the severity of obstruction in COPD nor has it been shown to be useful in diagnosing asthma.[20,21]

Inspiratory wheezing on physical examination is not specific for extrathoracic upper airway conditions, and it is not a sensitive sign of extrathoracic UAO. While inspiratory wheezing frequently accompa-

## expiration

## inspiration

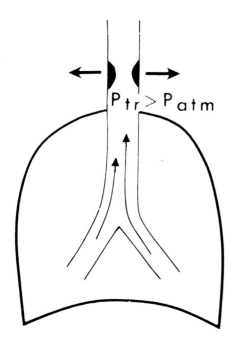
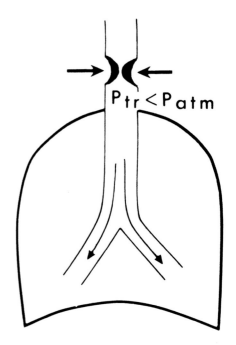

**Figure 1.** The effect of transmural pressure changes during inspiration and expiration on the severity of obstruction at different airway sites. The direction of airflow is indicated by the long thin arrows. **A.** Extrathoracic variable upper airway obstruction. During forced expiration, intrapleural pressure ($P_{pl}$) and subsequently intratracheal pressure ($P_{tr}$) are greater than atmospheric pressure ($P_{atm}$). Therefore, the site of the obstruction widens. During forced inspiration, since $P_{pl}$ and $P_{tr}$ are less than $P_{atm}$, the site narrows. *continued*

nies expiratory wheezing during acute asthma, wheezing during asthma also may be heard only during inspiration.[19] Once symptoms and physiologic abnormalities are present due to extrathoracic UAO, the obstruction is usually far advanced. Patients will develop dyspnea on exertion when the site of UAO is less than 8 mm in diameter, and stridor when the diameter is less than 5 mm.[22,23]

On the basis of the above considerations, it is clinically most useful to appreciate that a wheeze is caused by obstruction of an airway. While it is a common adage in pulmonary medicine that "all that wheezes is not asthma," a more appropriate aphorism is that "all that wheezes is obstruction." This statement serves as the basis for the evaluation of wheezing and provokes a search for the site of obstruction and a consideration of the specific disease. This approach provides a conceptual framework of evaluation that should be especially useful for evaluating the patient with wheeze of unknown or uncertain causes or the patient with wheeze that is not responding to treatment as expected.

## Pulmonary Function Testing (PFT) in the Evaluation of Wheeze

Unless the patient history and initial physical examination have been able to

# expiration

# inspiration

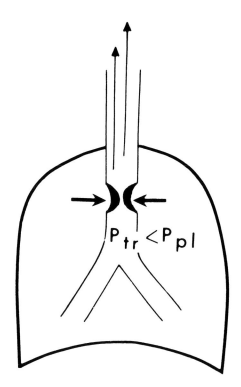
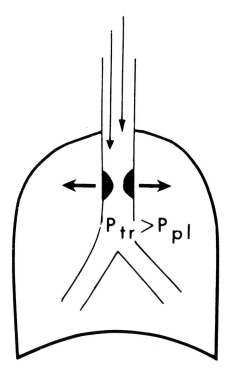

**Figure 1.** *(continued)* **B.** Intrathoracic variable upper airway obstruction. During forced expiration, since $P_{pl}$ is greater than $P_{tr}$, the site narrows. During forced inspiration, since $P_{tr}$ is greater than $P_{pl}$, the site widens. (Reprinted by permission of the publisher from Diagnosis of Obstruction of the Upper and Central Airway and Kryger M et al., American Journal of Medicine, Vol. 61, pp 85–93. Copyright 1976 by Excerpta Medica Inc.)

suggest the origin of the wheeze, the airways should be systematically evaluated to discover the site of obstruction. Since the airway can be divided into three anatomic areas with different physiologic characteristic, obstructions in these three areas can be physiologically differentiated (Figure 2). The three areas are as follows: (1) the extrathoracic upper airway that includes the nose, mouth, pharynx, larynx, and extrathoracic trachea; (2) the intrathoracic upper airways, including the intrathoracic trachea and bronchi down to the level of the 2 mm airways; and (3) the small airways that are less than 2 mm in diameter (ie, airways that are beyond the 8th and 9th branching generations from the trachea).[24] From a physiological standpoint, the distinguishing characteristics of these anatomic areas are as follows: (1) the extrathoracic and intrathoracic large upper airways undergo different and opposite transmural pressure changes during the respiratory cycle (Figure 1); (2) air flow is turbulent through large airways and laminar through small airways[25;] and (3) obstruction in the large airways impedes all of the air in a uniform manner when there is one point of narrowing, while obstruction in small airways, which is almost always in multiple scattered sites, impedes in a nonuniform manner. Be-

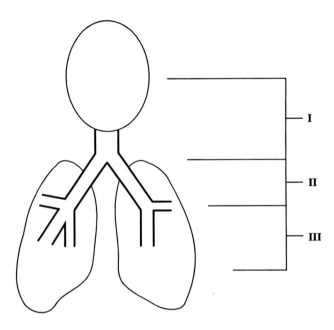

**Figure 2.** The airway can be divided anatomically into 3 regions. I.) extrathoracic upper airway; II.) intrathoracic upper airway from the trachea to the level of the 9th branching generation from the trachea; III.) small airways less than 2 mm in diameter.

cause spirometry and flow-volume loops are influenced by these phenomena, they can be routinely utilized to localize airway obstruction.

Upper airway obstructing lesions are best identified by flow-volume loops (Figure 3). When there is only one site of obstruction, as usually occurs in the trachea, airflow is likely to remain constant during the middle portion of a maximum respiratory effort. If the obstruction is variable (ie, it allows the airway to respond to the normal transmural pressure changes), it will be possible to distinguish an extrathoracic from an intrathoracic location. A variable extrathoracic obstruction will typically only be seen during a maximal inspiratory effort (Figure 3b). Since the extrathoracic airway will dilate during expiration, the maximum expiratory flow-volume curve and spirometry, tests traditionally performed during expiration, will typically be normal. It follows that a variable intrathoracic obstruction will only be observed during a maximal expiratory effort (Figure 3c) and spirometry will reveal values consistent with expiratory airflow obstruction. Spirometry alone cannot distinguish large from small intrathoracic airway diseases since $FEV_1$, peak expiratory flow rate

(PEFR), and $FEV_1/FVC\%$ will be reduced in both situations.

Since inspiratory flow rates are normally always greater than expiratory flow rates when compared at the same lung volume, the ratio of the two may distinguish variable extrathoracic from intrathoracic upper airway lesions.[26] When a variable extrathoracic lesion is present, inspiratory flow rates are less than expiratory flow rates (eg, $FIF_{50\%}/FEF_{50\%}$ and $FIF_{25\%-75\%}/FEF_{25\%-75\%}$ are less than 1).

If the UAO is fixed (ie, it does not allow the airway to respond to normal transmural pressure changes), it cannot be localized physiologically to an extrathoracic or intrathoracic location. Nevertheless, the flow-volume loop will have a characteristic shape (Figure 3d) that will suggest that the obstruction is in large, rather than in small, airways (Figure 3e). In the former, airflow is uniformly impeded during inspiration and expiration because there is no difference between the amount of narrowing in inspiration and expiration. Since expiratory as well as inspiratory flow rates are decreased in a fixed UAO, spirometry will reflect the expiratory flow limitation.

While spirometry is the primary way

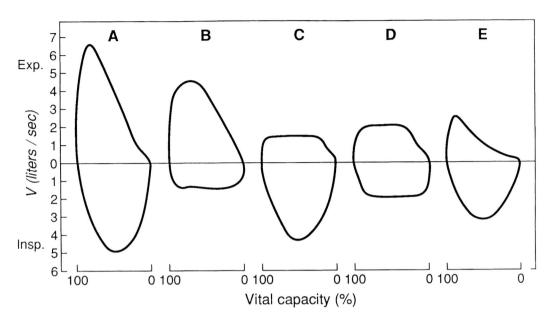

**Figure 3.** Flow-volume loop configurations. A) Normal state. B) Variable extrathoracic upper airway obstruction (UAO). C) Variable intrathoracic UAO. D) Fixed UAO. E) Small airways obstruction.

of identifying intrathoracic airway obstruction, flow-volume loops can also help differentiate small from large airway intrathoracic diseases. Airflow obstruction in small airways causes distinctive changes in the configuration of the maximum expiratory flow-volume curve. Unlike the single obstructing lesion through which all air flows in a tracheal lesion, small airway diseases impede air flow at multiple, unevenly distributed sites. In addition, obstruction in small airways has a greater impact on flow at effort-independent lower lung volumes. Consequently, expiratory flow decreases with volume in an exponential, curvilinear pattern (Figure 3e).

By comparing maximum expiratory flow-volume curves while patients first breathe room air and then breathe a 20% oxygen and 80% helium mixture, it may also be possible to detect coexisting large and small airway intrathoracic obstructions. The relationship between expiratory flows under these two conditions can be quantitated by measuring the volume of isoflow (VisoV). This term describes the percentage of the FVC that is exhaled at

an identical flow rate after inhaling both gases. Expiratory flow will substantially increase with the oxygen-helium mixture when an obstruction occurs in large airways since the turbulent flow that occurs in this region improves with the less dense helium mixture.[17] On the other hand, laminar flow in the small airways will be unaffected by the less dense gas.[25] When intrathoracic airflow limitation is due to combined large airway and small airway diseases (eg, tracheal stenosis superimposed on COPD), flow-volume loops obtained with both air and the helium-oxygen mixture will show improved flow after the patient has breathed the helium-oxygen mixture. If the component of UAO is large, the expiratory flow curves will be dissimilar and the VisoV will be smaller (Figure 4). If the component of UAO is small, then the expiratory flow curves will be more alike, and the VisoV will be larger.[25]

When adult patients present with wheeze and a reduced $FEV_1/FVC$ and the flow-volume loop is consistent with intrathoracic small airway disease, the differ-

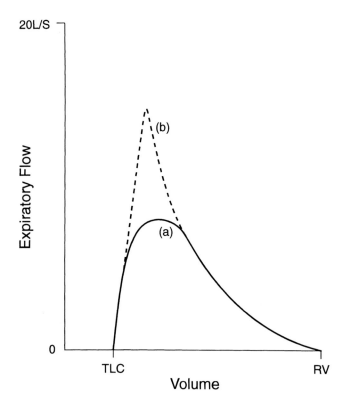

**Figure 4.** The effects of air (A) and oxygen-helium mixture (B) on the maximum expiratory flow-volume curve in a mixed upper and lower airway obstruction. Flow limitation due to the upper airway obstructing component of tracheal stenosis (A) is improved when a less dense gas such as oxygen-helium mixture is passed through an area of turbulent flow (B). TLC = total lung capacity; RV = residual volume.

ential diagnosis often lies between COPD and chronic asthma. Spirometry repeated after bronchodilator can, at times, help to distinguish between the two. For instance, if $FEV_1$ and $FEV_1/FVC$ normalize, the diagnosis of asthma is certain. If $FEV_1$ or FVC improve at least 200 mL and 12% from pre-bronchodilator values, the presence of a component of reversible airways disease consistent with asthma has been uncovered.[27] Failure to observe improvement after bronchodilator does not rule out a reversible component to the patient's disease since airflow obstruction solely or predominantly due to inflammation may improve over time or during anti-inflammatory therapy.[28]

Lastly, in patients with a history of wheeze who have normal or nearly normal baseline spirometry, bronchoprovocation challenge testing with the nonspecific pharmacological agents, methacholine or histamine, can reveal clinically significant bronchial hyperreponsiveness. A positive test suggests that symptomatic asthma may be present and the cause of the wheeze.[29] A favorable response to specific asthma medication will be necessary to prove the diagnosis since a positive pharmacologic bronchoprovocation challenge can also be associated with other conditions.[29]

## Differential Diagnosis of Wheeze

The spectrum and frequency of causes of wheeze have been studied only once. In that study of patients presenting to a pulmonary outpatient clinic at a university hospital with a history of wheeze, postnasal drip syndrome (PNDS) was found to be the most common cause of wheezing and accounted for 47% of all causes of wheeze.[18] (Figure 5) Since (1) wheezing can occur in 11% of patients presenting with the common cold[30]; (2) the common cold is the most common disease that affects mankind; (3) the common cold causes PNDS; (4) PNDS can cause a vari-

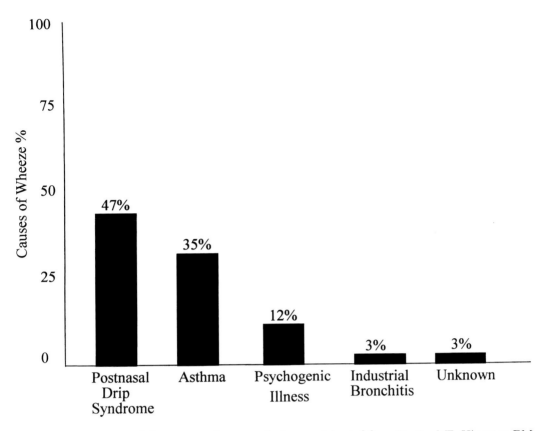

**Figure 5.** Spectrum and frequency of causes of wheeze. Adapted from Pratter MR, Hingston DM, Irwin RS. Diagnosis of bronchial asthma by clinical evaluation: an unreliable method. Chest 1983; 84:42–47.

able extrathoracic UAO; and (5) UAO can cause wheezing, it is not surprising that PNDS makes up a large percentage of cases of wheezing. For additional reading about PNDS beyond what is found here, the reader should see chapter on "Cough." Asthma, which has classically been considered to be the disease most commonly associated with wheezing, comprised only 35% of cases of wheezing.[18] While these results are interesting, they have not been repeated in other settings. A discussion of the more common causes of wheeze follows. Table I includes a more complete listing of causes.

## Upper Airway Conditions

The diagnosis of upper airway obstruction (UAO) may be suspected from patient history and physical examination. A history of shortness of breath, fever, chills, sore throat, frequent throat clearing, difficulty swallowing, recent intubation, weight loss, or voice change is consistent with UAO. The presence of symptoms implies that the disease is advanced since early UAO is frequently asymptomatic.[17] Similarly, physical findings, (eg, fever, tonsillar exudate, cobblestoned pharyngeal mucosa, goiter, deviated trachea, hoarseness, severe obesity, or mucus in the oropharynx) may be invaluable diagnostic clues. Wheezing can be either inspiratory or expiratory with an extrathoracic UAO, although inspiratory wheeze (ie, stridor) is typical.[17] When high-pitched wheezing is heard best on inspiration, is loudest over the trachea, and is accentuated by in-

**Table I**
Causes of Wheeze

Upper airway obstruction
  Extrathoracic causes
    Anaphylaxis[102]
    Postnasal drip syndrome[18]
    Vocal cord dysfunction syndrome[32]
    Hypertrophied tonsils[150]
    Epiglottitis[31]
    Laryngeal edema[115]
    Retropharyngeal abscess[31]
    Malignancy[151]
    Obesity[150]
    Klebsiella rhinoscleroma[152]
    Mobile supraglottic soft tissue[153]
    Relapsing polychondritis[154]
    Vagus nerve compression due to increased
      intracranial pressure[155]
    Laryngocele[156]
    Abnormal arytenoid movement[157]
    Hemorrhagic vocal cord obstruction[158]
    Bilateral vocal cord paralysis[159,160]
    Cricoarytenoid arthritis[161,162]
    Wegener's granulomatosis[163]
  Intrathoracic causes
    Tracheal stenosis due to intubation[21]
    Foreign body aspiration[164]
    Benign bronchial tumors[67]
    Malignancies[26]
    Intrathoracic goiter[165]
    Tracheobronchomegaly[150,166]
    Acquired tracheomalacia[166]
    Tracheal chondroma[167]
    Tracheal leiomyoma[168]
    Herpetic tracheobronchitis[169]
    Right-sided aortic arch[170]
Lower airways obstruction
  Asthma[18]
  Chronic obstructive pulmonary disease[56]
  Pulmonary edema[63]
  Aspiration[67]
  Pulmonary embolism[82,83]
  Bronchiolitis[95]
  Cystic fibrosis[97]
  Anaphylaxis[102]
  Carcinoid syndrome[67]
  Bronchiectasis[29]
  Lymphangitic carcinomatosis[68]
  Parasitic infections[110]
  Pseudomembranous aspergillus tracheobron-
    chitis[171]

creased flow, extrathoracic UAO should be strongly suspected.[17]

Pulmonary function tests with flow-volume loops can detect the presence of a UAO, but cannot diagnose its cause. A chest roentgenogram may demonstrate narrowing of the tracheal air column. A lateral view can localize lesions in the mediastinum. A lateral view of the neck may detect conditions that reduce the antero-posterior diameter of the airway (Figures 6a and 6b). In suspicious cases a computer-assisted tomographic (CT) scan of the neck and chest may be helpful. Finally fiberoptic laryngoscopy and/or bronchoscopy can visualize airway structures directly and tissue may be obtained for the histologic diagnosis of potentially malignant lesions.

There are many potential causes of wheezing due to UAO. Table I gives an extensive list of causes of extrathoracic and intrathoracic UAO. However, several of these entities deserve further mention. Since anaphylaxis can lead to wheezing as a cause of lower airway obstruction as well as upper airway obstruction (eg, angi-oedema of vocal cords), it is discussed in detail in the section entitled "Lower Airway Conditions."

### Postnasal Drip Syndrome

Postnasal drip syndrome is the most common cause of UAO with or without wheezing. It may be either acute or chronic. In the acute setting, the vast majority of cases of PNDS are due to a viral nasopharyngitis, the common cold. In the chronic situation, there are a variety of causes of PNDS, including allergic, perennial nonallergic, postinfectious, environmental irritant, as well as vasomotor rhinitis and sinusitis. Postnasal drip should be considered when patients describe a sensation of having something drip down into the throat, a frequent need to clear the throat, and/or frequent nasal discharge. It should also be considered when physical examination of the oropharynx reveals mucoid or mucopurulent secretions or a cobblestone appearance of the mucosa.

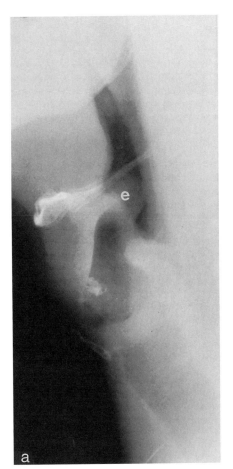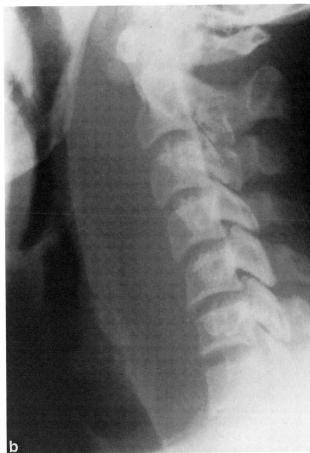

**Figure 6.** Lateral roentgenograms of the neck demonstrating (A) epiglottitis with a characteristic "thumb sign"(e) and (B) retropharyngeal abscess.

## Epiglottitis (Supraglottitis)

Epiglottitis is an acute infection of the supraglottic region, including the arytenoids, epiglottis, aryepiglottic folds, and posterior tongue. It is more common (and frequently more dangerous) in children because of differences in the anatomy of the upper airway during childhood that make the development of UAO more likely. In adults, epiglottitis should be suspected when a patient presents with a sore throat that is out of proportion to the severity of the pharyngitis seen. Occasionally respiratory distress, fever, drooling, and muffled voice can be seen. Diagnosis is made by directly visualizing the supraglot-tic area, in contrast to the approach taken in children which emphasizes avoiding the manipulation of that region. Lateral neck radiographs (Figure 6a) are also helpful in the diagnosis, especially if epiglottic thickening (ie, the thumb sign), swelling of the aryepiglottic folds, or narrowing of the vallecula are seen.[31] Epiglottitis may be caused by a variety of agents, including fungi and viruses, although bacterial infection with *Hemophilus influenzae* is by far the most common cause.

## Vocal Cord Dysfunction Syndrome

Vocal cord dysfunction syndrome has gained a great deal of attention in recent years as a cause of wheeze and stridor. Patients suffering from an attack of this syndrome demonstrate paradoxical movement of their vocal cords during inspiration.[32] The result of this movement is near complete adduction of the cords during inspiration, leading to dyspnea and wheezing. A helpful indicator in identifying these patients is the absence of an increased alveolar-to-arterial oxygen tension gradient [P(A-a)O$_2$], which distinguishes their condition from asthma and other intrapulmonary causes of wheezing. There is no evidence that these patients willfully cause UAO. Instead, this syndrome is thought to be a conversion disorder in response to emotional distress or trauma.[33] A characteristic flow-volume curve with early closure in inspiration is very suggestive of this syndrome. These patients may be diagnosed by laryngoscopy performed during an attack. By directly visualizing the unanesthetized cords in an unsedated patient, the physician can see the cords close during inspiration and thereby confirm the diagnosis.

### Retropharyngeal Abscess

Retropharyngeal abscess is a severe infection of the neck that usually arises in the lymph nodes that drain the pharynx and sinuses. In adults there may be a history of trauma to the posterior pharynx such as endotracheal intubation or a foreign body. Common symptoms include dyspnea, stiff neck, noisy breathing, as well as symptoms directly associated with infection such as fever and sore throat.[31] Lateral films of the neck (Figure 6b) and/or CT scan are valuable in making the diagnosis.

### Laryngotracheal Injury Due to Endotracheal Intubation

Upper airway damage due to endotracheal intubation is also a common cause of UAO. This may be due either to damage caused acutely at the time of intubation or

to the extended presence of a foreign body in the trachea. This includes edema of the supraglottic region and vocal cords (seen with translaryngeal intubation) to near complete obstruction of the trachea, either by granulation tissue or by fibrous connective tissue, that causes circumferential narrowing. The locations most commonly affected are the sites where the foreign body comes into contact with the mucosa (eg, at the vocal cords, at the site of the tube cuff, at the tip of the tube, or at the tracheostomy stoma site). Injury may occur in as short a period of time as the time necessary to perform an appendectomy, although it is thought that longer intubation predisposes the patient to a higher likelihood of injury. These lesions usually require laryngoscopy or bronchoscopy for diagnosis, and the clinician should maintain a high index of suspicion in any patient intubated for an extended period of time.

## Lower Airway Conditions

### Asthma

Asthma is a common and potentially fatal disease. The prevalence of asthma is estimated at 10.6 per 100 people, but it is more common among men, blacks, residents in the south and west, and poor people.[34] The mortality rate from asthma is calculated as 1.8 per 100,000 cases and is suspected to be higher among minorities.

Asthma is defined as being a disease with the following characteristics: airway obstruction that is at least partly reversible, either with treatment or spontaneously; airway inflammation; and airway hyperresponsiveness.[35] Obstruction is caused by muscle spasm associated with hyperresponsiveness, mucus, sloughed bronchial epithelium, and bronchial wall edema related to inflammation. Hyperresponsiveness itself appears to be caused by inflammation, as evidenced by the role of inflammatory mediators such as histamine in early asthma responses and by the salutary effect of anti-inflammatory medications such as inhaled corticosteroids on the level of hyperresponsiveness and degree of inflammation.[36,37] An initial trigger releases inflammatory mediators from epithelial cells, mast cells, and macrophages. The released substances stimulate the infiltration of additional inflammatory cells, such as eosinophils and neutrophils, which perpetuate and exacerbate the tissue damage done and lead to the pathologic changes seen.[38] While airway resistance in the large intrathoracic airways of asthmatic patients may be increased, the major site of airflow limitation is in the small airways. Wheeze in patients with asthma may be constant or may disappear during times of remission.

There is also an uncommon syndrome of reversible restrictive lung disease that is clinically indistinguishable from asthma.[39,40] Patients with this syndrome manifest episodic dyspnea and wheezing that is treatable with bronchodilators and corticosteroids. Pulmonary function testing shows a reduction in lung volumes and increased elastic recoil, but normal airway resistance and flow rates.[39,40] Whether this is a variant of asthma or a separate disease entirely is unclear.

Patients in whom asthma is suspected should be evaluated with PFT. In patients with a clinical picture consistent with asthma, a reduction of the $FEV_1/FVC$ ratio with normalization of pulmonary function and improvement in symptoms following therapy with bronchodilators and/or steroids is diagnostic of asthma. Patients suspected of asthma but who do not have airflow obstruction at baseline are appropriate candidates for pharmacologic bronchoprovocation challenge. Whether methacholine or histamine is used, virtually all symptomatic asthmatic patients will have a decrease of their $FEV_1$ of 20% or greater following administration of standard doses of these medications.[29] Improvement in symptoms with specific asthma medications must then be demonstrated to confirm the diagnosis.

## Chronic Obstructive Pulmonary Disease

"Chronic Obstructive Pulmonary Disease (COPD) may be defined as a process characterized by the presence of chronic bronchitis or emphysema that may lead to the development of airway obstruction; airway obstruction need not be present at all stages of the process and may be partially reversible."[41] The term COPD is used in a general sense to include a variety of conditions that have in common the characteristic of chronic airflow obstruction within the lungs. Most often the term COPD is taken to mean cigarette smoke-induced lung disease which leads to airflow obstruction. While there are hereditary diseases (eg, alpha-1-antiprotease inhibitor deficiency) as well as alternative environmental exposures (eg, raw cotton dust leading to chronic byssinosis) that may cause COPD, this working definition is helpful in placing the disease to be discussed into context.

Chronic obstructive pulmonary disease is a disease that afflicts older, white men most often. This epidemiological pattern may reflect the long latency period for the development of the disease and the fact that until the past several years, cigarette smoking was primarily a habit of white men. Therefore, the common picture of the COPD patient may change over the years as the effects of long-term cigarette smoking are seen more commonly in women and nonwhite people. Patients with COPD also tend to be from lower socioeconomic groups and have increased exposure to occupational pollutants.[42] Since only about 15% of habitual cigarette smokers develop disabling COPD,[43] there must also be a host component to the development of COPD that is separate from alpha-1-antiprotease deficiency since this deficiency state is very uncommon.

The initial lesion of cigarette smoke-induced lung disease is respiratory bronchiolitis.[44] In susceptible individuals, this inflammatory process can progress to cause the glandular enlargement and mucous plugging in bronchi, goblet cell metaplasia, smooth muscle hypertrophy, inflammation in the walls of membranous bronchioles and a worsening respiratory bronchiolitis, and emphysema.[41,45] Although pathologic changes in bronchi or bronchioles correlate weakly with chronic airflow obstruction, they are almost never associated with irreversible obstruction in the absence of emphysema. Emphysema is the major determinant of severe airflow obstruction.

The pathophysiologic consequences of severe chronic airflow obstruction in the lung include (1) markedly restricted flow rates that set a limit on minute ventilation,[46] (2) maldistributed ventilation, resulting in both wasted ventilation (ie, high ventilation-perfusion mismatch) and impaired gas exchange (low ventilation-perfusion mismatch),[46,47] and (3) markedly elevated frictional resistance, which causes an increased work of breathing (ie, the work of the respiratory muscles is excessive),[48] and air trapping and hyperinflation, which alter the geometry of the respiratory muscles and shorten resting fiber lengths, thereby decreasing the maximum force the patients are capable of generating and predisposing them to fatigue.[49,50]

The patient history and physical examination serve an important purpose in the diagnosis of COPD by helping to select those patients who should undergo objective laboratory testing.[51-53] A chronic productive cough and dyspnea on exertion are the two symptoms most commonly associated with COPD. Unfortunately, these symptoms are nonspecific. A history of chronic productive cough is of limited value in the diagnosis of COPD because: (1) the presence of a cough-phlegm syndrome may be due to a variety of other causes, such as asthma, bronchiectasis, postnasal drip from sinusitis, and gastroesophageal reflux with aspiration[54] and (2) there is little correlation between the presence of cigarette smoke-induced, chronic, productive cough (ie, a manifestation of large airway mucous hypersecretion) and the development of significant airflow limitation (ie, predominantly a manifestation of disease of the small airways less than 2 mm in diameter)[55]. The finding of chronic dyspnea on exertion, the cardinal symptom of COPD, is also limited in its diagnostic value because it is associated with a large variety of other respiratory and nonrespiratory causes. Wheezing is slightly less common than cough and dys-

pnea. However it has been found to be associated with an approximately equal annual rate of decline in $FEV_1$ as the other two symptoms.[56] The three most useful physical findings of chronic airflow obstruction are (1) a forced expiratory time greater than 4 seconds measured during auscultation, [57] (2) a definite decrease in breath-sound intensity,[58] and (3) the presence of unforced wheezing audible during auscultation.[20] Therefore, a history or physical examination finding of wheezing in a heavy cigarette smoker should always raise the possibility of COPD, which can then be evaluated by PFT.

Because findings on clinical evaluation are often subjective, difficult or impossible to quantitate, and nonspecific, PFT ultimately determines the diagnosis of COPD. They are objective, quantifiable, and most important, reflect the key physiologic parameters involved. A decrease in the ratio of $FEV_1/FVC$ with little improvement after bronchodilators and corticosteroids is the hallmark of COPD. The decrease in $FEV_1$ in established COPD is linearly related to the number of cigarettes smoked per day in the interval between the two measurements. [56] The rate of decline of $FEV_1$ decreases when smoking is stopped. Patients with COPD may also demonstrate an increased total lung capacity and residual volume and a decrease in diffusion capacity of carbon monoxide. Arterial blood gases may be normal, show mild hypoxemia, or more severe hypoxemia associated with hypercapnia.

## Pulmonary Edema

Cardiac asthma, or wheezing associated with congestive heart failure (CHF), was first described over a century ago. Wheezing can be due to airflow obstruction secondary to peribronchial edema presumably at the small airway level. It can occur when edema is superimposed upon preexisting asthma. Studies performed on a dog model indicate that increased pulmonary capillary pressures may be associated with a reduction in dynamic compliance and increases in airway resistance and closing volume and that these effects can be eliminated by performing a vagotomy.[59] This implies that wheezing associated with pulmonary edema may be under vagal control. Finally, there is evidence to suggest that airway edema can be responsible for causing bronchial hyperresponsiveness.[60,61] The clinician must be aware of all four of these possibilities to treat the patient appropriately.

Results of studies describing PFT data in patients with congestive heart failure provide the strongest support for the peribronchial edema mechanism of wheezing in pulmonary edema. Mid–expiratory flow rate ($FEF_{25-75\%}$), $FEV_1$, and FVC have been shown to be reduced in correlation with the degree of pulmonary congestion found after myocardial infarction and other causes of pulmonary edema.[62–65] The wheezing associated with congestive heart failure has been shown to correlate with increases in extravascular lung water.[63] Increases in left ventricular end-diastolic pressures lead to increased pulmonary vascular pressures, which cause extravasation of fluid into the interstitium of the lung. This fluid accumulates initially in the peribronchial interstitium and can cause early airway closure, increased ventilation-to-perfusion mismatch, and increased airway resistance.[64,66] The extrinsic compression of the airways due to fluid is exacerbated by mucosal edema and a decrease in the normal transmural distending pressure.

Any cause of increased pulmonary interstitial fluid can cause the abnormalities described above. Therefore, noncardiogenic pulmonary edema can lead to similar pulmonary function abnormalities and wheezing.[67] In addition, patients whose primary abnormality is a decreased clearance of fluid should theoretically have similar findings. For instance, patients with impaired lymphatic drainage due to malignancy have been described to have wheezing due to pulmonary edema and they may respond to diuretic therapy.[68]

The diagnosis of pulmonary edema as a cause of wheezing may be suspected by patient history, physical examination, and chest roentgenogram. Pulmonary edema should not be excluded even if the patient has a normal cardiac examination because the clinical diagnosis of congestive heart failure is unreliable. Patients whose wheezing is either unexplained or refractory to therapy may require more sophisticated evaluation such as echocardiography, radionuclide ventriculography, or cardiac catheterization.[69,70] For instance, wheezing that occurs in the setting of an acute myocardial infarction should be suspected to be due to edema even when the chest roentgenogram and cardiac examination are normal.[63,64]

There are a modest number of studies that attempted to evaluate the role of bronchial hyperresponsiveness in pulmonary edema states.[60,61,71] Although these studies have evaluated small groups of patients with varying classes of congestive heart failure and found conflicting results, two of these studies suggest that bronchial hyperresponsiveness may play some role in the pathogenesis of obstruction in some of these patients.[60,61]

## Aspiration

Aspiration is a common event. Almost everyone aspirates some of their oral contents during sleep.[72] This rarely causes a problem in healthy, young people.[73] Respiratory problems arise when there is an excessive volume or frequency of aspiration, when the content of the aspirate is particularly noxious, or when normal defense mechanisms are inadequate to detoxify and clear what has been aspirated. Inspiratory wheezing is likely to be due to laryngeal irritation or laryngospasm. Expiratory wheezing may occur secondary to tracheobronchitis, obstruction of airways from aspirated material, or peribronchial edema associated with noncardiogenic pulmonary edema. Lastly, micro as well as macroaspiration may contribute to the wheezing of asthmatic patients by increasing their bronchial hyperresponsiveness.

There are several medical conditions that predispose a patient to frequent, large-volume aspirations. Hiatal hernia, Zenker's diverticulum, esophageal dysmotility, nasogastric feeding tubes, gastroesophageal reflux disease (GERD), and reduced lower esophageal sphincter pressure due to medications (eg, calcium channel blockers, nitrates, methylxanthines) can all contribute to the increased presence of food and gastric contents in the esophagus which predisposes to aspiration. Stroke, sedative-hypnotic drug use, neuropsychiatric disorders, ethanol abuse, and neuromuscular disorders all reduce a patient's ability to protect his or her airway. In addition, there is an age-dependent reduction in the reflex ability to close the vocal cords to protect against aspiration.[74]

Aspiration should be considered in the differential diagnosis of wheeze under certain circumstances. When the aspiration event is witnessed, the association is obvious. However, the presence of any of the predisposing factors listed above is a clue that aspiration may have occurred. The association of wheezing with diffuse infiltrates, especially in a posterior or inferior location, can be helpful. Nocturnal symptoms can be a clue to the presence of occult aspiration. Symptoms of GERD, such as heartburn, regurgitation, and a bitter taste in the mouth, can be helpful.

A variety of diagnostic steps can be taken when a patient is suspected of aspirating. The physician should watch the patient swallow a glass of water. A pharyngeal problem may be uncovered by watching the patient cough and sputter and tilt his or her neck and head in an unnatural posture. A cricopharyngeal problem may be suggested by the inability to swallow despite repeated attempts. A chest roentgenogram will occasionally detect a large hiatal hernia with an air-fluid level and can reveal infiltrates consistent with aspiration pneumonitis. A contrast cine-esophagram (ie, barium swallow) can help in the diagnosis of aspiration several ways. This study can detect silent aspiration associated with abnormal swallowing due to neuromuscular dysfunction, and it can reveal structural lesions, such as a stricture, that may predispose the patient to aspirate.[75] Even though barium swallow is an insensitive and nonspecific test in the diagnosis of GERD, it may detect reflux to

the hypopharynx with aspiration. The most sensitive and specific test for linking GERD and pulmonary disease is 24-hour esophageal pH probe monitoring.[76] This test is well tolerated by patients.[77,78]

Standard methods for diagnosing aspiration as a cause of wheeze may not be feasible in critically ill patients. A variety of methods have been proposed to help document aspiration in intubated patients. Fat stains performed on unfixed sputum and bronchoalveolar lavage specimens may reveal numerous lipid-laden macrophages consistent with aspiration of exogenous lipid, but are not specific for this diagnosis since they may also represent nothing more than a nonspecific response of the lung to acute injury of any nature.[79] Radionuclide scintiscanning using $^{99m}$Tc-sulfur colloid also appears to be an insensitive technique for documenting pulmonary disorders as a consequence of GERD. Winterbauer et al.[80] have advocated using an indicator, such as glucose or food coloring, placed into the enteral feeding formula as a tracer. If a glucose level of greater than 25 mg/dL, as measured with glucose oxidase reagent strips, or any of the food coloring is discovered in the sputum during endotracheal suctioning, then aspiration or the presence of a tracheoesophageal fistula is implied. However, a more recent study found that the average concentration of glucose in the tracheal secretions of patients fed by either the enteral or parenteral route was considerably higher (66 mg/dL and 105 mg/dL, respectively) even without clinical or roentgenographic evidence of aspiration.[81] In fact, the tracheal concentrations of glucose were higher than the concentrations in most of the enteral feeding solutions used. Therefore, this method is unlikely to be helpful in diagnosing aspiration.

## Pulmonary Embolism (PE)

Pulmonary embolism (PE) can result in wheezing.[82,83] This wheezing can be very marked and may at times mimic the acute presentation of asthma.[83,84] In many patients the diagnosis of asthma is suspected so strongly that therapy with bronchodilators is begun.

The wheezing associated with PE is thought to be due to bronchoconstriction and increased airway resistance presumably in small airways. This has been demonstrated in both animal and human models. In dogs, there are transient increases in airway resistance and decreases in lung compliance following experimental emboli.[85] Alterations in pulmonary function have also been documented in humans. Forced vital capacity, $FEV_1$, peak flow, and maximum voluntary ventilation are all reduced in patients with PE in comparison with the population at large.[82,86]

Some investigators postulate that PE causes wheezing because of the release of mediators, such as thromboxanes, serotonin, and histamine, from platelets.[86,87] These mediators are potential stimulants for bronchial smooth muscle contraction and therefore bronchoconstriction. In addition, patients with symptomatic PE have been found to be more susceptible to the bronchoconstricting effects of platelet activating factor than those with asymptomatic emboli.[88] These patients demonstrated increased airway resistance following a dose of platelet activating factor that was independent of bronchial hyperresponsiveness to methacholine. If it can be demonstrated subsequently that platelet activating factor is released in PE, these findings may help explain why some patients develop symptoms while others remain asymptomatic even when experiencing large emboli.

The changes in pulmonary function associated with PE have not been reversible with conventional bronchodilator therapy.[83] However some have observed the reversal of symptoms and the improvement of airflow obstruction when heparin is administered.[86] Heparin may block the release of mediators by preventing the incorporation of platelets into the clot. This would eliminate or at least minimize the resulting airflow obstruction and wheezing.

## Bronchiolitis

Bronchiolitis has been reported to occur in association with a wide range of clinical settings and diseases.[89–92] These include toxic fume inhalation, infection (eg, adenovirus, legionella, mycoplasma), connective tissue disease (eg, scleroderma, systemic lupus, rheumatoid arthritis, Sjögren's syndrome), transplantation (eg, bone marrow, lung, heart-lung), and ulcerative colitis. In each of these settings, patients can present with wheeze by history and physical examination. Pathogenetically, these diverse conditions somehow injure airway epithelium, primarily at the bronchiolar level, leading to inflammation. The process may result in irreversible fibrotic and obliterative changes.

Idiopathic bronchiolitis is probably the most common form. From a diagnostic standpoint, the most important clinical feature is its natural history.[91] Unlike most lung disorders characterized by chronic airflow limitation, obstruction in idiopathic bronchiolitis develops over a shorter interval of several months to a few years rather than over many years. It should also be suspected when chronic airflow limitation develops in patients who are nonsmokers and who are determined not to have asthma, cystic fibrosis (CF), bronchiectasis, or emphysema. Diagnostic confusion is most likely to occur in prior or present smokers since bronchiolitis may not be suspected. However, it is important to consider bronchiolitis since it may respond favorably to prolonged high-dose corticosteroid therapy.

A syndrome of "diffuse panbronchiolitis" was originally described in Japan and has subsequently been reported in the United States.[93] It is manifested by chronic inflammation of the respiratory bronchioles. Pulmonary function tests exhibit a mixed obstructive and restrictive defect.[93] Roentgenograms of the chest demonstrate hyperinflation and fine nodular densities. The cause of this entity is not known.

Obliterative bronchiolitis associated with lung and heart-lung transplantation was first reported in heart-lung transplant patients in 1984,[94] but has also been reported in lung transplant recipients.[95] This syndrome is considered to be a manifestation of chronic rejection which occurs usually between 3 and 15 months following transplantation.[96] It may occur in the absence of rejection of the transplanted heart in heart-lung patients. Patients may demonstrate an insidious onset, possibly following a viral infection.[89] Typically cough, sputum production, dyspnea, and recurrent lower respiratory tract infections are the early manifestations. Both crackles and wheezes may be heard on auscultation of the chest.[95] Pulmonary function tests show evidence of small airway disease initially, but will progress subsequently to overt airflow obstruction, frequently combined with restriction.[95] Hypoxemia and respiratory failure develop after only months. Biopsy specimens reveal inflammation of the respiratory and terminal bronchioles, injury to the respiratory epithelium, intraluminal granulation tissue, and severe surrounding fibrosis. The disease is thought to progress consistently to respiratory failure in the absence of therapy.

## Cystic Fibrosis

Cystic fibrosis is an autosomal recessive genetic disorder that is characterized by abnormal chloride ion transport in a variety of organs. The genetic abnormality seen in CF is found on the long arm of chromosome 7 and codes for the CF transmembrane conductance regulator.[97] Abnormalities of this protein can lead to dysfunction of the lungs, sinuses, pancreas, liver, gastrointestinal tract, and male (and possibly female) reproductive tract. In addition, patients with CF develop problems with drug metabolism, nutritional status, and psychosocial adjustment that cannot be attributed to dysfunction in one particular organ.

Wheezing in CF is caused by airway obstruction, which is a result of hypersecretion of thick, tenacious mucous and hypertrophy of goblet cells and submucosal glands. Then, bronchiectasis results as a consequence of the chronic obstruction and infection. There is also evidence of

bronchial hyperresponsiveness, which can cause obstruction and lead to wheezing. Although lung function in CF is thought to be normal at birth, there is a steady deterioration throughout life beginning with small airways obstruction progressing to obstruction of larger airways, and subsequently to a mixed obstructive and restrictive picture.[98]

Cystic fibrosis is the most common genetic disease seen in Caucasians. One in 25 Caucasians carries the gene and 1 in approximately 2500 infants born have CF. Therefore, physicians must have a high index of suspicion for this disease. While presentations, such as meconium ileus, at birth are diagnostic for CF, the physician must also consider the diagnosis in children who present with failure to thrive, recurrent sinopulmonary infections, chronic cough, and steatorrhea. In addition, some patients with CF are not diagnosed until adulthood, in one instance as late as age 69.[99] Therefore, internists and family physicians as well as pediatricians must consider this diagnosis. The CF Foundation's diagnostic criteria for the diagnosis of CF are: (1) clinical features consistent with CF, such as chronic obstructive lung disease with *Pseudomonas* infection of airways, obstructive azoospermia confirmed by scrotal exploration and testicular biopsy, family history, and pancreatic insufficiency, and (2) two sweat chloride tests with results greater than 60 mEq/L.[97] In addition, being homozygous for (delta)F508, the most common allele of the CF gene, is also diagnostic. However, there are patients who have a clinical syndrome very similar to CF but have nondiagnostic sweat chloride tests and are not homozygous for (delta)F508. Recently, a specific mutation at the site of the CF gene has been found to be associated with this scenario.[100] In the future, genotyping may be an even more important component of the evaluation of CF, especially if more genotype/phenotype relationships are established.

## Anaphylaxis

Wheezing can also be seen in patients with anaphylaxis. This typically occurs as an allergy to stinging insects, drugs, or sensitivity to contrast agents. Patients may also develop anaphylaxis in response to exercise.[101] Anaphylaxis is typically an abrupt onset of wheezing and dyspnea associated with urticaria, angioedema, nausea, diarrhea, and hypotension.[102]

Wheeze in anaphylaxis can be inspiratory, expiratory, or both and can be caused by either upper or lower airway obstruction. Upper airway obstruction is caused by edema of the tongue, larynx, and/or vocal cords. A variety of chemical mediators, including histamine, serotonin, eosinophilic chemotactic factor of anaphylaxis, heparin, neutrophil chemotactic factor, and trypsin, are released from preformed granules in mast cells and basophils and are involved in this reaction.[103] Lower airway obstruction is caused by bronchoconstriction, mucosal edema, and mucous hypersecretion. These findings can occur together or separately and can occur with or without cardiovascular collapse.

## Carcinoid Syndrome

Patients with the carcinoid syndrome can also develop wheeze. The syndrome can occur with either a primary lung tumor or metastatic disease of the liver. Wheezing can be related to the systemic bronchoconstricting effects of the mediators released or a local phenomenon due to obstruction from an endobronchial carcinoid.[67] Pulmonary carcinoid tumors usually originate endobronchially. Therefore, they are frequently detected by bronchoscopy when the local airway obstruction they cause creates an abnormality on chest roentgenogram and prompts further evaluation. The diagnosis is often supported by detecting an elevated 5-hydroxyindoleacetic acid level in a 24-hour urine specimen obtained from a patient with an appropriate clinical presentation.

## Bronchiectasis

Bronchiectasis can also be associated with wheeze. Bronchiectasis is the chronic dilatation of one or several bronchi. It may be seen in bronchi of any size, although medium-sized bronchi seem to be most commonly effected. Bronchiectasis may be caused by a number of entities, including inadequately treated pneumonia, abnormalities of ciliary function, bronchial obstruction, CF, allergic bronchopulmonary aspergillosis, various immune deficiencies, alpha-1-antiprotease deficiency, defects of bronchial anatomy, chronic sarcoidosis, toxic inhalations, obstructing neoplasms, yellow nail syndrome, and tuberculosis.[104]

Several mechanisms have been proposed in the pathogenesis of bronchiectasis. Of these, the one that is most appealing and has the most popular support is the combination of bronchial wall damage and a dilating force.[105] Bronchial wall damage occurs usually as a result of a necrotizing infection, while the dilating force is usually provided by the elastic recoil of surrounding consolidated tissue. If these forces are temporary, the lung and bronchial tissue may return to its original configuration once they are removed. However, if these forces cause permanent damage to the airway, bronchiectasis will persist.

Bronchiectasis can produce a variety of clinical syndromes. It may cause a syndrome of chronic airflow obstruction with wheezing due to lack of supporting structure, mucosal edema, or bronchial hyperresponsiveness.[29] Exacerbations of bronchiectasis are typically associated with cough, expectoration, and fever. Bronchiectasis may also cause massive hemoptysis associated with abnormal blood flow to the bronchiectatic region. In addition, bronchiectasis may be associated with increased risk of malignancy.[105]High-resolution CT scan of the lung has become the standard for diagnosis of bronchiectasis. Chest roentgenogram has been used, but many of the findings associated with bronchiectasis on plain films of the chest are nonspecific. Prior to the development of high-resolution CT scan, bronchography was considered the gold standard. However, bronchography is an uncomfortable procedure for the patient, can be dangerous in some settings, and does not provide information about the surrounding lung tissue. High-resolution CT scan protocols that combine thin cuts through the abnormal areas with high-resolution reconstruction algorithms are needed for accurate diagnosis. Typical findings associated with bronchiectasis on CT scan include bronchial dilatation (including the classic signet ring sign), lack of bronchial tapering, bronchial wall thickening, and the presence of visible bronchi in the periphery.[105]

### Lymphangitic Carcinomatosis

Wheezing can develop as a result of pulmonary lymphangitic carcinomatosis. In one study, stomach, breast, prostate, and pancreatic cancers accounted for 70% of these tumors.[106] Obstruction can theoretically occur in these patients for a variety of reasons, including direct compression of the bronchi due to peribronchial involvement, the associated inflammatory response, and possibly resultant interstitial edema that accumulates due to inadequate clearance of normal lung water.

### Parasitic Infections

Wheeze can occasionally be the result of parasitic infection. Several different parasites have been reported to cause wheeze, including *Strongyloides stercoralis*, *Ascaris lumbricoides*, *Ancylostoma duodenale*, *Necator americanus*, *Toxocara canis*, *Schistosoma* species, the filarial species *Wuchereria bancrofti*, *Brugia malayi,* and *Dirofilaria immitis*.[107–110] Cases associated with filarial infection often exhibit a marked eosinophilia and

are referred to as tropical pulmonary eosinophilia. The mechanism of wheezing in these cases may be bronchial hyperresponsiveness due to hypersensitivity to filarial infection.[110] Important clinical features include symptoms of wheeze and/or cough in a nonasthmatic patient, travel to endemic areas, fatigue, weight loss, low-grade fever, and infiltrates on chest roentgenogram.

## Approach to the Diagnosis of Wheeze

A large number of conditions located in a variety of anatomic airway locations can produce airway obstruction and present with expiratory or inspiratory wheezing, or both. The basis of evaluating this symptom is to localize the site of the obstruction to either large or small intrathoracic, or extrathoracic airways using the patient history, physical examination, and the knowledge of the most common causes of wheeze. When the physician is unable to diagnose wheeze using this information, specialized testing such as PFT, chest roentgenogram, computed axial tomographic scans of the chest, and bronchoscopy may then be helpful in arriving at a specific diagnosis. Figure 7 illustrates our suggested diagnostic protocol for the evaluation of the adult patient with wheeze of unknown or uncertain etiology or wheeze that is not responding to treatment as expected. The main points of this protocol are as follows:

1. For all patients a patient history and physical examination should be performed, concentrating on the anatomy of the entire extent of the airways.

2. If the patient history and physical

---

**Figure 7.** Suggested diagnostic protocol for the evaluation of wheeze. In general, the approach involves: (1) addressing whatever is found in the patient history and physical examination; (2) looking for common causes of wheezing; and (3) further evaluation for less common causes in a physiologically oriented approach when common causes do not explain the patient's symptoms. ARDS = acute respiratory distress syndrome; CF = cystic fibrosis; COPD = chronic obstructive pulmonary disease; CXR = chest roentgenogram; GERD = gastroesophageal reflux disease; LV = left ventricle; MI = myocardial infarction; PBC = pharmacologic bronchoprovocation challenge test; PNDS = postnasal drip syndrome; VTE = venous thromboembolism.

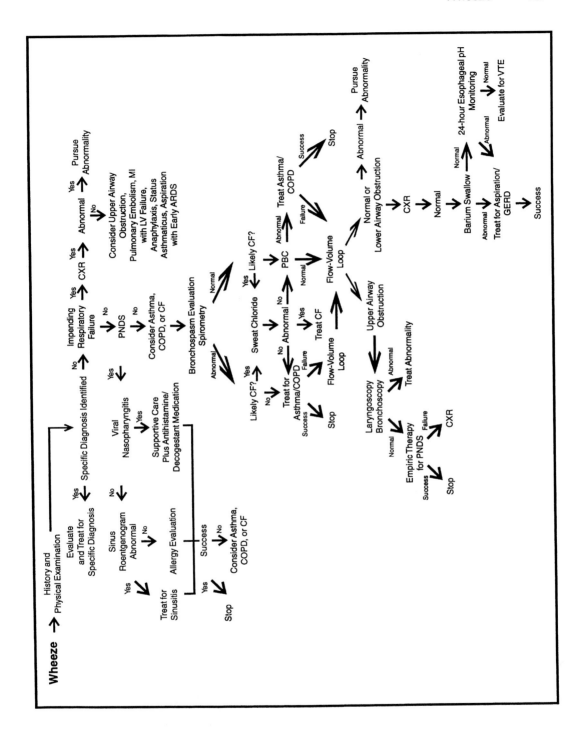

examination suggest a specific diagnosis, confirmatory testing or therapy should be ordered for that diagnosis.

3. If the patient history and physical examination do not identify a definite diagnosis and the patient is not in impending respiratory failure, the physician should first consider PNDS, which is the most common cause of wheezing. If the patient has evidence for PNDS and the PNDS is thought to be due to a viral nasopharyngitis (the common cold), a trial of supportive care and oral antihistamine/decongestant medication should be attempted.[30] If there is no suggestion of a viral nasopharyngitis but PNDS is still suspected, sinus roentgenograms should be performed. If these indicate sinusitis, treatment should be given. If the sinus x-rays are not diagnostic, an allergy evaluation should be pursued.

4. If the patient history and physical examination do not suggest PNDS, the physician should consider the other most common causes of wheeze including asthma, COPD, and CF (in some populations). In most of these cases, the initial evaluation of adults with these conditions would begin with spirometry before and after bronchodilator. Based on the result of the spirometry, patients will usually be divided into two groups: (1) those with normal spirometry results and (2) those with abnormal spirometry results (Figure 7). Further evaluation from that point may begin with either therapy for asthma/COPD, a pharmacologic bronchoprovocation challenge test, or sweat chloride iontophoresis, depending on the specific circumstances of that patient.

5. In those patients for whom these measures have not led to a diagnosis, a flow-volume loop should be performed. The flow-volume loop may help distinguish between upper and lower airway causes of obstruction. Further testing may be directed at the anatomic area implicated.

6. If a diagnosis has not been made to this point, a chest roentgenogram should be performed. If the chest roentgenogram reveals an abnormality, that abnormality should be pursued with appropriate testing and therapy. If the abnormality is consistent with either infection or malignancy, expectorated sputum studies or fiberoptic bronchoscopy, or both should be considered.

7. If a cause still has not been discovered, tests for aspiration and GERD should be ordered. If a cineradiographic barium swallow is nondiagnostic, 24-hour esophageal pH probe monitoring should be considered. In the critically ill patient, aspiration may be suspected if gastrointestinal contents are suctioned from the endotracheal tube or if enteral feedings are uniquely colored with a nontoxic dye, such as food coloring, and that coloring is subsequently discovered in the tracheobronchial secretions.

8. If the above-mentioned studies do not distinguish a cause for the wheezing, then an evaluation for recurrent pulmonary emboli should be undertaken. In the situation where wheezing is of acute onset and there is no clear-cut diagnosis, the evaluation for PE may take place sooner in the protocol.

## Therapy

### Upper Airway Conditions

Therapy for wheeze due to upper airway conditions has two components: (1) nonspecific management to ensure adequacy of the airway and (2) specific therapy, which addresses the presumed pathophysiologic process causing airway obstruction.

Patients with severe UAO require immediate attention to assure the adequacy of their airways. In general, these patients must be observed in an intensive care unit. While some cases will require endotracheal intubation or tracheostomy, there are measures short of these interventions that can be used in many situations. The most effective of these measures is the inhalation of the helium-oxygen mixture, which has been used in UAO from a variety of causes with improvement in air flow and relief of hypercapnia.[111–114] While racemic epinephrine has also been used with success in acute laryngeal edema, it is associated with a rebound worsening of edema when the medicine wears off.[115]

## Postnasal drip syndrome

Specific therapy for PNDS is discussed in detail in Chapter 1 on "Cough".

## Epiglottitis

Medical treatment of epiglottitis begins with humidification of the air and close observation. Cultures of blood and occasionally of the epiglottis should be obtained. Antibiotics should be given which cover the most common pathogens, particularly *H influenzae*. Cefuroxime, cefotaxime, and ceftriaxone are the agents most frequently used in this situation. Organisms which have been reported to cause this disease include infection by *H influenzae*, *S pneumoniae*, beta-hemolytic streptococci, *Staphylococcus aureus*, *K pneumonia*, *Bacteroides* species, *Hemophilus parainfluenzae*, *Candida albicans*, and *P multocida*[31]. Antibiotics should be given intravenously for the first several days and a 10- to 14-day course should be completed with oral medication. Some experts advocate giving intravenous corticosteroids to help reduce inflammation, but this is not universally accepted.

All adults with epiglottitis should be admitted to an intensive care unit for close observation and intubation as needed. As opposed to the situation in children, in which immediate intubation upon diagnosis is often advocated, adults may be closely observed until there are early signs of UAO.

When conservative measures fail, endotracheal intubation is the procedure of choice. Tracheostomy is an acceptable alternative if intubation is unsuccessful.

## Vocal Cord Dysfunction Syndrome

The most important component in the management of wheezing due to vocal cord dysfunction is its recognition. This allows the physician to discontinue nonessential and potentially dangerous therapies, such as corticosteroids. In an acute attack, a helium-oxygen mixture may help relieve the obstruction because the less dense gas can pass more easily through an area of turbulent flow. After the acute attack has passed, the most important component of treatment is speech therapy with a trained speech pathologist.[116] During therapy, patients with this syndrome are taught techniques that will allow them to relax their laryngeal muscles during an attack and hopefully terminate the episode. Much of this effort revolves around getting them to focus on expiration rather than inspiration. The patients are also taught general relaxation techniques with or without psychotherapy.

## Retropharyngeal Abscess

Potential treatments for retropharyngeal space abscess include airway management, medications, and surgery. Airway management can be accomplished with tracheostomy, cricothyroidotomy, or endotracheal intubation with or without a fiberoptic laryngoscope. The decision of which of these methods to use must take into account the unique circumstances of each situation. Antibiotics are given intravenously and should cover upper airway anaerobes in all cases. High-dose intravenous penicillin and metronidazole are the drugs of choice in most cases except for patients with allergy to either medication. When penetrating trauma or vertebral disease is involved, antibiotics directed against *S. aureus* infection should also be used. Additional antibiotics may be added if the individual circumstances implicate additional potential pathogens. Surgical drainage of retropharyngeal space abscesses is almost always necessary.

## Endotracheal intubation

In most cases, the edema and granulation tissue associated with the presence of a foreign body in the trachea will respond to the removal of that foreign body.[117] This means that a difficult decision must be made each time, weighing the risks of losing control of the airway with the risks of continued irritation of the upper airway mucosa by the tube. Adjunctive therapies that have been tried include inhaled and systemic corticosteroids and antibiotics. There are no conclusive data to support the use of either of these modalities. In rare cases, the structure of the defect may be such that the lesion can be removed by laser surgery. Finally, in some situations of localized tracheal narrowing resection of a segment of trachea has been performed with good success. This should be done only by a thoracic surgeon with extensive experience in performing the procedure.

## Lower Airway Conditions

### Asthma

The National Heart, Lung, and Blood Institute created the National Asthma Education Program (NAEP) to increase public and professional awareness of asthma and to improve the overall care of asthmatic patients. The NAEP convened a panel of experts to develop guidelines for the diagnosis and therapy of asthma.[35] The basis of their approach is a four-component process involving: (a) objective measures of lung function to assess severity and monitor therapy; (b) pharmacologic therapy to reverse and prevent airway inflammation as well as to treat airway narrowing; (c) environmental control measures to eliminate factors that cause asthma exacerbations; and (d) patient education. What follows is a summary of those recommendations.

**Objective Measures:** Spirometry is the first objective measure recommended. If spirometry is abnormal or clinical conditions suggest a "complex" situation, then specialized PFT is recommended. (This may include the previously discussed broncho-provocation challenge testing.) Once a di-

agnosis of asthma has been established, therapy may be monitored by the use of PEFR. Peak flows are interpreted in comparison to the patient's own "personal best" values obtained over a 2- to 3-week baseline period while the patient's disease is stable. Subsequent values can be placed into "zones" labeled as green (80% to 100% of baseline), yellow (50% to 80% of baseline), and red (below 50% of baseline). Specific actions to take can be worked out by the patient and his or her physician based on these values.

**Pharmacologic Therapy:** Three major conditions are identified for treatment in the Guidelines. They are: (i) chronic asthma, (ii) exercise-induced asthma, and (iii) acute asthma.

*Chronic Asthma:* Treatment should be tailored to the individual patient. The physician should be prepared to develop a treatment plan for each patient and to change treatment as indicated by changes in the patient's symptoms and peak flow measurement. Asthma triggers, such as viral and bacterial upper respiratory infections, allergen exposures, rhinitis, chemical irritants, sulfites, tartrazine dye, aspirin, beta-blocking medications, climatic conditions, and GERD, should be sought and either treated or avoided.

Medication should be administered in the following step-care fashion:

1. All patients should have a beta-2 agonist inhaler to be used every 3 to 4 hours as needed for symptoms or variabilities in peak flow.

2. Should medication be required frequently for either reason, or should symptoms interfere with the patient's normal activities or require occasional emergency care, an inhaled anti-inflammatory medication, such as a corticosteroid, cromolyn, or nedocromil, should be given.

3. If symptoms are not controlled or exacerbations persist on standard doses of anti-inflammatory medications (2 to 4 puffs, bid), higher doses of inhaled corticosteroids (2 to 6 puffs, bid to qid) should be administered.

4. In addition to higher doses of inhaled corticosteroids, sustained-release theophylline preparations and/or oral beta-2 agonists may be given at this stage of therapy. A longer acting inhaled beta-2 agonist (eg, salmeterol) may also be considered.

5. Patients who do not respond to this level of therapy should be evaluated by a specialist in asthma management.

6. Inhaled beta-2 agonists should be increased in frequency and dose (up to 4 puffs, as needed for short periods).

7. In addition to combinations of the medications listed above, short courses (1 to 2 weeks) of oral corticosteroids should be used intermittently when symptoms are poorly controlled. A consideration should be given to daily or alternate day chronic use in the most severe cases.

*Exercise-induced Asthma:* Although many asthmatic patients have other symptoms with exercise, for some exercise is the only trigger. These patients will typically experience cough, wheeze, or dyspnea upon exercising, and when spirometry is measured before and after an exercise challenge, they exhibit at least a 15% decrease in $FEV_1$. In those patients, a management strategy should be developed that allows them to participate in the activities of their choosing without medicating them unnecessarily at other times. This goal can usually be accomplished by pretreating them with 2 puffs of either cromolyn sodium or a beta-2 agonist inhaler approximately 20 to 30 minutes prior to exercise. This can be repeated after 2 hours if exercise continues. Alternatively, inhaled salmeterol seems to provide an extended duration of protection when compared to albuterol.[118] This advantage may disappear in patients who are chronically treated with salmeterol since tachyphylaxis has been reported to develop.[119] In those patients who continue to have symptoms despite treatment with a beta-2 agonist or cromolyn, the dose of either medication can be doubled or the two medications can be combined.

*Acute Asthma:* The goals in managing exacerbations of asthma include: (1) rapid reversal of airflow obstruction and relief of dyspnea, (2) correction of hypoxemia, and (3) prevention of relapse. The response to therapy of an asthma exacerbation should be monitored by observing clinical signs and symptoms as well as by objective measurements such as PEFR or $FEV_1$.

The initial management of a mild asthma attack is usually accomplished in the home. The patient should be instructed to take 2 to 4 puffs of the inhaled beta-2 agonist medication every 20 minutes for up to 1 hour. If the patient has a good response, including relief of symptoms and return of the PEFR to a stable level of greater than 70% of the baseline, he or she may continue to administer beta-2 agonist therapy up to every 3 hours as needed for 24 to 48 hours. The need for follow-up should be determined by the physician.

Asthma attacks that are severe from the start or have an incomplete response to the previously described regimen require more aggressive therapy. Patients whose symptoms persist at rest or with mild exertion and whose PEFR is between 50% to 70% of baseline should be treated with oral corticosteroids and hourly beta-2 agonist therapy. If the patient fails to improve after 2 to 6 hours of this regimen or if the PEFR begins at or drops to below 50% of baseline, the patient should seek emergency medical treatment from his or her physician. At that point, the physician may choose to either treat the patient with 4 to 6 puffs of beta-2 agonist inhaler every 10 minutes for 30 minutes or to refer the patient to the emergency department. Any patient who has not improved on the regimen described should go to the emergency department.

***Environmental Control:*** Asthma is characterized by hyperresponsiveness of the airways. The stimuli for this hyperresponsiveness include both nonspecific irritants and specific airborne allergens. Among the nonspecific irritants that may cause asthma exacerbations are tobacco and other smoke, strong odors and sprays, and air pollutants. In addition, a large percentage of patients with asthma demonstrate positive skin test reactions to common inhalant antigens. Common antigens causing these reactions are outdoor allergens, such as ragweed, grass, pollens, molds; house dust components, such as animal materials, dust mites, and cockroach allergen; and indoor molds. Indoor allergens can be made more offensive by mobilizing them with vacuum cleaners or humidifiers. Environmental control consists primarily of eliminating exposure to these triggers, either by physically avoiding them or by eliminating them from the environment. Air conditioning, high-efficiency particulate air filters (ie, HEPA filters), and electrostatic precipitators can be helpful to this end. If these measures and an appropriate medical regimen do not succeed in controlling symptoms, immunotherapy may be helpful.

**Patient Education:** Since much of the responsibility for the day-to-day management of asthma falls upon the patients, it is important to enlist them in a cooperative role in their own care. One way of doing this is to educate patients in all aspects of their disease. Important topics to be covered in a complete asthma education program include: (1) the definition of asthma, (2) important signs and symptoms, (3) the role of inflammation in asthma pathogenesis, (4) the effects of medications, (5) asthma triggers and techniques for avoidance, (6) treatment strategies, premedication, and appropriate use of medications, (7) patient fears and feelings regarding the disease and treatment, (8) the role of family and other support systems, (9) the role of home peak flow monitoring, (10) the role of written guidelines and diaries, and (11) how to evaluate the success or failure of treatment. One way of achieving these goals is by enrolling patients in a structured asthma comanagement program. While it is still not clear whether these programs consistently can decrease emergency department visits, hospitalizations, and cost of health care, they have been found to help identify new triggers, improve patients' sense of self-control, and educate patients.[120]

## Chronic Obstructive Pulmonary Disease

The therapy of COPD can be discussed from physiological and symptomatic standpoints. Smoking cessation is crucial; it affects both standpoints. While it has been shown to significantly reduce the rate of decline of lung function, it also can result in marked improvement of symptoms, particularly cough.[121–123]

Inhaled bronchodilator therapy may also be helpful. Ipratropium bromide is usually the first bronchodilator given to a patient with COPD because some studies have shown a better effect than beta-2 agonists in improving flow rates in these patients.[124] An acceptable alternative is to use a less costly beta-2 agonist as initial therapy. A combination of ipratropium bromide and beta-2 agonists can be tried on patients who fail to improve substantially, since at least one recent study has indicated a better effect with both than either agent alone.[125]

Alternatively, while inhaled bronchodilators may decrease airway resistance and improve symptoms, the improvement is modest and is not consistent. In addition, prophylactic inhaled ipratropium does not appear to have any effect on the long-term rate of decline of lung function.[123] In other words, therapy with ipratropium bromide does not have a disease modifying effect. Therefore, if a COPD patient notes no improvement in symptoms despite a 5% to 10% improvement in $FEV_1$, it is reasonable to stop the medications rather than expose the patient to side effects.

Another bronchodilator that has been used in many patients with COPD is theophylline. Theophylline appears to act directly on the bronchial smooth muscle, although the biochemical mechanism of its action is controversial. In addition, theophylline may have an effect on the respiratory muscles, airway cilia, and central nervous system. Multiple studies have shown theophylline to be an effective bronchodilator.[126] While theophylline has a narrow therapeutic window for the development of side effects (eg, nausea, vomiting, anxiety, insomnia, tremor, and cardiac dysrhythmia) it continues to be valuable in the management of COPD, particularly in those patients with severe disease, nocturnal symptoms, and those who have difficulty with or adverse reactions to inhaler administration.

Chronic oxygen therapy is a mainstay of the therapy for hypoxemic patients with COPD. Two randomized controlled clinical trials have shown convincingly that long-term oxygen therapy can improve the survival of these patients.[127,128] The goals of oxygen therapy are to reduce the cardiovascular and neuropsychiatric complications of hypoxemia, although patients frequently report symptomatic improvement as well.

Multiple studies strongly suggest that pulmonary rehabilitation also has a role in the management of disabled COPD patients.[129,130] Comprehensive programs appear to reduce (1) use of medical resources, (2) hospitalizations, (3) emergency department visits, (4) physician visits, (5) dyspnea, and (6) depression/fear; and improve (1) quality of life, (2) exercise tolerance, (3) activities of daily living, (4) return to work, (5) knowledge about the disease, (6) independence, and (7) control of symptoms. Additional large, randomized controlled clinical trials will be required to substantiate the results of these studies and better define the benefits of pulmonary rehabilitation.

In addressing the issue of corticosteroid therapy in COPD, we must distinguish between chronic or short-term use. In the acute setting, one prospective double-blind randomized, placebo-controlled study showed that a group of COPD patients in acute hypercapnic decompensation given 0.5 mg/kg of methylprednisolone intravenously every 6 hours for 72 hours exhibited more improvement in indices of airflow obstruction over the entire study period compared to the placebo-treated control group.[131] On the basis of this study, therefore, the short-term administration of corticosteroids in patients with exacerbations of COPD appears reasonable. Additional studies to confirm these beneficial effects would be desirable.

In regard to chronic use, both inhaled administration and systemic administration have been evaluated. A 6-week trial of inhaled beclomethasone resulted in reduced indices of airway inflammation and improved spirometry when compared to placebo.[132] In another study that included patients with either asthma or COPD, the rate of decline in $FEV_1$ was slower when patients received inhaled beclomethasone.[133] However, a concurrent control group was not studied. In addition, most of the difference was seen in the asthmatic patients in this study. On the other hand, long-term administration of at least 7.5 mg per day of oral prednisolone caused a stabilization or a slowing of the decline of pulmonary function in a group of COPD patients studied in the Netherlands.[134] However, many patients developed severe side effects from the treatment. Those side effects were so significant that many patients were unable to continue on the minimum dose necessary to see a therapeutic effect. The severity of the side effects precludes the long-term use of systemic corticosteroids in anything but the most severe cases. However, given these clinical results and the previously discussed pathophysiology of COPD, it seems reasonable to give inhaled corticosteroids to: (1) moderate or severe COPD patients, (2) those with evidence of bronchial hyperresponsiveness on PFT, (3) patients whose function declines rapidly over time, and (4) patients whose symptoms are inadequately controlled on bronchodilators alone.

The importance of bacterial infection in COPD exacerbations is still open to debate. Traditional indicators of bacterial infection, such as core body temperature and white blood cell count are usually normal. Serological studies have failed to link *H. influenzae* and *S. pneumoniae* to exacerbations, and expectorated sputum studies are notoriously poor in defining the cause of lower bacterial infection. Finally, the results of studies evaluating the effect of antibiotics in routine exacerbations of COPD have been conflicting. A major criticism voiced by those who doubt the efficacy of antibiotics is that many of the studies supporting their use have failed to effectively exclude patients with bronchiectasis, pneumonia, or sinusitis. Therefore, because of the risks of toxicity and allergy, the cost of expensive antibiotics, and the increasing incidence of antibiotic resistance, we feel that the use of antibiotics in exacerbations of COPD that are mild in severity and do not show clinical or radiographic evidence of bronchiectasis, pneumonia, or sinusitis is unwarranted. The limited number of patients with routine exacerbations who would benefit from antibacterial therapy will declare themselves by failing to improve with closely observed therapy that includes bronchodilators, corticosteroids, and oxygen where necessary. For exacerbations that are other than routine, the physician should search for specific diseases such as pneumonia, sinusitis, PE, left ventricular failure, or gastroesophageal reflux with aspiration and treat these entities accordingly.

## Pulmonary Edema

When wheeze occurs in a patient with known or suspected asthma the patient should be treated initially as described above for asthma. There are conflicting reports as to whether obstruction entirely due pulmonary edema is responsive to bronchodilator therapy.[64,135] Therefore, effective treatment of wheezing in this situation consists of both inhaled bronchodilator medication and left ventricular preload reduction with diuretics and nitrates. In addition, afterload reduction can improve forward flow and reduce lung water. In some situations a cardiac inotrope may also improve left ventricular output and minimize edema.

## Aspiration

Patients may aspirate because of pharyngeal dysfunction, esophageal dysfunction, and/or gastroesophageal reflux. Swallowing abnormalities must be addressed specifically by a certified speech pathologist and any predisposing factors

must be eliminated. One common problem is inadequately fitting dentures that must be corrected to eliminate aspiration of large pieces of food. Sedative-hypnotic drugs must be eliminated, and ethanol abuse must be curbed. Any neuropsychiatric or neuromuscular disorders must be treated whenever possible. Esophageal function can be assisted with physical measures, such as appropriate timing of meals and elevation of the head of the bed. Occasionally, surgical therapy of a Zenker's diverticulum is necessary to prevent recurrent aspiration. GERD is treated with special diet, a prokinetic agent, and/or $H_2$ blockers. A more complete discussion of the therapy of GERD is described in Chapter 1, "Cough."

## Pulmonary Embolism

A full discussion of the treatment of PE is beyond the scope of this text. Recent in depth reviews of this topic have been published elsewhere. [136,137] While wheezing due to PE may be unresponsive to bronchodilator therapy, anticoagulation with heparin has been observed to reverse bronchoconstriction and reduce wheezing as rapidly as 5 minutes after the administration of a heparin bolus.[86] Subsequent therapy with warfarin should proceed after the patient has been evaluated carefully for conditions that may predispose to poor outcomes, such as poor compliance, a history of falls, gait abnormalities, or peptic ulcer disease.[138]

## Bronchiolitis

Idiopathic bronchiolitis has been shown to respond to high-dose corticosteroid therapy. In one study, 11 of 15 patients demonstrated a significant (>15%) improvement in their $FEV_1$ following 3 months of therapy with prednisone (1 mg/kg per day).[91] Therefore, it is important to distinguish these patients from other patients with chronic airflow obstruction.

Diffuse panbronchiolitis is treated with erythromycin. Erythromycin acts as an anti-inflammatory agent on this condition, possibly by inhibiting neutrophil chemotactic activity.[93] The long-term prognosis for patients with this disease treated with erythromycin is uncertain.

Post-transplantation bronchiolitis obliterans is treated best by preventing its occurrence using an immunosuppressive regimen that includes corticosteroids, cyclosporine A, and azathioprine. This regimen has reduced the incidence and severity of obliterative bronchiolitis seen in these patients.[95] Cases that do develop may be treated with high doses of corticosteroids. Despite these regimens some patients inexorably progress to respiratory failure. In those cases, some have advocated repeat heart-lung transplantation or single-lung transplantation, even in patients who originally received heart-lung units.[139] This approach requires further study with larger groups of patients before firm recommendations can be made.

## Cystic fibrosis

A large number of therapeutic modalities have been used in CF. While some methods remain unproven, others have clearly contributed to the increasing life span of CF patients and yet others are effective in reducing symptoms and improving quality of life. In addition, intensive research into CF treatment appears to be yielding other promising therapies that may become available over the next several years.

**Antibiotics:** Antibiotics may be used for acute exacerbations of CF or as prophylaxis/maintenance. Intravenous antibiotics, directed against *Pseudomonas aeruginosa, S aureus,* and *H influenzae* are firmly recommended by most experts for use during exacerbations of CF although randomized, placebo-controlled studies have never been done. As a general rule, CF patients require very high doses of antibiotics because of abnormalities in the metabolism of the drugs. Antibiotics directed against the same pathogens, nasal decongestants, and drainage procedures are also used for the treatment of sinus infections associated with CF. Short-term administration of inhaled tobramycin is associated with an increase in pulmonary function, including $FEV_1$ and FVC, and with a decrease in the amount of *Pseudomonas* organisms in the sputum.[140] The clinical effects of this are uncertain and the long-term effects on pulmonary function and bacterial resistance have not been described. Other uses of antibiotics, including intravenous administration for maintenance and inhaled administration for acute management, do not enjoy consensus support.

**Chest Physiotherapy:** Methods to assist the removal of thick secretions from the lungs have become the standard of care for CF patients. Chest percussion, deep breathing, forced cough, and postural drainage are all methods advocated by physicians who treat CF. Newer techniques, including high-frequency chest compression, autogenic drainage, and positive expiratory pressure, have been tried but have not been proven to be superior to traditional methods.[141–143] However, they may be easier to perform and therefore enhance compliance. No method has been shown definitively to be the best.

**Inhaled Bronchodilators:** Patients with bronchial hyperresponsiveness, wheezing, and/or positive bronchodilator responses on PFT should be treated with standard doses of inhaled beta-2 agonists on an as needed basis. Studies that have looked at the effectiveness of bronchodilators in CF have not attributed a benefit to their use on the group as a whole, but may reveal a benefit in the subgroup of patients most likely to be hyperresponsive.[144,145]

**Inhaled Corticosteroids:** Patients who are candidates for treatment with inhaled bronchodilator may also be candidates for treatment with inhaled corticosteroids, although there is little evidence to support the use of these medications in CF.

**Inhaled Recombinant Human Deoxyribonuclease [I(DNAse)]:** Dead and dying airway inflammatory cells release large amounts of polymerized deoxyribonucleic acid (DNA) into the airways of patients with CF. The DNA causes the sputum to be very thick and tenacious. Inhalation of DNAse can lyse the DNA strands and make the sputum more watery and more easily expectorated. Studies of this drug administered to CF patients have shown small improvements in $FEV_1$ and FVC and possible improvements in quality of life measures, including reduced hospitalization, antibiotic use, and sensation of well being. However the cost of administering the drug daily approaches $12,000 per year for the drug alone. In addition, no long-term benefits have yet been proven.

**Lung Transplantation:** Patients with CF may be candidates for double-lung or heart-lung transplantation. Patients with CF are subject to the same qualifying restrictions and seem to have similar outcomes as other patients under consideration for these procedures.

**Mechanical Ventilation:** Some patients with CF may require mechanical ventilation for life support. This is a topic that has generated many ethical discussions, although firm recommendations have never been developed. Patients may be ventilated if they are failing due to a correctable acute problem, providing they or their surrogates understand the prognosis for their particular problem. The prognosis of patients with long-term home mechanical ventilation for CF has never been evaluated.

**Other:** The treatment of the pancreatic, hepatobiliary, gastrointestinal, reproductive, orthopedic, and psychosocial complications of CF are beyond the scope of this book. An excellent review of the topic has recently been published.[97] In addition, while gene therapy, ion transport modulators, anti-inflammatory agents, and immunotherapy are all under investigation, there has not been sufficient research into

their effects to consider them standard therapy.[146]

## Anaphylaxis

The therapy of anaphylaxis has been discussed extensively elsewhere.[103] General treatment involves airway management, cardiopulmonary function support, tourniquet use to impede absorption of the inciting antigen when appropriate, fluids, medications to counteract the effects of released chemical mediators (eg, antihistamines), and continuous monitoring. Upper airway obstruction should be managed first by establishing a patent airway. Oxygen should be administered. Intubation, cricothyrotomy or tracheotomy may be necessary in some cases. Lower airway obstruction should be treated initially with subcutaneous epinephrine. Inhaled metaproterenol or albuterol, aminophylline, and intravenous corticosteroids may also be beneficial.

## Carcinoid Syndrome

The most important component of therapy for carcinoid-induced wheezing is appropriate antitumor therapy. Management of localized or regionally extensive gastrointestinal carcinoids consists of surgical excision.[147] Bronchial carcinoid tumors can also be surgically removed with excellent results.[148] A variety of different cytotoxic medications are available for treatment of metastatic carcinoid tumors. However, since all of these therapies are potentially toxic and none have shown dramatic success, chemotherapy is usually reserved for patients with advanced disease or symptoms that interfere with activities of daily living.[147] Symptomatic treatment of carcinoid-induced wheeze should be undertaken with caution since catecholamines are known to induce symptoms. Corticosteroids and inhaled beta-2 agonists may provide some relief, although there is no clear evidence to support their use.

## Bronchiectasis

The therapy of bronchiectasis is discussed in Chapter 1, "Cough" and Chapter 4, "Hemoptysis."

## Lymphangitic Carcinomatosis

Antitumor therapy is the mainstay of treatment for wheeze due to lymphangitic carcinomatosis. Surgery is not an option in this situation because of the extent of the metastases. Several of the malignancies capable of causing this condition may respond to cytotoxic or hormonal therapy. Corticosteroids have also been used to decrease inflammation. In addition, diuretics may provide the best, albeit short-term, relief in inevitably fatal disease since they will help to remove edema not cleared by compromised lymphatic vessels.

## Parasitic infections

Patients who wheeze due to parasitic infections may show dramatic response to antiparasite therapy. Antiparasitic agents are selected according to the specific parasite detected, but frequently include thiabendazole, mebendazole, diethylcarbamazine, and/or praziquantel.[149]

## Conclusions

Wheezes are continuous musical lung sounds that last longer than 250 milliseconds. They may occur during inspiration, as well as during expiration. They may prompt a visit to a physician when they are heard by the patient, or they may be auscultated by the physician when he or she is listening to the lungs for another reason. Wheezes occur only when there is obstruction of an airway. They are caused by the oscillation of the walls of airways that have been narrowed almost to the point of closure.

Wheezes are not synonymous with asthma; they may occur with a variety of clinical diseases and syndromes. In fact, only about one-third of the patients who presented to a pulmonary outpatient clinic with a history of wheezing were found to have asthma. Among the clinical entities in addition to asthma that have been associated with wheezing are UAO, COPD, pulmonary edema, aspiration, PE, bronchiolitis, anaphylaxis, carcinoid syndrome, lymphangitic carcinomatosis, bronchiectasis, CF, and parasitic infections of the lungs.

The protocol for evaluation of wheeze places great emphasis on findings during patient history and physical examination. Unless the patient appears in imminent danger of respiratory failure, the physician should address (1) whatever is found in the patient history and physical examination; (2) common causes of wheezing; and (3) less common causes in a physiologically oriented approach when common causes do not explain the patient's symptoms. That evaluation may involve spirometry before and after bronchodilator, pharmacologic bronchoprovocation challenge, flow-volume loops, chest roentgenograms, and other specialized testing.

The treatment of wheezing depends on its cause. Because the differential diagnosis of wheezing includes diseases which are potentially life-threatening, it is important that the physician arrive at a specific diagnosis and institute specific therapy. The specific treatments for the various causes of wheezing have been described. The failure of a therapy to correct wheezing should prompt the physician to either adjust the therapy or search for an additional cause of wheezing. The number of patients who have more than one simultaneous cause for wheezing is unknown.

## *References*

1. Hudson LD, Conn RD, Matsabura RS, et al. Rales: Diagnostic usefulness of qualitative adjectives. Am Rev Respir Dis 1976; S113:187.
2. Fletcher CM. The clinical diagnosis of pulmonary emphysema. An experimental

study. Proceedings of the Royal Society of Medicine 1952;45:577.

3. Schilling RSF, Hughes JPW, Dingwall-De-Fordyce I. Disagreement between observers in an epidemiological study of respiratory disease. Br Med J 1955;1:65.

4. Burrows B, Huang N, Hughes R, et al. Pulmonary terms and symbols—a report of the ACCP-ATS Committee on Pulmonary Nomenclature. Chest 1975;67:583–593.

5. Loudon R, Murphy RLH. Lung Sounds. Am Rev Respir Dis 1984;130:663–673.

6. Acres JC, Kryger MH. Upper airway obstruction. Chest 1981;90:207–211.

7. Forgacs P. The functional basis of pulmonary sounds. Chest 1978;73:399–405.

8. Pasterkamp H, Carson C, Daien D, et al. Digital respirosonography. Chest 1989; 96:1405–1412.

9. Munakata M, Ukita H, Doi I, et al. Spectral and waveform characteristics of fine and coarse crackles. Thorax 1991;46:651–657.

10. Sparrow D, O'Connor GT, Basner RC, et al. Predictors of the new onset of wheezing among middle-aged and older men—the normative aging study. Am Rev Respir Dis 1993;147:367–371.

11. Senthisselvan A, Chen Y, Dosman JA. Predictors of asthma and wheezing in adults: grain farming, sex, and smoking. Am Rev Respir Dis 1993;148:667–670.

12. Luyt DK, Burton PR, Simpson H. Epidemiological study of wheeze, doctor diagnosed asthma, and cough in preschool children in Leicestershire. Br Med J 1993; 306:1386–1390.

13. Speight ANP, Lee DA, Hey EN. Underdiagnosis and undertreatment of asthma in childhood. Br Med J 1983;286: 1253–1256.

14. Anderson HR, Bailey PA, Cooper JS, et al. Morbidity and school absence caused by asthma and wheezing illness. Arch Dis Childhood 1983;58:777–784.

15. Akasaka K, Konno K, Ono Y, et al. Acoustical studies on respiratory sounds in asthmatic patients. Tohoku J Exp Med 1975;117:323–333.

16. Takezawa Y, Shira F, Sawaki S, et al. Presented at the Fifth International Lung Sounds Conference. Boston: International Lung Sounds Association, 1980.

17. Kryger M, Bode F, Antic R, et al. Diagnosis of obstruction of the upper and central airways. Am J Med 1976;61:85–93.

18. Pratter MR, Hingston DM, Irwin RS. Diagnosis of bronchial asthma by clinical evaluation: an unreliable method. Chest 1983; 84:42–47.

19. Shim CS, Williams MH. Relationship of wheezing to the severity of obstruction in asthma. Arch Intern Med 1983; 143: 890–892.

20. Marini JJ, Pierson DJ, Hudson LD, et al. The significance of wheezing in chronic airflow obstruction. Am Rev Respir Dis 1979;120:1069–1072.

21. King DK, Thompson T, Johnson DC. Wheezing on maximal forced exhalation in the diagnosis of atypical asthma. Ann Intern Med 1989;110:451–455.

22. Al-Bazzaz F, Grillo H, Kazemi H. Response to exercise in upper airway obstruction. Am Rev Respir Dis 1975;111: 631–640.

23. Geffin B, Grillo HC, Pontoppidian H. Stenosis following tracheostomy for respiratory care. JAMA 1971;216:1984–1988.

24. Macklem PT. Airway obstruction and collateral ventilation. Physiol Rev 1971;51: 368–436.

25. Gelb AF, Klein E. The volume of isoflow and increase in maximal flow at 50% of forced vital capacity during helium-oxygen breathing as tests of small airways dysfunction. Chest 1977;71:396–399.

26. Miller RD, Hyatt RE. Obstruction lesions of the larynx and trachea: clinical and physiologic characteristics. Mayo Clin Proc 1969;44:145–161.

27. Crapo RO. Pulmonary function testing. N Engl J Med 1994;331:25–30.

28. Webb J, Clark TJH, Chilvers C. Time course of response to prednisolone in chronic airflow obstruction. Thorax 1981; 36:18–21.

29. Irwin RS, Pratter MR. The clinical value of pharmacologic bronchoprovocation challenge. Med Clin North Am 1990;74: 767–778.

30. Curley FJ, Irwin RS, Pratter MR, et al. Cough and the common cold. Am Rev Respir Dis 1988;138:305–311.

31. Jacobs TJ, Irwin RS, Raptopoulos V. Severe Upper Airway Infections. In: Rippe JM, Irwin RS, Fink MP, Cerra FB, eds. *Intensive Care Medicine*, 3rd ed. Boston, Ma: Little Brown and Company. 1996: 883–903.

32. Christopher KL, Wood RP, Eckert C, et al. Vocal-cord dysfunction presenting as asthma. N Engl J Med 1983;308: 1566–1570.

33. Sokol W. Vocal cord dysfunction presenting as asthma. West J Med 1993;158: 614–615.

34. Weiss KB, Wagener DK. Asthma surveillance in the United States-a review of current trends and knowledge gaps. Chest 1990;98:179s–184s.
35. Sheffer AL, Bailey WC, Bleecker ER, and the Expert Panel on the Management of Asthma. *Guidelines for the Diagnosis and Management of Asthma*. Bethesda, Md: U.S. Department of Health and Human Services; 1991.
36. Lemanske RF. Mechanisms of airway inflammation. Chest 1992;101:372S-377S.
37. Cockcroft DW. Airway hyperresponsiveness: therapeutic implications. Ann Allergy 1987;59:405–414.
38. Holgate ST, Beasley R, Twentyman OP. The pathogenesis and significance of bronchial hyperresponsiveness in airways disease. Clin Sci 1987;73:561–572.
39. Kaminsky DA, Irvin CG. Anatomic correlates of reversible restrictive lung disease. Chest 1993;103:928–931.
40. Hudgel D, Cooper D, Souhrada J. Reversible restrictive lung disease simulating asthma. Ann Intern Med 1976;85:328–332.
41. Snider GL. Chronic obstructive pulmonary disease: a definition and implications of structural determinants of airflow obstruction for epidemiology. Am Rev Respir Dis 1989;140:S3-S8.
42. Snider GL. Emphysema: the first two centuries and beyond. A historical overview, with suggestions for future research: Part 1. Am Rev Respir Dis 1992;146:1334–1344.
43. Lopata M, Evanich MJ, Opal E, et al. Airway occlusion pressure and respiratory nerve and muscle activity in studies of respiratory control. Chest 1978;73(Suppl):285–286.
44. Niewohner DE, Kleinerman J, Rice DB. Pathologic changes in the peripheral airways of young cigarette smokers. N Engl J Med 1974;291:755–758.
45. Hogg JC, Macklem PT, Thurlbeck WM. Site and nature of airway obstruction in chronic obstructive lung disease. N Engl J Med 1968; 278:1355–1360.
46. West JB. *Pulmonary Pathophysiology: The Essentials*. Baltimore, Md: Williams and Wilkins, 1982.
47. Davidson FF, Glazier JB, Murray JF. The components of the alveolar-arterial oxygen tension difference in normal subjects and in patients with pneumonia and obstructive lung disease. Am J Med 1972;52:754–762.
48. Roussos C, Macklem PT. The respiratory muscles. N Engl J Med 1982;307:786–797.
49. Luce JM, Culver BH. Respiratory muscle function in health and disease. Chest 1982;81:82–90.
50. Janoff A, Carp H. Possible mechanisms of emphysema in smokers:cigarette smoke condensate suppresses protease inhibition in vitro. Am Rev Respir Dis 1977;116:65–72.
51. Pardee NE, Winterbauer RH, Morgan EH, et al. Combinations of four physical signs as indicators of ventilatory abnormality in obstructive pulmonary syndromes. Chest 1980;77:354–358.
52. Schneider IC, Anderson AE Jr. Correlation of clinical signs with ventilatory function in obstructive lung disease. Ann Intern Med 1965;62:477–485.
53. Stubbing DG, Mathur PN, Roberts RS, et al. Some physical signs in patients with chronic airflow obstruction. Am Rev Respir Dis 1982;125:549–552.
54. Irwin RS, Corrao WM, Pratter MR. Chronic persistent cough in the adult: the spectrum and frequency of causes and successful outcome of specific therapy. Am Rev Respir Dis 1981;123:413–417.
55. Peto R, Speizer FE, Cochrane AL, et al. The relevance in adults of airflow obstruction,but not of mucus hypersecretion,to mortality from chronic lung disease. Results from 20 years of prospective observation. Am Rev Respir Dis 1983;128:491–500.
56. Sherman CB, Xu X, Speizer FE, et al. Longitudinal lung function decline in subjects with respiratory symptoms. Am Rev Respir Dis 1992;146:855–859.
57. Rosenblatt G, Stein M. Clinical value of the forced expiratory time measured during auscultation. N Engl J Med 1962;267:432–435.
58. Pardee NE, Martin CJ, Morgan EH. A test of the practical value of estimating breath sound intensity. Breath sounds related to measured ventilatory function. Chest 1976;70:341–344.
59. Jones JG, Lemen R, Graf PD. Changes in airway caliber following pulmonary venous congestion. Br J Anaesth 1978;50:743–751.
60. Nishimura Y, Maeda H, Yokoyama M, et al. Bronchial hyperreactivity in patients with mitral valve disease. Chest 1990;98:1085–1090.
61. Sasaki F, Ishizaki T, Mifune J, et al. Bronchial hyperresponsiveness in patients

with chronic congestive heart failure. Chest 1990;97:534–538.

62. Frank NR, Cugell DW, Gaensler EA, et al. Ventilatory studies in mitral stenosis: a comparison with findings in primary pulmonary disease. Am J Med 1953;15:60–76.

63. Hales CA, Kazemi H. Pulmonary function after uncomplicated myocardial infarction. Chest 1977;72:350–358.

64. Interiano B, Hyde RW, Hodges M, et al. Interrelation between alterations in pulmonary mechanics and hemodynamics in acute myocardial infarction. J Clin Invest 1973;52:1994–2006.

65. Light RW, George RB. Serial pulmonary function in patients with acute heart failure. Arch Intern Med 1983;143:429–433.

66. Staub NC. Pulmonary edema. Phys Rev 1995;54:678–811.

67. Hollingsworth HM. Wheezing and stridor. Clin Chest Med 1987;8:231–240.

68. Mendeloff AI. Severe asthmatic dyspnea as the sole presenting symptom of generalized endolymphatic carcinomatosis. Ann Intern Med 1945;22:386–397.

69. Chakko S, Waska D, Martinez H, et al. Clinical, radiographic, and hemodynamic correlations in chronic congestive heart failure: conflicting results may lead to inappropriate care. Am J Med 1991;90:353–359.

70. Stevenson LW, Perloff JK. The limited reliability of physical signs for estimating hemodynamics in chronic heart failure. JAMA 1989;261:884–888.

71. Eichacker PQ, Seidelman MJ, Rothstein MS, et al. Methacholine bronchial reactivity testing in patients with chronic congestive heart failure. Chest 1988;93:336–338.

72. Huxley EJ, Viroslav J, Gray WR, et al. Pharyngeal aspiration in normal adults and patients with depressed consciousness. Am J Med 1978;64:564–568.

73. Bartlett JG, Borback SL. The triple threat of aspiration pneumonia. Chest 1975;68:560–566.

74. Pontopiddian H, Beecher HK. Progressive loss of protective reflexes in the airway with the advance of age. JAMA 1960;174:2209–2213.

75. Horner J, Massey EW. Silent aspiration following stroke. Neurology 1988;38:317–319.

76. Mattox HE III, Richter JE. Prolonged ambulatory esophageal pH monitoring in the evaluation of gastroesophageal reflux disease. Am J Med 1990;89:345–356.

77. Irwin RS, Zawacki JK, Curley FJ, et al. Chronic cough as the sole presenting manifestation of gastroesophageal reflux. Am Rev Respir Dis 1989;140:1294–1300.

78. DeMeester TR, Wang CI, Wernly JA, et al. Technique, indications, and clinical use of 24 hour esophageal pH monitoring. J Thoracic Cardiovasc Surg 1980;79:656–670.

79. Corwin RW, Irwin RS. The lipid-laden alveolar macrophage as a marker of pulmonary aspiration in parenchymal lung disease. Am Rev Respir Dis 1985;132:576–581.

80. Winterbauer RH, Durning RB, Barron E, et al. Aspirated nasogastric feeding solution detected by glucose strips. Ann Intern Med 1981;95:67–68.

81. Kinsey GC, Murray MJ, Swensen SJ, et al. Glucose content of tracheal aspirates: implications for the detection of tube feeding aspiration. Ann Intern Med 1994;22:1557–1562.

82. Sasahara AA, Cannilla JE, Morse RL, et al. Clinical and physiologic studies in pulmonary thromboembolism. Am J Cardiol 1967;20:10–20.

83. Windebank WJ, Boyd G, Moran F. Pulmonary thromboembolism presenting as asthma. Br Med J 1973;1:90–94.

84. Webster JR, Saadeh GB, Eggum PR, et al. Wheezing due to pulmonary embolism—treatment with heparin. N Engl J Med 1966;274:179s-184s.

85. Stein M, Alkalay I, Bruderman I. Pulmonary function after experimental autologous pulmonary emboli. J Clin Invest 1962;41:1402.

86. Gurewich V, Thomas D, Stein M, et al. Bronchoconstriction in the presence of pulmonary embolism. Circulation 1963;27:339–345.

87. Gurewich V, Cohen ML, Thomas DP. Humoral factors in massive pulmonary embolism: an experimental study. Am Heart J 1968;76:784–794.

88. Ruiz J, Monreal M, Sala H, et al. Effects of inhaled platelet activating factor on bronchial responsiveness in patients with symptomatic and asymptomatic pulmonary embolism. Chest 1992;102:819–823.

89. Allen MD, Burke CM, McGregor CGA, et al. Steroid-responsive bronchiolitis after human heart-lung transplantation. J Thoracic Cardiovasc Surg 1986;92:449–451.

90. Hakala M, Paakko P, Sutinen S, et al. As-

sociation of bronchiolitis with connective tissue disorders. Ann Rheum Dis 1986;45: 656–662.

91. Kindt GC, Weiland JE, Davis WB, et al. Bronchiolitis in adults. Am Rev Respir Dis 1989;140:483–492.

92. Lahdensuo A, Mattila J, Vilppula A. Bronchiolitis in rheumatoid arthritis. Chest 1984;85:705–708.

93. Oda H, Kadota J, Kohno S, et al. Erythromycin inhibits neutrophil chemotaxis in bronchoalveoli of diffuse panbronchiolitis. Chest 1994;106:1116–1123.

94. Burke C, Theodore J, Dawkins K, et al. Post-transplant obliterative bronchiolitis and other late sequelae in human heart-lung transplantation. Chest 1984;86: 824–829.

95. Theodore J, Starnes VA, Lewiston NJ. Obliterative bronchiolitis. Clin Chest Med 1990;11:309–321.

96. Scott JP, Higenbottam TW, Sharples L, et al. Risk factors for obliterative bronchiolitis in heart-lung transplant recipients. Transplant 1991;51:813–817.

97. Aitken ML, Fiel SB. Cystic fibrosis. DM 1993; 39:1–52.

98. Boat TF. Cystic Fibrosis. In: Murray JF, Nadel JA, eds. *Textbook of Respiratory Medicine.* Philadelphia, Pa: W B Saunders Company; 1988:1126–1152.

99. Brown RF, Dibenedetto R, Russell D, et al. Variant cystic fibrosis in an elderly man. S Med J 1986;79:1430–1432.

100. Highsmith WE, Burch LH, Zhou Z, et al. A novel mutation in the cystic fibrosis gene in patients with pulmonary disease but normal sweat chloride concentrations. N Engl J Med 1994; 331:974–980.

101. Kyle JM. Exercise-induced pulmonary syndromes. Med Clin North Am 1994;78: 413–421.

102. Bochner BS, Lichtenstein LM. Anaphylaxis. N Engl J Med 1991; 324:1785–1790.

103. Hollingsworth HM, Giansiracusa DS, Upchurch KS. Anaphylaxis. J Intensive Care Med 1991;6:55–70.

104. Luce JM. Bronchiectasis. In: Murray JF, Nadael JA , eds, *Textbook of Respiratory Medicine.* Philadelphia, Pa: W B Saunders Company, 1994:1398–1417.

105. Westcott JL. Bronchiectasis. Radiol Clin North Am 1991; 29:1031–1042.

106. Wu TT. Generalized lymphatic carcinosis (lymphangitis carcinomatosa) of the lungs. J Pathol Bac 1936;13:61.

107. Chhabra SK, Gaur SN. Airway hyperactivity in tropical pulmonary eosinophilia. Chest 1988;93:1105–1106.

108. Marshall J, Altman D, Lauber M, et al. COPD exacerbation associated with a skin rash. Chest 1991;99:1016–1017.

109. Neva FA, Ottensen EA. Current concepts in parasitology—tropical (filarial) eosinophilia. N Engl J Med 1978;298: 1129–1131.

110. Peterson C, Slutkin G, Mills J. Parasitic Infections. In: Murray JF, Nadel JA, eds. *Textbook of Respiratory Medicine.* Philadelphia, Pa:W B Saunders Company, 1988:950–986.

111. Duncan PG. Efficacy of helium-oxygen mixtures in the management of severe viral and post-intubation croup. Can J Anaesth 1979;26:206–212.

112. Lu TS, Omhura A, Wong KC, et al. Helium-oxygen in treatment of upper airway obstruction. Anesthesiology 1976;45: 678–681.

113. Pingleton SK, Bone RC, Ruth WC. Helium-oxygen mixtures during bronchoscopy. Crit Care Med 1980;8:50–53.

114. Houck JR, Keamy MF, McDonough JM. Effect of helium concentration on experimental upper airway obstruction. Ann Otol Rhinol Laryngol 1990;99:556–561.

115. Hollingsworth HM, Irwin RS. *Extrapulmonary Causes of Respiratory Failure.* In: Rippe JM, Irwin RS, Fink MP, Cerra FB, eds. 2nd edition. Intensive Care Medicine, 3rd ed. Boston, MA: Little, Brown and Company. 1996:628–641.

116. Newman KB. Vocal cord dysfunction: an asthma mimic. Pulmonary Perspectives 1993; 10:3–5.

117. Colice GL. Resolution of laryngeal injury following translaryngeal intubation. Am Rev Respir Dis 1992;145:361–364.

118. Anderson SD, Rodwell LT, DuToit J, et al. Duration of protection by inhaled salmeterol in exercise induced asthma. Chest 1991;100:1254–1260.

119. Ramage L, Lipworth BJ, Ingram CG, et al. Reduced protection against exercise induced bronchoconstriction after chronic dosing with salmeterol. Respir Med 1994; 88:363–368.

120. Irwin RS, Curley FJ, French CF, et al. Efficacy of an asthma self-management program (abstract). Am Rev Respir Dis 1993; 147:A775.

121. Wynder EL, Kaufman PL, Lesser RL. A short-term follow-up study on ex-cigarette smokers. Am Rev Respir Dis 1967; 96:645–655.

122. Fletcher C, Peto R, Tinker C, et al. *The Natural History of Chronic Bronchitis and Emphysema.* Oxford: Oxford University Press: 1976.

123. Anthonisen NR, Connett JE, Kiley JP, et al. Effects of smoking intervention and the use of an inhaled anticholinergic bronchodilator on the rate of decline of $FEV_1$: The Lung Health Study. JAMA 1994; 272:1497–1505.

124. Gross NJ. Ipratropium bromide. N Engl J Med 1988; 319:486–494.

125. Combivent Inhalation Aerosol Study Group. In chronic obstructive pulmonary disease, a combination of ipratropium and albuterol is more effective than either alone. Chest 1994;105:1411–1419.

126. Vaz Fragaso CA, Miller MA. Review of the clinical efficacy of theophylline in the treatment of chronic obstructive pulmonary disease. Am Rev Respir Dis 1993; 147:S40-S47.

127. Nocturnal Oxygen Therapy Trial Group. Continuous and nocturnal oxygen therapy in hypoxemic chronic obstructive lung disease: a clinical trial. Ann Intern Med 1980;93:391–398.

128. Medical Research Council Working Party. Long term domiciliary oxygen therapy in chronic cor pulmonale complicating chronic bronchitis and emphysema. Lancet 1981;1:681–685.

129. Ries RL. Pulmonary rehabilitation:rationale,components,and results. J Cardiopulmon Rehabil 1991;11:23–28.

130. Goldstein RS, Gort EH, Stubbing D, et al. Randomised controlled trial of respiratory rehabilitation. Lancet 1994;344: 1394–1397.

131. Albert RK, Martin TR, Lewis SW. Controlled clinical trial of methylprednisolone in patients with chronic bronchitis and acute respiratory insufficiency. Ann Intern Med 1980;92:753–758.

132. Thompson AB, Mueller MB, Heires AJ, et al. Aerosolized beclomethasone in chronic bronchitis: improved pulmonary function and diminished airway inflammation. Am Rev Respir Dis 1992;146: 389–395.

133. Dompeling E, van Schayck CP, van Grunsven P, et al. Slowing the deterioration of asthma and chronic obstructive pulmonary disease observed during bronchodilator therapy by adding inhaled corticosteroids. Ann Intern Med 1993;118: 770–778.

134. Postma DS, Steenhuis EJ, Van Der Weele LT, et al. Severe chronic airflow obstruction: can corticosteroids slow down progression? Eur J Respir Dis 1985;67:56–64.

135. Snashall PD, Chung KF. Airway obstruction and bronchial hyperresponsiveness in left ventricular failure and mitral stenosis. Am Rev Respir Dis 1991;144: 945–956.

136. Stein PD. Acute Pulmonary Embolism. *DM* 1994;40:467–523.

137. Dalen JE. When can treatment be withheld in patients with suspected pulmonary embolism? Arch Intern Med 1993; 153:1415–1418.

138. Montamat SC, Cusack BJ, Vestal RE. Management of drug therapy in the elderly. N Engl J Med 1989;321:303–309.

139. Adams DH, Cochrane AD, Khagani A, et al. Retransplantation in heart-lung recipients with obliterative bronchiolitis. J Thorac Cardiovasc Surg 1994;107: 450–459.

140. Ramsey BW, Dorkin HL, Eisenberg JD, et al. Efficacy of aerosolized tobramycin in patients with cystic fibrosis. N Engl J Med 1993;328:1740–1746.

141. Arens R, Gozal D, Omlin KJ, et al. Comparison of high frequency chest compression and conventional chest physiotherapy in hospitalized patients with cystic fibrosis. Am J Respir Crit Care Med 1994; 150:1154–1157.

142. Mortensen J, Falk M, Groth S, et al. The effects of postural drainage and positive expiratory pressure physiotherapy on tracheobronchial clearance in cystic fibrosis. Chest 1991;100:1350–1357.

143. Lannefors L, Wollmer P. Mucus clearance with three chest physiotherapy regimes in cystic fibrosis: a comparison between postural drainage, PEP, and physical exercise. Eur Respir J 1992;5:748–753.

144. Eggleston PA, Rosenstein BJ, Stackhouse CM, et al. A controlled trial of bronchodilator therapy in cystic fibrosis. Chest 1991;99:1088–1092.

145. Shapiro GG, Bamman J, Kanarele P, et al. The paradoxical effect of adrenergic and methylxanthine drugs in cystic fibrosis. Pediatrics 1976;58:740–743.

146. Fiel SB. Clinical management of pulmonary disease in cystic fibrosis. Lancet 1993; 341:1070–1074.

147. Moertel CG. Treatment of the carcinoid tumor and the malignant carcinoid syndrome. J Clin Oncol 1983;1:727–740.

148. Arrigoni MG, Woolner LB, Bernatz PE. Atypical carcinoid tumors of the lung. J

Thorac Cardiovasc Surg 1994;64: 413–421.

149. Mandell GL, Douglas RG, Bennett JE. *Principles and Practice of Infectious Diseases: Antimicrobial Therapy.* New York, NY: Churchill Livingstone, 1992:57–81.

150. Fesmire FM, Pesce RR. Tracheal obstruction presenting as new-onset wheezing. Am J Emerg Med 1989;7:173–176.

151. Owens GR, Murphy DMF. Spirometric diagnosis of upper airway obstruction. Arch Intern Med 1983;143:1331–1334.

152. Colt HG, Gumpert BC, Harrell JH. Tracheobronchial obstruction caused by klebsiella rhinoscleromatis: diagnosis, pathologic features, and treatment. J Bronchol 1994;1:31–36.

153. Kletzker GR, Bastian RW. Acquired airway obstruction from histologically normal, abnormally mobile supraglottic soft tissues. Laryngoscope 1990;100:375–379.

154. Hussain SSM. Relapsing polychondritis presenting with stridor from bilateral vocal cord palsy. J Laryngol Otol 1991; 105:961–964.

155. Chaten FC, Lucking SE, Young ES, et al. Stridor: intracranial pathology causing postextubation vocal cord paralysis. Pediatrics 1991;87:39–43.

156. Griffin JL, Ramadan HH, Wetmore SJ. Laryngocele: a cause of stridor and airway obstruction. Otolaryngol Head Neck Surg 1993; 108:760–762.

157. Bittleman DB, Smith RJH, Weiler JM. Abnormal movement of the arytenoid region during exercise presenting as exercise induced asthma in an adolescent adult. Chest 1994; 106:615–616.

158. Duong TC, Burtch GD, Shatney CH. Upper-airway obstruction as a complication of oral anticoagulation therapy. Crit Care Med 1986; 14:830–831.

159. Job A, Rama R, Gnanamuthu C. Laryngeal stridor in myasthenia gravis. J Laryngol Otol 1992;106:633–634.

160. Moralee SJ, Reilly PG. Metabolic stridor: bilateral vocal cord abductor paralysis secondary to hypokalemia. J Laryngol Otol 1992; 106:56–57.

161. Libby DM, Schley WS, Smith JP. Cricoarytenoid arthritis in ankylosing spondylitis: a cause of acute respiratory failure and cor pulmonale. Chest 1981;80:641–643.

162. Polisar IA, Burbank B, Levitt LM, et al. Bilateral midline fixation of cricoarytenoid joints as a serious medical emergency. JAMA 1960;172:901–906.

163. Case records of the Massachusetts General Hospital. N Engl J Med 1986; 315: 378–387. Case 31–1986.

164. Caglayan S, Erkin S, Coteli I, et al. Bronchial foreign body vs asthma. Chest 1989; 96:509–511.

165. Karbowitz SR, Edelman LB, Nath S, et al. Spectrum of advanced upper airway obstruction due to goiters. Chest 1985; 87: 18–21.

166. Hunter JH, Stanford W, Smith JM, et al. Expiratory collapse of the trachea presenting as worsening asthma. Chest 1993; 104:633–635.

167. Streider DJ, Kanarek DJ, Ferrucci JT, et al. Case records of the Massachusetts General Hospital. N Engl J Med 1975; 293: 866–871.

168. Paludette G, Rosignobi M. Leiomyoma of the trachea: report of case and review of the literature. J Laryngol Otol 1984;98: 947–951.

169. Sherry MK, Klainer AS, Wolff M, et al. Herpetic tracheobronchitis. Ann Intern Med 1988; 109:229–233.

170. Bose S, Hurst TS, Cockcroft DW. Right-sided aortic arch presenting as refractory intraoperative and postoperative wheezing. Chest 1991;99:1308–1310.

171. Tait RC, O'Driscoll BR, Denning DW. Unilateral wheeze caused by pseudomembranous aspergillus tracheobronchitis in the immunocompromised patient. Thorax 1993;48:1285–1287.

# 4

# Hemoptysis

Meyer S. Balter, M.D.

## Introduction

Hemoptysis is derived from the Greek word "haima" (blood) and "ptysis" (spitting). It refers to the coughing of blood that arises from the lungs or airways below the larynx. Hemoptysis, even in tiny amounts, alarms most patients who then seek early medical care. It is a symptom in 7% to 15% of patients attending chest clinics.[1-4] Hemoptysis may range from simple blood-streaking of purulent sputum, as seen frequently with infectious flares of chronic bronchitis,[5] to massive hemorrhage from an aortobronchial fistula leading to exsanguination.[6] The amount of expectorated blood does not lead to a specific diagnosis but does relate to prognosis. Therefore, when discussing the approach and therapy to hemoptysis, we divide the conditions into mild, moderate, and massive subcategories. Unfortunately, the exact definitions vary quite widely from study to study making comparisons difficult.[4, 7-22] Mild hemoptysis refers to blood-streaked sputum, with less than 20 mL in 24 hours. Moderate hemoptysis is the production of more than 20 mL and as much as 200 to 600 mL in 24 hours. Massive hemoptysis is defined as at least 200 mL in 24 hours,[10,18,22] but more commonly refers to production of greater than 600 mL of blood in 24 hours.[9,11,13-15,17]

The rate of blood loss appears to be more important than the total blood loss with rates of 150 mL or more per hour greatly increasing the risk of sudden death due to asphyxiation or exsanguination.[16]

Hemoptysis may be confused with lesions of the gingival mucosa or tongue that cause spitting of blood. Lesions in the nose, pharynx, and gastrointestinal tract may all lead to pooling of blood in the oropharynx, triggering the cough reflex and pseudohemoptysis.[23] Finally, the possibility of factitious hemoptysis must be considered when there are unusual aspects to the patient's medical history or behavior.[24]

## Anatomy and Pathophysiology

### The Pulmonary Vascular Supply

The respiratory system is unique in having a dual blood supply. The pulmonary arterial trunk originates from the base of the right ventricle and divides into a right and left main pulmonary artery after 4 to 5 cm. The individual main pulmonary arteries tend to travel adjacent to the bronchial tree and branch with the correspond-

From Irwin RS, Curley FJ, Grossman RF (eds): Diagnosis and Treatment of Symptoms of the Respiratory Tract. Armonk, New York, Futura Publishing Company, Inc., © 1997.

ing division. Numerous accessory branches penetrate the lung parenchyma.[25] Normal pulmonary arterial systolic pressure is 15 to 20 mm Hg with diastolic pressures of 5 to 10 mm Hg. The pulmonary arterioles branch into a capillary network surrounding the alveoli, from which the pulmonary veins subsequently arise. Larger venous branches run within the interlobular septa, separate from the bronchoarterial network, and then empty into the left atrium. The major role of the pulmonary circulation is gas exchange but the capillary network also serves as a blood filter and has a number of metabolic functions.[26]

Unlike the pulmonary circulation, the bronchial circulation is a high-pressure system. Whereas the pulmonary circulation receives the entire cardiac output, flow through the bronchial circulation is only about 1% to 3% of the cardiac output under normal conditions. This may increase significantly during cardiopulmonary bypass.[27] The bronchial vascular anatomy is highly variable in humans, but arteries generally originate from the aorta or intercostal arteries.[28] There are usually 2 to 4 bronchial arteries, with the average being 2.7, and there are almost always more arteries on the left side than on the right side.[29,30] Many variations of bronchial anatomy have been described but in a study of 150 cadavers, four patterns made up 93% of cases: (1) 41% had two left-side and one right-side arteries, most arising as separate trunks from the aorta; (2) 21% had one left-side and one right-side arteries; (3) 21% had two left-side and two right-side arteries; and (4) 10% had one left-side and two right-side bronchial arteries.[29] The bronchial artery on the right is more likely to come off of an intercostal artery, whereas the two on the left tend to arise slightly lower and directly from the descending aorta.[30] Nonetheless, marked variations of these patterns have been demonstrated by bronchial angiography.[31] Rarely, bronchial vessels arise from the subclavian, innominate, internal mammary, or even the coronary arteries.[32] It is important to note that the spinal artery of Adamkiewicz arises from a bronchial artery in up to 5% of individuals.[29] Possible embolization therapy is contraindicated in these patients because of the risk of spinal artery infarction.

The extrapulmonary bronchial arteries travel to the hila, from which at least two branches course along the bronchial tree with each bronchus. The arteries continue as far as the terminal bronchioles and have numerous communications within the bronchiole adventitia with a rich submucosal capillary network. The bronchial circulation also supplies the peribronchial and perivascular connective tissue; the tracheal wall; the middle third of the esophagus; the visceral diaphragmatic and mediastinal pleura; paratracheal and hilar lymph nodes; vagus and bronchopulmonary lymph nodes; and the vasa vasorum of the aortic arch, pulmonary arteries, and pulmonary veins.

The venous blood from the proximal tracheobronchial tree drains into the azygous and hemiazygous veins through bronchial veins and subsequently enters the right atrium. However, the major portion of the venous return from the intrapulmonary airways drains into the left atrium via the pulmonary veins.[32, 33]

## Bronchopulmonary Anastomoses

Although bronchial artery-to-pulmonary artery anastomoses can occur in the normal lung, their extent and significance in health are debated. They appear to be more common in neonates but decrease with age.[34, 35] Bronchopulmonary anastomoses become more common as the number of bronchioles increases as one moves closer to the lung periphery.[32] There are subpleural and intrapleural anastomoses between precapillary-sized bronchial arteries and the pulmonary veins that may increase in diseased states.[36] Anastomoses between bronchial and pulmonary veins are much more common, as discussed above, and represent the normal pathway of bronchial venous return. This does not represent as much of a shunt as previously thought because the intrapulmonary bronchial blood flow can exchange gas as it passes along the airways.[32]

The extensive anastomoses between the bronchopulmonary circulations provide a physiologic advantage in certain clinical situations. The bronchial circulation is not routinely re-established at the time of lung transplantation surgery. This is of little consequence for the intrapulmonary airways which can derive nutrition from pulmonary vessel anastomoses. However, because there are minimal bronchopulmonary anastomoses in the larger airways, breakdown of the anastomotic site is a frequent problem after transplantation unless other anastomoses are surgically created.[37] This problem is largely overcome by new surgical techniques. The bronchial circulation has a much greater capacity to expand than the pulmonary circulation. In cases of surgical ligation of the pulmonary artery, bronchial circulation is capable of assuming gas exchange responsibilities.[38]

Pulmonary infarction is rare after pulmonary vascular obstruction unless the bronchial blood flow is also decreased. This most commonly occurs in the face of left ventricular failure[39] probably because the intrapulmonary bronchial blood flow is decreased by high pulmonary venous pressure.

## Pathophysiology

Hemoptysis originates from the bronchial circulation in approximately 90% of cases. Exceptions include Rasmussen's aneurysm,[40] arteriovenous malformations,[41] pulmonary artery tears during right heart catheterization,[42] necrotic pulmonary infarcts, and occasionally, pyogenic lung abscess,[43] and congestive heart failure. In response to inflammation, the pulmonary circulation vasoconstricts, develops in situ thrombosis or, being a low-pressure system, is compressed by local edema. The bronchial circulation, on the other hand, vasodilates and expands in response to chronic inflammation as occurs in chronic bronchitis and bronchiectasis. These vessels are part of the high-pressure

systemic circulation and have a greater propensity to bleed.

## Etiology And Pathogenesis

There are more than 140 causes of hemoptysis (Table I).[5,6,24,44–175] An extensive review of the literature is not helpful in determining the exact frequency of the major causes of hemoptysis due to (1) occasional exclusion of patients with only blood-streaked sputum; (2) changing incidence and prevalence of certain diseases over the past few decades (eg, tuberculosis and bronchiectasis); (3) different local infectious pathogens in various countries where reviews of the topic have been written; and (4) patients' age and medical history. It is helpful to consider hemoptysis under nonmassive and massive subcategories, despite the fact that there is considerable overlap between the two.

### Nonmassive Hemoptysis

Causes of nonmassive hemoptysis can be broken down into large categories as illustrated in Table I. Only the most important common causes of hemoptysis will be discussed in any detail.

### *Infections*

Infections, both airway and parenchymal, are by far the most common causes of hemoptysis. Chronic inflammation of the airways, as occurs in chronic bronchitis, increases vascular supply to the airways through the bronchial circulation. This is not related to loss of pulmonary function.[176] The hyperemia of the airways makes them quite friable, resulting in bleeding, particularly following viral or bacterial infections that increase epithelial cell desquamation. If patients with blood streaked sputum are included, chronic bronchitis has become the leading cause of hemoptysis in North America.[177] Bronchiectasis, from any cause (Table II), has

**Table I**
Causes of Hemoptysis

**1. INFECTIOUS**
*Bronchial*
  Bronchiectasis[43]*
  Bronchitis[5]*
*Parenchymal*
  *Bacterial*
  Actinomycosis[44]
  Leptospirosis[46]
  Lung Abscess[47]
  Necrotizing Pneumonia*
    Klebsiella[48]
    Legionella[49]
    Melioidosis[50]
    Staphylococcus[51]
    Nocardiosis[52]
  *Fungal*
  Aspergilloma[53]
  Aspergillosis[54]
  Candidiasis[55]
  Coccidioidomycosis[56]
  Cryptococcosis[57]
  Exophilia dermatitis[58]
  Histoplasmosis[59]
  Mucormycosis[60]
  Paracoccidioidomycosis[61]
  Pseudoallescheriasis[62]
  Sporotrichosis[63]
  *Helminthic/Protozoal*
  Amebiasis[64]
  Ancylostomiasis[65]
  Ascariasis[66]
  Dirofilariasis[67]
  Echinococcosis[68]
  Malaria[69]
  Paragonimiasis[70]*
  Pneumocystis carinii[71]
  Schistosomiasis[72]
  Strongyloidosis[73]
  *Mycobacterial*
  Mycobacterium Avium Complex[74]
  Mycobacterium tuberculosis[75]*
  Mycobacterium xenopi[76]
  *Viral*
  Influenza[77]
  Varicella[78]
**2. NEOPLASTIC**
  *Benign*
  Bronchial carcinoids[79]*
  Hamartoma[80]
  Inflammatory polyps[81]
  Lymphangioma[82]
  *Malignant*
  Bronchogenic carcinoma[83]*
  Choriocarcinoma[84]
  Epithelioid hemangioendothelioma[85]

Fibrous histiocytoma[86]
Hemangiopericytoma[87]
Melanoma[88]
Metastatic carcinoma[89]
Osteogenic sarcoma[90]
Thyroid carcinoma[91]
**3. CARDIAC**
  Bacterial endocarditis[92]
  Congenital heart disease[93]
  Congestive heart failure[94]*
  Left ventricular pseudoaneurysm[95]
  Mitral stenosis[96]
  *Tumors*
  Angiosarcoma[97]
  Liposarcoma[93]
  Malignant fibrous histiocytoma[98]
**4. VASCULAR/EMBOLIC**
  Abdominal aortic aneurysm[99]
  Arteriovenous malformation
    Cirrhosis[100]
    Osler-Weber-Rendu[101]
    Systemic-to-pulmonary[102]
  Atresia of pulmonary veins[103]
  Bronchial artery rupture[104]
  Fat embolism[105]
  IVC absence[106]
  Pulmonary artery aneurysm[107]
    Behcet's syndrome[108]
    Hughes-Stovin syndrome[109]
    Mycotic[109]
  Pulmonary artery stenosis[111]
  Pulmonary embolism[112]
  Pulmonary hypertension[113]
  Septic emboli[114]
  Subclavian artery aneurysm[115]
  SVC syndrome[116]
  Thoracic aortic aneurysm[6]
  Tumor emboli[117]
**5. CONGENITAL**
  Cystic fibrosis[118]*
  Cystic lung disease[119]
  Duplication cyst[120]
  Pulmonary sequestration[121]
**6. TRAUMA**
  Pulmonary contusion[122]
  Pulmonary hematoma[122]
  Pulmonary laceration[122]
  Pulmonary pneumatocele[122]
  Thoracic splenosis[123]
  Tracheobronchial injury[124]
**7. IATROGENIC**
  Hickman catheter[125]
  Irradiation[126]
  Lymphangiography[127]
  Pulmonary artery catheter[128]
  Tracheostomy[129a]
  Transbronchial biopsy[130]
  Transthoracic needle aspirate[131]

## Table I
### (*continued*)

**8. SYSTEMIC DISEASES**
  Amyloidosis[130]
  Bullous Pemphigoid[131]
  Endometriosis[132]
  Goodpasture's syndrome[133]
  Idiopathic pulmonary hemosiderosis[134]
  Idiopathic rapidly progressive GN[126]
  Vasculitides and Collagen Vascular Disease
    Cryoglobulinemia[137]
    Hemolytic uremic syndrome[138]
    Henoch-Schönlein purpura[139]
    IgA nephropathy[140]
    Microscopic polyarteritis[141]
    Mixed connective tissue disease[142]
    Polyarteritis nodosa[127]
    Progressive systemic sclerosis[143]
    Rheumatoid arthritis[144]
    Systemic lupus erythematosis[145]
    Takayasu's arteritis[146]
    Wegener's granulomatosis[147]

**9. HEMATOLOGIC**
  DIC[148]
  Hemophilia[149]
  Leukemia[150]
  Thrombocytopenia[151]
  von Willebrand's disease[152]

**10. DRUGS/TOXINS**
  Amiodarone[153]
  Anticoagulants[154]
  Charcoal lighter fluid[155]
  Cocaine[156]
  Inhaled isocyanates[157]
  Liquor[158]
  Moxalactam[159]
  Oxyphenbutazone[151]
  Penicillamine[160]
  Thrombolysis[161]
  Trimellitic anhydride[162]

**11. MISCELLANEOUS**
  Broncholithiasis[163]
  Cryptogenic[164]*
  Foreign body aspiration[165]
  Gastric acid aspiration[166]
  Hypersensitivity pneumonitis[167]
  Lung torsion[168]
  Lymphangiomyomatosis[169]
  Pheochromocytoma[170]
  Pulmonary alveolar proteinosis[171]
  Sarcoidosis[172]
  Tracheoesophageal fistula[173]

**12. FACTITIOUS**
  Clofazimine[174]
  Malingering[24]
  Serratia marcescens[175]

* = common causes.
IVC = inferior vena caval; GN = glomerulonephritis; SVC = superior vena caval; DIC = disseminated intravascular coagulopathy.

## Table II
### Causes of Bronchiectasis

| Focal | Diffuse |
| --- | --- |
| Post-infectious | Cystic fibrosis |
|   Bacterial pneumonia | Ciliary Dyskinetic Syndromes (Kartagener's, Young's) |
|   Tuberculosis | Impairment of Humoral Defense |
|   Pertussis, measles, adenovirus |   Panhypogammaglobulinemia |
| Airway Obstruction |   Selective IgA or IgG subclass deficiency |
|   Neoplasm—benign or malignant |   Chronic granulomatous disease |
|   Foreign body | Congenital Disorders |
|   Enlarged lymph nodes |   Williams-Campbell syndrome |
| Allergic Bronchopulmonary Aspergillosis |   Alpha$_1$ antitrypsin deficiency |
| Recurrent Aspiration |   Mounier-Kuhn syndrome |
| |   Yellow nail syndrome |
| |   Ehler-Danlos syndrome |
| |   Marfan's syndrome |
| | Recurrent Aspiration |

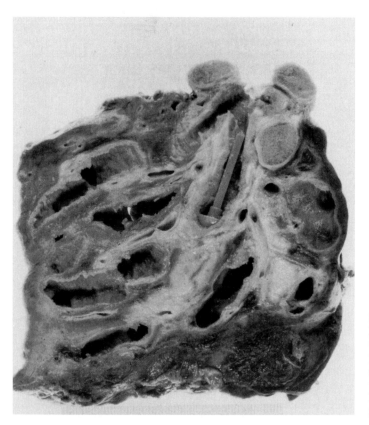

**Figure 1.** Severe right lower lobe bronchiectasis secondary to an inhaled foreign body. Note enlarged lymph nodes caused by chronic inflammation. Courtesy of Dr. B. Mullen, Mount Sinai Hospital, Toronto.

traditionally been one of the most common causes of hemoptysis.[178] However, recent series suggest its declining role.[179] This is partially due to earlier and better treatment of bacterial lung infections since the advent of antibiotic therapy. In bronchiectasis, the bronchial arteries proliferate and enlarge, forming new precapillary anastomoses with the pulmonary circulation.[180] These enlarged vessels are susceptible to injury from the products of local inflammation or repeated infections that characterize the disease (Figure 1).

Tuberculosis remains a prevalent cause of hemoptysis. Early in the course of the disease, hemoptysis may be caused by local mucosal ulceration and necrosis of adjacent bronchial vessels. Early bleeding during the course of tuberculous pneumonitis tends to be relatively minor. Later complications of tuberculosis that can cause hemoptysis include the development of bronchiectasis, broncholithiasis,

and chronic cavitary disease. Tuberculous lymph nodes calcify when healing. They may impinge on a bronchial wall and eventually erode into the bronchial lumen, causing streaky hemoptysis by disrupting vessels in the peribronchial and submucosal bronchial plexi.[181] Rarely, the hemoptysis may be massive if a larger bronchial artery lies in the path of the broncholith.[182] Histoplasmosis is the other common cause of broncholithiasis.

Hemoptysis accompanied by chronic tuberculous cavitary disease may be due to a Rasmussen's aneurysm or a mycetoma within a healed tuberculous cavity. Rasmussen described the incorporation of normal pulmonary vessels into expanding thick-walled tuberculous cavities.[40] Exposure of these vessels to the chronic inflammation of the tuberculous cavities weakens the elastic components of the vessels. The tuberculous organisms themselves invade the vessel adventitia and media caus-

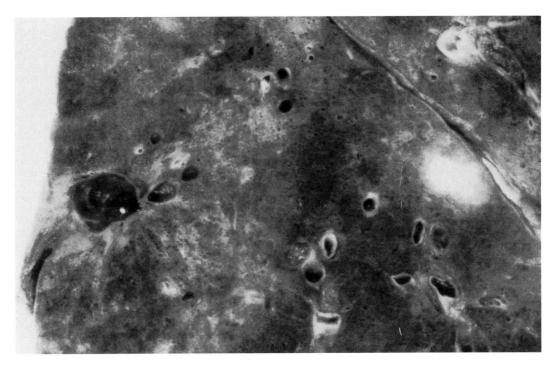

**Figure 2.** (a) Mycetoma in superior segment, left lower lobe cavity caused by chest tube trauma.

ing the vessel to become ectatic and to bulge into the lumen of the cavity. Eventually the vessel is eroded by inflammatory byproducts, which lead to massive, often fatal, hemorrhage.

Mycetomas, classically due to *Aspergillus* species, develop within any pre-existing cavity (Figure 2). The latter are most commonly due to tuberculosis but may also complicate histoplasmosis, sarcoidosis, vasculitis, emphysematous bulla, cavitary neoplasm, pulmonary fibrosis, lung abscess, bronchial cyst, asbestosis, ankylosing spondylitis, or pulmonary infarction.[52] Hemoptysis complicates the conditions of 50% to 85% of patients with aspergilloma and has an overall estimated incidence of 74%.[53] The pathogenesis of hemorrhage from a mycetoma remains unknown. Possible mechanisms include friction caused by movement of the fungus ball against the highly vascular wall of the cavity, direct vascular damage caused by endotoxin, or release of anticoagulant and trypsin-like proteolytic enzymes from the fungus.[183, 184]

Paragonimiasis is one of the leading causes of hemoptysis worldwide, particularly in southeast Asia, but is extremely rare in North America. Humans acquire the fluke by ingesting raw or undercooked crabs or shellfish. The adult parasite resides in 1- to 3-cm cystic spaces near large bronchioles or bronchi. Bronchial arteries adjacent to the cysts undergo hypertrophy, which may lead to hemoptysis as the cysts erode into a draining airway. Hemoptysis occurs in the majority of patients, but is irregular and rarely severe.[69, 70]

## Neoplasms

Hemoptysis is the presenting symptom in 7% to 10% of patients with bronchogenic carcinoma[83] but will eventually be seen in up to 60% of afflicted individuals.[185] There is an increase in the bronchial arterial blood flow to the region of the tumor, and local tumor necrosis or mucosal ulceration leads to mild, streaky hemoptysis. Approximately 10% of patients

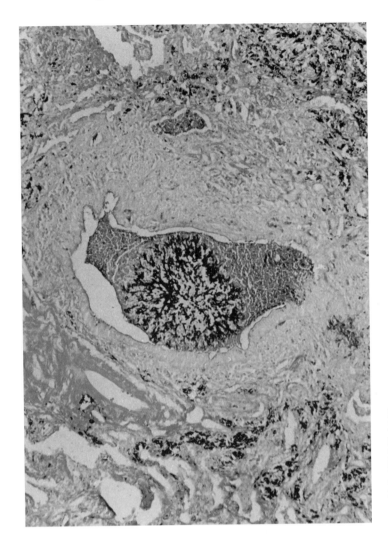

**Figure 2.** *(continued)* (b) high-power photomicrograph of cavity showing aspergillus hyphae with Gomori's Methenamine Silver stain (original magnification x400). Courtesy of Dr. B. Mullen, Mount Sinai Hospital, Toronto.

with bronchogenic carcinoma develop massive hemoptysis during the course of their disease.[83] The majority of these cases are due to cavitary squamous cell carcinoma or a tumor in the mainstem bronchus adjacent to a larger vessel.

Bronchial carcinoids account for approximately 5% of primary pulmonary neoplasms. They are extremely vascular tumors so that hemoptysis is seen as a presenting symptom in approximately one-third of cases, although the reported incidence varies widely.[186–188] Hemoptysis is more common with central, rather than peripheral, tumors.

## Cardiac

Congestive heart failure is a common cause of mild hemoptysis due to rupture of low-pressure pulmonary veins or capillaries distended by elevated intravascular pressure. Although it is now mostly of historical interest, mitral stenosis was a very important cause of hemoptysis. This symptom developed in up to 36% of patients before early detection and surgical therapy of mitral stenosis became common.[189] In this cardiac disease, high left atrial pressure can lead to a reversal of blood flow from the pulmonary circulation to the bronchial veins via the azygous and intercostal veins. The bronchial veins subsequently dilate and form submucosal varices in the bronchial walls which are prone to rupture.[190]

## Vascular/Embolic

Pulmonary embolism leads to hemoptysis in up to one-third of patients although this figure may rise to more than 50% in patients with pre-existing heart disease.[191–193] Hemoptysis in this setting implies infarction, congestive atelectasis, or hemorrhagic consolidation.[191, 192] Hemoptysis occurs more commonly in mild-to-moderate embolic disease as compared to massive emboli. Tissue infarction caused by septic emboli, vasculitis, or invasion of blood vessels by *Pseudomonas* or *Aspergillus* species may also lead to hemoptysis.[5] Infarction following pulmonary vascular obstruction is more common where there is concomitant reduced bronchial blood flow such as in congestive heart failure.[39] Pulmonary arteriovenous malformations are an uncommon cause of hemoptysis but are important to consider because of the propensity for massive bleeding. The majority that bleed are due to hereditary hemorrhagic telangiectasia (Osler-Weber-Rendu syndrome), are often multiple and are occasionally bilateral.[41, 194, 195] The fistulas may be supplied by more than one branch of the pulmonary artery. The draining veins distend and develop varicosities, leading to degenerative changes of the vessel walls. These, as well as the fistulas, are prone to rupture leading to hemoptysis in a minority of patients.

Aneurysms of the pulmonary arteries not only complicate tuberculosis but may be due to other bacterial and fungal diseases, congenital heart disease, Marfan's syndrome, vasculitis, pulmonary hypertension, trauma, or be an idiopathic illness.[107] They often present with hemoptysis which is a marker of instability of the lesion and a strong indicator of the need for intervention.[107]

## Congenital

Cystic fibrosis is the most common lethal genetic disease in Caucasians. Hemoptysis occurs in approximately 60% to 75% of cystic fibrosis patients and the risk of bleeding increases with age.[196, 197] There are numerous reasons for the high rate of hemoptysis in cystic fibrosis. The lungs are diffusely involved with pulmonary abscesses, bronchopneumonias, and bronchiectasis. There is an increase in vascularity of the bronchial circulation supplying the endobronchial and peribronchial circulation tissue as well as bronchopulmonary shunts in areas of bronchiectasis.[118] The frequent development of pulmonary arterial hypertension with age contributes to the risk of bleeding and may increase the incidence of massive hemoptysis.

## Trauma

Blunt chest trauma and penetrating injuries may both lead to hemoptysis. Pulmonary contusion results in hemorrhage and edema formation in the alveoli and interstitium but does not cause major parenchymal disruption and is rarely associated with hemoptysis. Pulmonary laceration, pulmonary hematoma, and traumatic pulmonary pneumatocele are all caused by blunt chest trauma and indicate varying degrees of damage to the pulmonary parenchyma or small bronchi.[122] Each is frequently complicated by hemoptysis, which in these cases is rarely severe. Injuries to the large airways are less common than parenchymal injuries and may initially be asymptomatic. Presenting symptoms early on may include hemoptysis, which may be massive in up to 14% of patients with penetrating trauma.[198]

Hemoptysis may follow a penetrating wound to the chest when there is a communication between the missile track and the bronchial tree.[5]

## Iatrogenic

Hemoptysis may complicate any of the procedures outlined in Table I, but iatrogenic causes are relatively rare. Pulmonary infarction following insertion of a pulmonary artery catheter was initially reported to occur in as many as 7.2% of cases,[199] but more recent studies have shown a much lower incidence of infarction ranging from 0% to 1.3%.[200, 201] Pulmonary artery rupture only occurs in 0.1% to 0.2% of patients,[200] but is catastrophic and usually rapidly fatal. Pulmonary arterial hypertension and recent cardiopulmonary bypass are recognized risk factors for this complication.

Hemoptysis following transbronchial biopsy was reported to be as high as 9% in some older series,[130] but more recent studies place the risk at approximately 2%.[202] Hemoptysis is usually mild and self-limited, however hemorrhage leading to exsanguination has been reported. Patients at increased risk for bleeding include those with thrombocytopenia and uremia, immunocompromised patients, and patients on positive-pressure ventilation. Minor hemoptysis occurs in up to 10% of percutaneous transthoracic needle biopsies but is rarely severe unless needles of 18 gauge or larger are used.[131] Risk factors for bleeding include coagulopathies, pulmonary hypertension, and use of a large-bore needle.

Tracheoarterial fistula is an unusual, but rapidly fatal, complication of tracheostomy if unrecognized.[129] It occurs following approximately 0.7% of tracheostomies.

### Systemic Disease

Numerous systemic diseases cause diffuse alveolar hemorrhage with hemoptysis as a prominent, presenting symptom. When no associated disease can be found, the term idiopathic pulmonary hemosiderosis is used [136]; however, a number of these patients later develop Goodpasture's syndrome[203] or evidence for a systemic vasculitis.[204] Anti-glomerular basement membrane antibody disease (Goodpasture's syndrome) is probably the most common of the alveolar hemorrhage syndromes to present with hemoptysis, which is the initial symptom in 80% of patients. The vast majority of these patients also have glomerulonephritis. The mechanism of damage to the alveolo-capillary basement membrane leading to alveolar hemorrhage has not yet been elucidated but may be due to antibody binding to shared epitopes on type IV collagen molecules in the lung and kidney.[205]

The alveolar hemorrhage associated with Wegener's granulomatosis, idiopathic rapidly progressive glomerulonephritis, systemic lupus erythematosus, and the various specific and nonspecific necrotizing vasculitides are immune-mediated and due to damage to capillaries, rather than larger vessels, in the lung.[206] Hemoptysis in these diseases is almost always associated with glomerulonephritis, but variable involvement of the skin, joints, nervous system, or gastrointestinal tract separates them from Goodpasture's syndrome.

Ectopic endometrial implants may lead to catamenial hemoptysis although the rare patient has coughed up blood unrelated to her menstrual period.[207] Usually patients present with recurrent hemoptysis within 48 to 72 hours of the onset of menses. Pelvic endometriosis need not be present. The ectopic implants most commonly involve distal pulmonary parenchyma but rarely are seen in major bronchi.[134] The implants may enter the thoracic cavity via retrograde flow from the fallopian tubes via diaphragmatic fenestrations, but more commonly arrive through lymphatic or hematogenous seeding in women who have undergone uterine manipulation.[134]

### Drugs/Toxins

Exogenous agents are very rarely the cause of hemoptysis. Some, such as penicillamine[160] or trimellitic anhydride,[162] may cause alveolar hemorrhage via possible immune mechanisms. Others, such as oxyphenbutazone, may lead to drug-induced thrombocytopenia, increasing the likelihood of hemoptysis.[151] By far the most common cause of drug-induced hemoptysis is the use of anticoagulants[154] or thrombolytic therapy.[161] Both of these classes of drugs are much more likely to lead to bleeding from puncture sites, the gastrointestinal tract, or the genitourinary tract than they are to cause occult alveolar hemorrhage. They more often cause hemoptysis in patients with pre-existing lung conditions, such as chronic bronchitis or bronchiectasis, who have a propensity to bleed anyway.[208] Aside from underlying pulmonary disease, pulmonary artery catheterization and pulmonary edema may increase the risk of anticoagulant-related or thrombolytic-related hemoptysis.

### Cryptogenic

Cryptogenic or idiopathic hemoptysis is the term used when no specific abnormalities can be found on physical examination, roentgenographic studies, or bronchoscopy. Some series report an incidence of idiopathic hemoptysis as high as 29% to 30%,[164, 209] but these include patients who most likely have chronic bronchitis with a recent infectious flare.[164] The true incidence of cryptogenic hemoptysis is probably closer to 10% to 15% of patients. Men are reported to have a higher incidence than women although recent series[164] do not support a gender preference. Generally, these patients have an excellent prognosis with clearing of the hemoptysis, although approximately 10% of patients continue to have intermittent episodes of small hemoptysis.[210] If initial investigations are negative 5-year survival for patients with cryptogenic hemoptysis is 85% to 95%.[164, 210–215]

## Massive Hemoptysis

Virtually all of the causes of hemoptysis listed in Table I can lead to massive bleeding. The most common causes of massive hemoptysis are listed in Table III. Tuberculosis, bronchiectasis from any cause, bronchogenic carcinoma, bronchitis, and lung abscess cause the vast major-

### Table III
#### Common Causes of Massive Hemoptysis

Bronchogenic carcinoma
Bronchiectasis
Bronchitis
Tuberculosis
Fungus ball
Pyogenic lung abscess
Cystic fibrosis

ity of massive hemoptysis.[7–22, 177] Idiopathic causes of massive hemoptysis are quite unusual and account for less than 5% of cases.[177] Massive hemoptysis is rare, accounting for only 1.5% to 4.5% of cases of hemoptysis,[2, 4] but, importantly, accounting for significant mortality. Patients are less likely to die from blood loss but are likely to asphyxiate, making the volume of hemoptysis less critical than the rate of blood loss.

The risk of massive hemoptysis is directly related to the pathogenesis of the bleeding in any particular disorder. Most patients with lung cancer have mild streaky hemoptysis due to local mucosal erosion. Patients with squamous cell carcinoma have almost 10 times the risk of massive hemoptysis than other patients with bronchogenic carcinoma. Lesions in these patients have a propensity to cavitate or be mainstem bronchial lesions that can erode into a larger, systemic artery.[83, 216] Certain diseases that are much less common than bronchogenic carcinoma have a much higher likelihood of causing massive hemoptysis when they bleed. As many as 25% of patients with aspergilloma will develop moderate-to-massive hemoptysis[217] and it is the cause of death in 2% to 26% of patients.[53] Other diseases with a relatively high risk for massive hemoptysis include cystic fibrosis,[118] lung abscess,[47] and broncholithiasis.[163]

## Diagnostic Approach

In approaching the patient with presumed hemoptysis, one must first ascertain that the blood is coming from the lower respiratory tract and then try to localize the site of bleeding. Standard evaluation includes a careful history and physical examination, some simple laboratory tests, a chest roentgenogram and, often, flexible fiberoptic bronchoscopy. Subsequent evaluation and therapy will be directed by clues obtained during the initial evaluation. When the patient is hemodynamically stable and bleeding at a rate slower than 200 mL/24 h, the workup can proceed at a more leisurely pace; however, in patients with massive hemoptysis the site of bleeding must be quickly and accurately established to allow immediate therapeutic intervention.

## History

Sources of bleeding other than the respiratory tract must be ruled out by asking questions about gingival disease, epistaxis, or problems in the larynx or pharynx. The features separating hemoptysis from hematemesis were originally suggested by Lyons[23] and are modified in Table IV. Coughing versus vomiting up blood is often helpful in separating these two entities; however, more excessive hemoptysis can cause nausea and retching by irritating pharyngeal receptors. Patients with brisk gastrointestinal hemorrhage, particularly from esophageal varices, often describe a sensation of blood welling up in the back of the throat with no true nausea, vomiting, or coughing. Rarely, patients sense a gurgling sensation in their chests and feel that they can localize the site of bleeding. In a study of 105 patients with hemoptysis, only 10 believed that they could localize the side of bleeding, and, of these, 7 were correct.[4]

Younger patients are more likely to have inflammatory conditions such as bronchiectasis or acute bronchitis accounting for their symptoms. Less than 1% of bronchogenic carcinomas occur in patients younger than 40 years; however, the possibility of metastatic germ cell tumors or bronchial adenomas must be kept in mind in these patients. Smoking history is important to consider because it predisposes to chronic bronchitis and bronchogenic carcinoma. The chronicity of the symptoms may be helpful, but can occasionally be misleading as in the case of a patient with chronic bronchitis who has developed lung cancer. Although hemoptysis is a common complaint in patients with bronchogenic carcinoma, it is rarely the initial symptom of the disease particularly when the tumor is more peripheral.[3] An acute onset of hemoptysis, chest pain, and fever suggests infection or infarction.

A description of the appearance of the sputum is occasionally helpful. Pink frothy sputum is seen in pulmonary edema. Gritty, white material mixed with blood suggests the possibility of broncholithiasis complicating tuberculosis or histo-

---

**Table IV**
Differentiating Hemoptysis from Hematemesis

| Hemoptysis | Hematemesis |
|---|---|
| Blood coughed | Blood vomited |
| Frothy blood | Not frothy blood |
| Often bright red blood | Usually dark colored blood |
| Blood-tinged sputum for days | No blood-tinged sputum |
| History of lung disease | History of stomach, esophageal, or liver disease |
| Alkaline pH | Acid pH |
| Blood mixed with macrophages, neutrophils, or bacteria | Blood mixed with food particles |
| Anemia uncommon | Anemia common |

plasmosis. Blood mixed with purulent sputum suggests an acute infection such as pneumonia or a chronic infection such as bronchiectasis. Occasionally, red sputum contains no blood but is due to an organism that produces red pigment such as Serratia,[175] expectoration of a drug containing red dye such as clofazimine,[174] or due to ingestion of red beets.

A history of hematuria suggests the presence of a vasculitic process or a systemic disease such as Goodpasture's syndrome. Bleeding from the gastrointestinal tract, genitourinary tract, the skin, or the nose often accompanies a major bleeding diathesis induced by anticoagulants, thrombocytopenia, or disseminated intravascular coagulation (DIC). A history of oral contraceptive use, which increases the risk for pulmonary embolic events, or narcotic abuse, which may lead to pulmonary edema or frank hemoptysis, should be ascertained.

Travel history is important to consider in determining exposure to various fungi, bacteria, protozoa, and mycobacteria that can lead to hemoptysis. For example, patients who have travelled to or come from Southeast Asia are at increased risk for developing tuberculosis, melioidosis, paragonimiasis, and strongyloidiasis. Patients from South America are more likely to be exposed to schistosomiasis and paracoccidioidomycosis, whereas patients from the southwest United States are more likely to be exposed to coccidioidomycosis. The timing of symptoms is occasionally helpful. Hemoptysis coinciding with menses suggests pulmonary endometriosis.[134] Hemoptysis developing during sexual intercourse suggests left ventricular dysfunction.[94] Hemoptysis developing after dental work or an alcoholic binge raises the possibility of aspiration of a foreign object.

Some of the important points of patient history are summarized in Table V.

## Physical Examination

A carefully performed, complete physical examination is mandatory. Spe-

### Table V
#### Hemoptysis—Important Points in Patient History

Age of Patient
History of smoking
History of gum, nose, laryngeal, or gastrointestinal disease
Patient localization of bleeding source
Appearance of sputum
History of hematuria
History of cardiopulmonary disease
Acute vs. chronic hemoptysis
History of drug/medication use
Travel history
Inhalation of foreign matter/recent dental work

cial attention should be paid to the nose, gums, and pharynx to exclude nonpulmonary bleeding sources. Nasal disease is frequently encountered in Wegener's granulomatosis. Telangiectasias on the lips or buccal mucosa may be seen in Osler-Weber-Rendu disease. Clubbing of the fingers and toes is seen in bronchiectasis, tuberculosis, lung abscess, bronchogenic carcinoma, cirrhosis, bacterial endocarditis, pulmonary arteriovenous malformations, and congenital heart disease.

Cardiovascular examination may reveal evidence for mitral stenosis or congestive heart failure. Extensive lymphadenopathy and hepatomegaly suggest lymphoma or metastatic malignancy. Diffuse ecchymoses, petechiae, and purpura may suggest an underlying coagulopathy or hematologic malignancy, but may also be seen secondary to collagen vascular diseases or vasculitic processes. The lower limbs are examined to look for signs of deep venous thrombosis such as edema, venous distension, and pain on forced dorsiflexion of the foot (Homans' sign). Unfortunately, these findings are neither sensitive nor specific, and clinical judgement is correct less than 50% of the time.

Examination of the lung fields is crucial but may occasionally be misleading. Localized wheezing suggests an endobronchial lesion, and stridor suggests an extrathoracic lesion. Localized inspiratory crackles suggest focal airspace disease, but

**Table VI**
Hemoptysis: Laboratory Evaluation

Complete blood count, platelet count
Coagulation studies
Urinalysis
Sputum for AFB, fungus, bacteria, and parasites
Sputum cytology
BUN, creatinine
ANA, rheumatoid factor, serum complement
Anti-glomerular basement membrane antibodies
Antineutrophil cytoplasmic antibodies

AFB = acid-fast bacillus; BUN = blood urea nitrogen;
ANA = antinuclear antibody.

may be secondary to pneumonitis caused by aspirated blood in an area separate from the primary disorder. Pursel and Lindskog determined that focal physical findings were helpful in localizing the bleeding site in 45 of 105 patients with hemoptysis, but findings were misleading in 2 patients and not helpful or equivocal in 58 patients.[4] Therefore, although frequently helpful in determining the cause of hemoptysis, physical examination is often unreliable in localizing the site of bleeding, which often requires more invasive investigations.

## Laboratory Evaluation

Table VI lists some of the routine and less common laboratory tests that may be helpful in elucidating the cause of hemoptysis. The use of these tests should be guided by clues obtained on history and physical examination.

The complete blood count may reveal evidence for unexpected anemia as may occur in Goodpasture's syndrome or idiopathic pulmonary hemosiderosis; a leukocytosis in acute infection; or leukopenia as part of an underlying hematologic malignancy or systemic lupus erythematosus. The platelet count may be low due to drug ingestion, hematologic disease, or collagen vascular disease. A coagulation profile is necessary to rule out a generalized bleeding disorder that may lead to hemoptysis.

The urinalysis and renal function studies may be abnormal in any of the pulmonary-renal syndromes that lead to alveolar hemorrhage[218] including bacterial endocarditis[219] and *Legionella pneumophila* infection.[49]

Sputum for cytology, gram-stain, acid-fast bacilli, and mycobacterial cultures should be performed in most cases, but examination of the sputum for fungi, ova, and parasites should only be done if a history of travel to a relevant area is obtained. Expectorated sputum gram-stain for bacteria is only helpful if it shows overwhelming numbers of one morphotype in areas of excessive numbers of neutrophils. Blood for antiglomerular basement membrane and antineutrophil cytoplasmic antibodies should be obtained when Goodpasture's syndrome, Wegener's granulomatosis, or polyarteritis are clinically suspected.

## Chest Roentgenogram

The chest roentgenogram is the single most important initial investigation in patients with hemoptysis. A well-penetrated posteroanterior (PA) film and left lateral film are required to visualize the lung fields and the proximal tracheobronchial tree. Roentgenographic evaluation will be normal in 20% to 30% of patients with hemoptysis.[220–223] Other patients may have bilateral lesions and therefore the source of hemoptysis cannot be localized in up to 40% of patients with this clinical complaint.[4] In addition, one must be careful about attributing the hemoptysis to the roentgenographic abnormality. Bronchoscopy may occasionally reveal bleeding sources separate from the area of radiographic abnormality.[143, 178, 224] Nonetheless, the chest roentgenogram remains an invaluable tool in the evaluation of the patient with hemoptysis.

Hemoptysis in a patient with a normal chest roentgenogram should raise the possibility of a large airway lesion, such as carcinoma, bronchial adenoma, amyloidosis, or small angiomas. Iatrogenic or systemic causes of coagulopathies may also

**Table VII**
Hemoptysis with Cavitary Lesions

| | |
|---|---|
| *Infectious* | *Thromboembolic* |
| Bacteria |     Cavitary pulmonary infarct* |
|     Lung abscess |     Septic emboli |
|     Meliodosis | *Congenital* |
|     Mycobacterium |     Bronchial cyst* |
| Fungal |     Pulmonary sequestration* |
|     Aspergillosis (invasive) | *Trauma* |
|     Coccidiodomycosis |     Pulmonary laceration* |
|     Histoplasmosis | *Vasculitis* |
|     Paracoccidiodomycosis |     Wegener's granulomatosis* |
|     Sporotrichosis | |
| Parasitic | |
|     Amebiasis | |
|     Echinococcus | |
|     Paragonimiasis | |
|     Strongyloidosis | |
| *Neoplastic* | |
|     Bronchogenic carcinoma* | |
|     Metastatic malignancy* | |

\* = may become secondarily infected.

cause hemoptysis in patients with normal roentgenograms and may increase the risk of bleeding from pre-existing chronic bronchitis or bronchiectasis.[208]

Various diseases can present with hemoptysis and cavitary or cystic lesions on chest roentgenogram (Table VII). Infectious causes are more common in younger people, particularly if they are from an appropriate endemic area. Aspergillomas do not cause cavitation, but are a common cause of hemoptysis following colonization of a pre-existing cavity (Figure 3). On the other hand, cavitation often precedes the start of massive hemoptysis in patients with invasive pulmonary aspergillosis.[225] Malignancy is more common in elderly patients; although metastatic testicular carcinoma and melanoma may present as cavitary hematogenous metastases causing hemoptysis. Of the primary lung neoplasms, squamous cell carcinoma is most likely to cavitate, adenocarcinoma and large-cell carcinomas are less likely to cavitate, and small-cell carcinomas cavitate rarely, if ever.

Multiple nodules suggest hematogenous spread of malignancy, septic emboli, granulomatous disease, or Wegener's granulomatosis.

Hilar and mediastinal adenopathy are seen most commonly in malignancy but may be present in infectious diseases or amyloidosis.

Diffuse, ground-glass opacities, especially if sparing the apices and costophrenic angles, suggest alveolar hemorrhage, but are hardly diagnostic for this condition.

Occasionally, a feeding vessel to an arteriovenous malformation or a calcification suggesting a broncholith can be seen on chest roentgenogram.

A pleural-based density in a patient with chest pain and new hemoptysis should raise the possibility of pulmonary embolism with infarction.

Thick, dilated bronchi with air fluid levels may be seen in patients with bronchiectasis. However, this does not necessarily correlate with the site of bleeding because the airway lesions are often more extensive than suggested by plain roentgenograms and the bleeding source is often not localized without more invasive procedures.

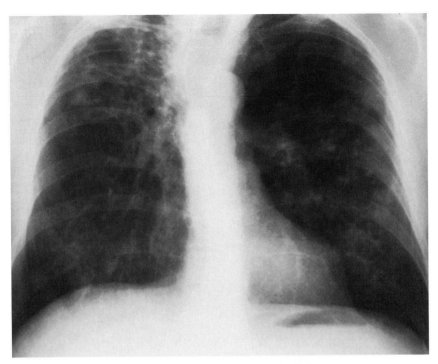

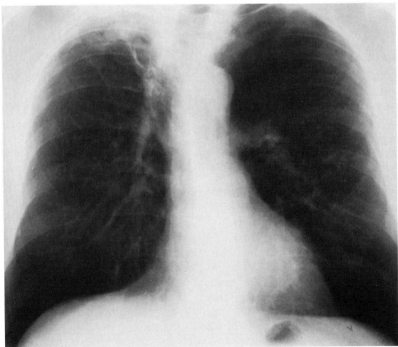

**Figure 3.** A 54-year-old man with previous history of nontuberculous mycobacterium infection. (a) Posteroanterior (PA) chest roentgenogram showing irregular, thin-walled, right upper lobe cavity with adjacent airspace disease. (b) Posteroanterior chest roentgenogram 3 years later, at time of hemoptysis, showing right upper lobe cavitary lesion with adjacent solid density.

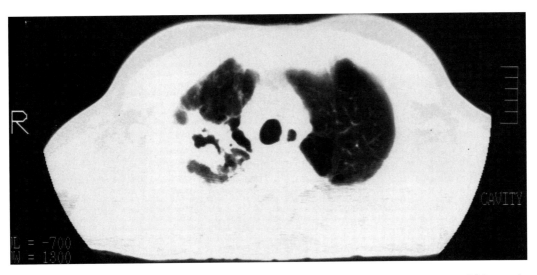

**Figure 3.** *(continued)* (c) Computed tomography (CT) scan showing mycetoma within cavity with characteristic air crescent or meniscus sign. Courtesy of Dr. M. Steinhardt, Mount Sinai Hospital, Toronto.

The presence of Kerley B lines and cardiac enlargement suggest congestive heart failure.

## Bronchoscopy

Bronchoscopy is the procedure of choice for localizing the bleeding source within the lung and often for providing a specific diagnosis. The major questions associated with the use of bronchoscopy are (1) Does everybody with hemoptysis require the procedure? (2) Should a fiberoptic or rigid scope be used? and (3) Should bronchoscopy be performed early or late? There is a great debate about which patients with hemoptysis do not require bronchoscopy. Clearly, patients with acute infarction or infection diagnosed by other means do not require bronchoscopy. Weaver and colleagues suggested four low-risk groups of patients that can safely forego bronchoscopy.[220] The first group consists of patients with strong clinical evidence for nonneoplastic pulmonary disease, such as bronchiectasis. The concern when applying the same rationale to patients with chronic bronchitis is that this is the same group at risk of developing bronchogenic carcinoma so that a high level of suspicion must be maintained in the face of a changing clinical picture. A recent survey of physicians attending a national conference determined that 91% would bronchoscope a 55–year-old, heavy smoker with a 1-week history of hemoptysis and a nonlocalizing chest roentgenogram.[226] This is due to the discovery of bronchogenic carcinoma in 3% to 11% of patients with hemoptysis and a normal or nonlocalizing chest roentgenogram.[164, 209, 212–214, 227–229] The second group comprises patients with documented extrapulmonary source or sources of bleeding. The third group of patients are those whose clinical state is so poor that no action will be taken no matter what is found on bronchoscopy. The availability of localized bronchoscopic techniques as well as radiologic interventions to, at least, temporarily control bleeding should make this a very small group. The fourth and last group of patients are those younger than 40 years old who have had mild hemoptysis lasting less than 1 week. The debate in this latter group is the most contentious.

Despite the fact that bronchogenic carcinoma is quite rare in younger age groups, approximately 0.8% do occur in patients younger than 40 years of age.[230] The younger the patient was when starting smoking as well as the total amount smoked increases the risk of bronchogenic carcinoma.[230] The value of performing bronchoscopy in virtually all patients with unexplained hemoptysis lies not only in detecting an occult, potentially resectable neoplasm, but also in providing useful prognostic information. Patients with normal or nonlocalizing chest roentgenograms and nondiagnostic bronchoscopy have an excellent prognosis with only a very small chance of developing a lung malignancy.[164, 213, 227] This may not be true in older, men smokers.[214]

The issue of flexible versus rigid bronchoscopy appears to be due to a difference of opinion between thoracic surgeons and pulmonologists. Older, primarily surgical, series tended to promote the use of the rigid bronchoscope,[4, 9, 13, 14, 16, 22, 231–233] whereas more recent, primarily medical series, preferred the use of the flexible fiberoptic bronchoscope.[164, 178, 209, 212–214, 226, 227, 234, 235] There has never been a head-to-head comparison of these two techniques; therefore, it is difficult to be dogmatic about recommendations regarding their usage. Both have distinct advantages and disadvantages and occasionally a combination of both procedures is helpful.[236] The major advantages of the rigid bronchoscope include its large lumen ensuring airway control and room to introduce packing materials or even a fiberoptic scope, in addition to providing excellent suctioning capability. This is of greatest importance in the case of massive hemoptysis, extensive necrotic tissue within the airways, or for removal of foreign objects causing hemoptysis. The major problems with the rigid scope include the need for patient transport to the operating room, use of a general anesthetic with its inherent risks, and visual range limited to only the major airways.

The advantages of the flexible fiberoptic bronchoscope include its portability so that procedures can be done at the bedside if necessary, use of local rather than general anesthetic, and greatly improved visualization of the airways. Nonetheless, the flexible scope can usually only be passed to the fourth generation and, occasionally, up to the sixth generation airways so that the source of hemoptysis cannot always be found and other techniques must be used (eg, chest computed tomography [CT] scan). The major disadvantage to the flexible bronchoscope is that its suction capability is limited and does not always guarantee good control of the airway. More frequently, the tip of the scope becomes obscured by blood. One potential solution is to intubate patients who are actively bleeding, both to gain control of the airway and to allow repeated removal and re-insertion of the scope to clean the viewing tip. With fiberoptic bronchoscopy, isolated bronchoalveolar lavage can be performed and may be particularly useful in diagnosing various infectious lung diseases. On the basis of the above discussion, I believe that the flexible fiberoptic scope has become the instrument of choice in evaluating hemoptysis[226] although the rigid scope still has an important role to play, particularly in patients with massive hemoptysis.

When should bronchoscopy be carried out? Initial concerns were raised about the use of rigid bronchoscopy during or shortly after moderate-to-massive bleeds because of the risk of aggravating or renewing bleeding.[221] The two issues to be considered are whether early bronchoscopy, as compared with delayed bronchoscopy, increases the diagnostic accuracy of the test and if the improved diagnostic capability changes management or affects survival. Only three studies have directly compared early (within 24 to 48 hours of onset) versus delayed bronchoscopy. Pursel and Lindskog were able to identify the site of bleeding in 86% of patients undergoing early rigid bronchoscopy as compared to only 52% of patients undergoing delayed bronchoscopy.[4] Using flexible fiberoptic bronchoscopy, others were able to localize bleeding in 34% to 91% of patients undergoing early procedures and only 11% to 50% of patients in whom bronchoscopy was delayed.[209, 237] Other series in which only early bronchoscopy was carried out identified the source of bleeding in 68% to 100% of patients.[7, 16, 178, 234] These data suggest an improved diagnostic rate if bronchoscopy is carried out during active bleeding. The risk of aggravating bleeding appears to be small, although one should be careful not to disturb a forming clot because this may precipitate massive hemorrhage.

There is some debate about the importance of making an early diagnosis. Despite the fact that Gong and Salvatierra noted a significant improvement in diagnostic yield with early versus late bronchoscopy, they felt that this rarely altered patient management.[209] However, earlier diagnosis and localization may allow for therapeutic interventions that improve short-term outcome.[22]

## Computed Tomography

The development of newer generation, high-resolution CT scanners has virtually rendered the roles of lung tomography and bronchography obsolete in evaluating chest disease. Nonetheless, the role for CT scanning for evaluating patients with hemoptysis remains unclear. Computed tomography has been shown to be superior to plain roentgenograms in detecting both airway and parenchymal lesions (Figure 3).[238,239]

Early comparisons of CT and fiberoptic bronchoscopy suggested that CT was inferior in predicting the nature of endobronchial mucosal abnormalities.[240] Although recent studies have shown comparable results between the two, bronchoscopy remains superior in identifying central lesions.[241–243] A number of studies have compared CT scanning versus bronchoscopy in the evaluation of patients with hemoptysis.[244–248] Summarizing the results is difficult because of different underlying diseases, use of both regular- and thin-cut CT scans, and different outcome measurements. Computed tomography scanning has the ability to pick up many abnormalities not detected on plain roentgenograms and after bronchoscopy,[249] although it is argued that this rarely influences patient outcome or management strategies.[244] More recent series suggest an expanding role for CT.

Millar and colleagues[246] performed CT in 40 patients with hemoptysis, normal chest roentgenograms, and normal fiberoptic bronchoscopy. They found abnormalities in 50% of the patients. Bronchiectasis was discovered in 7 patients, 4 of these patients had parenchymal abnormalities—2 of which due to underlying malignancy—and 3 patients had arteriovenous malformations.

Despite the fact that the authors concluded that CT should precede bronchoscopy to direct the procedure, there is little evidence that CT significantly affected outcome in the group as a whole. Similar findings and conclusions using high-resolution CT scans were made by McGuiness and colleagues.[248] They found that the diagnostic yield of CT scans was 61% compared to 43% for bronchoscopy. In addition, they discovered a specific cause for hemoptysis in 50% of patients with nondiagnostic bronchoscopy. The major value of CT scanning appears to be the detection of a peripheral malignant nodule amenable to surgical resection. However, the presence of an occult malignancy is quite low, approximating 1% to 8%, in the population with cryptogenic hemoptysis following evaluation by fiberoptic bronchoscopy.[164, 210–215]

In my opinion, patients who are actively bleeding should be referred directly to bronchoscopy to identify the bleeding site rather than be delayed until a CT scan is performed. In the time taken to perform the CT scan the active bleeding may cease, decreasing the diagnostic yield of the bronchoscopy.[4, 209, 237] In addition, early CT scan results may be misleading by directing bronchoscopy to an area of aspirated blood separate from the primary lesion. Bronchoscopy is superior to CT in diagnosing localized mucosal abnormalities such as bronchitis, telangiectasias, early carcinoma, squamous metaplasia, benign papillomas, and Kaposi's sarcoma. The major role for CT is in the nonactively bleeding patient with a normal or nondiagnostic chest roentgenogram. It is superior to bronchoscopy in the diagnosis of bronchiectasis (Figure 4), aspergilloma (Figure 3), broncholithiasis and peripheral carcinoma, and, in certain cases, may obviate the need for bronchoscopy or help direct the procedure to a previously unsuspected, involved part of the lung.

## Bronchography

Bronchography is mostly of historical interest given the development of high resolution CT scanning and fiberoptic bronchoscopy.[250] It is an excellent technique for demonstrating bronchiectasis although it is technically demanding and difficult for patients to tolerate. It is of no value during active hemoptysis because the intraluminal contrast may lead to hypoxemia and airflow obstruction, further aggravating the problems induced by blood in the airways.[251] In addition, results of bronchography performed during acute bleeding may be misleading because clots within the airways may be misinterpreted as endobronchial lesions. Bronchography previously had a major role in detecting and defining the extent of bronchiectasis and particulary in planning surgical resections of involved areas. Earlier reports stated that CT was inferior to bronchography in detecting bronchiectasis, particularly of the cylindric and varicose type[252, 253]; however, more recent series conclude that its less invasive nature and improved resolution make CT scanning the procedure of choice (Figure 5).[254–256] Bronchography remains slightly more sensitive than CT, particularly for limited bronchiectasis[257, 258]; but it is only very rarely requested prior to surgery and is now obsolete in the investigation of hemoptysis.

## Radionuclide Scanning

Initial studies in dogs suggested that bleeding rates as low as 0.1 mL/min could be detected with technetium-labelled sulfur colloid.[259] Studies in humans have shown less consistent results even with higher rates of bleeding, and this technique has rarely been shown to add any information to that obtained by bronchoscopy.[260, 261] False-positive results may be seen with rib pathology, increased bone marrow production, and increased reticuloendothelial activity of the pulmonary capillary bed. Use of radio-labelled red blood cells may help to localize the bleeding site but requires active bleeding at a rate of at least 6 mL/min.[262] In addition, time is required to label the erythrocytes, which may delay the time to diagnostic bronchoscopy. Radionuclide studies should be reserved for situations where CT scanning is unavailable and patients are too ill for bronchoscopy.

Ventilation-perfusion scintigraphy remains the screening procedure of choice in assessing patients with hemoptysis for pulmonary embolism. Despite its approximately 98% sensitivity in detecting pulmonary embolism, the specificity of an abnormal scan is only around 10% so that other investigations, such as noninvasive studies of the deep veins of the thigh or pulmonary angiograms, are frequently required.[263] The major value of the ventilation-perfusion scan is that it can exclude the diagnosis of pulmonary embolism with a high degree of certainty with a normal scan and diagnose emboli with 97% specificity in patients with a high-probability scan.[263]

Radionuclide angiography can be used to detect the presence of a right-to-left shunt in cases of pulmonary arteriovenous malformations.[264] However, a positive result is not specific for these disorders nor does it help localize the abnormality if small. Therefore, it has no role in the evaluation of patients with hemoptysis.

## Bronchial Angiography

The major role of angiography is in planning therapeutic embolization in some patients with hemoptysis. Occasionally, angiography may provide diagnostic information when the site of bleeding has not been localized when using the combination of bronchoscopy and simpler radio-

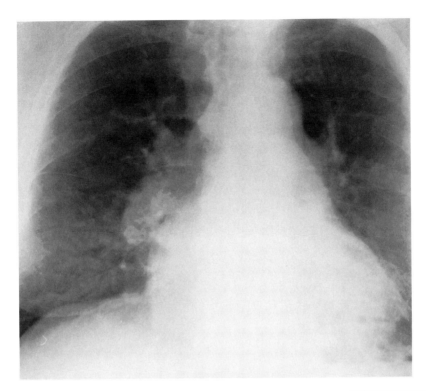

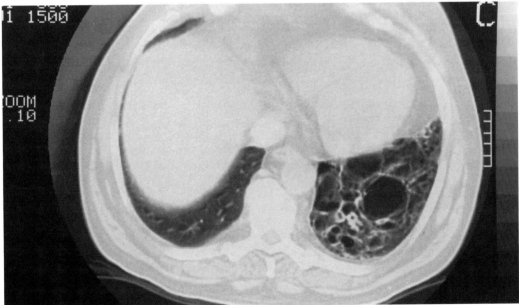

**Figure 4.** A 65-year-old male with recurrent purulent sputum and hemoptysis. (a) Posteroanterior (PA) chest roentgenogram showing increased interstitial markings in both lower lobes. (b) Computed tomography (CT) scan revealing extensive, cystic bronchiectasis in left, lower lobe. Courtesy of Dr. M. Steinhardt, Mount Sinai Hospital, Toronto.

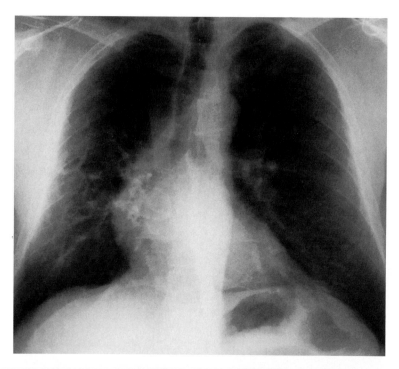

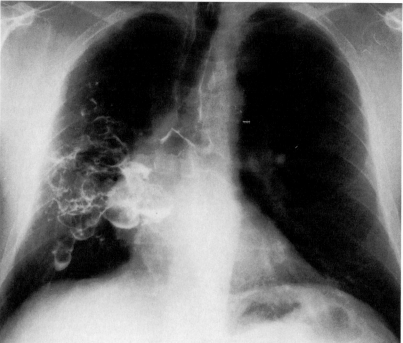

**Figure 5.** A 48-year-old man with hemoptysis. (a) Posteroanterior (PA) chest roentgenogram revealing cystic changes in the right mid-lung field. (b) Bronchogram showing huge, saccular bronchiectasis predominantly in the middle lobe and superior segment of the right lower lobe.

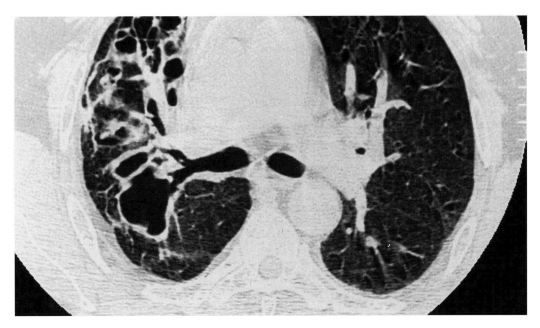

**Figure 5.** *(continued)* (c) Computed tomography (CT) scan 19 years later showing extensive cystic bronchiectasis in the right middle and lower lobes with pleural thickening. Courtesy of Dr. M. Steinhardt, Mount Sinai, Toronto.

logic techniques. Hemoptysis represents bleeding from the bronchial arterial system in the majority of cases; therefore, bronchial angiography is usually the initial angiographic procedure. The angiographic features of abnormal bronchial arteries were reviewed by Roberts[265] and include (1) hypertrophy, with increased number, size, and tortuosity of branches, and increased vascularity; (2) systemic-to-pulmonary shunting; (3) occasionally, bronchial artery aneurysms; and (4) very rarely, extravasation of contrast into the pulmonary parenchyma (Figure 6). This is the only pattern providing direct evidence of a bleeding site.

Complications of bronchial arteriography alone are uncommon if the procedure is carefully performed by an experienced invasive radiologist. Injection of contrast into a bronchial artery may trigger coughing, which potentially may worsen hemoptysis. Cases of transverse myelitis have been reported with the use of nonionic contrast material,[266] but this risk is minimized with the use of low-osmolality contrast material.

Katoh and colleagues compared the bronchoscopic and angiographic features of bronchial artery lesions.[267] They found that an intrabronchial bulge corresponded to a vascular aneurysm and an intrabronchial mass corresponded to a hypervascular area on angiography. They cautioned about the potential for massive or fatal hemorrhage if one of these lesions are brushed or biopsied. Because they only studied seven patients, they could not recommend the use of routine bronchial angiography prior to bronchoscopy. Occasionally bleeding arises from nonbronchial systemic collateral vessels, such as the subclavian, axillary, intercostal, or phrenic arteries. This may rarely be responsible for massive hemoptysis.[268]

## Pulmonary Angiography

Approximately 10% of cases of hemoptysis arise from pulmonary arterial causes. This most commonly happens in the case of pyogenic lung abscess, tubercu-

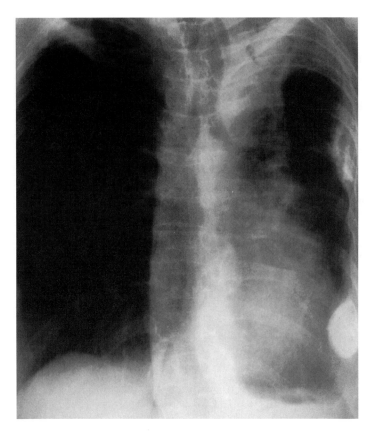

**Figure 6.** A 65-year-old woman with a history of tuberculosis treated with recurrent pneumothorax therapy 39 years previously presents with massive hemoptysis. (a) Posteroanterior (PA) chest roentgenogram showing left-sided pleural thickening and calcification. Tomograms (not shown) did not reveal a cavitary lesion.

losis complicated by Rasmussen's aneurysm formation, pulmonary arteriovenous malformations (Figure 7), or the rare case of pulmonary artery tears.[269] One of these risk factors or failure to control the bleeding following bronchial artery embolization therapy should lead to consideration of pulmonary angiography if embolization therapy is felt to be practical.[270]

The other pulmonary arterial source of bleeding is from pulmonary embolism. Pulmonary angiography is the gold standard for diagnosis, although false-negative results are reported in approximately 1% of cases.[271] The use of pulmonary angiography in the diagnosis of pulmonary embolism should be reserved for patients in whom the diagnosis is still in doubt following ventilation/perfusion scanning and noninvasive studies of the leg veins.

## Miscellaneous Tests

Pulmonary function testing has no role in specifically diagnosing the cause of hemoptysis but measurement of the diffusion capacity may help detect alveolar hemorrhage.[272] Erythrocytes in the alveolar spaces and interstitium will bind inhaled carbon monoxide so that serial measurements of the diffusion capacity allow for monitoring of alveolar hemorrhage. Lack of baseline values, particularly in patients with other diseases that reduce diffusion capacity (eg, emphysema) can make

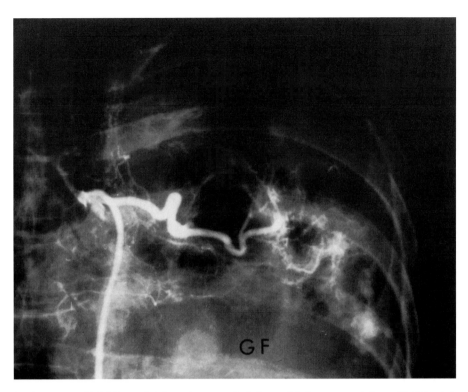

**Figure 6.** *(continued)* (b) Bronchial angiogram. Left bronchial artery, arising off of the intercostal artery, shows serpiginous, hypervascular branches and extravasation of dye, which is pathognomonic for active bleeding. Bleeding was subsequently controlled by the injection of Gelfoam particles. Courtesy of Dr. KW. Sniderman, The Toronto Hospital, Toronto.

interpretation of the results difficult. In addition, some patients with alveolar hemorrhage are too ill to perform the diffusion capacity measurement.

Echocardiography is helpful in diagnosing left ventricular dysfunction and valvular lesions, although these are usually readily apparent by the time the underlying problem is severe enough to precipitate hemoptysis. Contrast echocardiography can be useful in diagnosing the presence of right-to-left shunting but rarely can make a specific diagnosis of pulmonary arteriovenous malformation.[273]

Percutaneous needle aspiration biopsy is a very valuable procedure for determining the cause of a peripheral nodule recognized radiographically but beyond reach of the bronchoscope.[131] The technique is particularly good for diagnosing

malignancy but does not frequently give a specific diagnosis in benign diseases except for some infections and hamartoma. Before performing this procedure, it must be determined that the nodule is not an arteriovenous malformation. Complications of needle biopsy include pneumothorax, severe enough to require chest tube drainage in 1% to 10% of patients, bleeding, air embolism, and the potential for tumor seeding.[274]

## Management Algorithm

An algorithm summarizing the diagnostic and therapeutic approach to the patient with hemoptysis is presented in Figure 8.

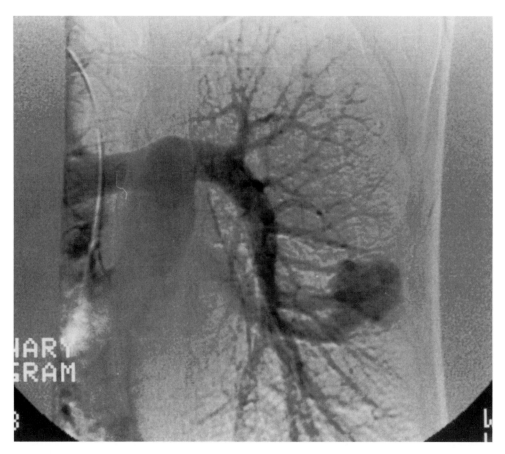

**Figure 7.** Digital subtraction pulmonary angiography showing left lower lobe pulmonary arterio-venous malformation. Courtesy of Dr. M. Asch, Mount Sinai Hospital, Toronto.

## Treatment

The main objectives of therapy in patients with hemoptysis include preventing aspiration and asphyxiation, localizing the site of bleeding, determining the primary cause, and stopping the bleeding. Certain general supportive measures apply to most patients and specific therapies vary from antibiotic therapy to surgical resection. The amount and rate of bleeding determines the rapidity and order of both investigations and therapy. An overview of the therapeutic approach is outlined in Table VIII.

### General Measures

Patients who cough up more than 20 mL of blood should be placed on bed rest. If the site of the bleeding is known, patients should be placed with the involved lung down to minimize aspiration into the normal lung. The role of sedatives and cough suppressants is contentious. Although violent coughing that may dislodge formed clots and worsen bleeding should be controlled with low doses of narcotics such as codeine, significant depression of the cough reflex should be avoided unless the patient is intubated. Other measures to prevent increases in intrathoracic pressure, such as stool softeners to prevent straining and avoidance of chest physiotherapy, make theoretical sense although their true importance is not known.

Patients with massive hemoptysis should be admitted to an intensive care unit and consultation with experts in pulmonary medicine, thoracic surgery, and

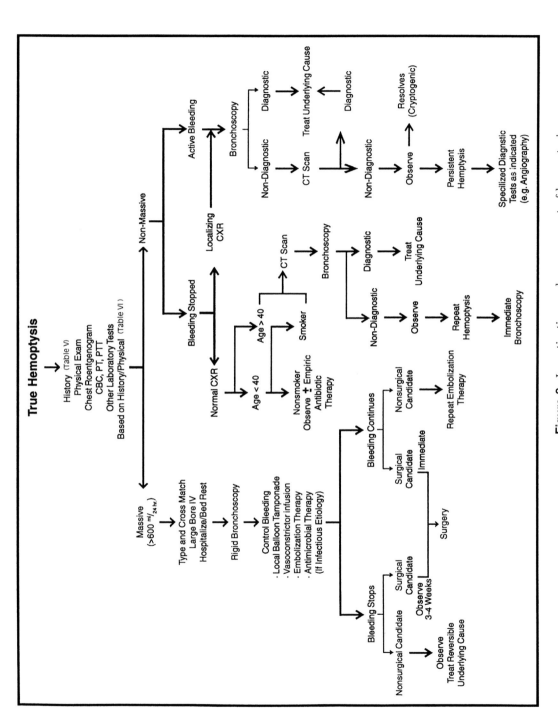

**Figure 8.** Investigation and management of hemoptysis.

**Table VIII**
Treatment of Hemoptysis

General Measures
  Bed rest with bad side down
  Fluid resuscitation
  Correct coagulopathy
  Oxygen supplementation
  Cough suppression—mild
  Stool softeners
  Endotracheal intubation—single vs double
    lumen
Topical Treatments
  Balloon bronchial tamponade
  Cold saline lavage
  Topical coagulants, vasoconstrictors
  Laser therapy
  Positive end-expiratory pressure (PEEP)
  Radiation therapy
Pharmacologic Therapy
  Antibiotics
  Steroids
  Vasoconstrictors—vasopressin,
    desmopressin
  Antifibrinolytic Agents
Interventional radiology
  Bronchial artery embolization
  Other systemic artery embolization
  Pulmonary artery embolization
Surgery
  Lobectomy
  Pneumonectomy
  Cavernostomy
  Mitral valve repair/commissurotomy

interventional radiology be considered. Any associated coagulopathy or thrombocytopenia should be corrected with the use of fresh frozen plasma and platelets, respectively. Large-bore venous access for fluid resuscitation should be standard for patients with moderate-to-massive hemoptysis. Arterial blood gases or oxygen saturation should be carefully monitored and oxygen supplementation titrated accordingly. Patients who cannot protect their airways, or in whom rapid hemoptysis is continuing and the risk of aspiration is high, should be intubated with a number 8 or larger endotracheal tube. This allows for subsequent bronchoscopy through the tube.

Some physicians routinely advocate placing a double-lumen Carlen's tube to allow the two lungs to be isolated and ventilated separately. However, because the tube is difficult to insert, the procedure occasionally requires the patient to be under general anesthesia. Additionally, the tube has a small, internal lumen that makes suctioning difficult and bronchoscopy impossible.[231] Once bleeding has been lateralized by bronchoscopy, a Carlen's tube can be placed to protect the unaffected lung. Even in this setting the small lumen may be blocked by clot and blood may still be aspirated into the normal lung.[17] A newer plastic double-lumen tube (Broncho cath, Mallinckrodt Inc.), which is somewhat easier than a Carlen's tube to insert and has a larger internal diameter allowing insertion of either a 14F suction catheter or a 4.8 mm diameter bronchoscope, has been introduced but its role remains undefined.[275]

If the patient is intubated, applying positive-end expiratory pressure (PEEP) of 20 cm $H_2O$ may decrease bleeding by lessening the pressure gradient between the pulmonary artery and the airway.[276] Stoller suggests that PEEP is most likely to help control hemoptysis when bleeding is coming from the low-pressure pulmonary arterial system.[277]

## Topical Bronchoscopic Measures

The bronchoscope is not only useful in localizing the bleeding site but can be used to help tamponade bleeding directly or guide instillation of either mechanical or pharmacological products to stop bleeding.

### Local Infusion Therapy

Hemorrhage induced by bronchoscopy brushing or biopsy is usually mild and can easily be stopped by tamponade of the bleeding site with the bronchoscope and/or infusion of 2 to 3 cc of 1:10,000 to 1:20,000 dilutions of epinephrine.[130, 278] Conlan and colleagues advocate instillations of 50 mL aliquot of cold saline (4°C) to arrest massive bleeding.[13, 231, 232] The presumed mechanism is similar to that exerted by epinephrine, that is, local vasoconstriction reducing blood flow and promoting subsequent hemostasis.

### Topical Coagulants

Attempts at increasing local hemostasis have led to trials of intrabronchial instillation of thrombin,[279, 280] fibrinogen-thrombin,[280, 281] fibrin precursors,[282] and various enzymes derived from snake venom.[283, 284] These procedures have been successful in 60% to 100% of patients; however, the numbers have been very small and endobronchial instillation therapy should only be considered when patients are too ill to undergo surgical therapy and local expertise in bronchial embolization therapy is not available.

### Balloon Tamponade

Use of mechanical tamponade has been practiced for years initially with rigid bronchoscope-guided packing of the bronchus with sponges.[285] Subsequently, use of Fogarty catheters inserted via the fiberoptic bronchoscope became popular and has been shown to be effective in temporarily controlling hemorrhage.[286–290] Generally, a 4F catheter can be inflated in a lobar or segmental bronchus and left in place for up to 24 hours. Use of a smaller pulmonary artery balloon catheter has been advocated to stop bleeding in subsegmental bronchi and, theoretically, to cause less gas exchange abnormalities than the larger Fogarty catheters.[291] The pulmonary artery catheter was left inflated for 48 hours with no mucosal damage noted. Recently a new double-lumen balloon catheter specifically designed to control airway hemorrhage was developed and reported to successfully control bleeding in 19 of 20 patients, although no further details were provided.[292]

## Laser Therapy

Photocoagulation with the neodymium-yttrium-aluminum-garnet (Nd-YAG) laser has been used to control bleeding in patients with massive hemoptysis from endobronchial tumors.[293, 294] Because of brisk bleeding, clots, and necrotic tumor, this procedure should only be done through a rigid bronchoscope.

## Pharmacologic Measures

Treatment of the underlying cause should be the primary goal once the patient with hemoptysis is stabilized. This includes the use of antibiotics for bacterial and mycobacterial infections as well as for therapy of flares of bronchiectasis. Exacerbations of chronic bronchitis should be treated with bronchodilators, antibiotics, and systemic steroids (see Chapter 3, Wheeze).

The use of steroids has been shown to reduce bleeding in patients with alveolar hemorrhage,[295] although occasionally the addition of immunosuppressive drugs, particularly for Wegener's granulomatosis, or plasmapheresis for Goodpasture's syndrome, is required.[295] Treatment of patients with immune alveolar hemorrhage should begin before the underlying disease is specified because of the high morbidity and mortality associated with the presentation. Therapy with pulse methylprednisolone (1 gram daily for 3 days) should be promptly initiated.[290] For patients who also have evidence of glomerulonephritis, it is reasonable to add cyclophosphamide (2 to 3 mg/kg) and consider a trial of plasmapheresis pending the results of specific antibody testing (eg, anti-glomerular basement membrane) and a kidney biopsy.

Similar to its use in controlling bleeding from esophageal varices, vasopressin at an infusion rate of 0.2 to 0.4 U/min has been used to temporarily control hemoptysis.[296] It functions as a potent systemic arterial vasoconstrictor agent and, as such, may cause problems in patients with underlying coronary artery disease or hypertension. In addition, if therapeutic bronchial artery embolization is planned, vasopressin may prevent angiographic visualization of the vessels.[297] Bilton and colleagues used a combination of desmopressin (DDAVP) and vasopressin to control hemoptysis in a patient with cystic fibrosis.[298] Desmopressin has the added advantage of being a procoagulant by virtue of its effects on von Willebrand's factor and plasminogen activator release from endothelial cells; however, it is a weaker vasoconstrictor agent than vasopressin.

Percutaneous intracavitary injection with various antifungal agents including sodium iodide, nystatin, and amphotericin B has been reported to be helpful in the therapy of pulmonary aspergillomas.[299, 300] Success rates of approximately 76% in controlling hemoptysis have been achieved,[300] although the long-term results have not been well studied and do not appear to be nearly as good. Shapiro and colleagues also infused N-acetylcystine with Amphotericin in an attempt to clear the mass of fungus, fibrin, mucus, and blood making up the mycetoma.[299]

Damaged lung tissue has been reported to release fibrinolysis activators which may worsen hemoptysis.[301] Therefore, a number of authors have suggested adding an antifibrinolytic agent, such as aminocaproic acid to treat hemoptysis caused by mycetoma[299] or tranexamic acid in combination with topical fibrin precursor therapy.[282]

## Radiation

A single case report describes a patient with massive hemoptysis from an aspergilloma in whom bleeding was controlled with 2000 rads of external beam radiotherapy fractionated over 7 days.[302] A subsequent recurrence 2 months later was controlled with an additional 1000 rads. The authors hypothesized that radiation caused swelling, necrosis, and endothelial cell hyperplasia leading to thrombosis and subsequent fibrosis of vessels.

## Embolization Therapy

Over the past 20 years, therapeutic embolization therapy has consistently been proven to give excellent short-term control of moderate-to-massive hemoptysis. Interventional radiologists may target bronchial arteries, other systemic vessels, or pulmonary arteries.

### Bronchial Artery Embolization

Remy and colleagues introduced the technique of bronchial artery embolization in 1974 and reported their first large series of 104 patients in 1977.[297] Forty-nine patients were treated during active bleeding, and of these, 84% had immediate arrest of bleeding. Of these, 15% had recurrent hemoptysis within 2 to 7 months from the initial procedure. Longer periods of follow-up, albeit in a smaller group of patients, revealed a recurrence rate of 27%.[31] A review of large, recent series reveals success rates of approximately 90% to 100% in immediately controlling hemorrhage, early recurrence in 5% to 14% of patients, (many are amenable to repeat procedures) and late recurrence in up to 23% of patients followed for up to 5 years.[20, 265, 270, 297, 303, 304]

Bronchial embolization therapy is primarily reserved for patients with massive hemoptysis, but should also be considered for patients with chronic, bilateral inflammatory diseases, such as cystic fibrosis or bronchiectasis, that are likely to bleed recurrently and cannot be resected; for patients with poor pulmonary reserve who could not tolerate resection of lung tissue; and for patients with multiple bleeding sites. Operative cure, although advocated as the procedure of choice by some, has as high as a 33% mortality if performed during a period of active hemoptysis.[17] Therefore, bronchial embolization therapy is a particularly attractive alternative for short-term stabilization of the underlying inflammatory cause and allows for surgical resection of localized disease at a later date when the patient is in better physiologic shape. In patients with moderate-to-massive hemoptysis in whom the bleeding source is unclear following initial workup bronchial arteriography can serve not only as a diagnostic test but can play a therapeutic role as well (Figure 6).[270] There are many different types of embolic material that can be used including liquids, powder, sponges, and coils. The material used should be tailored to the specific clinical situation. In the case of chronic inflammatory diseases, one wants to occlude peripherally because proximal occlusion will allow distal bleeding secondary to extensive bronchial and mediastinal collaterals. Therefore coils are avoided because they cause central occlusion and preclude re-embolization in the future.

Materials that occlude too distally may cause necrosis of the bronchial or pulmonary arterial wall by passing into excessively small vessels within the capillary bed, thereby compromising the bronchopulmonary collaterals.[305] These substances include liquids, such as alcohol and isobutyl-2 cyanoacrylate, or fine Gelfoam powder. Gelfoam particles are useful for embolization (Figure 6). However, they are reabsorbed by the body, which allows for recanalization that in turn may contribute to rebleeding. Polyvinyl alcohol (Ivalon) has become the particulate matter of choice for bronchial embolization. It has low antigenicity, is relatively nonbiodegradable, and produces long-term vascular occlusion with minimal recanalization or inflammation.[265]

Initial causes of failure of bronchial embolization therapy include (1) extensive, bilateral disease with repeated episodes of hemoptysis; (2) technical difficulties, such as inability to visualize or cannulate the bronchial vessels or takeoff of the anterior spinal artery from the bronchial artery, contraindicating embolization therapy (technical failures can occur in 4 to 13 of attempted embolization [20, 31, 297]); and (3) bleeding from other systemic collateral vessels or from the pulmonary arterial system.[306]

Recurrence of hemoptysis following initial successful embolization is due to (1) incomplete embolization due to unrecognized systemic collaterals; (2) recanalization of the embolized vessels; or (3) progression of the underlying disease.[306]

Rare complications of bronchial artery embolization include paralysis from embolization of branches of the spinal artery,[29] transverse myelitis,[266] cough, and mainstem bronchus necrosis.[305] Complications related to embolization of material too distally or reflux of embolic material into the systemic circulation include esophagobronchial fistula[31] and bowel, renal, arm, or leg ischemia.[265, 277] Fortunately, these are all exceptionally rare. A very common side effect of bronchial artery embolization therapy that may last for 2 to 7 days is the so-called "postembolization syndrome," which includes retrosternal pain, dysphagia, intercostal pain, and fever.[265]

## Systemic Collateral Embolization

If hemoptysis persists after the initial bronchial embolization attempt, a search should begin for nonbronchial systemic collaterals to the diseased lung. These are more likely to be present in chronic inflammatory diseases such as tuberculosis and mycetomas. Nonbronchial systemic collaterals may be the major source of hemoptysis in patients who have undergone previous embolization therapy.[268] They may originate from the phrenic, intercostal, internal mammary, thyrocervical, and other branches of the subclavian and axillary arteries.[265, 268] A thoracic aortogram will pick up most systemic arterial collaterals to the lung.

## Pulmonary Artery Embolization

The pulmonary arterial tree may be the source of hemoptysis in less than 10% of cases.[269] Therefore, when bronchial and systemic collateral angiography has failed to locate the bleeding site or embolization therapy has not controlled the hemoptysis, a pulmonary angiogram should be performed. When a pulmonary arterial source of bleeding is discovered embolization or balloon occlusion therapy has been successful in abolishing hemoptysis.[20, 269, 270, 307]

## Surgery

Surgery has an important role to play in the management of hemoptysis, but the questions of which patients benefit from surgery and when the surgery should be performed remain unanswered. Most series addressing the role of surgery look at early results in patients with massive hemoptysis.[7, 9–18, 21, 22, 308, 309] It is very difficult to compare results from one center to the next because of different definitions for massive hemoptysis and different underlying diseases. Nonetheless, of all patients in the above-mentioned studies, 469 patients were treated surgically and 406 were treated medically. Overall mortality in the surgically treated group was a mean of 13% (range 0% to 33%) and in the medically treated group it was 30% (range 18% to 85%). Series that reported good survival in medically treated groups generally defined massive hemoptysis as 150 to 200 cc/day,[7, 10, 12, 18, 22] whereas series with poor nonsurgical outcomes defined massive hemoptysis as greater than 600 cc/day.[9,14,15,17] It is important to note that none of these series were randomized so that the decision to operate or not was often based on other patient characteristics. Therefore, patients with poor pulmonary reserve, inoperable diseases or diffuse bleeding were often placed in the nonsurgical group. It only makes sense that their mortality would be very high. In fact, some series looked separately at surgical candidates who were managed medically and found mortality rates of only 1.6% to 11%,[7, 11] although the number of patients falling into these subsets was relatively small. The rate and initial control of bleeding were also important in surgically treated patients. Patients who continued to bleed briskly at the time of surgery had a 37% mortality compared to 8% in patients whose bleeding had stopped or was minimal by the time of the operation.[17]

Patients who survive surgery have a high rate of major postoperative complications. In the series where complication rates were able to be evaluated, 41% of patients had major complications,[10, 12, 17, 21, 309] The most common postoperative complication was a persistent bronchopleural fistula, occurring in 10% to 14% of patients and often requiring surgical repair.[217] Other, less common, complications included postoperative hemorrhage, empyema, hemothorax, wound infection, pulmonary infarction, and respiratory failure leading to prolonged mechanical ventilation. The latter was more likely to occur in patients with poor pulmonary reserve. Ideally, one would like to have some idea of pre-operative pulmonary function and limit resection to patients who will have predicted postoperative forced expiratory volume in 1 second ($FEV_1$) of greater than 0.8 L. Unfortunately, patients requiring emergency surgery can rarely perform pulmonary function tests.

In some of the series reporting good short-term survival in patients treated nonsurgically, there was a high incidence of rebleeding. Knott-Craig and colleagues[22] found that more than 36% of patients treated medically had recurrent hemoptysis during a 6–month follow-up. Mortality among those patients who re-bled was 45%. None of the surgically treated patients in their series re-bled during the 6-month follow-up.

One of the major limitations, aside from lack of randomization, of the studies comparing medical to surgical therapy is the fact that medical therapy did not include interventional radiology and often did not include local attempts at endobronchial tamponade. Given that (1) the very successful short-term results now reported with embolization therapy[20, 265, 297, 303, 304]; (2) the early recurrence of bleeding of up to 45% in medically treated patients[22]; (3) the late recurrence of bleeding in up to 23% of patients undergoing embolization therapy; and (4) the higher mortality rate in patients undergoing emergency versus elective surgery,[22] some general guidelines to the therapy of massive hemoptysis can be stated. Patients should be stabilized medically and bleeding controlled with local balloon tamponade or embolization therapy, or both. Underlying bronchiectasis or infectious diseases should be treated with appropriate antimicrobial therapy and the patients pre-operative medical status optimized. If localized disease amenable to surgical resection is responsible for the hemoptysis, the patient should be brought back to hospital within the next few weeks for curative surgery assuming that he or she has sufficient pulmonary reserve to withstand either a lobectomy or pneumonectomy. A recent preliminary report tends to support this type of approach.[310] Emergency surgery should be carried out when embolotherapy is not available, technically unfeasible, or has failed in the patient with massive hemoptysis. Other situations where emergency surgery may be appropriate include trauma,[198] and iatrogenic rupture of the pulmonary artery.[128]

Two other surgical approaches are mostly of historic interest. Gourin and Garzon[14, 17] described the technique of cavernostomy for patients with poor pulmonary reserve and large cavitary lesions. The cavity is opened to allow cauterization of bleeding sites and is then packed. Bronchocutaneous fistula is a common complication of this approach and frequently requires thoracoplasty to close the fistula.[14] Massive hemoptysis due to mitral stenosis should be treated with emergent mitral commissurotomy[192] or valve replacement.[311]

## References

1. Chaves AD. Hemoptysis in chest clinic patients. Am Rev Tuberc 1951;63:194–201.
2. Johnston RN, Lockhart W, Ritchie RT. Hemoptysis. Br Med J 1960;1:592–595.
3. Moersch HJ. Clinical significance of hemoptysis. JAMA 1952;148:1461–1465.
4. Pursel SE, Lindskog GE. Hemoptysis: a clinical evaluation of 105 patients examined consecutively on a thoracic surgical service. Am Rev Respir Dis 1961;84:329–336.
5. Wolfe JD, Simmons DH. Hemoptysis: diagnosis and management. West J Med 1977;127:383–390.
6. Coblontz CL, Sallee DS, Chiles C. Aorto-bronchopulmonary fistula complicating aortic aneurysm: diagnosis in four cases. AJR 1988;150:535–538.
7. Bobrowitz ID, Ramakrishna SD, Shim Y-S. Comparison of medical v surgical treatment of major hemoptysis. Arch Intern Med 1983;143:1343–1346.
8. Ehrenhaft JL, Taber RE. Management of massive hemoptysis not due to pulmonary tuberculosis or neoplasm. J Thorac Cardiovasc Surg 1955;30:275–287.
9. Crocco JA, Rooney JJ, Fankushen DS, et al. Massive hemoptysis. Arch Intern Med 1968;121:495–498.
10. Yeoh CB, Hubaytor RT, Ford JM, et al. Treatment of massive hemoptysis in pulmonary tuberculosis. J Thorac Cardiovasc Surg 1967;54:503–510.
11. Corey R, Hla KM. Major and massive hemoptysis: reassessment of conservative management. Am J Med Sci 1987;294:301–309.
12. Amirana M, Frater R, Tirschwell P, et al. An aggressive surgical approach to significant hemoptysis in patients with pulmonary tuberculosis. Am Rev Respir Dis 1968;97:187–192.
13. Conlan AA, Hurwitz SS, Krige L, et al. Massive hemoptysis: review of 123 cases. J Thorac Cardiovasc Surg 1983;85:120–124.
14. Garzon AA, Gourin A. Surgical management of massive hemoptysis. A ten year experience. Ann Surg 1978;187:267–271.
15. Sehhat S, Oreizie M, Moindedine K. Massive pulmonary hemorrhage: surgical approach as choice of treatment. Ann Thorac Surg 1978;25:12–15.
16. Garzon AA, Cerruti MM, Golding ME. Exsanguinating hemoptysis. J Thorac Cardiovasc Surg 1982;84:829–833.
17. Gourin A, Garzon AA. Operative treatment of massive hemoptysis. Ann Thorac Surg 1974;18:52–60.
18. Yang CT, Berger HW. Conservative management of life-threatening hemoptysis. Mt Sinai J Med 1978;45:329–333.
19. Stern RC, Wood RE, Boat TF, Mathews LW, et al. Treatment and prognosis of massive hemoptysis in cystic fibrosis. Am Rev Respir Dis 1978;117:825–828.
20. Rabkin, JE, Astafjev VI, Gothman LN, et al. Transcatheter embolization in the

management of pulmonary hemorrhage. Radiology 1987;163:361–365.

21. McCollum WB, Mattox KL, Guinn GA, et al. Immediate operative treatment for massive hemoptysis. Chest 1975; 67: 152–155.

22. Knott-Craig CJ, Oostuizen JG, Rossouw G, et al. Management and prognosis of massive hemoptysis: recent experience with 120 patients. J Thorac Cardiovasc Surg 1993;105:394–397.

23. Lyons HA. Differential diagnosis of hemoptysis and its treatment. Basics of RD 1976;5:26–30.

24. Baktari JB, Tashkin DP, Small GW. Factitious hemoptysis: adding to the differential diagnosis. Chest 1994;105:943–945.

25. Elliott FM, Reid L. Some new facts about the pulmonary artery and its branching pattern. Clin Radiol 1965;16:193–198.

26. Junod AF. Metabolism, production and release of hormones and mediators in the lung. Am Rev Respir Dis 1975;112: 93–108.

27. Baile EM, Ling H, Heyworth JR, et al. Bronchopulmonary anastomotic and noncoronary collateral blood flow in humans during cardiopulmonary bypass. Chest 1985;87:749–754.

28. Pump KK. The bronchial arteries and their anastomoses in the human lung. Dis Chest 1963;43:245–255.

29. Cauldwell EW, Seikert RG, Lininger RE, Anson BJ. The bronchial arteries: an anatomic study of 150 human cadavers. Surg Gynecol Obstet 1948;86:395–412.

30. Liebow AA. Patterns of origin and distribution of the major bronchial arteries in man. Am J Anat 1965;117:19–32.

31. Uflacker R, Kaemmerer A, Picon PD, et al. Bronchial artery embolization in the management of hemoptysis: technical aspects and long-term results. Radiology 1985; 157:637–644.

32. Deffebach ME, Charan NB, Lakshminarayan S, et al. The bronchial circulation: small, but a vital attribute of the lung. Am Rev Respir Dis 1987;135:463–481.

33. Murara K, Itoh H, Todo G, et al. Bronchial venous plexus and its communication with pulmonary circulation. Invest Radiol 1986;21:24–30.

34. Wagenvoort CA, Wagenvoort N. Arterial anastomoses, bronchopulmonary arteries, and pulmobronchial arteries in perinatal lungs. Lab Invest 1967;16:13–24.

35. Tobin CE. The bronchial arteries and their connections with other vessels in the human lung. Surg Gynecol Obstet 1952; 95:741–750.

36. Turner-Warwick M. Precapillary systemic-pulmonary anastomoses. Thorax 1963;18:225–237.

37. Mills NL, Boyd AD, Gheranpong C. The significance of bronchial circulation in lung transplantation. J Thorac Cardiovasc Surg 1970;60:866–878.

38. Tabakan BS, Hanson JS, Adhikari PK, et al. Physiologic studies in congenital absence of the left main pulmonary artery. Circulation 1960;22:1107–1111.

39. Tsao M-S, Schraufnagel D, Wang N-S. Pathogenesis of pulmonary infarction. Am J Med 1982;72:599–606.

40. Rasmussen V. Hemoptysis, especially when fatal, in its anatomical and clinical aspects. Edinb Med J 1868;14:385–404.

41. Burke CM, Safai C, Nelson DP, et al. Pulmonary arteriovenous malformation: a critical update. Am Rev Respir Dis 1986; 134:334–339.

42. Thoms NW, Wilson RF, Puro HE, et al. Life-threatening hemoptysis in primary lung abscess. Ann Thorac Surg 1972;14: 347–358.

43. Bartter T, Irwin RS, Phillips DA, et al. Pulmonary artery pseudoaneurysm: a potential complication of pulmonary artery catheterization. Arch Intern Med 1988; 148:471–473.

44. Moll HH. A clinical and pathological study of bronchiectasis. Q J Med 1932;25: 457–469.

45. Hamer DH, Schwab LE, Gray R. Massive hemoptysis from thoracic actinomycosis successfully treated by embolization. Chest 1992;101:1442–1443.

46. Turner JS, Wilcox PA. Respiratory failure in leptospirosis. Q J Med 1989;72: 841–847.

47. Philpott NJ, Woodhead MA, Wilson AG, et al. Lung abscess: a neglected cause of life threatening haemoptysis. Thorax 1993;48:674–675.

48. Reyes MP. The aerobic gram-negative bacillary pneumonias. Med Clin NA 1980; 64:363–383.

49. Case Records of the Massachusetts General Hospital. Case 17–1978. N Engl J Med 1978;298:1014–1021.

50. Le HQ, Sapico FL, Davidson PT. Pulmonary melioidisis. Semin Respir Med 1991; 12:28–34.

51. Musher DM, McKenzie SO. Infections due to Staphylococcus aureus. Medicine (Baltimore) 1977;56:383–409.

52. Van Kralingen KW, Hekker TAM, Bril H, et al. Haemoptysis and an abnormal x-ray after prolonged treatment in the ICU. Eur Respir J 1994;7:419–420.

53. Glimp RA, Bayer AS. Pulmonary aspergilloma: diagnostic and therapeutic considerations. Arch Intern Med 1983;143:303–308.

54. Rinald MG. Invasive aspergillosis. Rev Infect Dis 1983;5:1061–1077.

55. Masur H, Rosen PP, Armstrong D. Pulmonary disease caused by candida species. Am J Med 1977;63:914–925.

56. Case Records of the Massachusetts General Hospital. Case 21–1994. N Engl J Med 1994;330:1516–1522.

57. Kerkering TM, Duma RJ, Shadomy S. The evolution of pulmonary crypotococcosis: clinical implications from a study of 41 patients with and without compromising host factors. Ann Intern Med 1981;94:611–616.

58. Barenfanger J, Ramirez F, Tewari RP, et al. Pulmonary phaeohyphomycosis in a patient with hemoptysis. Chest 1989;95:1158–1160.

59. Wheat LJ, Slama TG, Eitzen HE, et al. A large urban outbreak of histoplasmosis: Clinical features. Ann Intern Med 1981;94:331–337.

60. Bigby TD, Serota ML, Tierney LM Jr, et al. Clinical spectrum of mucormycosis. Chest 1986;89:435–439.

61. Bethlem NM, Lemle A, Bethlem E, et al. Paracoccidioidomycoses. Semin Respir Med 1991;12:81–97.

62. Alture-Werber E, Edberg SC, Singer JM. Pulmonary infection with Allescheria boydii. Am J Clin Pathol 1976;66:1019–1024.

63. Pluss JL, Opal SM. Pulmonary sporotrichosis: review of treatment and outcomes. Medicine (Baltimore) 1986;65:143–153.

64. Ibarra-Perez C. Thoracic complications of amebic abscess of the liver: report of 501 cases. Chest 1981;70:672–677.

65. Fraser RG, Paré JAP, Paré PD, et al. Diagnosis of diseases of the chest. Philadelphia: W.B. Saunders Company. Third Edition. 1989:1097.

66. Gelpi AP, Mustafa A. Ascaris pneumonia. Am J Med 1968; 44:377–389.

67. Goodman ML, Gore I. Pulmonary infarct secondary to dirofilaria larvae. Arch Intern Med 1964;113:702–705.

68. Xanthakis D, Efthimiadis M, Papadakis G, et al. Hydatid disease of the chest: report of 91 patients surgically treated. Thorax 1972;27:517–528.

69. Barrett-Connor E. Parasitic pulmonary disease. Am Rev Respir Dis 1982;126:558–563.

70. Nana A, Bovornkitti S. Pleuroplumonary paragonimiasis. Semin Respir Med 1991;12:46–54.

71. Mascarenhas DAN, Vasudevan VP, Vaidya KP. Pneumocystis carinii pneumonia: rare cause of hemoptysis. Chest 1991;99:251–253.

72. Shimazu C, Pien FD, Parnell D. Bronchoscopic diagnosis of Schistosoma japonium in a patient with hemoptysis. Respir Med 1991;85:331–332.

73. Bruno P, McAllister K, Mathews JI. Pulmonary strongyloides. South Med J 1982;75:363–365.

74. Prince DS, Peterson DD, Steiner RM, et al. Infection with Mycobacterium Avium complex in patients without predisposing conditions. N Engl J Med 1989;321:863–868.

75. Plessinger VA, Jolly PN. Rasmussen's aneurysm and fatal hemorrhage in pulmonary tuberculosis. Am Rev Tuberc 1949;60:589–603.

76. Shamsuddin D, Tuazon CU. Massive hemoptysis caused by Mycobacterium xenopi. Tubercle 1984;65:201–204.

77. Louria DB, Blumenfield HL, Ellis JT, et al. Studies on influenza in the pandemic of 1957–1958. II. Pulmonary complications of influenza. J Clin Invest 1959;38:213–265.

78. Davidson RN, Lynn W, Savage P, et al. Chickenpox pneumonia: experience with antiviral treatment. Thorax 1988;43:627–630.

79. Davila DG, Dunn WF, Tazelaar HD, et al. Bronchial carcinoid tumors. Mayo Clin Proc 1993;68:795–803.

80. Kleinman J. Zirkin H, Feuchtwanger MM, et al. Benign hamartoma of the lung presenting as massive hemoptysis. J Surg Oncol 1986;33:38–40.

81. Mittelman M, Fink G, Mor R, et al. Inflammatory bronchial polyps complicated by massive hemoptysis. Eur J Respir Dis 1986; 69:63–66.

82. Holden WE, Morris JF, Antonovic R, et al. Adult intrapulmonary and mediastinal lymphangioma causing haemoptysis. Thorax 1987;42:635–636.

83. Miller RR, McGregor D. Hemorrhage from carcinoma of the lung. Cancer 1980;46:200–205.

84. Benditt JO, Farber HW, Wright J, et al. Pulmonary hemorrhage with diffuse alveolar infiltrates in men with high-volume choriocarcinoma. Ann Intern Med 1988;109: 674–675.

85. Carter EJ, Bradburne RM, Jhung JW, et al. Alveolar hemorrhage with epithelioid hemangioendothelioma: a previously unreported manifestation of a rare tumor. Am Rev Respir Dis 1990;142:700–701.

86. Case Records of the Massachusetts General Hospital. Case 14–1994. N Engl J Med 1994;330:997–1002.

87. Yousem S, Hochholzer L. Primary pulmonary hemangiopericytoma. Cancer 1987; 59:549–555.

88. Bagwell SP, Flynn SD, Cox PM, et al. Primary malignant melanoma of the lung. Am Rev Respir Dis 1989;139:1543–1547.

89. Baumgartner WA, Mark JBD. Metastatic malignancies from distant sites to the tracheobronchial tree. J Thorac Cardiovasc Surg 1980;79:499–503.

90. Fitzgerald RH. Endobronchial metastases. South Med J 1977;40:440–441.

91. Weiland JE, de los Santos ET, Mazzaferri EL, et al. Hemoptysis as the presenting manifestation of thyroid carcinoma: a case report. Arch Intern Med 1989; 149: 1693–1694.

92. Cosmo LY, Risi G, Nelson S, et al. Fatal hemoptysis in acute bacterial endocarditis. Am Rev Respir Dis 1988;137: 1223–1226.

93. Black MD, Masters RG, Walley VM, et al. Hemoptysis:two unusual causes. Can J Cardiol 1990;6(1)27–30.

94. Bansal S, Day JA Jr, Braman SS. Hemoptysis during sexual intercourse: unusual manifestation of coronary artery disease. Chest 1988;93:891–892.

95. Adkins MS, Laub GW, Pollock SB, et al. Left ventricular pseudoaneurysm with hemoptysis. Ann Thorac Surg 1991;51: 476–478.

96. Wood P. An appreciation of mitral stenosis. I. Clinical features. Br Med J 1954;1: 1051–1063.

97. Zwaveling JH, Teding van Berkhout F, Hanevald GT. Angiosarcoma of the heart presenting as pulmonary disease. Chest 1988;94:216–218.

98. Dinardo-Ekery D, Lau K-Y, Spicer MJ, et al. Malignant fibrous histiocytoma of the heart presenting as hemoptysis: association with pseudothrombocytopenia. Chest 1988;93:1099–1100.

99. Villar MT, Wiggins J, Corrin B, et al. Recurrent and fatal haemoptysis caused by an atheromatous abdominal aortic aneurysm. Thorax 1990;45:568–569.

100. Rydell R, Hoffbauer FW. Multiple pulmonary arteriovenous fistulas in juvenile cirrhosis. Am J Med 1956;21:450–460.

101. Hodgson CH, Kaye RL. Pulmonary arteriovenous fistula and hereditary hemorrhagic telangiectasia: a review and report of 35 cases of fistula. Dis Chest 1963;43: 449–455.

102. Powels HMM, Janevski BK, Penn OCKM, et al. Systemic to pulmonary vascular malformation. Eur Resp J 1992;5: 1288–1291.

103. Cabrera A, Vazquez C, Lekuona I. Isolated atresia of the left pulmonary veins. Int J Cardiol 1985;7:298–302.

104. Sheffield EA, Moore-Gillon J, Murday AR, et al. Massive hemoptysis caused by spontaneous rupture of a bronchial artery. Thorax 1988;43:71–72.

105. Benatar SR, Ferguson AD, Goldschmidt RB. Fat embolism-some clinical observations and a review of controversial aspects. Q J Med 1972;41:85–98.

106. Ashour MH, Jain SK, Kattan KM, et al. Massive haemoptysis caused by congenital absence of a segment of inferior vena cava. Thorax 1993;48:1044–1045.

107. Bartter T, Irwin RS, Nash G. Aneurysms of the pulmonary arteries. Chest 1988;94: 1065–1075.

108. Salamon F, Weinberger A, Nili M, et al. Massive hemoptysis complicating Behcet's syndrome: the importance of early pulmonary angiography and operation. Ann Thorac Surg 1988;45:566–567.

109. Hughes JP, Stovin PGI. Segmental pulmonary artery aneurysms with peripheral venous thrombosis. Br J Dis Chest 1959;53: 19–27.

110. Morgan JM, Morgan AD, Addis B. Bradley GW, Spiro SG. Fatal haemorrhage from mycotic aneurysms of the pulmonary artery. Thorax 1986;41:70–71.

111. Matsumoto AH, Delany DJ, Parker LA, et al. Massive hemoptysis associated with isolated peripheral pulmonary artery stenosis. Cath Cardiovasc Diag 1987;13: 313–316.

112. Rosenow EC III, Osumundson PJ, Brown ML. Pulmonary embolism. Mayo Clin Proc 1981;56:161–178.

113. Olivari M-T. Southwestern Internal Medicine Conference: Primary pulmonary hypertension. Am J Med Sci 1991;302: 185–198.

114. Webb DW, Thadepalli H. Hemoptysis in patients with septic pulmonary infarcts from tricuspid endocarditis. Chest 1979; 76:99–100.

115. Wu MH, Lai WW, Lin MY, et al. Massive hemoptysis caused by a ruptured subclavian artery aneurysm. Chest 1993;104: 612–613.

116. Parish JM, Marschke RF, Dines DE, et al. Etiologic considerations in superior vena cava syndrome. Mayo Clin Proc 1981;56: 407–413.

117. Case Records of the Massachusetts General Hospital. Case 25–1991. N Engl J Med 1991;324:1795–1804.

118. Porter DK, Van Every MJ, Anthracite RF, et al. Massive hemoptysis in cystic fibrosis. Arch Intern Med 1983;143:287–290.

119. Panos RJ, Kumpe DA, Samara N, et al. Recurrent cryptogenic hemoptysis associated with bronchial artery-pulmonary artery anastomoses and cystic lung disease. Am J Med 1989;87:683–686.

120. Faerber EN, Balsara R, Vinocur CD, et al. Gastric duplication cyst with hemoptysis: CT findings. AJR 1993;161:1245–1246.

121. Koyama A, Sasou K, Nakao H, et al. Pulmonary intralobar sequestration accompanied by aneurysm of an anomalous arterial supply. Intern Med 1992;31: 946–950.

122. Shackford SR. Blunt chest trauma: the intensivist's perspective. J Intensive Care Med 1986;1:125–136.

123. Cordier JF, Gamondes JP, Marx P, et al. Thoracic splenosis presenting with hemoptysis. Chest 1992;102:626–627.

124. Baumgartner R, Sheppard B, de Virgilio C, et al. Tracheal and main bronchial disruptions after blunt chest trauma: presentation and management. Ann Thorac Surg 1990;50:569–574.

125. Winkler TR, Hanlin RJ, Hinke TD, Clouse LH, et al. Unusual cause of hemoptysis: Hickman-induced cava-bronchial fistula. Chest 1992; 102:1285–1286.

126. Isaacs RD, Wattie WJ, Wells AU, et al. Massive haemoptysis as a late consequence of pulmonary irradiation. Thorax 1987, 42:77–78.

127. Leatherman JW, Davies SF, Haidal JR. Alveolar hemorrhage syndromes: diffuse microvascular lung hemorrhage in immune and idiopathic disorders. Medicine (Baltimore) 1984;63:343–361.

128. Feng WC, Singh AK, Drew I, et al. Swan-Ganz catheter-induced massive hemoptysis and pulmonary artery false aneurysm. Ann Thorac Surg 1990;50:644–646.

129. Schaefer OP, Irwin RS. Tracheo-arterial fistula: an unusual complication of tracheostomy. J Intensive Care Med 1995;10: 64–75.

130. Zavala DC. Pulmonary hemorrhage in fiberoptic transbronchial biopsy. Chest 1976;70:584–588.

131. Westcott JL. Percutaneous transthoracic needle biopsy. Radiology 1988;169: 593–601.

132. Road JD, Jacques J, Sparling JR. Diffuse alveolar septal amyloidosis presenting with recurrent hemoptysis and medial dissection of pulmonary arteries. Am Rev Respir Dis 1985;132:1368–1370.

133. Kariya ST, Stern RS, Schwatzstein RM, et al. Pulmonary hemorrhage associated with bullous pemphigoid of the lung. Am J Med 1989;86:127–128.

134. Bateman ED, Morrison SC. Catamenial hemoptysis from endobronchial endometriosis—a case report and review of previously reported cases. Respir Med 1990;84:157–161.

135. Briggs WA, Johnson JP, Teichman S, et al. Antiglomerular basement membrane antibody—mediated glomerulonephritis and Goodpasture's syndrome. Medicine (Baltimore) 1979;58:348–361.

136. Soerge KH, Sommers SC. Idiopathic pulmonary hemosiderosis and related syndromes. Am J Med 1962;32:499–511.

137. Bombardieri S, Paoletti P, Ferri C, et al. Lung involvement in essential mixed cryoglobulinemia. Am J Med 1979;66: 748–756.

138. Green J, Brenner B, Gery R, et al. Case report:adult hemolytic uremic syndrome associated with nonimmune deposit crescentic glomerulonephritis and alveolar hemorrhage. Am J Med Sci 1988;296: 121–125.

139. Kathuria S, Cheifec G. Fatal pulmonary Henöch-Schonlein syndrome. Chest 1982;82:654–656.

140. Border WA, Baehler RW, Bhathena D, et al. IgA antibasement membrane nephritis with pulmonary hemorrhage. Ann Intern Med 1979;91:21–25.

141. Zashin S, Fattor R, Fortin D. Microscopic polyarteritis: a forgotten aetiology of haemoptysis and rapidly progressive glomerulonephritis. Ann Rheum Dis 1990; 49:53–56.

142. Germain MJ, Davidman M. Pulmonary hemorrhage and acute renal failure in a

patient with mixed connective tissue disease. Am J Kidney Dis 1984;3:420–424.

143. Kim JH, Follett JV, Rice JR, et al. Endobronchial telangiectasias and hemoptysis in scleroderma. Am J Med 1988;84:173–174.

144. Smith B. Idiopathic pulmonary hemosiderosis and rheumatoid arthritis. Br Med J 1966;1:1403–1405.

145. Carette S, Macher AM, Nussbaum A, et al. Severe, acute pulmonary disease in patients with systemic lupus erythematosis: ten years of experience at the National Institutes of Health. Semin Arthritis Rheum 1984;14:52–59.

146. Lopez AJ, Brady AJ, Jackson JE. Case report: therapeutic bronchial artery embolization in a case of Takayasu's arteritis. Clin Radiol 1992;45:415–417.

147. Hoffman GS, Kerr GS, Leavitt RY, et al. Wegener's granulomatosis: an analysis of 158 patients. Ann Intern Med 1992;116:488–498.

148. Robboy SJ, Minna JD, Colman RW, Birndor NI, Lopas H. Pulmonary hemorrhage syndrome as a manifestation of disseminated intravascular coagulation: analysis of ten cases. Chest 1973;63:718–721.

149. Connolly JP. Hemoptysis as a presentation of mild hemophilia A in an adult. Chest 1993;103:1281–1282.

150. Smith LJ, Katzenstein AL. Pathogensis of massive pulmonary hemorrhage in acute leukemia. Arch Intern Med 1982;142:2149–2152.

151. Fireman Z, Yust I, Abramov AL. Lethal occult pulmonary hemorrhage in drug-induced thrombocytopenia. Chest 1981; 73:358–359.

152. Milman N, Rossel K. Recurrent haemoptysis and pulmonary haemosiderosis associated with granulomatous lung disease and von Willebrand's coagulopathy. Eur J Respir Dis 1986;69:192–194.

153. Vizioli LD, Cho S. Amiodarone-associated hemoptysis. Chest 1994;105:305–306.

154. Finley TN, Aronow A, Cosentino AM, et al. Occult pulmonary hemorrhage in anticoagulated patients. Am Rev Respir Dis 1975;112:23–29.

155. Vaziri ND, Jeminson-Smith P, Wilson AF. Hemorrhagic pneumonitis after intravenous injection of charcoal lighter fluid. Ann Intern Med. 1979;90:794–795.

156. Murray RJ, Albin RJ, Mergner W, et al. Diffuse alveolar hemorrhage temporally related to cocaine smoking. Chest 1988;93:427–429.

157. Patterson R, Nugent KM, Harris KE, et al. Immunologic hemorrhagic pneumonia caused by isocyanates. Am Rev Respir Dis 1990;141:226–230.

158. Conetta R, Tamarin FM, Wogalter D, et al. Liquor lung (letter). N Engl J Med 1987;316:348–349.

159. Brandstetter RD, Tamarin FM, Rangraj MS, et al. Moxalactam disodium—induced pulmonary hemorrhage. Chest 1984;86:644–645.

160. Matloff DS, Kaplan MM. D-penicillamine-induced Goodpasture's-like syndrome in primary biliary cirrhosis-successful treatment with plasmapheresis and immunosuppressives. Gastroenterology 1980;78:1046–1049.

161. Nathan PE, Torres AV, Smith AJ, et al. Spontaneous pulmonary hemorrhage following coronary thrombolysis. Chest 1992;101:1150–1152.

162. Ahmad D, Morgan WKC, Patterson R, et al. Pulmonary haemorrhage and haemolytic anemia due to trimellitic anhydride. Lancet 1979;2:328–330.

163. McLean TR, Beall AC Jr, Jones JW. Massive hemoptysis due to broncholithiasis. Ann Thorac Surg 1991; 52:1173–1175.

164. Adelman M, Haponik EF, Bleecker ER, et al. Cryptogenic hemoptysis: clinical features, bronchoscopic findings and natural history in 67 patients. Ann Intern Med 1985; 102:829–834.

165. Pattison CW, Leaming AJ, Townsend ER. Hidden foreign body as a cause of recurrent hemoptysis in a teenage girl. Ann Thorac Surg 1988;45:330–331.

166. Wynne JW, Modell JH. Respiratory aspiration of stomach contents. Ann Intern Med 1977;87:466–474.

167. Salvaggio JE. Hypersensitivity pneumonitis. J Allergy Clin Immunol 1987;79:558–571.

168. Ghio AJ, Elliott CG, Crapo RO, Collins MP, et al. A migratory infiltrate in a patient with hemoptysis and chest pain. Chest 1989;96:195–196.

169. Fliegel E, Chitkara RK, Azueta V, et al. Fatal hemoptysis in lymphangiomyomatosis. NY State J Med 1991:91:66–67.

170. Frymoyer PA, Anderson GH Jr, Blair DC. Hemoptysis as a presenting symptom of pheochromocytoma. J Clin Hypertension 1986;2:65–67.

171. Prakash UBS, Barham SS, Carpenter HA, et al. Pulmonary alevolar phospholipo-

proteinosis: experience with 34 cases and a review. Mayo Clin Proc 1987;62: 499–518.

172. Chang JC, Driver AG, Townsend CA, et al. Hemoptysis in sarcoidosis. Sarcoidosis 1987;4:49–54.

173. Akgun S, Lee DE, Weissman PS, et al. Hemoptysis and tracheoesophageal fistula in a patient with esophageal varices and Sengstaken-Blakemore tube. Am J Med 1988;85:450–452.

174. Girdhar A, Venkatesan K, Chauhan SL, et al. Red discoloration of the sputum by clofazimine simulating haemoptysis—a case report. Leprosy Rev 1992; 63:47–50.

175. Meltz DJ, Grieco MH. Characteristics of Serratia marcescens pneumonia. Arch Intern Med. 1973;132:359–363.

176. Boushy SF, North LB, Trice JA. The bronchial arteries in chronic obstructive pulmonary disease. Am J Med 1969;46: 506–515.

177. Johnston H, Reisz G. Changing spectrum of hemoptysis: underlying causes in 148 patients undergoing diagnostic flexible fiberoptic bronchoscopy. Arch Intern Med 1989:149:1666–1668.

178. Smiddy JF, Elliott RC. The evaluation of hemoptysis with fiberoptic bronchoscopy. Chest 1973;64:158–162.

179. Santiago S, Tobias J, Williams AJ. A reappraisal of the causes of hemoptysis. Arch Intern Med; 1991:2449–2451.

180. Liebow AA, Hales MR, Lindskog GE. Enlargement of the bronchial arteries and their anastomoses with the pulmonary arteries in bronchiectasis. Am J Pathol 1949;25:211–231.

181. Groves LK, Effler DB. Broncholithiasis: a review of twenty-seven cases. Am Rev Tuberc 1955;73:19–30.

182. Lin CS, Becker WH. Broncholith as a cause of fatal hemoptysis. JAMA 1978; 239:2153.

183. Varkey B, Rose HD. Pulmonary aspergilloma—a rational approach to treatment. Am J Med 1976;61:626–631.

184. Joynson DHM. Pulmonary aspergilloma. Br J Clin Pract 1977;31:207–221.

185. Filderman AE, Shaw C, Matthay RA. Lung cancer: part I. Etiology, pathology, natural history, manifestations, and diagnostic techniques. Invest Radiol 1986;21: 80–90.

186. Hurt R. Bates M. Carcinoid tumors of the bronchus: a 33-year experience. Thorax 1984;39:617–623.

187. McCaughan BC, Martini N, Bains MS. Bronchial carcinoids: review of 124 cases. J Thorac Cardiovasc Surg 1985;89:8–17.

188. Lawson RM, Ramanathan L, Hurley G, et al. Bronchial adenoma: review of an 18-year experience at the Brompton Hospital. Thorax 1976;31:245–253.

189. Lunger M, Abelson DS, Elkind AH, et al. Massive hemoptysis in mitral stenosis: control by emergency mitral commissurotomy. N Engl J Med 1959;261:393–395.

190. Ferguson FC, Kobilack RE, Deitrick JE. Varices of the bronchial veins as a source of hemoptysis in mitral stenosis. Am Heart J 1944;28:445–446.

191. Moser KM. State of the Art. Pulmonary embolism. Am Rev Respir Dis 1977;115: 829–852.

192. Dolan JE, Haffajee CI, Alpert JS, et al. Pulmonary embolism, pulmonary hemorrhage and pulmonary infarction. N Engl J Med 1977;296:1431–1435.

193. Bell WR, Simon TL, DeMets DL. The clinical features of submassive and massive pulmonary emboli. Am J Med 1977;62: 355–360.

194. Bosher LH Jr, Blake DA, Byrd BR. An analysis of the pathologic anatomy of pulmonary arteriovenous aneurysms with particular reference to the applicability of local excision. Surgery 1959;45:91–104.

195. Ference BA, Shannon TM, White Jr RI, et al. Life-threatening pulmonary hemorrhage with pulmonary arteriovenous malformations and hereditary hemorrhagic telangiectasias. Chest 1994;106:1387–1390.

196. di Sant'Agnese PA, Davis PB. Cystic fibrosis in adults. Am J Med 1979;66:121–132.

197. Lloyd-Still JD, Wessel HU. Advances and controversies in cystic fibrosis. Semin Respir Med 1990;11:197–210.

198. Wilson RF, Soullier GW, Wiencek RG. Hemoptysis in trauma. J Trauma 1987;27: 1123–1126.

199. Foote GA, Schabel SI, Hodges M. Pulmonary complications of flow-directed balloon-tipped catheters. N Engl J Med 1974; 290:927–931.

200. Boyd KD, Thomas SJ, Gold J, et al. A prospective study of complications of pulmonary artery catheterization in 500 consecutive patients. Chest 1983;84:245–249.

201. Sise MJ, Hollingsworth P, Brimm JE, et al. Complications of the flow-directed pulmonary artery catheter: a prospective analysis of 219 patients. Crit Care Med 1981;9:315–318.

202. Ahmad M, Livingston DR, Golish JA, et

al. The safety of outpatient transbronchial biopsy. Chest 1986;90:403–405.

203. Case Records of the Massachusetts General Hospital. Case 16–1993. N Eng J Med 1993;328:1183–1190.

204. Leaker B, Cambridge G, du Bois RM,et al. Idiopathic pulmonary haemosiderosis: a form of microscopic polyarteritis? Thorax 1992;47:988–990.

205. Crouch EC. Molecular diversity of basement membrane collagen: elucidation of the Goodpasture's epitope. Am J Respir Cell Mol Biol 1991;5:99–100.

206. Mark EJ, Ramirez JF. Pulmonary capillaritis and hemorrhage in patients with systemic vasculitis. Arch Pathol Lab Med 1985;109:413–418.

207. Di Palo, Mari G, Castoldi R, et al. Endometriosis of the lung. Respir Med 1989; 83: 255–258.

208. O'Reilly SC, Taylor PM, O'Driscoll BR. Occult bronchiectasis presenting as streptokinase-induced haemoptysis. Respir Med 1994;88:393–395.

209. Gong H, Salvatierra C. Clinical effiacy of early and delayed fiberoptic bronchoscopy in patients with hemoptysis. Am Rev Respir Dis 1981;124:221–225.

210. Barret R, Tuttle W. A study of essential hemoptysis. J Thorac Cardiovasc Surg 1960;40:468–473.

211. Douglas BE, Carr DT. Prognosis in idiopathic hemoptysis. JAMA 1952;150: 764–765.

212. Jackson CV, Savage PJ, Quinn DC. Role of fiberoptic bronchoscopy in patients with hemoptysis and a normal chest roentgenogram. Chest 1985;87:142–144.

213. Poe RH, Israel RH, Marin MG, et al. Utility of fiberoptic bronchoscopy in patients with hemoptysis and a nonlocalizing chest roentgenogram. Chest 1988;92: 70–75.

214. Lederle FA, Nichol KC, Parenti CM. Bronchoscopy to evaluate hemoptysis in old men with nonsuspicious chest roentgenograms. Chest 1989;95:1043–1047.

215. Santiago SM, Lehrman S, Williams AJ. Bronchoscopy in patients with haemoptysis and normal chest roentgenograms. Br J Dis Chest 1987;81:186–188.

216. Costarangos C, Fletcher EC. Bronchogenic carcinoma, massive hemoptysis and systemic air embolus. Chest 1986;90: 140–141.

217. Winter SM, Ingbar DH. Massive hemoptysis: pathogenesis and management. J Intensive Care Med 1988;3:171–188.

218. Albelda SM, Gefter WB, Epstein DM, et al. Diffuse pulmonary hemorrhage: a review and classification. Radiology 1985;154: 289–297.

219. Simon MW, Mitchell BL, O'Connor WN, et al. Glomerulonephritis, pulmonary hemorrhage and coagulopathy associated with Haemophilus parainfluenzae endocarditis. Pediatr Infect Dis 1985;4: 183–188.

220. Weaver LJ, Solliday N, Cugell DW. Selection of patients with hemoptysis for fiberoptic bronchoscopy. Chest 1979;76: 7–10.

221. Jackson CL, Diamond S. Hemorrhage from the trachea, bronchi and lungs of non-tuberculous origin. Am Rev Tuberc 1942: 46:126–138.

222. Schneider L. Bronchogenic carcinoma heralded by hemoptysis and ignored because of negative chest x-ray results. NY State Med J 1959;59:637–642.

223. Kallenbach J, Song E, Zwi S. Haemoptysis with no radiological evidence of tumor—The value of early bronchoscopy. S Afr Med J 1981;59:556–558.

224. Holsclaw DS, Grank RJ, Schwachman H. Massive hemoptysis in cystic fibrosis. J Pediatr 1970;76:829–838.

225. Albelda SM, Talbot GH, Gerson SL, et al. Pulmonary cavitation and massive hemoptysis in invasive pulmonary aspergillosis: influence of bone marrow recovery in patients with acute leukemia. Am Rev Respir Dis 1985;131:115–120.

226. Haponik EF, Chin R. Hemoptysis: clinicians' perspective. Chest 1990;97: 469–475.

227. Heimer D, Bar-Ziv J, Scharf SM. Fiberoptic bronchoscopy in patients with hemoptysis and nonlocalizing chest roentgenograms. Arch Intern Med 1985;145: 1427–1428.

228. Peters J, McClung HC, Teague RB. Evaluation of hemoptysis in patients with a normal chest roentgenogram. Arch Intern Med 1984;141:624–626.

229. O'Neill KM, Lazarus AA. Hemoptysis: indications for bronchoscopy. Arch Intern Med 1991;151:171–174.

230. Snider GL. When not to use the bronchoscope for hemoptysis. Chest 1979;76:1–2.

231. Conlan AA. Massive hemoptysis—diagnostic and therapeutic implications. Surg Ann 1985;17:337–354.

232. Conlan AA, Hurwitz SS. Management of massive haemoptysis with the rigid bron-

choscope and cold saline lavage. Thorax 1980;35:901–904.

233. Tucker GF Jr, Olsen AM, Andrews AH Jr, et al. The flexible fiberscope in bronchoscopic perspective. Chest 1973;64: 149–150.

234. Rath GS, Schaff JT, Snider GL. Flexible fiberoptic bronchscopy: techniques and review of 100 bronchoscopies. Chest 1973;63:689–693.

235. Imgrund SP, Goldberg SK, Walkenstein MD, et al. Clinical diagnosis of massive hemoptysis using the fiberoptic bronchoscope. Crit Care Med 1985;13:438–443.

236. Anonymous. Life-threatening haemoptysis. Lancet 1987; i:1354–1356.

237. Saumench J, Escarrabill J, Padró L, et al. Value of fiberoptic bronchoscopy and angiography for diagnosis of the bleeding site in hemoptysis. Ann Thorac Surg 1989;48:272–274.

238. Aberle DA, Brown K, Young DA, et al. Imaging techniques in the evaluation of tracheobronchial neoplasms. Chest 1991;99: 211–215.

239. Woodring JH. Determining the cause of pulmonary atelectasis: a comparison of plain radiography and CT. AJR 1988;150: 757–763.

240. Colice GL, Chappel GJ, Frenchman SM, et al. Comparison of computerized tomography with fiberoptic bronchoscopy in identifying endobronchial abnormalities in patients with known or suspected lung cancer. Am Rev Respir Dis 1985;131: 397–400.

241. Henschke CL, Davis SD, Auh PR, et al. Detection of bronchial abnormalities: comparison of CT and bronchoscopy. J Comput Assist Tomogr 1987;11:432–435.

242. Naidich DP, Lee JJ, Garay SM, et al. Comparison of CT and fiberoptic bronchoscopy in the evaluation of bronchial disease. AJR 1987;148:1–7.

243. Mayr B, Ingrisch H, Haussinger K, et al. Tumors of the bronchi: role of evaluation with CT. Radiology 1989;172:647–652.

244. Haponik EF, Britt EJ, Smith PL, et al. Computed chest tomography in the evaluation of hemoptysis: impact on diagnosis and treatment. Chest 1987;91:80–85.

245. Naidich DP, Funt S, Ettenger NA, et al. Hemoptysis: CT-bronchoscopic correlations in 58 cases. Radiology 1990;177: 357–362.

246. Millar AB, Boothroyd AE, Edwards D, et al. The role of computed tomography (CT)

in the investigation of haemoptysis. Respir Med 1992;86:39–44.

247. Set PAK, Flower CDR, Smith IE, et al. Hemoptysis: comparative study of the role of CT and fiberoptic bronchoscopy. Radiology 1993;189:677–680.

248. McGuiness G, Beacher JR, Harkin TJ, et al. Hemoptysis: prospective high-resolution CT/bronchoscopic correlation. Chest 1994;105:1155–1162.

249. Elliot DL, Barker AF, Dixon LM. Catamenial hemoptysis: new methods of diagnosis and therapy. Chest 1985;87:687–688.

250. Forrest JV, Sagell SS, Omell GH. Bronchography in patients with hemoptysis. AJR 1976;126:597–600.

251. Christoforidis AJ, Nelson SW, Tomashefski JF. Effects of bronchography on pulmonary function. Am Rev Respir Dis 1962:85:127–129.

252. Muller NL, Bergin CJ, Ostrow DN, et al. Role of computed tomography in the recognition of bronchiectasis. AJR 1984;143: 971–976.

253. Cooke JC, Currie DC, Morgan AD, et al. Role of computed tomography in the diagnosis of bronchiectasis. Thorax 1987;42: 272–277.

254. Joharjy IA, Bashi SA, Abdullah AK. Value of medium-thickness CT in the diagnosis of bronchiectasis. AJR 1987;149: 1133–1137.

255. Silverman PM, Goodwin JD. CT/bronchographic correlations in bronchiectasis. J Comput Assist Tomogr 1987;11:52–56.

256. Mootoosamy IM, Reznek RH, Osman J, et al. Assessment of bronchiectasis by computed tomography. Thorax 1985;40: 920–924.

257. Jones DK, Cavanagh P, Shneerson JM, et al. Does bronchography have a role in the assessment of patients with haemoptysis. Thorax 1985;40:668–670.

258. Munro NC, Cooke JC, Currie DC, et al. Comparsion of thin section computed tonography with bronchography for identifying bronchiectatic segments in patients with chronic sputum production. Thorax 1990;45:135–139.

259. Barry J, Alazraki HP, Heaphy JH. Scintigraphic detection of intrapulmonary bleeding using technetium—99m sulfur colloid:concise communication. J Nucl Med 1981;22:777–780.

260. Haponik EF, Rothfeld B, Britt EJ, Bleeker ER. Radionuclide localization of massive pulmonary hemorrhage. Chest 1984;86: 208–212.

261. Winzelberg GG, Wholey MH. Scintigraphic detection of pulmonary hemorrhage using Tc—99m—sulfur colloid. Clin Nucl Med 1981;6:537–540.

262. Coel MN, Druger G. Radionuclide detection of the site of hemoptysis. Chest 1982; 81:242–243.

263. The PIOPED Investigators. Value of the ventilation/ perfusion scan in acute pulmonary embolism: results of the prospective investigation of pulmonary embolism diagnosis (PIOPED). JAMA 1990;263: 2753–2759.

264. Salimi Z, Thomasson J, Vas W, et al. Detection of a right-to-left shunt with radionuclide angiocardiography in refractory hypoxemia. Chest 1985;88:784–786.

265. Roberts AC. Bronchial artery embolization therapy. J Thorac Imaging 1990;5: 60–72.

266. Feigelson HH, Ravin HA. Transverse myelitis following selective bronchial arteriography. Radiology 1965;85:663–665.

267. Katoh O, Yamada H, Hiura K, et al. Bronchoscopic and angiographic comparison of bronchial arterial lesions in patients with hemoptysis. Chest 1987;91: 486–489.

268. Keller FS, Rosch J, Loflin TG, et al. Nonbronchial systemic collateral arteries: significance in percutaneous embolotherapy for hemoptysis. Radiology 1987;164: 687–692.

269. Remy J, Lemaitre L, Lofitte JJ, et al. Massive hemoptysis of pulmonary arterial origin: diagnosis and treatment. AJR 1984; 143:963–969.

270. Ferris EJ. Pulmonary hemorrhage. Vascular evaluation and interventional therapy. Chest 1981;80:710–714.

271. Bertucci V, Asch MR, Balter MS. Prognosis in a patient with an initial normal pulmonary angiogram. Chest 1994;105: 1257–1258.

272. Ewan PW, Jones HA, Rhodes CG, et al. Detection of intrapulmonary hemorrhage with carbon monoxide uptake. N Engl J Med 1976;296:1391–1396.

273. Hernandez A, Strauss AW, McKnight R, et al. Diagnosis of pulmonary arteriovenous fistula by contrast echocardiography. J Pediatr 1978; 93:258–261.

274. Macfarlane J. Lung biopsy. BMJ 1985;290; 97–98.

275. Shivaram U, Finch P. Nowak P. Plastic endobronchial tubes in the management of life-threatening hemoptysis. Chest 1987;92:1108–1110.

276. Scuderi PE, Prough DS, Price JD, et al. Cessation of pulmonary artery catheter-induced endobronchial hemorrhage associated with the use of PEEP. Anest Analg 1983;62:236–238.

277. Stoller JK. Diagnosis and management of massive hemoptysis: a review. Respir Care 1992;37:564–581.

278. Cordasco EM Jr, Mehta AC, Ahmad M. Bronchoscopically induced bleeding: a summary of nine years' Cleveland Clinic experience and review of the literature. Chest 1991;100:1141–1147.

279. Kinoshita M, Shiraki R, Wagai F, et al. Thrombin instillation therapy through the fiberoptic bronchoscope in cases of hemoptysis. Japan J Thorac Dis 1982;20: 251–254.

280. Tsukamoto T, Sasaki H, Nakamura H. Treatment of hemoptysis patients by thrombin and fibrinogen-thrombin infusion therapy using a fiberoptic bronchoscope. Chest 1989;96:473–476.

281. Takagi O, Sakamoto K, Tohda Y, et al. Fibrinogen and thrombin infusion therapy of hemoptysis. J Japan Bronchology 1983; 5:45–51.

282. Bense L. Intrabronchial selective coagulative treatment of hemoptysis:report of three cases. Chest 1990,97:990–996.

283. Bhambure NM, Abhyankar NY, Gandhi Y, et al. Hemoptysis after Batroxobin infusion using a fiberoptic bronchoscope (letter). Chest 1991;99:1313.

284. Nakano S. Use of Reptilase with an endoscope against bronchial hemorrhage. Clin Rep 1986;20:229–235.

285. Wilson HE. Control of massive hemorrhage during bronchoscopy. Dis Chest 1969;56:412–417.

286. Hiebert CA. Balloon catheter control of life-threatening hemoptysis. Chest 1974; 66:308–309.

287. Saw EC, Gottlieb LS, Yokoyama T, et al. Flexible fiberoptic bronchoscopy and endobronchial tamponade in the management of massive hemoptysis. Chest 1976; 70:589–591.

288. Faloney JP, Balchum OJ. Repeated massive hemoptysis: successful control using multiple balloon-tipped catheters for endobronchial tamponade. Chest 1978;74: 683–685.

289. Gottlieb LS, Hillberg R. Endobronchial tamponade therapy for intractable hemoptysis. Chest 1975;67:482–483.

290. Swersky RB, Chang JB, Wisoff BG, et al. Endobronchial balloon tamponade of he-

moptysis in patients with cystic fibrosis. Ann Thorac Surg 1979;27:262–264.

291. Jolliet P, Soccal P, Chevrolet JC. Control of massive hemoptysis by endobronchial tamponade with a pulmonary artery balloon catheter. Crit Care Med 1992;20: 1730–1732.

292. Freitag L. Development of a new balloon catheter for management of hemoptysis with bronchofiberscopes. Chest 1993; 103:593.

293. Edmonstone WM, Nanson EM, Woodcock AA, et al. Life threatening haemoptysis controlled by laser photocoagulation. Thorax 1983;38:788–789.

294. Lang N, Maners A, Broadwater J, et al. Management of airway problems in lung cancer patients using the Nd-YAG laser and endobronchial radiotherapy. Am J Surg 1988;156:463–465.

295. Leatherman JW. Immune alveolar hemorrhage. Chest 1987;91:891–897.

296. Magee G. Williams MH Jr. Treatment of massive hemoptysis with intravenous pitressin. Lung 1982;160:165–169.

297. Remy J, Arnaud A, Fardou H, et al. Treatment of hemoptysis by embolization of bronchial arteries. Radiology 1977;122: 33–37.

298. Bilton D, Webb AK, Foster H, et al. Life-threatening haemoptysis in cystic fibrosis: an alternative therapeutic approach. Thorax 1990;45:975–976.

299. Shapiro MJ, Albelda SM, Mayock RL, et al. Severe hemoptysis associated with pulmonary aspergilloma: percutaneous intracavitary treatment. Chest 1988;94: 1225–1231.

300. Lee KS, Kim HT, Kim YH, et al. Treatment of hemoptysis in patients with cavitary aspergilloma of the lung: value of percutaneous instillation of amphotericin B. AJR 1993;161:727–731.

301. Khandekar JD. Effect of hemoptysis on blood fibrinolysis. Am Rev Respir Dis 1972;105:457.

302. Shneerson JM, Emerson PA, Phillips RH. Radiotherapy for massive haemoptysis from an aspergilloma. Thorax 1980;35: 953–954.

303. Lampmann LEH, Tjan TG. Embolization therapy in haemoptysis. Eur J Radiol 1994;18:15–19.

304. Cremaschi P, Nascimbene C, Vitub P, et al. Therapeutic embolization of bronchial artery: a successful treatment in 209 cass of relapse hemoptysis. Angiology 1993; 44:295–299.

305. Ivanick MJ, Thorwait W, Donahue J, et al. Infarction of the left main bronchus: a complication of bronchial artery embolization. AJR 1983;141:535–537.

306. Nath H. When does bronchial arterial embolization fail to control hemoptysis? Chest 1990;97:515–516.

307. Bredin CP, Richardson PR, King TKC, et al. Treatment of massive hemoptysis by combined occlusion of pulmonary and bronchial arteries. Am Rev Respir Dis 1978;117:969–973.

308. Mattox KL, Guinn GA. Emergency resection for massive hemoptysis. Ann Thorac Surg 1974;17:377–383.

309. Solit RV, McKeown JJ Jr, Smullens S, et al. The surgical implications of intracavity mycetomas (fungus balls). J Thorac Cardiovas Surg 1971;62:411–422.

310. Shamji FM, Vallieres E, Todd ER, et al. Massive or life-threatening hemoptysis (abstract).Chest 1991;100(Suppl):78S.

311. Diamond MA, Genovese PD. Life-threatening hemoptysis in mitral stenosis: emergency mitral valve replacement resulting in rapid, sustained cessation of pulmonary bleeding. JAMA 1971;215: 441–444.

# Chest Pain: Pathophysiology and Differential Diagnosis

Frederick J. Curley, M.D.
Mark M. Wilson, M.D.

## Introduction

Virtually every person experiences chest pain at some time in their life. Mild chest pain frequently occurs due to trauma, musculoskeletal overuse or injury, or indigestion. The clear cause and self-limited nature of these pains rarely prompt physician visits. Episodes of chest pain, however, do account for 10% of new symptoms,[1] 8% of emergency department evaluations, and 2.8% of adult primary care encounters[2]; lead to 500,000 cardiac catheterizations per year in the United States[3,4]; and result in millions of hospital admissions per year in the United States. Estimates of the cost of evaluating and managing cardiac chest pain alone reach levels of billions of dollars per year.[5,6]

Despite the cost and prevalence of chest pain many physicians do not have an organized, systematic approach for diagnosing and treating this symptom. Because of its ominous implications, physicians focus on chest pain of cardiac causes. However, at least 50% of patients admitted with chest pain initially suspected of being of cardiac cause are discharged with the descriptive but nonspecific diagnosis of "myocardial infarction (MI) ruled out."[7–15] Between 6% and 31% of cardiac catheterizations reveal normal coronaries or coronaries with insignificant abnormalities.[3] The absence of a systematic approach for evaluating these noncardiac chest pain patients remains unfortunate. Data indicate that although the mortality in these patients over the subsequent decade is low, pain frequently recurs, has significant morbidity, and results in frequent, extensive, costly evaluation.[1]

By utilizing a protocol based on the locations of pain receptors in the thorax when the patients do not present with a "classic" chest pain syndrome (see Table I), the clinician should be able to more consistently diagnose and successfully treat the cause of a patient's chest pain. This chapter will focus on a discussion of the pathophysiology and differential diagnosis of chest pain. The next chapter will review the diagnostic strategies for evaluating chest pain and the treatment of specific chest pain syndromes.

From Irwin RS, Curley FJ, Grossman RF (eds): Diagnosis and Treatment of Symptoms of the Respiratory Tract. Armonk, New York, Futura Publishing Company, Inc., © 1997.

**Table I**
Causes of Chest Pain

**Aorta**
  Aortic Dissection
  Aortic Aneurysms
  Aortic Arteritis Syndromes
**Cardiovascular**
  Myocardium
    Myocardial Infarction (MI)
    Myocardial Ischemia
      Stable Angina Pectoris
      Unstable Angina
      Variant Angina
      Syndrome X
      Rocky Mounting Spotted Fever
    Myocarditis
      Infectious: syphilis, TB, fungi, parasites
      Collagen Vascular: SLE, RA, scleroderma,
        dermatomyositis, polyarteritis nodosa
  Pericardial and Myocardial Trauma
    Pericardial Injury
    Myocardial Contusion
    Cardiac Tumors
    Cardiomyopathy
      Dilated
      Hypertrophic
  Pericardial Disease
    Pericarditis: rheumatic, TB, SLE, uremic
    Postpericardiotomy Syndrome
    Pericardial Tumors
    Post–Myocardial Infarct Syndrome (Dressler's
      Syndrome)
  Valvular Disease
    Aortic Stenosis
    Mitral Stenosis
    Mitral Valve Prolapse (MVP, Barlow's
      Syndrome)
**Pulmonary: Lung and Pleura**
  Viral Pleuritis
  Pneumonia
  Neoplastic Pleurisy
  Asbestos-related Diseases
  Pleurisy and Connective Tissue Disorders
  Radiation Pleuritis
  Pneumothorax
  Pulmonary Embolism
  Pulmonary Hypertension
  Panic/Hyperventilation/Anxiety Syndromes
**Gastrointestinal**
  Esophageal disease
    Gastroesophageal Reflux Disease (GERD)
    Esophageal Motility Disorders and Achalasia
    Diverticula
    Rupture/Perforation
    Diaphragmatic Hernia
    Vascular Ring Dysphagia
    Cancer

Pancreas
  Pancreatitis
  Carcinoma
  Cyst
Spleen
  Hypersplenism
  Infarct
  Rupture
Biliary Tract Disease
  Biliary Colic
  Cholecystitis
  Choledocholithiasis
Stomach
  Peptic Ulcer/Gastritis
  Aerophagia
  Diverticula
  Cancer
**Musculoskelatal Disease**
  Fibromyalgia
  Pectoral Girdle Syndrome
  Benign Overuse
  Xyphoidynia, Xyphoidalgia
  Sternoclavicular Joint Disease
  Precordial Catch
  Tietze's Syndrome and Costochondritis
  Ankylosing Spondylitis
  Rib Pain
  Spine
    Infection
    Cervical Disease
  Shoulder
    Acromioclavicular Joint
    Rotator Cuff
  Thoracic Outlet Syndrome
  Diaphragm: flutter, hiccup, rupture
  Myositis: viral, bacterial, parasitic, polymyositis,
    dermatomyositis
**Neck**
  Tumors
  Cysts
  Thyroid
  Pyogenic and Subacute Granulomatous
    Thyroiditis
**Skin**
  Burns
  Inflammatory Lesions: Panniculitis, neurotic
    excoriations
  Infiltrative Diseases
  Infections: Herpes Zoster, bacterial cellulitis
  Tumors: glomus, malignant
**Breast**
  Mastitis
  Mammary Duct Ectasia
  Fibrocystic Disease
  Breast Cancer
  Trauma
  Breast Implants
  Gynecomastia

## Table I
### (*continued*)

| | |
|---|---|
| **Mediastinum** | **Kidneys** |
| Traumatic Hematoma | Pyelonephritis |
| Substernal Thyroid | Renal Infarct |
| Lipoma | Renal Calculi |
| Cancer | **Drugs** |
| Lymphoma | 5-fluorouracil |
| Cysts: hygromas, dermoid | Bleomycin |
| Epicardial Pacing Wires | Methotrexate |
| Mediastinitis | Ranitidine |
| Pneumomediastinum | Corticotropin-releasing hormone |
| **Nerves** | Apraclonidine |
| Spinal Subarachnoid Hermorrhage | Odansetron |
| Epilepsy | 100% Oxygen |
| Intercostal Nerve Injury Due to Internal Mammary | Vancomycin |
|    Artery Grafting | Sertraline |
| Sternal Wires | Sumatriptan |
| Neuroma | Cocaine |

RA = rheumatoid arthritis; SLE = systemic lupus erythematosus; TB = tuberculosis

## Definition

Chest pain is pain that the patient localizes to the thorax. The thorax includes all structures bounded by the diaphragm, ribs/spine and connective tissues, the shoulders, and the neck. Pain may arise from the mediastinal structures, heart, lungs, pleura, esophagus, ribs, muscles, skin, shoulder girdle, breasts, or thoracic nerves. Pain arising from the neck, arms, or abdomen may also be referred to the chest and be perceived by the patient as arising from the thorax.

Chest pain is a sensory phenomenon. As such, it possesses characteristics of intensity and quality. Intensity is usually measured on a scale of 0 to 10, with 0 indicating no pain and 10 maximally imaginable pain. Patients choose numerous descriptors for pain which include temperature, timing, or other characteristics of pain, such as burning, squeezing, sharp, deep, cool, pricking, numbing, or knifelike. The sensation of pain also has a cognitive or affective component. Pain may be described as suffering or torturing. Several instruments have been developed which rate and describe pain. Although some indices, such as the McGill-Melzack pain rating index,[16] have been widely used in research protocols, no pain index has achieved routine acceptance or demonstrated utility in the routine clinical evaluation of chest pain. Unfortunately, the description of a patient's pain by itself rarely indicates the cause of the pain.

## Anatomy

The clinician must understand the anatomy and physiology of pain in order to best understand and evaluate the chest pain syndromes. Anatomy and physiology explain why gall bladder distention may be perceived as parasternal or shoulder pain or why carrying a heavy object on the shoulder may result in anterior chest pain. Pain from superficial structures may be grouped according to the dermatomes involved in generating the pain. Pain from visceral structures arises via more overlapping afferent groupings. Knowledge of the visceral and dermatomal afferent pathways may help the clinician identify structures responsible for initiating the pain. This section will briefly review the anatomy of the main afferent pathways, the physiology of pain in general, and our specific knowledge of thoracic pain.

## Afferent Pain Pathways

The primary pain afferents in the chest are the cutaneous nerves, the vagus and recurrent laryngeal nerves, the phrenic nerves, and the sympathetic trunk. Recent electron microscopic studies have confirmed that afferent fibers predominate numerically in the vagus nerve.[17] The vagus and recurrent laryngeal nerves are found in the superior mediastinum, the phrenic nerves in the middle mediastinum, and the superior cervical ganglions of the sympathetic nervous system are located in the posterior mediastinum. Each of these large nerve groups carries impulses from pain fibers to the brainstem or spinal cord and then to higher centers.

### Cutaneous Nerves

The cutaneous nerves are organized in dermatomes. Each cervical and thoracic segment of the spinal cord sends and receives a bundle of cutaneous nerves which typically innervate a well-circumscribed surface of cutaneous tissue. The segment of tissue innervated, the dermatome, is named for the spinal segment receiving the afferent nerves. Figure 1[18] displays the thorax with each dermatome clearly labelled. Sensation from the cutaneous and subcutaneous tissues in each dermatome may be poorly localized so that pain arising in any portion of the dermatome may be perceived as pain from another portion of the same dermatome. Thus, pain arising near the shoulder may be perceived as left anterior chest pain.

### Vagus Nerves

The vagus nerve is embryologically formed by the fusion of the fourth and sixth bronchial arches.[19] Figure 2 indicates the structures innervated by the

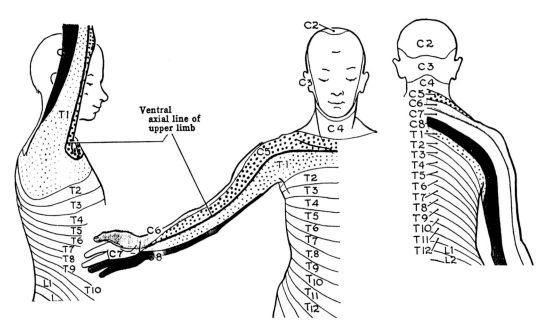

**Figure 1.** The dermatomes are displayed as contour lines in the anterior, posterior, and lateral views. Each segment between two lines is a dermatome and is labelled to indicate the spinal level involved in innervation. Pain is frequently radiated from somatic structures within a dermatome to other areas of the dermatome. (Modified from *Grant's Atlas of Anatomy*, Grant, JCB, ed. Baltimore, Md: Williams & Wilkins Company; 1972.[18])

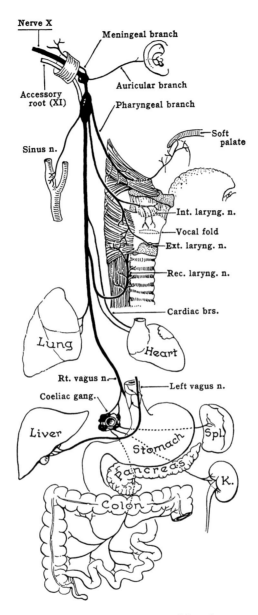

Nerve X

Meningeal branch

Accessory
root (XI)

Auricular branch

Pharyngeal branch

Soft
palate

Sinus n.

Int. laryng. n.

Vocal fold

Ext. laryng. n.

Rec. laryng. n.

Cardiac brs.

Lung

Heart

Rt. vagus n.

Left vagus n.

Coeliac gang.

Liver

Spl

Stomach

Pancreas

K.

Colon

**Figure 2.** Schematic drawing of the organs innervated by the vagus nerves. (Modified from *Grant's Atlas of Anatomy*, Grant, JCB, ed. Baltimore, Md: Williams & Wilkins Company; 1972.[18])

vagus nerves. On the left, the vagus nerve descends from the neck along the posterolateral aspect of the left common carotid artery and adjacent to the left subclavian artery. The vagus innervates the esophagus along its entire thoracic course and then it continues along the esophagus into the abdomen after giving off branches that will traverse into the lung and the heart. At the level of the aortic arch, the left recurrent laryngeal nerve arises from the left vagus nerve and passes beneath the arch through the aortopulmonary window as it travels cephalad to the larynx along the left side of the trachea. The abdominal vagus innervates the esophagus, stomach, small intestine, and at least the proximal colon and cecum.

The cell bodies of vagal afferents lie in the nodose ganglion in the medulla. Anatomical studies suggest that the majority of visceral sensory receptors exist as free-nerve endings. These **mucosal receptors** are generally responsive to direct mechanical stimulation and to various chemicals (ie, are polymodal) and are relatively insensitive to distension, contraction, or compression. Some receptors show a high degree of specificity for such substances as glucose or acid. Receptors located in the **muscle layers** of the viscera, conversely, are activated by distension, contraction, or compression of that viscus.

Neuropeptides found in vagal afferents include substance P, cholecystokinin, vasoactive intestinal peptide (VIP), somatostatin, calcitonin gene-related peptide (CGRP), and prodynorphin-derived peptides.[20] These neuropeptides are localized in neurons with the classical neurotransmitters, such as acetylcholine, noradrenaline, and serotonin. The physiological significance of neuropeptides outside of the brainstem and spinal cord is unclear, but populations of peripheral fibers with each specific neuropeptide do exhibit a distinctive pattern of termination sites. These neuropeptides may function as peripheral neuromodulators or act as mediators of local tissue responses.

Afferent impulses from the gastrointestinal (GI) tract, lungs and heart, carried in the vagus nerves, are conveyed to the nucleus tractus solitarious in the dorsomedial medulla. Interneurons then project to discrete pools of neurons in the ventrolateral medulla, just dorsal to the inferior olive in the region of the nucleus ambiguous. In the absence of any identifiable pathology, nerve injury, neuralgia, or demyelinating process, the mechanism of "central crosstalk" has been proposed to explain the noted cardiovascular and respiratory reflex responses to stimulation of the larynx, pharynx, or esophagus[21] (eg, hiccoughs, laryngospasm, or hypotensive bradycardia). According to this theory, aberrant synaptic contacts within the brainstem are responsible for an overlapping or misrouting of interneurons responsible for separating signals from the GI tract, heart, and lungs. Central crosstalk could presumably occur at either the sensory nucleus in the dorsomedial medulla, the motor nuclei in the ventrolateral medulla, or both. Although the theory of medullary crosstalk has never been documented in humans or experimental animals, it is felt to be a plausible mechanism analogous to the type of spinal cord crosstalk that underlies referred pain and it has been proposed that the term "referred vagal reflexes" be used to identify such phenomena.

## Phrenic Nerves

The phrenic nerves arise from the ventral portions of the third, fourth, and fifth cervical nerves and are the only motor supply to the diaphragm. They also provide visceral afferent pathways from the diaphragm, liver, gallbladder, pericardium, and pancreas.[22] The left phrenic nerve descends from the neck between the left subclavian artery and vein. It subsequently passes anterior to the hilum of the left lung after crossing the aortic arch. The left phrenic nerve reaches the diaphragm after traversing along the left side of the pericardial sac. The right phrenic nerve follows a similar course along the predominantly venous structures of the right side of the mediastinum—it enters the thorax adjacent to the right brachiocephalic vein and runs along the lateral wall of the superior vena cava. It then passes anteriorly to the hilum of the (right) lung before travelling across the pericardial sac to finally innervate the right hemidiaphragm. Figure 3 indicates the structures innervated by the phrenic nerves.

## Sympathetic Nervous System

The sympathetic nervous system is composed of bilateral chains of ganglia that are segmentally arranged and interconnected by longitudinal nerve fibers called sympathetic trunks. These struc-

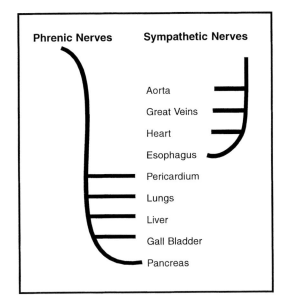

**Figure 3.** Schematic drawing of the organs innervated by the phrenic and sympathetic nerves.

sensation (ie, sharp, pricking, stinging) that lasts as long as the acute stimulus is acting. The threshold for this first pain is uniform from person to person.[23] In contrast, polymodal nociceptors are recruited when a painful stimulus is sufficiently strong and this information is transmitted via C (unmyelinated) axons. Polymodal nociceptors transmit the sensation of "second pain," a more diffuse and persistent burning sensation that lasts beyond the termination of an acutely painful stimulus. Second pain is also associated with the affective-motivational aspects of pain and tolerance to it is seen to vary from person to person. The composite sensory message to the central nervous system induced by an acute noxious stimulus, then, can be understood as a complex interaction of activated A-$\delta$, C fibers, and also some low-threshold fibers.[23] In acute cutaneous pain, both first and second pain may apply depending on the noxious stimulus and its intensity. In chronic pain and pain of visceral origin, second pain pathways clearly predominate.

Both high-threshold mechanoreceptors and polymodal nociceptors use L-glutamate as a transmitter. Polymodal C fibers also contain a variety of other potential neuropeptide transmitters, especially substance P and CGRP. How nociceptors are activated by various stimuli is incompletely understood. Some of the activation is likely the result of direct stimulation, while under different circumstances intermediary substances may take a more active role (eg, potassium, hydrogen ions, serotonin, histamine, prostaglandins, bradykinin, and adenosine triphosphate). These intermediary substances may be released into tissue as a result of the noxious stimulus itself or as byproducts of any induced inflammatory states. All of these substances have the potential to further activate or sensitize additional nociceptors and to have local vasodilatory and increased capillary permeability properties to cause further release of mediators. Sensitization may occur in any neurons throughout the pain pathways and consists of a decreased threshold for activation, increased intensity of response to a

tures are located in the posterior mediastinum and can be seen to cross the heads of ribs two through nine, eventually coming to lie on the lateral border of the lower thoracic vertebrae. A convoluted series of interconnections can be traced out as this system provides its contribution to the innervation of the great vessels of the thorax, the lung, the heart, the esophagus, and more caudal aspects of the GI system.

## The Spinal Column, Ascending Tracts, and Brain

The dorsal horn of the spinal column receives the sympathetic and cutaneous afferents. Peripheral sensation of pain occurs via two main classes of neurons whose cell bodies lie within the dorsal root ganglia and whose axons project to the dorsal horn of the spinal cord. Both types of axons have naked nerve endings. High-threshold mechanoreceptors transmit impulses with A-$\delta$ axons, which are recruited first and send information of "first pain"—a well-localized discriminative stimulus, and/or emergence of sustained spontaneous activation.

Axons of second-order dorsal horn neurons cross the spinal cord via the anterior white commissure and then ascend the spinal cord in the anterolateral quadrant, which contains several ascending and descending pathways. The two major pain pathways of the anterolateral quadrant include the spinothalamic tract and the spinoreticular tracts.[23] Of the axons that will ascend to the thalamus, approximately 50% are capable of responding to "gentle stimuli" and then increase their responses as the stimuli becomes more intense, 30% respond exclusively to noxious stimuli, 10% are activated by stimulation of visceral tissue, and 2% are stimulated by innocuous tactile sensations.[24]

**Spinothalamic tract** pain neurons are destined to synapse in two main groups of nuclei in the thalamus. Those axons that proceed to the lateral nuclei (ie, the ventroposterolateral nucleus and the posterior nuclear group) originate in laminae I and V in the dorsal horn and are primarily involved with fine discrimination of pain signals from the periphery. Those axons projecting to thalamic medial nuclei (ie, the central lateral nucleus of the intralaminar complex and the nucleus submedius) originate from laminae I, IV, and VI of the dorsal horn and relay signals from widespread areas and have been implicated in the affective-motivational aspects of pain perception.[23] Communication between these two major groups of thalamic afferents is presumed to occur. Third-order neurons from the lateral thalamic nuclei then project to the somatosensory cortex where conscious localization of pain occurs. Neurons from the medial nuclei of the thalamus then project to the cingulate gyrus, where the emotional reaction to pain and the perception of "suffering" is thought to originate.[25]

Axons of pain fibers that ascend via the **spinoreticular tract** project to the reticular formation of the brainstem in two major subgroups—the bulbopontine group and the mesencephalic group. The bulbopontine fibers synapse in a variety of nuclei located in the medulla and pons (ie,

nucleus gigantocellularis, nucleus paragigantocellularis, nuclei reticularis pontis caudalis and oralis, and the nucleus subcaeruleus). Axons subserving the mesencephalic group terminate in the periaqueductal gray, the deep layers of the superior colliculi and the nucleus cuneiformis.[24] The entire reticular formation is a core system of primitive origin that allows for homeostasis and the integration of affective-motivational aspects of motor, sensory, and visceral pain functions. It is also the source of a descending neural pathway that allows for modulation of the pain pathways described above.

***Descending pathways*** that influence the transmission of pain originate in at least three major areas—the cerebral cortex, the thalamus, and the brainstem. Neurotransmitters found in these pathways are generally inhibitory in nature and include epinephrine, norepinephrine, serotonin, and various opioid compounds. A similar pharmacology is operative on both somatic and visceral input. Stimulation of the somatosensory cortex can lead to inhibitory, excitatory, or mixed signals to the dorsal horn neurons of the spinal cord via direct descending pathways or through mediation of the brainstem structures. Descending pathways also originate from the reticular formation in the brainstem, the dorsal raphe nucleus (ie, the ventral portion of the periaqueductal gray) in the midbrain, and the nucleus raphe centralis superior and nucleus raphe magnus in the medulla. These nuclei then project fibers down through the dorsolateral funiculus to the dorsal horn of the spinal cord. Some of these connections are direct while others are via interneurons.

## Physiology of Chest Pain Syndromes

Chest pain syndromes can be physiologically separated into somatic and visceral pain syndromes. Pain from the skin, subcutaneous tissues, and the bones and muscles of the chest wall and spine generally presents with a more localized, richer quality of pain than from the deeper visceral structures. This somatic pain group has pain along dermatomal lines and includes descriptions of pain in cutaneous terms, such as hot, cool, burning, pricking, or stabbing. Pain typically arises from focal inflammation and can frequently be localized to a 1-cm focus.

Visceral pain is more often described as a type of "discomfort" rather than being a true "pain." Many forms of tissue injury are frequently not painful. Moreover, pain may arise from some stimuli (ie, distension of a hollow organ) that does not damage or even threaten to damage that tissue. The end-sensation is usually of a dull, aching, or boring quality and will be described by the patient as being a pressure, tightness, or squeezing. Generally, the discomfort is poorly localized, perceived over an area much larger than the precipitating stimulus, and may be felt in areas away from the site of origin (ie, so-called "referred pain"). Visceral pain, in particular, can show a wavelike quality, presumably waxing and waning with contractions of smooth muscle. In addition, visceral pain is usually accompanied by malaise, anxiety, and strong autonomic reflexes.

Visceral tissues may exhibit varying sensitivities. Some viscera, notably the parenchymatous portions of the lung, liver, and kidney do **not** give rise to pain sensations with any stimulus, iincluding gross destruction from malignancy or surgical manipulation. Perhaps the best-described sensitivity of viscera is that produced by distension of hollow, muscular walled organs. The distending pressures associated with pain are generally not damaging to the tissues, but estimates of the threshold pressures to produce pain in particular viscera often vary considerably in the literature. The most important theory offered to explain this discrepancy is that of spatial summation—the volume or area of tissue being stimulated is the crucial determinant of the threshold-of-pain perception. Other effective stimuli for visceral pain are ischemia, via accumulation of pain-producing substances in the ischemic tissue (ie., bradykinin, adenosine) and inflammation, due to mediator-induced hyperalgesia.

The apparent lack of specificity for "noxious" stimuli to produce pain in the viscera has led to the intensity theory for an encoding mechanism for noxious visceral events by afferent fibers.[22,26] Here, the same fibers will respond to innocuous events by encoding at some low-discharge frequency and then with higher discharge frequencies for noxious stimuli. Considerable electrophysiological evidence exists in support of this theory for some visceral tissues. An additional factor of great importance is that the majority of visceral structures have an extremely low innervation density. The total number of visceral afferents for the entire thoracic and abdominal contents amounts to only 5% to 15% of the total pool of spinal afferents.[22,26] Consequently, as mentioned above, the summation of afferent information is very likely an important, if not necessary, factor in visceral sensation. Experimental studies again are in agreement and suggest that individual afferent fibers exhibit a continuum of mechanical thresholds.

Evidence also exists for the presence in some viscera of an appreciable number of afferent fibers that do not normally respond to any level of mechanical stimulation. Instead, some of these fibers respond specifically to chemical stimuli and have been termed "silent" or "sleeping" afferents. These fibers, then, would appear to be ideally suited to respond to local changes occurring as the result of inflammation. Moreover, once activated by the presence of chemical mediators, these same fibers then become capable of responding to mechanical events such as distension. The presence of these fibers further reinforces the concept that the mechanisms involved in the generation and perception of visceral pain may dramatically change as the local environment transforms from normal healthy tissue to diseased pathologic states. Evidence supports a slowly developing recruitment of C fibers that exhibit a sustained increase in excitability and responsiveness in the setting of inflammatory states.

For visceral pain, two distinct patterns of localization have been described:

(1) the so-called "true" visceral pains which are perceived as arising from deep inside the body in the midline, either anterior or posterior, and which may occasionally radiate over considerable distances, and (2) the so-called "referred pain" (or perhaps more appropriately as *ubertragener schmerz* in German for "transferred pain") which localizes in a generally dermatomal distribution to more superficial structures. Other notable features of referred pain are its ability to mask the initial "true" visceral pain and for the area of referral to become hyperalgesic with time.

A number of mechanisms have been proposed over the years to explain the origins of these referred sensations.[26] Current opinion appears to favor a combination of at least three of the following theories: projection-convergence, convergence-facilitation, and psychological. Referred pain in the projection-convergence model arises from primary somatic and visceral afferents having axons that converge onto common dorsal horn interneurons. According to this theory, ascending visceral sensory information from the spinal cord is ultimately misconstrued as arising from somatic structures. There is now a large body of experimental evidence that shows somatovisceral convergence in spinal neurons to be a common occurrence; however, it is still unknown whether signal-processing itself or the integration of somatic and visceral reflexes is the primary mode for the generation of the referred pain sensation. Referred hyperalgesia is not adequately explained by this theory, but the concept of convergence-facilitation does and is coming into more favor as our understanding of the molecular mechanisms involved is advancing. This latter theory proposes that activity in visceral afferent neurons does not give rise to the sensation of pain directly, but instead induces a state of "irritability" within the spinal cord that allows other segmentally appropriate somatic neurons to produce the actual sensation of referred pain. Lastly, the psychological mechanism of referred pain suggests that inputs from supraspinal levels are important forces in the generation of the referred pain sensation.

The anatomy of pain appears to promote a somatic-visceral interaction. The sympathetic afferents and efferents to and from the spinal cord lie in close physical proximity to afferent nociceptors and allow for a peripheral somatic-visceral interaction. Segmental reflexes between the systems are responsible for some somatic responses to primary visceral pain, such as guarding or muscle-splinting, and for visceral responses to primary somatic pain, such as local vasodilation. In addition, the autonomic nervous system participates in another type of sympathetically maintained pain cascade known as reflex sympathetic dystrophy. This phenomenon is felt to be the result of a close regulation of the excitability of mechanoreceptors, such that even mild stimulation is capable of activating nociceptors.[27] This phenomena is capable of extending across contiguous axons and their neurons in the central nervous system and periphery.

The **physiology of the visceral pain syndromes** has been best described for the GI viscera and much less clearly for the thoracic viscera. Visceral pain from the GI tract is mediated by free-nerve endings that have specialized sensory receptors and are located in the mucosa, muscle, and serosa. Mechanoreceptors in the muscle respond to both distension and contraction, and would thus appear to be tension receptors.

Most pain syndromes from the lungs result from inflammation of the pleura. None of the visceral fibers innervating the lungs appear to directly mediate a sensation of pain.

## Etiology and Classic Presentations

The causes of the chest pain syndromes can be categorized according to the organ system producing the pain. This anatomic classification parallels both the physiology of the thoracic pain syndromes and the traditional clinical approach to chest pain. This section will focus on the classic pain syndromes arising from the heart and great vessels, the lungs, the GI tract, and the thoracic muscles and bones. Pain arising from the neck, skin, breasts, mediastinum, nerves, and kidneys will also be briefly discussed. We will review the pathophysiology of pain (if known) and classic presentation for each syndrome. The subsequent section of diagnostic strategy will focus on how to discriminate among the pain syndromes.

## Aorta

### Aortic Dissection

Chest pain is the cardinal symptom of dissection, occurring in more than 90% of cases. Approximately 2000 new cases of this potentially catastrophic disease occur each year in the United States.[28,29] Pain starts in the midscapular region or anterior chest and migrates along the course of the dissection. Pain results from the release of inflammatory mediators due the traumatic disruption of vascular tissues and due to subsequent peripheral ischemia.

Aortic dissection might be more accurately described by the term "dissecting hematoma," which vividly depicts the underlying pathophysiology of this illness. Cystic medial necrosis of the aortic wall results from an expanding column of blood that is driven under arterial pressure to strip the intima from the adventitia.[30] The initial event of this process may be either the development of an acute tear in the intima, or a hemorrhage within the media that then expands and eventually causes a tear along the intima. More than 95% of all cases arise in one of two locations: (1) in the ascending aorta within several centimeters of the aortic valve, or (2) just beyond the origin of the left subclavian artery in the descending thoracic aorta.[29] One classification scheme in use is based upon the approach to therapy and divides dissections into two types—all dissections that involve the ascending aorta and/or arch (Type A or "proximal") and dissections involving only the descending thoracic aorta (Type B or "distal").[31] Proximal dissections account for at least two-thirds of all cases, according to autopsy studies.[32] Clinical series may report a larger percentage of distal dissections because proximal dissections are generally much more rapidly lethal.[33]

While occurring in all age groups, the peak incidence of aortic dissection is in the sixth and seventh decades of life, with men accounting for approximately two-thirds of all cases. The most common presenting symptom (seen in 90% of cases) is severe pain.[34] The minority of patients without pain are, for the most part, suffering from an alteration in the level of consciousness. The pain of dissection is usually severe from the outset and may be all but unbearable. These patients will typically be agitated, writhing in agony, or pacing about continuously in an attempt to find a more comfortable position. Patients will frequently describe the quality of their pain as tearing, stabbing, or ripping. With proximal dissections, the pain is generally felt maximally in the anterior chest. In distal dissections, an interscapular location for the pain is most common and is reported by more than 90% of these patients.[33] Dissections that involve the ascending aorta or arch may also manifest pain in the neck, throat, jaw, or teeth. Importantly, the majority (>70%) of patients with aortic dissection will report migration of the pain from its point of origin, following the path of the dissection as it progresses.[33] Vasovagal symptoms are also common at the outset and may include diaphoresis, anxiety, nausea, vomiting, or lightheadedness. With extensive dissections, other clinical manifestations may occur depending on the structures involved. These clinical manifestations can include congestive heart failure from dissection-induced severe aortic insufficiency; pain of cardiac ischemia from involvement of the coronary arteries; syncope or "cerebrovascular accidents" without focal neurologic deficits from involvement of the arterial branches off the aortic arch; or possibly even cardiac tamponade from rupture of the dissection into the pericardial space.

Physical exam alone is reasonably predictive of the diagnosis of aortic dissection. Generally, these patients will appear to be in a shock state; however, an elevated blood pressure can also be encountered. The reported "classic" findings for the diagnosis of aortic dissection are more characteristic of the proximal-type dissections, including pulse deficits, aortic insufficiency with an incidence of more than 50%, and neurologic manifestations. Other findings that occur occasionally include a notable pulsation of one of the sternoclavicular joints, Horner's syndrome, vocal cord paralysis, superior mediastinal syndrome, pulsating neck masses, hemoptysis, hematemesis, bronchospasm, or pleural effusions.[29,35,36]

Routine laboratory studies are not helpful in making the diagnosis. The electrocardiogram (ECG) will usually show changes consistent with left ventricular hypertrophy without signs of myocardial ischemia. The chest roentgenogram reveals a widened aortic contour in 40% to 50% of cases and comparison with previous films is most helpful. The so-called "calcium sign," defined as a greater than 1-cm separation of the intimal calcification in the aortic knob from the border of the adventitia, is virtually pathognomonic of aortic dissection.

Numerous imaging techniques are available to help the clinician with diagnosis and determination of appropriate therapy. Transthoracic echocardiography is diagnostic in only about one of three of these patients. Computed tomography (CT) of the chest with contrast enhancement is accurate in two-thirds of both proximal and distal dissections. Transesophageal echocardiography (TEE) combined with transthoracic echocardiography has a reported 99% sensitivity and a 98% specificity in the diagnosis of aortic dissections[37,38]; this is now the initial procedure of choice for rapid diagnosis. Aortography remains the single best method to establish the diagnosis, identify the site of origin, and to determine the extent of involvement and it has an overall sensitivity of 96% in experienced hands.

## Aortic Aneurysms

Aortic aneurysms are an uncommon cause of chest pain. The pain is usually gradual at onset, severe by the time of presentation, and localized to the right anterior chest or sternum in ascending aneurysms or the left posterior ribs and spine for descending aneurysms. Diagnosis can usually be established by patient history and chest roentgenogram.

Hypertension and arteriosclerosis are important cofactors in the development of aortic aneurysms. The structural changes that result may lead to accelerated medial degeneration of the aortic wall in excess of the "normal" aging process and localized dilation. Approximately 25% of all arteriosclerotic aneurysms involve the thoracic aorta,[39] especially the arch and/or the descending portion. Aneurysms of the aortic root and ascending portion may occur in the presence of syphilitic heart disease, Marfan's syndrome, and annuloaortic ectasia.

The natural history of thoracic aneurysms is one of gradual expansion of the aneurysm with clinical manifestations resulting from compression of surrounding structures,[40] such as dysphagia or superior vena cava syndrome. Chest pain syndrome that develops is due to compression and erosion of any adjacent musculoskeletal structures. Erosions of the sternum and right side of the thoracic cage may result from expanding aneurysms of the ascending aorta, while descending aortic aneurysms may erode into the vertebral column or left side of the posterior ribs. Patients will usually describe the pain as being steady, boring, occasionally pulsating, and exceptionally severe. Compression of the tracheobronchial tree and especially the left mainstem bronchus may lead to tracheal deviation, wheezing, cough, dyspnea, hemoptysis, or recurrent pneumonitis. A hoarse voice may develop with compression of the left recurrent laryngeal nerve. Rupture of the aneurysm, most commonly when larger than 7 cm, is associated with the onset of excruciating pain.

Most thoracic aneurysms are easily seen on chest roentgenograms. Fluoroscopy can be utilized to help differentiate them from mediastinal masses. Angiography is the definitive diagnostic procedure to assess the size, location, and other anatomical features of the aneurysm. Alternatively, CT with contrast media injection can be used.[41] Transesophageal echocardiography has also emerged as an excellent imaging technique for the thoracic aorta, and it compares favorably with results from CT scanning.[42,43]

### Aortic Arteritis Syndromes

Aortic arteritis is a rare cause of chest pain. However, arteritis syndromes can be fatal and should easily be diagnosed and effectively treated. Aortic arteritis occurs in 50% of patients with Takayasu's arteritis,[44] 15% of patients with giant cell (temporal) arteritis, and sporadically with ankylosing spondylitis, psoriatic arthritis, arthritis associated with ulcerative colitis, Reiter's syndrome, and relapsing polychondritis.[45,46]

The onset of clinical manifestations of Takayasu's arteritis is in the teenage years in as many as 75% of cases.[44,47,48] Nonspecific constitutional symptoms develop initially and may include fever, anorexia, malaise, weight loss, night sweats, arthralgias, pleuritic or anginalike chest pain, and fatigue. Localized pain over affected arteries may also be noted. These symptoms subside and after a variable latent period, patients exhibit signs and symptoms of diminished or absent pulses, bruits, hypertension, and heart failure.[44] True myocardial ischemia or infarction as well as manifestations of ischemia to various affected sites may also occur. Criteria have been proposed for the clinical diagnosis of Takayasu's arteritis, and are reviewed elsewhere.[49] The course of the disease is unpredictable, but slow progression over ensuing months to years is usual.

The classic presentation of giant cell arteritis is with the triad of fever, severe headache, and malaise. When arteritis involves the aorta or major aortic branches, symptoms are similar to those seen in Takayasu's arteritis and result from ischemia of any involved arteries. More rarely, aortic aneurysms, aortic insufficiency, and aortic dissection may occur.[50]

## Cardiovascular

### Myocardial Ischemia

The vast majority of ischemic heart disease is the result of atherosclerotic obstruction of the coronary arteries. There is also a small group of rare causes of "nonatheromatous" coronary obstruction that is listed in Table II. Conditions that impair coronary blood flow or upset the balance of coronary oxygen supply and demand may also produce symptoms of ischemia, and many of these will be discussed subsequently. In the emergency department setting, nearly 90% of patients presenting with acute ischemia are correctly identified. In order to achieve this high sensitivity, many patients who ultimately prove not to have ischemia are admitted to the hospital. The resulting false-positive rate for hospital admission averages around 40%.[51]

Cardiac pain is probably mediated by vagal and sympathetic afferents via several nociceptors. Thin myelinated or unmyelinated afferent axons innervating the ventricles of the heart and the coronary vessels travel with the sympathetic cardiac nerves. Both A$\delta$ and C fibers are present and exist as a homogeneous population without any specific nociceptive capacity. Most, if not all, primary afferents from the heart exhibit pulse-related or volume-related activity, indicating mechanosensitivity.[22] Coronary occlusion that results in cardiac ischemia is likely *not* a necessary nor a sufficient stimulus for pain.[22,26] While many afferent fibers can be seen to respond briskly to such an event, likely induced by some chemical mediator given the usual 10- to 30-second

**Table II**
Causes of Myocardial Infarction Without Coronary Atherosclerosis

| | |
|---|---|
| **Coronary Arter Disease Other Than Athero-sclerosis** | **Emboli to Coronary Arteries** |
| Arteritis | Infective Endocarditis |
| Luetic | Prolapse of Mitral Valve |
| Granulomatous (Takayasu's disease) | Mural Thrombus from Left Atrium, Left Ventricle |
| Polyarteritis Nodosa | |
| Mucocutaneous Lymph Node (Kawasaki's) Syndrome | Prosthetic Valve Emboli |
| | Cardiac Myxoma |
| Disseminated Lupus Erythematosus | Associated with Cardiopulmonary Bypass Surgery and Coronary Arteriography |
| Rheumatoid Arthritis | |
| Ankylosing Spondylitis | Paradoxical Emboli |
| **Trauma to Coronary Arteries** | Papillary Fibroelastoma of the Aortic Valve ("fixed embolus") |
| Laceration | |
| Thrombosis | **Congenital Coronary Artery Anomalies** |
| Iatrogenic | Anomalous Origin of Left Coronary from Pulmonary Artery |
| **Coronary Mural Thickening with Metabolic Diseases or Intimal Proliferative Disease** | |
| | Left Coronary Artery From Anterior Sinus of Valsalva |
| Mucopolysaccharidoses (Hurler's disease) | |
| Homocystinuria | Coronary Arteriovenous Fistulas |
| Fabry's Disease | Coronary Artery Aneurysms |
| Amyloidosis | **Myocardial Oxygen Demand-Supply Disproportion** |
| Juvenile Intimal Sclerosis (Idiopathic arterial calcification of infancy) | |
| | Aortic Stenosis: all forms |
| Intimal Hyperplasia Associated with Contraceptive Steroids or the Postpartum Period | Incomplete Differentiation of the Aortic Valve |
| | Aortic Insufficiency |
| Pseudoxanthoma Elasticum | Carbon Monoxide Poisoning |
| Coronary Fibrosis Caused by Radiation Therapy | Thyrotoxicosis |
| | Prolonged Hypotension |
| Luminal Narrowing by Other Mechansisms | **Hematological (in situ Thrombosis)** |
| Spasm of Coronary Arteries (Prinzmetal's angina with normal coronary arteries) | Polycythemia Vera |
| | Thrombocytosis |
| Spasm with nitroglycerin withdrawal | Disseminated Intravascular Coagulation |
| Dissection of the Aorta | Hypercoagulability |
| Dissection of the Coronary Artery | Hypercoagulability, Thrombosis, Thrombocytopenic Purpura |
| Mucocutaneous Lymph Node Syndrome (Kawasaki's disease) | |
| | **Miscellaneous** |
| | Cocaine Abuse |
| | Myocardial Contusion |
| | Myocardial Infarction with Normal Coronary Arteries |

Modified from Cheitlin M. et al.: Myocardial infarction without atherosclerosis. JAMA 1975;231:951. Copyright 1975, American Medical Association.

latency period, growing experimental and clinical evidence suggests that afferent chemosensitivity is frequently irrelevant in the origin of cardiac pain. Evidence that simple mechanical effects, such as direct coronary artery traction or vessel occlusion without ischemia cause pain and the absence of pain in the setting of myocardial ischemia with electrocardiographic changes poses a significant challenge to the notion that cardiac pain is mediated via specific nociceptors.

## The Anginal Syndromes

Angina (Latin, "to choke" or "to strangle") refers to any pain or discomfort that results from ischemic myocardium. Symptoms of myocardial ischemia other than angina have also been reported and include such things as breathlessness, lightheadedness, fatigue, and belching. These represent the so-called "anginal equivalents." Regardless of the anginal syndrome under discussion, the discomfort of myocardial ischemia may be reported to range from minimal distress at one extreme to severely incapacitating at the other extreme. Patients frequently will deny the descriptor "pain" as being an accurate representation of their discomfort, instead opting to describe their perceptions as crushing, tightness, pressure, squeezing, heaviness, constricting, burning, searing, bursting, or even "indigestion." Levine's sign (ie, the clenching of a fist over the sternum) is a frequently seen mannerism used by patients to express these sensations.

Classically, the discomfort or pain is located retrosternally and may radiate into the left arm, down the medial aspect of the forearm, and into the wrist and fingers. Less often, it may travel to the neck, jaw, shoulder, teeth, back, or into the right arm. Very rarely, it may be entirely epigastric in location. In classical descriptions, there is always at least a brief period, even if only for a few seconds, of mounting discomfort. The pain of angina does not begin at its maximal intensity. Further, angina is almost never so precisely localized that a patient can point to the site of pain with one finger. While angina may include a sensation of involvement of the surface of the skin, the experience of pain is usually deep-seated within the chest. Angina is almost never an exclusively superficial sensation.

Chest pain of myocardial ischemia that does not clearly match the above description has been referred to over the years as "atypical chest pain." Pain characteristics that have most often been described as representing a cause other than angina include pleuritic pain (ie, sharp or knifelike pain brought on by respiration or coughing), pain whose location can be precisely localized with one finger, pain that is reproducible with movement or palpation of the chest wall or arms, pain that is

constant or lasts for days, and pain that is exceptionally brief lasting a few seconds or less. While it is true that these descriptions are more apt to be found in clinical entities other than coronary ischemia, it must be remembered that these characteristics are by no means entirely "benign." Lee et al.[52] showed that patients with proven coronary artery atherosclerosis resulting in ischemia will present with "atypical pain" in up to 20% of cases overall. Of note, it was also shown that coronary ischemia can be present in 23% of those presenting with "burning or indigestion," 22% of those with "sharp" or "stabbing" pains, 13% of those with pleuritic pain, 7% of those with pain that is reproducible with palpation, and 24% of those with "other" atypical pain descriptions.

A separation of angina into distinct clinical syndromes is in popular usage, although it is somewhat arbitrary since considerable overlap exists. They are associated with a spectrum of pathophysiological settings; isolated fixed obstruction to isolated intermittent spasm is envisioned to exist with varying combinations of obstruction and spasm in between. Deliberately simplistic, this classification is nonetheless useful as a framework to devise diagnostic and therapeutic regimens.

***Stable Angina Pectoris (Angina of Effort):*** Exertion, emotion (particularly anger), meals, sexual intercourse, and exposure to cold or heat will predictably reproduce onset of angina. These episodes are short-lived, lasting a few seconds to 30 to 45 minutes and will resolve quickly with rest and/or administration of nitroglycerin in 2 to 10 minutes. "Pain" lasting less than a few seconds or longer than 30 to 45 minutes suggests the presence of unstable angina or MI.

***Unstable Angina (Acute Coronary Insufficiency, Preinfarction Angina):*** This category includes the following three anginal syndromes:

(a) Angina pectoris that occurs at rest or with minimal exertion. These attacks may be prolonged and occur without apparent provocation. Response to nitroglycerin may be disappointing, and these patients have the highest incidence of eventual MI of all the patterns of angina discussed.

(b) Angina pectoris of new (ie, within 1 month) onset that occurs after minimal provocation. These patients generally respond well to nitroglycerin, at least at first.

(c) Angina pectoris that changes from a previously well-established pattern of exertion-related discomfort to becoming more frequent, more prolonged, or more severe. Nitroglycerin that previously provided relief may cease to be of benefit for pain relief.

**Variant Angina (Prinzmetal's Angina, Vasospastic Angina):** The pain of variant angina is similar to that of classic angina in location, quality, pattern of referred pain, and any associated symptoms. This group is different from classic angina in three important respects: (1) the pain occurs almost exclusively at rest and is not provoked by exertion or strong emotions; (2) the pain tends to occur at the same time of day or night (characteristically in the early morning hours); and (3) an ECG will reveal striking ST segment elevations. The pain and ECG changes often respond to nitroglycerin. This syndrome is thought to be the result of coronary artery spasm, more commonly in combination with fixed stenosis of a proximal coronary artery (about two-thirds of the time). Patients in this category tend to be younger and to lack the risk factors associated commonly with classic effort angina. Attacks tend to occur in clusters and patients in this group are also more likely to have additional vasospastic disorders, such as migraine or Raynaud's disease. Interestingly, spontaneous remissions occur commonly and may be of prolonged duration.

**Syndrome X:** This label came into clinical usage to describe patients with the combination of classic angina, "normal" coronary artery anatomy by angiography, and ischemic appearing ST segment changes during exercise testing. This category is truly a syndrome complex encompassing many possible causes, but with spasm of small myocardial arteries (so-called "microvascular angina"), psychiatric disorders, and/or the esophagus as the most common origins.[53-57] Although these patients also appear to have a heightened cardiac pain sensitivity,[55,57] there is no increased myocardial morbidity or mortality in this group. In general, a favorable prognosis exists, though many of these patients continue to complain of frequent chest pain to the point that the symptoms may substantially interfere with the patient's lifestyle.[58-62]

## Myocardial Infarction

The overall prevalence of MI in patients presenting to the emergency department with chest pain is approximately 10% to 20%.[52, 63-66] Of these, 92% to 98% will be admitted to the hospital. On average only 18% to 42% (and typically around one-third) of the 1.7 million patients admitted to the intensive care unit each year will subsequently prove to have an MI.[51]

In the under-35-years-of-age group, coronary atherosclerosis is less commonly the underlying pathologic mechanism of acute MI. As demonstrated by autopsy studies or by coronary arteriography,[67] approximately 6% to 25% of this age group will not have demonstrable atherosclerosis. A variety of other coronary vessel or myocardial lesions will be seen in approximately one-half of these patients (see Table II), while the other half will have no coronary obstructive lesions identified.[68,69] Following recovery from the initial MI, the occurrence of recurrent MI, biventricular heart failure, or death is very unusual in this group with normal coronary arteries,[70,71] and only a small minority will ever develop anginal syndromes.

Although no precipitating factor can be identified in nearly 50% of patients experiencing an MI, heavy or modest exertion and emotional stress have been identified as clear triggers.[72,73] Other important predisposing factors for MI affect the balance of myocardial oxygen supply and demand, such as acute blood loss, hypotension, fever, tachycardia, hypoxemia of any cause, hypoglycemia, serum sickness, allergy, administration of vasoconstricting agents, stroke, and myocardial contusions.

*History:* The clinical history can contribute substantially to the diagnosis of acute MI. A prodrome of classic angina pectoris or unstable angina is characteristic in 20% to 60% of patients.[74] While the nature of the pain is similar to the anginal syndromes mentioned above, the quality of the pain is noted to be severe to intolerable by the majority of patients and is not relieved by rest or nitroglycerin. Also, the pain of MI is usually protracted, generally lasting more than 30 minutes and sometimes for a number of hours or days. The discomfort is usually most apparent retrosternally and often radiates down the ulnar aspect of the left arm. In some patients, however, the pain may begin in the epigastric region or radiate into the shoulders, right arm, jaw, or interscapular regions. In some patients, especially the elderly, the symptoms of acute MI may manifest as the so-called "anginal equivalents" of weakness, dyspnea, diaphoresis, or nausea. Pain is now recognized as a marker of continued ischemia to viable myocardium and reminds clinicians to never be complacent about ongoing cardiac pain under any circumstance.

Numerous studies have documented a significant periodicity for the onset of acute MI,[75,76] with 9 a.m. corresponding to the peak incidence. This correlates with the circadian rhythms of other important biophysiologic factors (eg, catecholamines, cortisol, platelet aggregation) that also peak in effect in the early morning hours. In support of this relationship is the increased incidence of other vasospastic/thrombotic disorders at this time of day, such as sudden death,[77] stroke,[78] and transient myocardial ischemia.[79,80]

Activation of vagal reflexes is thought to be responsible for the noted occurrence of nausea and vomiting in more than 50% of patients with severe chest pain and transmural MI.[81] These symptoms are more commonly seen in inferior wall MI than in anterior wall MI. Other associated "vagal" symptoms include palpitations, dizziness, cold perspiration, and the sense of impending doom.

The Framingham Heart Study and other population studies have suggested that between 20% to 60% of all nonfatal MIs may be unrecognized by the patient and are discovered only by chance on subsequent ECG testing or at autopsy.[82-84] These episodes of so-called "silent infarction" may be more common in patients with hypertension or diabetes.

*Physical Examination:* The general appearance of patients suffering an acute MI is often one of anxiety and substantial distress. Dyspnea is common, and in patients with evidence of left ventricular failure, the respiratory rate may correlate with the degree of failure. Patients with acute MI complicated by cardiogenic shock may be listless and make few respiratory efforts. They frequently have cool, mottled, and clammy skin as well as cyanosis of the nailbeds and lips. The patient's mental status depends on the adequacy of cerebral perfusion.

Most commonly, sinus tachycardia at 100 to 110 bpm is seen initially with some subsequent slowing as the patient's pain and anxiety are treated. The heart rate can vary widely, however, depending on the underlying rhythm. Premature ventricular contractions are seen in up to 95% of patients evaluated early after the onset of symptoms. During the initial presentation, more than half of those patients with an inferior wall MI will exhibit hypotension, bradycardia, or both (due to excess parasympathetic stimulation), while half of patients with an anterior wall MI will have hypertension, tachycardia, or both (due to excess sympathetic stimulation).[85] Low-grade fevers (ie, rectal temperatures of 101°F to 102°F) are seen commonly within 24 to 48 hours of the onset of MI and usually resolve within a week. Diffuse wheezing or cough productive of frothy, pink sputum may suggest patients with severe left ventricular failure.

Although the cardiac examination can be remarkably unrevealing despite extensive ischemic injury, patients may present with a variety of physical findings. Patients with marked ventricular dysfunction and/or left bundle branch block (LBBB) may exhibit paradoxical splitting of the second heart sound ($S_2$). A third heart sound ($S_3$) is said to represent extensive left ventricular dysfunction in the setting of large MIs; however, it is audible in only half of those patients with a pulmonary capillary wedge pressure (PCWP) greater than 18 mm Hg, as well as in half of those with PCWPs less than 18 mm Hg.[86] In those patients with acute MI in sinus rhythm, a fourth heart sound ($S_4$) is almost invariably present and is of little diagnostic value. Systolic murmurs may be heard commonly in acute MI patients and are usually the result of mitral regurgitation due to dysfunction of papillary muscles or as the result of decreased compliance of the left ventricle. Other systolic murmurs may be present and suggest the diagnoses of papillary muscle rupture, interventricular septal rupture, or tricuspid regurgitation. Short-lived pericardial friction rubs may be heard in up to 7% to 20% of all patients with an acute MI.[87] Rubs are noted most commonly on the second or third day after infarction. Of patients with acute MI who have a pericardial friction rub, 40% or so will have a pericardial effusion on echocardiography.[88] Occasionally, only the systolic component of the rub is audible and the sound may be misinterpreted as a systolic murmur.

**Serum Markers:** Damaged myocardial cells release a large number of cytosolic components into the circulation, resulting in certain enzyme levels that can be specifically measured. Currently, the activity of creatine phosphokinase (CPK), and more specifically its MB isoenzyme, and of lactic dehydrogenase (LDH), and its isoenzyme ratios, are used in the laboratory diagnosis of acute MI.

Elevated serum CPK levels are the most sensitive enzymatic markers of acute MI that are in routine use today.[89,90] Serum CPK levels rise within 4 to 8 hours after the onset of MI and fall back to normal levels within 3 to 4 days. Estimation of infarct size by enzyme analysis is problematic due to therapeutic emphasis on achieving rapid reperfusion. The time to peak CPK activity will occur earlier in patients who have had successful reperfusion as a result of thrombolytic therapy, early spontaneous thrombolysis, or mechanical recanalization. Normal CPK levels in women are generally about two-thirds of those in similarly aged men.

Cardiac muscle principally contains the MM and MB isoenzymes of CPK. Except in cases of trauma or surgery performed on the diaphragm, uterus, small intestine, tongue, or prostate (additional sources of CPK-MB), elevated serum activity of CPK-MB should be considered first to arise from an acute MI. Transient severe ischemia, without myocardial necrosis, has also been shown to increase CPK-MB levels.[91] If MI is suspected, total CPK level and CPK-MB levels should be measured at 0, 12, and 24 hours. If these levels are nondiagnostic or if the suspected MI may have occurred more than 24 hours earlier, a total LDH level should be obtained and later fractionated into its component isoenzymes if the total LDH is elevated. When measured serially, CPK-MB levels have a sensitivity of 100% and a specificity of 98% for MI. Levels of these enzymes do **not** detect unstable angina or imminent infarction.

Total LDH is a sensitive but not a very specific indicator of myocardial injury. Levels of LDH rise above the normal range within 24 to 48 hours after an MI, reach peak levels in 3 to 6 days after the MI, and then return to baseline levels within 8 to 14 days after the MI. Fractionation of LDH into its five isoenzymes increases the diagnostic accuracy of this test as the heart contains $LDH_1$ primarily whereas $LDH_4$ and $LDH_5$ are principally found in skeletal muscle and the liver. Elevated levels of total LDH and of $LDH_1$ occur in more than 95% of patients with acute MI.[89,92] Because $LDH_1$ levels are also raised by hemolysis, handling of blood specimens is an important issue. Another useful measurement is the $LDH_1/LDH_2$ ratio, which when greater than 1.0 has a more than 90% sensitivity and specificity for the diagnosis of acute MI.[90,93] These levels are of particular interest when a mild CPK-MB elevation has occurred in a setting that may also have produced gut ischemia,[94] and therefore may be confused with a MI, as well as for those patients who are suspected to have had their MI 2 to 4 days earlier after their CPK levels have already fallen back to the normal range.

Other laboratory measures are generally nonspecific and are not routinely used to establish the diagnosis. Current research suggests that some promising new assays may soon be available to aid with more rapid diagnosis of acute MI than is possible with traditional CPK-MB testing. Initial work along these lines involving cardiac troponin T (cTT)[95,96] and new assays for subforms of CPK-MB[97] are quite hopeful, and the day may not be long off where clinicians will have rapid and accurate bedside testing at their disposal for the diagnosis of acute MI in as little as 15 minutes.

***Electrocardiography:*** Electrocardiography changes can be diagnostically useful during episodes of chest pain and in the majority of patients with acute MI (Figures 4A and 4B). Standard 12-lead ECGs are diagnostic for acute MI in 18% to 65% of initial exams and in fully 83% to 93% of those with MI when tracings are obtained serially over hours to days.[12,98–104] A summary of the ECG patterns for the diagnosis of acute MI is shown in Table III. While the most specific finding for acute MI is ST segment elevations of greater than or equal to 1 mm in two or more contiguous leads,[64,65] only 50% of MI patients will have this presentation on initial ECG.[98,101,105] An ST segment depression of greater than or equal to 1 mm is less specific and may represent ischemia or Q wave infarction. Of those patients with both Q waves and ST segment elevation, 82% to 94% will have acute MI. Deep ($\geq$ 1 mm) and symmetrical inverted T waves generally have the same significance as ST segment depressions. Isolated inverted T waves, however, are generally not helpful in diagnosis since they are seen in 10% of patients admitted to the cardiac intensive care unit, of whom only 22% have actual MI. Interestingly, a "normal" ECG (occurring in 6% to 20% of patients with chest pain syndromes) does **not** exclude ischemic heart disease; 1% to 6% of emergency department presentations will have acute MI and another 4% will have unstable angina. There are a few conditions in which ECG features may mimic the patterns of acute MI, and many of these are also in the differential diagnosis of chest pain syndromes (see Table IV).

## Table III
### Electrocardiogram Criteria for the Diagnosis of Myocardial Infarction

| Location of MI | Leads of Q Waves, ST Elevation, and T Wave Inversion | Leads of ST Depression |
|---|---|---|
| Anterior | I, aVL | II, III, aVF |
| Interior | II, III, aVF | I, aVL |
| Anterolateral | $V_1$–$V_6$ | |
| Anteroseptal | $V_1$–$V_4$ | |
| Inferolateral | II, III, aVF, $V_5$–$V_6$ | |
| Inferoapical | $V_4$–$V_5$ | |
| RV | $V_4$R–$V_6$R | |

aVF = augmented lead, left foot; aVL = augmented lead, left arm; MI = myocardial infarction; RV = right ventricle.

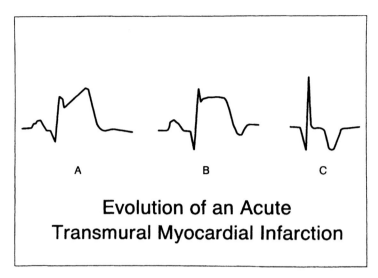

**Figure 4A.** This panel indicates the classic changes seen in the electrocardiogram during classic transmural myocardial infarction. (A) In the hyperacute stage, T waves are tall and peaked. A Q wave may be seen. (B) In the first 48 hours, the ST segment remains elevated and the T wave inverts. A Q wave is present by 48 hours. (C) Several days post-MI, the ST segment normalizes and the Q wave and inverted T wave persist. (Modified with permission from Davison R., *Electrocardiography in Acute Care Medicine*, St. Louis, Mo: Mosby-Year book Inc; 1995)

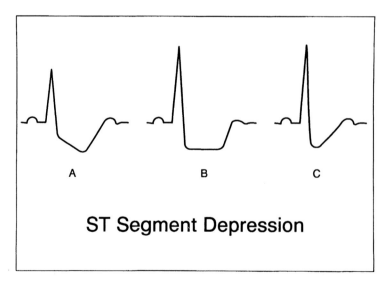

**Figure 4B.** This panel indicates the classic changes seen in the electrocardiogram during a non-Q wave or subendocardial myocardial infarction. Downsloping (A) or horizontal (B) ST segment depression are equally sensitive for myocardial ischemia. Upsloping ST segment depression (C) lacks specificity for ischemia. (Modified with permission from Davison R., *Electrocardiography in Acute Care Medicine*, St. Louis, Mo: Mosby-Year book Inc; 1995)

**Table IV**
Conditions Simulating Infarction on ECG

Ventricular Hypertrophy
  Right Ventricular (cor pulmonale)
  Left Ventricular
Condition Disturbances
Left Bundle Branch Block
Left Anterior Fascicular Block
Wolff-Parkinson-White Syndrome
Primary Myocardial Disease
Myocarditis
Dilated Cardiomyopathy (both obstructuve and
  nonobstructuve)
Friedreich's ataxia
Muscular Dystrophy
Pneumothorax
Pulmonary Embolism
Amyloid Heart Disease
Primary and Metastatic Tumors of the Heart
Traumatic Heart Disease
Intracranial Hemorrhage
Hyperkalemia
Pericarditis
Early Repolarization
Sarcoidosis Involving the Heart

ECG = electrocardiogram.
From Taussig AS et al. Misleading ECGs: Patterns of
infarction. J Cardiovasc Med 1983;9:1147.

*Imaging Studies:* Numerous imaging modalities are available to aid in the diagnosis of acute MI and will be discussed only briefly here. An initial study commonly used in the management of patients with chest pain is the chest roentgenogram. Two findings common in the setting of acute MI are cardiomegaly and signs of left ventricular dysfunction. Pulmonary vascular congestion and pulmonary edema exhibit diagnostic lag times of 12 or more hours for the radiographic findings to reflect the elevated left ventricular end-diastolic pressure. Cardiomegaly may signify other forms of cardiovascular disease such as chronic hypertension, prior MI, or valvular disease. Due to the low specificity of these findings, the major utility of the chest roentgenogram in this setting is its ability to confirm or disprove other diagnostic possibilities.

The detection of an acute MI, assessing the size of the infarct, determining the degree of ventricular dysfunction, and establishing a prognosis are all possible with magnetic resonance imaging and the various forms of nuclear cardiac imaging available today—perfusion scintigraphy, radionuclide angiography, infarct avid scintigraphy, and positron emission tomography. The application of these techniques is beyond the intended scope of this chapter and the interested reader is encouraged to review other sources of current information in this regard.[106,107] A new radiopharmaceutical agent, $^{99m}$Tc hexakis 2-methoxy-2-isobutyl isonitrile (technitium$^{99m}$sestamibi), is available for myocardial perfusion imaging and is useful for the early measurement of the extent of myocardium at risk and the recognition of salvaged myocardium after thrombolytic therapy.[108–111] Its use is being extensively evaluated for the rapid detection of those patients with chest pain syndromes who are suspected to have myocardial ischemia or MI.

Echocardiography has become an extremely useful and important imaging modality in all patients with cardiac disease. Used in both transthoracic and transesophageal locations, this technique is a very sensitive tool to assess for regional ventricular wall motion abnormalities which can be seen almost universally in patients with acute MI.[112,113] Two-dimensional echocardiography has been shown to be diagnostically useful as well as cost-efficient in the evaluation of emergency department patients with chest pain.[112,114] The addition of Doppler techniques to echocardiography allows for identification and assessment of valvular disease and the noninvasive estimation of cardiac output.[115,116]

## Myocarditis

Myocarditis remains a common problem in many areas of the world. Mild chest pain or discomfort frequently accompanies early myocarditis and may be the only symptom present until florid heart failure or dysrhythmias occur. The majority of patients will have no specific complaints referable to the cardiovascular system. Non-specific symptoms are common and may include fatigue, dyspnea, palpitations, and precordial discomfort. The chest pain is usually the result of associated pericarditis, but may on occasion be more suggestive of myocardial ischemia and simulate an acute MI (with anginalike pain, ECG abnormalities, regional wall motion abnormalities, and increased levels of myocardial enzymes).[117]

Numerous infectious agents (Table V)

may result in myocarditis, pathologically defined as an inflammation involving the myocytes, interstitium, or vascular elements of the heart. The specific diagnosis often depends on identifying the associated systemic illness and its characteristics.[118] The diagnosis of viral myocarditis is supported when virus can be identified in biologic specimens but cultures are usually negative and serologic testing is usually nondiagnostic.[119] even in fulminant and fatal cases. While endomyocardial bi-

---

**Table V**
**Principal Infectious Etiological Agents Associated with Myocarditis**

**Bacterial**

| | |
|---|---|
| Streptococcal | Diphtheria |
| Staphylococcal | Salmonellosis |
| Pneumococcal | Tuberculosis |
| Meningococcal | Tularemia |
| Hemophilus | Mycoplasma pneumoniae |
| Gonococcal | Psittacosis |
| Brucellosis | |

**Spirochetal Infections**

| | |
|---|---|
| Leptospirosis | Relapsing Fever |
| Lyme disease | Syphilis |

**Fungal Infections**

| | |
|---|---|
| Aspergillosis | Coccidiomycosis |
| Actinomycosis | Cryptococcosis |
| North American Blastomycosis | Histoplasmosis |
| Candidiasis | |

**Parasitic Infections**

| | |
|---|---|
| Cysticercosis | Trichinosis |
| Schistosomiasis | Trypanosomiasis |
| Toxoplasmosis | Visceral Larva Migrans |

**Rickettsial Infections**

| | |
|---|---|
| Rockey Mountain Spotted Fever | Scrub Typhus |
| Q Fever | Typhus |

**Viral Infections**

| | |
|---|---|
| Adenovirus | Mumps |
| Arbovirus | Poliomyelitis |
| Coxsackievirus | Respiratory Syncytial Virus |
| Cytomegalovirus | Rabies |
| Echovirus | Rubella |
| Encephalomyocarditis Virus | Rubeolla |
| Hepatitis | Vaccina |
| Human Immunodeficiency Virus | Varicella |
| Infectious Mononucleosis | Variola |
| Influenza | Yellow Fever |
| Mumps | |

Adapted from Marboe CC and Fenglio JJ. Pathology and natural history of human myocarditis. Pathol Immunopathol Res 1988;7:226.

opsy is frequently used to confirm the diagnosis of myocarditis, a borderline or negative biopsy does not exclude the diagnosis due to the patchy distribution of disease.

## Cardiac Tumors

The differential diagnosis of chest pain should include cardiac malignancy primarily in patients with tumors known to metastasize to the heart (eg, leukemia or melanoma) or to the pericardium (eg, lung, breast, leukemia, or lymphoma). The incidence of primary tumors of the heart is only 0.0017% to 0.28% in autopsy studies [120,121] and thus are far less common than metastatic tumors to the heart and pericardium.[122] The most common primary cardiac tumor is the benign myxoma and is usually solitary and occurs in the left atrium. Atypical chest pain from myocardial tumors may result from coronary artery obstruction or tumor embolism. Echocardiography (especially TEE), CT, and magnetic resonance imaging are all sensitive techniques to define location and extent of cardiac tumors. Cardiac catheterization with selective angiography is not necessary in all cases if adequate information can be garnered noninvasively.

## Cardiomyopathy

A group of diverse diseases, often of unknown causes, result in cardiomyopathy. The overall incidence of cardiomyopathy is increasing, and it is unclear if this is a reflection of the diseases themselves, or the result of better detection. A useful classification scheme for these varied disorders is based on the underlying functional impairment produced: (1) dilated cardiomyopathy, characterized by atrial and ventricular dilation and contractility problems (any ventricular hypertrophy is hemodynamically inadequate for the degree of dilation present.); (2) hypertrophic cardiomyopathy, so-called because of the inappropriate amount of ventricular hy-

pertrophy in the setting of a well-preserved contractile function, often with asymmetric involvement of the septum (formerly termed IHSS, or idiopathic hypertrophic subaortic stenosis, or also called ASH, or asymmetric septal hypertrophy); and (3) restrictive cardiomyopathy, characterized by the impairment to diastolic filling of the ventricle. This is not an absolute classification system since there is often clinical overlap in individual patients. Both the dilated and hypertrophic variants of cardiomyopathy commonly present with chest pain. The exact mechanism underlying chest pain in many cases remains unclear. Approximately 25% to 50% of these patients will experience chest pain symptoms suggestive of an ischemic nature, despite frequently normal coronary anatomy, both angiographically and at autopsy.[123,124] More than 80% of patients with hypertrophic cardiomyopathy experience an abnormally reduced lumen of their intramural coronary arteries, especially involving the ventricular septum.[125,126] These lesions may be responsible for the development of myocardial ischemia and are prominent in areas showing extensive myocardial fibrosis.[126] In the late stages of dilated cardiomyopathy, chest pain secondary to pulmonary emboli is thought to be frequent.[127] The diagnosis and treatment of cardiomyopathy is discussed in Chapter 2, Dyspnea.

## Pericardial and Myocardial Trauma

Blunt or penetrating injury to the heart remains a common cause of chest pain. In patients experiencing cardiac trauma, the most common symptom that resembles MI in character is precordial chest pain. The diagnosis usually is not difficult to establish when the history of trauma is present. Penetrating injuries to the heart, such as by a knife wound, are typically evident and catastrophic, requiring emergent surgical intervention to prevent death. As such, they are an uncommon cause of chest pain for most non-emergency department or nonsurgical physicians. The focus of this section will be on nonpenetrating cardiac injury.

Both direct compression (eg, the steering wheel squeezing the heart between the sternum and the spine) and indirect compression during automobile accidents may result in significant cardiac injuries. Other causes would include any physical forces that result in direct blows to the chest with blunt objects (eg, falls, sporting injuries, fists, kicks from large animals, cardiac resuscitation). Fractures of the thoracic cage are not necessary to sustain severe trauma and the clinical sequelae may not become apparent for days or even weeks after the incident. Those surviving the immediate trauma will be subject to myriad potential late consequences, such as MI, ventricular aneurysm or pseudoaneurysm, ventricular septal defect, injuries to the great vessels, valvular damage, cardiac tamponade, chronic recurrent pericarditis, and constrictive pericarditis.[128,129]

Pathologically, at least some degree of pericarditis is usually found after nonpenetrating chest trauma. The myocardium itself exhibits a range of findings from areas of small superficial ecchymoses to transmural contusions with areas of necrosis. Healing is in similar fashion to post-MI with scar formation and potential aneurysm formation.[130]

**Pericardial injury** ranges from mild contusions to large lacerations or rupture, and at least some degree of pericarditis can be found in the majority of patients regardless of whether the pericardium is torn. Herniation of all or a portion of the heart may occur through such rents in the pericardium, resulting in acute or delayed circulatory compromise.[131] Clinically, traumatic pericarditis presents in the same manner characteristic of nontraumatic pericarditis. In this setting, however, the major problem may not be the pericarditis itself but rather the complication of hemopericardium with resultant cardiac tamponade. Typically these patients will be agitated, hypotensive, oliguric, or anuric, and have distant heart sounds and an elevated pulsus paradoxus. The ECG will usually show diffuse low voltage and the presence of a pericardial effusion by echocardiogram.

**Myocardial contusion** generally produces insignificant symptoms and frequently goes unrecognized. The most common symptom is precordial chest pain that resembles MI. Chest pain also arises from the other areas of chest trauma and may confuse the clinical picture.[132] Some impairment of right or left ventricular function or both does occur, and this effect of blunt trauma may be potentiated by alcohol.[133,134] Various arrhythmias, including atrioventricular and intraventricular conduction defects, can be seen commonly after myocardial contusion.[135,136] In contrast to acute MI, severe heart failure rarely occurs after cardiac contusion unless there has also been massive valvular damage or rupture of the interventricular septum.[137] The ECG is a useful aid in the recognition of contusion of the left ventricle, commonly showing either nonspecific ST segment and T wave changes or the more classic changes of pericarditis. After the inflammation in pericarditis subsides, ECG signs of deeper injury to the myocardium (eg, Q waves) may become more evident. More important than any one isolated ECG analysis is the evolution of the abnormalities taken in context with additional testing. Today's reliable measures of the MB isoenzyme levels of total CPK can document the presence or absence of cardiac necrosis. An important caveat in this setting is that false-positive CPK-MB elevations can be seen with total CPK levels greater than 20,000 U, which may occur commonly in this setting if massive skeletal muscle injury has also occurred. Contused myocardium will exhibit reduced perfusion on radionuclide imaging studies, changes similar to those seen in patients with acute MI.[133] Echocardiography in this setting can be useful to identify significant pericardial effusions, abnormal wall motion, chamber enlargement, intracardiac shunts, and regurgitant valve lesions.[138]

## Pericardial Disease

Pain arising from the pericardium usually results from focal inflammation of the pericardium and adjacent structures. The most common and well-recognized pericardial chest pain syndromes include pericarditis, cardiac tamponade, the post-pericardiotomy syndromes, pericardial tumor, and the post-MI syndrome. Each of these will be discussed in detail below. Less frequent causes of chest pain include congenital defects in the pericardium, which can produce chest pain via herniation and incarceration of myocardium,[139] and pericardial cysts which may be large and cause chest pain by compression of surrounding structures.[140]

*Pericarditis:* Acute pericarditis is characterized by chest pain, a friction rub, and serial ECG abnormalities. Pericarditis accounts for 0.1% of hospital admissions and is found in 2% to 6% of autopsies. A vast number of medical and surgical conditions may be the cause of pericarditis (Table VI). All of these causes are more common in adults and in men. Coxsackievirus group B and echovirus 8 are the most common causes of acute viral pericarditis and are most commonly seen during spring and fall months.[141] Specific viral pathogens may also be seen with an increasing frequency in the early stages of the acquired immunodeficiency syndrome (AIDS).[142] The incidence of tuberculous pericarditis remains high in countries with endemic tuberculosis, but has decreased dramatically and is now an uncommon cause (ie, 0% to 7%) of acute pericarditis in the United States, except in patients with AIDS.[142,143]

*History:* With acute pericarditis, chest pain is often the patient's chief complaint. The location and quality of pain is variable, generally occurring in retrosternal and/or left precordial areas and frequently with radiation to the neck or trapezius ridge. On occasion, it will have a dull quality and radiate into the left arm, making the clinical separation from myocardial ischemia more difficult. The inflammatory process may also involve the adjacent pleura, resulting in a respirophasic (pleuritic) component to the pain. The pain is often aggravated by deep inspiration, cough, the

## Table VI
### Causes of Pericarditis

**Idiopathic** (nonspecific)

**Viral Infections:** Coxsackievirus Group A, Coxsackievirus Group B, echovirus, adenovirus, mumps virus, infectious mononucleosis, varicella, hepatitis B

**Tuberculosis**

**Acute Bacterial Infection:** pneumococcus, staphylococcus, streptococcus, Gram-negative septicemia, Neisseria Meningitidis, Neisseria gonorrhoeae, tularemia, *Legionella pneumophilia*, mycoplasma, *Nocardia species*, actinomycosis

**Fungal Infections:** histoplasmosis, coccidioidomycosis, *Candida* species, North American blastomycocis

**Other Infections:** toxoplasmosis, amebiasis, echinococcosis, Lyme disease

**Acute Myocardial Infarction**

**Uremia:** untreated uremia, in association with hemodialysis

**Neoplastic Disease:** lung cancer, breast cancer, leukemia, Hodgkin's disease, lymphoma

**Radiation**

**Immunological Disorders:** acute rheumatic fever, systemic lupus erythematosis, rheumatoid arthritis, scleroderma, mixed connective tissue disease, Wegener's granulomatosis, polyarteritis nodosa

**Other Inflammatory Disorders:** sarcoidosis, amyloidosis, inflammatory bowel diseases, Whipple's disease, temporal arteritis, Behçet's disease

**Drugs:** hydralazine, procainamide, diphenylhydantoin, isoniazid, phenylbutazone, dantrolene, doxorubicin, methysergide, penicillin (with hypereosinophilia)

**Trauma:** including chest trauma, hemopericardium following thoracic surgery, pacemaker insertion, cardiac diagnostic procedures—esophageal rupture, pancreatic-pericardial fistula

**Delayed Postmyocardial-Pericardial Injury Syndromes:** Postmyocardial infarction (Dressler's) syndrome, Postpericardiotomy syndrome

**Dissecting Aortic Aneurysm**

**Myxedema**

**Chylopericardium**

supine position, or swallowing. It may be alleviated somewhat by sitting upright and leaning forward. Patients who breathe more shallowly to avoid exacerbating their pain may also experience dyspnea. The presence of fever or large pericardial effusions may also contribute to the sensation of dyspnea.

*Physical Examiniation:* On physical examination, the pathognomonic sign of acute pericarditis is the high-pitched, grating or scratching sound of the pericardial friction rub. It is thought to arise from the chafing of the coarse surfaces of the epicardium and pericardium from the inflammatory process during cardiac motion, regardless of the size of any pericardial effusion. Prospective analysis[144] reveals the classic rub along the lower left sternal border in approximately half of the patients with pericarditis. The rub is classically described as having three components: (1) related to atrial systole, (2) ventricular systole, and (3) early diastole (ie, rapid ventricular-filling phase). The component resulting from ventricular systole is almost always present and is the loudest and most easily heard. The atrial systolic component is present in about 70% of the cases while the early diastolic segment is detectable much less frequently. Importantly, the friction rub may change in quality and intensity from one exam to the next. In order to optimize detection of a pericardial rub, firm pressure on the diaphragm side of the stethoscope should be applied as one listens over the lower left sternal border with the patient sitting upright and leaning forward. Rubs are sometimes confused with systolic murmurs, particularly mitral regurgitation, and skill in the use of bedside maneuvers to augment or alter cardiac sounds can prove useful.

*Diagnostic Testing:* Electrocardiography can be very helpful to confirm the diagnosis of acute pericarditis.[145,146] Epicardial injury and/or superficial inflammation of the myocardium are thought to give rise to the currents of injury seen and generally occur within a few hours to days of the onset of chest pain. Classically, there is an evolution of ST segment and T wave abnormalities through four stages (Figure 5). Overall, 90 % of patients with acute pericarditis will manifest ECG abnormalities, with less than 50% showing variations in the patterns described below.

Occurring with the onset of pericardial pain, stage I ECG changes are characterized by ST segment elevation and can be essentially diagnostic for acute pericarditis (Figure 5). Except for leads aVR and $V_1$, a diffuse elevation of the ST segment occurs with a concave upward aspect and T waves remain upright. Stage I changes must also be distinguished from the early repolarization changes that can be seen as a variant of normal. A useful tool to discriminate between these two ECG patterns is the finding of an ST segment/T wave ratio of greater than 0.25 in lead $V_6$ in cases of pericarditis, but not with early repolarization.[147,148] Stage II begins after several days, with the ST segments returning to baseline, followed by T wave flattening. In stage III, the T waves now characteristically become inverted in most leads. During the early course of ST segment elevation and T wave inversion, limb and precordial leads reveal a characteristic depression of the PR segment in up to 80% of the cases of acute pericarditis.[145] Over weeks to months, stage IV changes occur with the T waves returning to normal. In some conditions associated with chronic inflammation of the pericardium (eg, uremia, neoplasm, tuberculosis), T wave inversion may persist indefinitely. In contrast to the pattern of ECG changes occurring with an evolving acute MI, loss of R wave voltage or new Q waves do not develop in acute pericarditis. In addition, with acute MI, inversion of T waves generally occurs prior to normalization of the ST segment and the elevated ST segments usually have a convex upward configuration.

Sinus tachycardia is common in acute pericarditis, but other dysrhythmias are very infrequent and would suggest coexisting myocardial disease if present.[149]

Chest roentgenography may reveal (1) enlargement of the cardiac silhouette that may be seen when pericardial effusion is

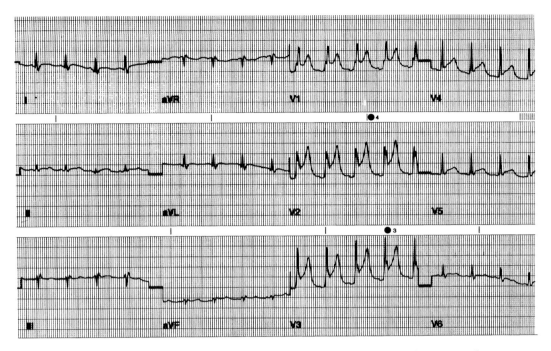

**Figure 5.** These panels indicate the classic changes seen in the electrocardiogram in the presence of acute pericarditis. Typical changes include ST segment elevation in most leads and PR segment depression (arrows). aVF = augmented lead, left foot; aVL = augmented lead, left arm; aVR = augmented lead, right arm. (Modified with permission from Davison R., *Electrocardiography in Acute Care Medicine*, St. Louis, Mo: Mosby—Year book Inc; 1995)

present, (2) clues to the underlying causes of tuberculosis or malignancy, and (3) pleural effusions, usually left-sided[150] and occurring in 25% of the patients.

Cardiac isoenzymes are normal in the majority of the cases; however, they may not be useful to help differentiate acute pericarditis from acute MI as modest CPK-MB fraction elevations may occur as the result of epicardial inflammation.[151] Nonspecific indicators of underlying inflammation, such as leukocytosis and elevation of the erythrocyte sedimentation rate, are often seen in conjunction with acute pericarditis. More extensive blood testing or serologies should be dictated by the possible causes (Table VI). Echocardiography is a sensitive and accurate method for the detection, localization, and quantification of any pericardial effusion.

Uncomplicated acute pericarditis in the immunocompetent host generally does not warrant diagnostic pericardiocentesis or pericardial biopsy due to the low diagnostic yield in this situation. One prospective study has addressed this issue [152] and showed a diagnostic yield of only 5% to 14% in patients with pericardial effusions lasting longer than 1 to 3 weeks. The diagnostic yield was substantially better if a procedure was necessary for the relief of cardiac tamponade, 39% for pericardiocentesis, and 54% for pericardiectomy with biopsy.

***Cardiac Tamponade:*** Almost any cause of pericarditis may cause tamponade in either acute or chronic forms. Approximately 15% of the patients with acute pericarditis will go on to develop tamponade.[152] Symptomatic tamponade is typically a catastrophic hemodynamic event, and chest pain is frequently a minor part of the symptom complex. The reader is referred elsewhere for a more detailed discussion of the pathophysiology, diagnosis, and treatment of tamponade.[153,154]

**Postpericardiotomy Syndromes:** After incision and manipulation of the pericardium, a syndrome of fever, pericarditis, and pleuritis will occur in 10% to 40% of patients 1 week or more after cardiac surgery.[155] Analogous to the Dressler's syndrome (see below), an autoimmune reaction against the epicardium is hypothesized, possibly with a new or reactivated viral infection serving as a triggering or permissive factor.[156] The incidence of this syndrome is generally higher in children than in adults. However, it is very rare in patients under 2 years of age. A pericardial friction rub is often present on physical exam. The chest roentgenogram shows noncardiogenic pulmonary edema or pleural effusion, which is left-sided or bilateral, in two-thirds of cases.[157,158] The ECG will reveal atrial tachyarrhythmias and nonspecific ST segment and T wave changes. Cardiac tamponade is a well-recognized complication of the postpericardiectomy syndrome and occurs in approximately 1% of adults after surgery.[159] Constrictive pericarditis is a rare complication that may occur months to years later.

**Pericardial Tumors:** While primary malignancies of the pericardium (eg, mesothelioma, fibrosarcoma, angiosarcoma, and benign and malignant teratomas[160]) are rare, chest pain due to neoplastic disease of the pericardium is most often due to metastatic disease. The pericardium is involved in 5% to 15% of patients with malignant neoplasms.[161,162] Dyspnea is the more common symptom at the time of presentation but patients frequently present with chest pain as the only cardiopulmonary symptom.[163] Pain arises due to pericardial inflammation. Lung cancer, breast cancer, leukemia, and lymphoma together account for approximately 80% of the reported cases of malignant pericarditis.[161,163] Neoplastic pericarditis is often asymptomatic during life and discovered only incidentally at autopsy. In the majority of patients, the diagnosis is only made after there is evidence of a cardiac compression syndrome. More than 90% of these patients will have an abnormal chest roentgenogram showing pleural effusions, cardiomegaly, widening of the mediastinum, a hilar mass, or sometimes an irregular and nodular contour of the cardiac silhouette.[163] The ECG changes in these patients are generally nonspecific, but if atrioventricular conduction abnormalities are present, malignant extension to the myocardium is suggested.

Pericardiocentesis should be performed in patients with large pericardial effusions or suspected cardiac tamponade. Subsequent cytological analysis is diagnostic of a malignancy in approximately 85% of cases.[163,164] Open pericardial biopsy may be required for diagnosis in some cases and has an accuracy of up to 90%, depending on the size of tissue removed for review.

**Post-Myocardial Infarction Syndrome (Dressler's Syndrome):** This syndrome is reported to occur in up to 4% of patients following MI.[165,166] Possibly of autoimmune origin, this acute illness is characterized by fever, pleuritis, and pericarditis that usually begin 2 to 3 weeks after infarction (range 1 week to several months).[166,167] The resultant chest pain may be severe enough to be confused with a repeat MI or postinfarction angina.[168] Occasionally, this may represent the first episode of chest pain after an initially "silent" episode of infarction. Objective evidence, such as the presence of friction rubs (pericardial or pleural), chest roentgenographic findings of a pericardial effusion and a pleural effusion, ECG abnormalities, or blood testing abnormalities, is unfortunately nondiagnostic in this setting. Dressler's syndrome can usually be distinguished from recent MI with the following three criteria: (1) the chest pain is "atypical" for angina and frequently pleuritic in nature, and fails to respond to nitroglycerin; (2) new Q waves are not seen on the ECG; and (3) there is not a significant rise in the CPK-MB isoenzyme level.

## Valvular Diseases

Although stenosis or insufficiency of each of the cardiac valves has been reported to cause chest pain, a chest pain syndrome occurs commonly only with aortic stenosis (AS), mitral stenosis (MS), and mitral valve prolapse (MVP).

***Aortic Stenosis:*** Isolated aortic stenosis (AS) is the most common of the valvular heart diseases,[169] occurs more commonly in men and is generally congenital or degenerative in origin.[170,171]

*History:* Pain occurs in two-thirds of patients with critical AS, usually defined as a valve area of less than 0.4 cm$^2$/m$^2$. Inadequate myocardial oxygenation may occur in severe AS, even in the absence of any significant degree of coronary artery disease due to an increase in myocardial oxygen consumption. Myocardial ischemia results from this relative underperfusion and may be responsible for the anginal complaints of these patients.[172,173]

The natural history of AS is one of gradually increasing obstruction to left ventricular outflow, with patients generally remaining asymptomatic during this latent phase. Symptoms typically begin around the sixth decade of life and characteristically include angina pectoris, syncope, and heart failure.[174] Once symptoms are manifest, prognosis is poor for those in whom the obstruction to flow is not corrected: 5 years for those with angina, 3 years in the presence of syncopal attacks, and 2 years for those with overt heart failure.[175] Classically dyspnea is the most common initial complaint and "typical" angina occurs in approximately two-thirds of those with critical AS (only 50% of whom will have significant coronary artery obstruction).[176]

*Physical Examination:* Physical examination typically reveals arterial pulses that rise slowly, peak at a reduced amplitude late in systole, and are sustained (ie, pulsus parvus et tardus).[177] Palpation of the carotid arterial pulse readily reveals a coarse systolic thrill, termed the carotid shudder. Palpation of the carotid arteries simultaneously with the cardiac impulse at the apex reveals a distinct lag time in patients with severe AS.[178] With resultant pulmonary hypertension and secondary right ventricular failure with tricuspid regurgitation, prominent v or c-v waves may be present in the jugular venous pulse. The precordial impulse is generally sustained in the presence of left ventricular failure with an inferolateral displacement on the chest wall. A hyperdynamic impulse, on the other hand, suggests a concomitant regurgitant lesion, either aortic or mitral. A precordial systolic thrill can be felt generally in the second intercostal space parasternally or in the suprasternal notch and can be augmented by having the patient lean forward in full expiration. On auscultation, the first heart sound (S$_1$) is generally normal or soft and a prominent S$_4$ (due to vigorous atrial contraction against a partially closed mitral valve) can be appreciated.[179] The systolic murmur of AS is best appreciated at the base of the heart and is often transmitted into the carotids and to the apex. In patients with calcified aortic valves the murmur is typically harsh and rasping in quality. In general, the more severe the stenosis, the greater the duration of the murmur and the more likely it is to peak around midsystole.[180] High-pitched decrescendo diastolic murmurs are common in patients with AS and represent coexisting aortic insufficiency (AI). The murmur of AS can be augmented by having the patient squat or lie supine, while the intensity of the murmur will diminish with Valsalva.

*Diagnostic Testing:* Approximately 85% of patients with severe AS will exhibit signs of left ventricular hypertrophy on ECG. In adults, there is no good correlation between the severity of obstruction and the absolute voltages, and the absence of left ventricular hypertrophy does not exclude the diagnosis of critical AS. Signs of a left ventricular "strain" pattern (ie, ST segment depressions greater than 0.3 mV) suggest extensive ventricular hypertrophy. More than 80% of those with severe

AS will have evidence of left atrial enlargement.[181] Various atrioventricular or intraventricular blocks may be present due to deposition of calcium in the conducting system.[182]

Isolated critical AS may have an entirely normal roentgenographic appearance unless left ventricular failure or coexisting AI lead to cardiomegaly. Poststenotic dilation of the ascending aorta is seen commonly. Almost all adults with significant AS will exhibit calcification of the aortic valve.

Echocardiography is useful to confirm the diagnosis as well as to determine the severity of the stenosis. Noninvasively determined valvular gradients correlate well with results of left heart catheterization.[183,184]

**Mitral Stenosis:** Chest discomfort with MS occurs in only 15% of patients and may be indistinguishable from angina pectoris.[185] The predominant cause of MS remains rheumatic fever.[186,187] Although rheumatic fever and mitral stenosis are both uncommon in the United States, they remain common in many countries. Approximately two-thirds of patients with MS are female. A minimum of 2 years is probably required before the progression from acute rheumatic fever to severe MS develops, with most of those patients in temperate climates remaining asymptomatic for 10 years or more.[186] Symptoms of MS begin most commonly in the third and fourth decades.[188] For unknown reasons, patients in underdeveloped areas in tropical climates may exhibit a more rapid progression to severe MS and can present symptomatically in their early teens.[189] Chronic MS may cause severe local complications, including left atrial enlargement, development of mural thrombi, and obliterative changes in the pulmonary vascular bed.

*History:* The principal symptom of MS is dyspnea resulting from decreased lung compliance and reduced vital capacity, presumably from interstitial edema and engorgement of the pulmonary vasculature. Chest pain may be the result of right ventricular hypertension, coexisting coronary atherosclerosis (25% with severe MS will have critical stenoses of one or more coronary arteries.[190,191]), or coronary embolization.[190,192] In a large fraction of patients, however, complete angiographic and hemodynamic studies are unable to reveal a totally satisfactory explanation for this symptom.

*Physical Examination:* Physical examination may reveal prominent a waves in the jugular venous pulse in those patients with elevated left atrial and pulmonary vascular pressures who are in normal sinus rhythm. With the onset of pulmonary hypertension, a palpable right ventricular lift is often present in the left parasternal region. In the left lateral recumbent position, the diastolic rumbling murmur of MS may be palpable as a thrill overlying the apex. On auscultation an accentuated $S_1$ will occur early in the course of the disease when the mitral valve leaflets are still flexible. With increasing pulmonary artery pressures, the $P_2$ component of the $S_2$ initially is accentuated and transmitted widely across the precordium. As pulmonary hypertension progresses, the splitting of $S_2$ narrows finally becoming single and accentuated. Other potential signs of pulmonary hypertension include the murmurs of tricuspid or pulmonic regurgitation or a right ventricular $S_4$. Unless there is coexisting significant mitral or aortic regurgitation, $S_3$ is generally absent. The classic opening snap of MS, caused by the abrupt termination of the movement of the partially pliable fused valve cusps, is heard best at the apex with the diaphragm of the stethoscope in early diastole and generally in association with an accentuated and delayed $S_1$.[193] The low-pitched, rumbling, diastolic murmur of MS is best heard with the bell of the stethoscope at the apex of the heart and may radiate into the axilla or lower left sternal area. The duration of the murmur, and not its intensity, can be used as a general estimate of the severity of the stenosis. Expiration augments both the diastolic murmur and the opening snap. Potentially useful maneuvers in auscultation include the Valsalva maneuver (ie, decreased transmitral valve blood flow) to reduce the MS murmur and coughing or sudden squatting to augment the murmur of MS.

*Diagnostic Testing:* Chest roentgenographic findings of hemodynamically significant MS invariably includes left atrial enlargement, best seen on the lateral view.[194] The severity of obstruction, however, does not correlate with the size of the left atrium. Extreme enlargement occurs rarely unless severe mitral regurgitation is also present. Severe MS will frequently manifest signs of enlarged pulmonary arteries, right atrium, and right ventricle. The presence of interstitial edema, manifested as Kerley B lines, is also an indication of severe obstruction and is seen in 70% of patients with pulmonary capillary wedge pressures greater than 20 mm Hg.[195]

The ECG is a relatively insensitive technique for the detection of mild MS, but with moderate or severe stenoses, characteristic changes are found.[196] Signs of left atrial enlargement are found in 90% of patients with significant MS. Sinus rhythm is the principal ECG finding of MS. Electrocardiographic criteria of right ventricular hypertrophy are late findings and are seen in approximately 50% of those patients with systolic right ventricular pressures of 70 to 100 mm Hg.[197] Once right ventricular systolic pressures exceeds 100 mm Hg, ECG evidence of right ventricular hypertrophy is found consistently. The axis of the QRS segment in the frontal plane has been shown to correlate with the degree of valvular obstruction and elevation of pulmonary vascular resistance.[197] A mean axis of 0° to +60° suggests a mitral valve area of greater than 1.3 cm$^2$. A mean QRS axis exceeding +110° is seen in patients with pulmonary vascular resistances that exceed 650 dynes·sec·cm$^{-5}$.

M-mode echocardiography readily identifies MS but does not allow determination of severity of disease. Two-dimensional echocardiography allows more accurate determination of the size of the orifice of the mitral valve, its suitability for balloon valvuloplasty, assessment of left atrial size, estimation of pulmonary artery pressure, and identification of any left atrial thrombi. Doppler echocardiography can be especially useful in assessing the severity of MS[198] and any coexisting mitral regurgitation or other valvular abnormalities. A detailed echocardiographic exam may provide enough information to formulate a treatment plan without requiring more invasive testing.

**Mitral Valve Prolapse (Barlow's Syndrome):** Now recognized as one of the most prevalent valve abnormalities, the MVP syndrome may affect as many as 5% to 10% of the general population.[199,200] This condition has been seen in patients of all ages and in both sexes, but especially in women. Echocardiographic criteria for MVP are met in 6% to 10% of presumably healthy, asymptomatic young females.[200] Mitral valve prolapse is now the most common cause of isolated mitral regurgitation requiring valve replacement.[201]

Chest discomfort may be "typical" for angina but more commonly is protracted, not clearly related to exertion, and characterized by transient episodes of severe stabbing pain over the left apex. Because MVP is sometimes associated with true angina pectoris from coronary atherosclerosis or other forms of heart disease (eg, atrial septal defect), chest pain may be produced from the latter conditions and may predominate. It has been suggested that many of the symptoms, including chest pain, are the result of increased adrenergic tone or related to dysfunction of the autonomic nervous system.[202,203] The vast majority of patients with MVP will have myxomatous degeneration of the valve, with a smaller proportion exhibiting postinflammatory changes that might also cause the characteristic fragmentation and disruption of the valvular collagen.[204] The valve leaflets eventually become redundant due to proliferation of the myxoid stroma, the middle layer of the leaflet, and this leads to failure in coaptation of the leaflet edges and prolapse of the mitral valves into the left atrium during systole, causing mitral regurgitation. The severity of the mitral regurgitation is determined by the extent of prolapse. Rupture of the chordae tendineae occurs commonly due to the myxomatous proliferation and may heighten the severity of mitral regurgitation. Similar changes are also common in the mitral annulus resulting in dilation, calcification, and worsened mitral regurgitation.

*History:* The clinical manifestations of MVP are varied with the overwhelming majority of patients being asymptomatic.[205] In addition to chest pain, other symptoms are generally nonspecific— anxiety, palpitations, easy fatigability, postural orthostasis, or other symptoms suggestive of autonomic dysfunction.

*Physical Examination:* The finding unique to MVP is a midsystolic click on auscultation, most readily apparent over the left lower sternal border. The click is thought to arise from the abrupt tensing of the lengthened chordae tendineae and the prolapsing mitral valve leaflets. The click is followed by a mid- to late-systolic crescendo murmur in approximately 10% of patients and is due to mitral regurgitation.[206] As the mitral regurgitation worsens, the murmur begins earlier in systole eventually becoming holosystolic in severe mitral regurgitation. These findings are very variable, even for the same individual examined serially. Confusion may arise when attempting to differentiate between the systolic murmurs of hypertrophic cardiomyopathy and MVP as both may exhibit midsystolic clicks and late systolic murmurs. Further, in both conditions the intensity of the murmur increases with standing and decreases with squatting.[207]

*Diagnostic Testing:* The ECG is normal in the majority of asymptomatic patients. In many symptomatic patients inverted or biphasic T waves and nonspecific ST-T segment changes can be found in leads II, III, and aVF, and sometimes in the anterolateral leads.[208] A spectrum of generally benign atrial and ventricular arrhythmias coexists with the MVP syndrome, most commonly paroxysmal supraventricular tachycardia. Ventricular fibrillation and refractory recurrent ventricular tachycar-

dia do occur and are significantly more common in those patients with resting ST segment and T wave abnormalities.[209] A relationship between the MVP syndrome and the occurrence of sudden death has been proposed but there are no clear data available to support this and generalizable interpretations are difficult.[210,211]

Echocardiography plays an important role in the diagnosis of MVP as well as identifying those at risk for the development of severe mitral regurgitation or infective endocarditis.[212]

The large majority of affected patients will remain asymptomatic for many years. Approximately 15% of patients, especially those with both clicks and murmurs initially, will experience progressive mitral regurgitation over the span of 10 to15 years. This same group also has a higher incidence of infective endocarditis.[213,214] Patients with the MVP syndrome also exhibit a greater propensity for thromboembolic complications, likely due to both the deformation of the valve and the occurrence of paroxysmal arrhythmias.[215,216]

## Pulmonary: Lung and Pleura

Since the majority of painful sensations from the respiratory system arise from the pleura, the differential diagnosis of pulmonary chest pain causes primarily involves those diseases that cause pleuritic chest pain (see Table VII). The parenchyma of the lung and the visceral surface of the pleura are innervated by visceral afferents and the resulting sensations from these regions are more vague and poorly localized pain (eg, asthma). Pleuritic chest pain results from the stretching or rubbing of the inflamed surface of the parietal pleura. This type of pain is usually described as sharp, "knifelike," and superficial in location. Characteristically, this pain is aggravated by changes in body position, coughing, or deep inspiration. The pain is also easily localized and is propagated by segmental thoracic nerves. Because the parietal pleura shares innervation with other somatic afferents, pain is often referred to more superficial regions,

## Table VII
### Differential Diagnosis of Pleuritic Chest Pain

| | |
|---|---|
| Viral Pleurisy | Mediastinitis |
| Pulmonary Embolism or Infarction | Ruptured Aortic Aneurysm |
| Pneumonia | Subdiaphragmatic abscess |
| Neoplasm | Splenic Infarction |
| Pneumothorax | Pancreatitis |
| Empyma | Boerhaave's Syndrome |
| Tuberculosis | Cholelithiasis/ |
| Rib Fractures | Cholecystitis |
| Connective Tissue Disorders | Osteoarthritis of the Thoracic Spine |
| Radiation Pneumonitis | Ruptured Cervical Discs |
| Sarcoidosis | Costochondritis |
| Uremia | |
| Pericarditis | |
| Mediastinal Tumors | |

those supplied by the intercostal nerves, and thoracic segments. If the diaphragmatic pleura (eg, levels C-3 to C-5) is inflamed, pain may be referred to the shoulder. Likewise, if the lower intercostal nerves are involved, the pain may be referred to the abdomen.

Data currently available on the frequency of the causes of pleuritic pain are based on two studies performed in the emergency department setting.[217,218] Generalizing from these studies, the most common cause responsible for pleuritic chest pain is viral or idiopathic pleurisy (ie, in 46% to 53% of cases). Pulmonary embolism (PE) accounts for 21% of cases, while infectious pneumonia is responsible for 8% to 18%. Lastly, a miscellaneous category, accounting for 8% to 25% of cases, includes chest-wall trauma, malignancy, systemic lupus erythematosus (SLE), tuberculosis, asthma, sickle cell disease, ruptured aortic aneurysm, and pancreatitis. There are other numerous, but rare, nonpulmonary conditions that may cause pleuritic chest pain, but they will not be discussed in detail here. The main point in the evaluation of these patients is to rapidly and accurately diagnose those conditions for which specific treatment regimens are required, as opposed to those for which symptomatic relief is all that is needed. A few of the more important and/or more common disorders are discussed in more detail below.

***Viral Pleuritis:*** This is generally a diagnosis of exclusion, although some viruses can be harvested from the pleural fluid to confirm the diagnosis. Viral pleurisy may result from a number of causes, including influenza; adenovirus; in children, respiratory syncytial virus and parainfluenza; and in immunocompromised hosts, cytomegalovirus, varicella-zoster virus, herpes simplex virus, Epstein-Barr virus, and enteroviruses. At least 20% to 30%[219,220] of cases will exhibit transient pleural effusions and up to 20% of that group will have pleuritic chest pain.[219]

Most commonly, viral pleurisy results from Coxsackievirus group B infection. Clinically, patients will usually present with a several-day history of pleuritic chest pain that was preceded by a generalized viral prodrome (eg, malaise and myalgia) and/or an upper respiratory tract infection.[221,222] A low-grade fever may be present and chest roentgenograms will usually appear normal, although they may also reveal a small pleural effusion. Parenchymal involvement with either infiltrate or atelectasis occurs rarely.[223] Pain may be abrupt, severe and easily mistaken for angina,[224] giving rise to the eponym "devil's grip." Although symptoms are most commonly confined to the chest after the viral prodrome, systemic involvement with meningitis, pericarditis, pancreatitis, or orchitis may occur. Any skeletal muscle, including the myocardium, may be infected with Coxsackievirus,[222] and pain may therefore also arise due to myositis as well as pleurisy. Epidemic infections were initially reported in Bamble, Norway in 1872 and later achieved medical prominence after an epidemic on the Danish island of Bornholm in 1930.[225] Epidemics are more common in the late summer and early fall months.[221,226] Spread is via oral-anal transmission.[222] Although the disease is usually self-limited, running its course within a few weeks, relapses are common.[222]

**Pneumonia:** Infectious pneumonitis often has associated pleuritic chest pain, especially in patients younger than 40 years old.[218] Parapneumonic effusions are the most common cause of an exudative pleural effusion and occur in 40% to 57% of patients with bacterial pneumonias.[227,228] Only a small percentage of these will go on to become complicated effusions, and only 5% will evolve into empyema.

**Tuberculous Pleurisy:** In many parts of the world, tuberculosis is the most common cause for pleural effusions in the setting of no demonstrable coexisting pulmonary disease.[229] In the United States, however, the annual incidence of tuberculous pleuritis is around 1000 cases, or approximately 3% to 5% of the total number of patients with tuberculosis.[230,231] Pleuritic chest pain may be seen in up to 75% of patients with tuberculous pleurisy. Slightly less than 10% of untreated skin test converters may develop tuberculous pleurisy. Tuberculous pleuritis may occur 6 to 12 weeks after the primary infection with Mycobacterium tuberculosis *or, more commonly, as reactivation disease.*[232] Tuberculous pleuritis presents most commonly as an acute illness characterized by nonproductive cough (in approximately 70% of cases), fever (86% of cases), and pleuritic chest pain (approximately 50% to 75% of cases).[232,233] The majority of these effusions will be unilateral and generally are small-to-moderate in size.[233,234]

The diagnosis of tuberculous pleuritis is dependent upon isolation of the tubercle bacillus in samples of sputum, pleural fluid, or pleural biopsy specimens or the demonstration of granulomas in the pleura. Pleural fluid analysis is generally very useful in the diagnostic evaluation and invariably reveals an exudate, frequently with protein levels greater than 5.0 g/dL. The white blood cell differential count of the pleural fluid typically shows a predominance of small lymphocytes (>50%) and a low fraction (<10%) of eosinophils.[234] The pleural fluid obtained in this setting will rarely contain more than 5% mesothelial cells. Other chemical tests of the pleural fluid may be suggestive of the diagnosis, such as adenosine deaminase levels above 70 U/L [235,236] or interferon-$\gamma$ levels exceeding 200 pg/mL.[236] Unfortunately neither of these tests is commercially available in the United States.

Except in the setting of a tuberculous empyema (very rare), routine acid-fast smears for mycobacteria on pleural fluid specimens are almost always unrevealing.[233,234] Similarly, the yield for pleural fluid cultures is low, generally around 25% to 30%.[170,231] Both of these facts are explainable by the underlying pathophysiology where it is noted that instead of a large bacterial load leading to an extensive inflammatory response, tuberculous pleuritis is the result of a delayed hypersensitivity response to a relatively small antigenic load. The diagnostic test with the greatest clinical utility is the histologic analysis of a pleural biopsy. This test has a diagnostic yield of approximately 60% to 80% [231,237,238] for granulomas. The yield can be increased to more than 90% when combined with cultures of biopsy material for acid-fast bacilli.[231,238] In those patients with exudative pleural effusions who have had a nondiagnostic work-up, pleural tissue can be obtained thoracoscopically or by open thoracotomy.

**Neoplastic Pleurisy:** Involvement of the pleura by tumor, either primary or metastatic, may cause pleural pain. The location of the neoplasm is more of a determining factor for the sensation of chest pain than for the cell type involved. Malignant pleural effusions are the second most common cause of exudative effusions, with lung and breast cancers representing approximately 60% of all cases and lymphoma another 10% of cases. Almost any tumor type can produce pleural effusion. The most common mechanism is blockage of lymphatics at the hilar lymph node level. Of primary lung malignancies, the frequency of malignant effusions is highest for large-cell carcinomas (67%), followed by adenocarcinoma (60%) and squamous cell carcinoma (34%). Due to the greater frequency of adenocarcinoma as a cell type in lung neoplasms, this cell type is most likely to be associated with a malignant pleural effusion. Malignant effusions may also account for 5% to 10% of all transudates.

**Asbestos-related Diseases:** Benign asbestos pleural effusions should be considered in the differential diagnosis of all idiopathic pleural effusions, especially with the appropriate occupational exposure history within the preceding 10 years. The clinical presentation is generally one of acute onset of pleuritic chest pain accompanied by fever, leukocytosis, nonspecific systemic symptoms, and an elevated erythrocyte sedimentation rate. Pleural fluid analysis usually reveals a blood-tinged exudate, but asbestos fibers are notoriously hard to find. Diffuse pleural thickening may be a sequela, but more often complete resolution occurs over several weeks to a few months and may recur several times over the ensuing months to years.

Pleuritic chest pain is also the dominant presenting complaint of patients who develop malignant mesothelioma many years after asbestos exposure. This is an uncommon malignancy (ie, a 1/1,000,000 incidence in the general population each year) with a lag time of 20 to 40 years from initial asbestos exposure to development. This malignancy characteristically spreads along serosal surfaces and commonly exhibits local invasion of adjacent structures. The roentgenographic features may be very subtle initially, showing a slowly enlarging pleural effusion. More characteristic is the encasement of the lung with masslike pleural densities. Pleural fluid analysis, closed-needle biopsy, and open biopsy techniques have a disappointingly low diagnostic yield. The yield is increased with immunohistochemical studies.

**Pleurisy and Connective Tissue Disorders:** Pleural involvement in this group of diseases occurs most commonly with SLE and rheumatoid arthritis.

*Pleurisy Due to SLE:* Of all the collagen vascular diseases, the pleura is involved most commonly (ie, 16% to 44%) in SLE.[239,240] A comparable incidence is noted in pleural effusions from drug-induced SLE.[240] In contrast to patients with rheumatoid arthritis-caused pleurisy, most affected patients in this group are female and may come from any age group.[241,242] Pleuritic chest pain is the most common symptom and is seen in 56% to 100% of patients with pleural inflammation.[241,243] More than half of these patients will also be febrile, and the majority will have had arthralgias or arthritis prior to the onset of pleuritis.

The pleural effusions seen in SLE are usually small in size and occur bilaterally in 50% of the patients.[242] In the remainder, they will be unilateral in 34% (ie, 17% right only, 17% left only) and will be seen to alternate from side to side in 17%. Frequently, the chest roentgenogram will also reveal an enlarged cardiac silhouette and/or basilar nonspecific alveolar infiltrates.[243]

Drug-induced SLE may result after administration of many different medications, but especially with hydralazine, procainamide, isoniazid, phenytoin, and chlorpromazine. These agents cause an increase in serum antinuclear antibody (ANA) levels and have a comparable clinical presentation to that of idiopathic SLE. There is, however, a lower incidence of renal involvement with drug-induced SLE and symptoms will typically resolve within 30 days of stopping the offending agent.[240]

Pleural fluid examination typically reveals an exudate with high ANA titers (ie, >1:320 and in a homogeneous pattern is very suggestive of SLE[244]). Analysis sometimes reveals an overlap between SLE and rheumatoid arthritis pleural effusions; however, typically pleuritis due to SLE will have higher glucose levels (>60 mg/dl), lower levels of lactic dehydrogenase (<500 IU/L), and more alkalotic pleural fluid pH (>7.35) than patients with pleurisy caused by rheumatoid arthritis.[241] Pleural biopsy with immunofluorescence studies and lupus erythematosus-cell preparations are felt to be only rarely helpful and are not recommended at the present time.[62]

*Pleurisy Due to Rheumatoid Arthritis:* Pleural effusions occur in approximately 3% to 5% of those patients with rheumatoid arthritis.[245,246] Classically, these effusions will occur in men (80%) over the age of 35 years and who have subcutaneous nodules (80%).[241,245,247,248] Typically, the effusion appears only after the patient has had arthritis for several years, and the degree of inflammatory activity in the joints and pleural space is not necessarily in parallel. The clinical presentation is somewhat variable, with 33% to 88% experiencing pleuritic chest pain,[241,245,249] 25% who are febrile,[241] and others who may complain of dyspnea. In most patients, the chest roentgenogram reveals a unilateral (in 75% of patients), small-to-moderate-sized effusion that occupies less than half of the hemithorax.[245] No predilection exists for one side over the other.

Pleural fluid analysis can be a valuable aid to establish the diagnosis. Characteristically, the fluid is exudative with a low glucose (<50 mg/dl in 83%[248]), increased lactic dehydrogenase levels (>700 IU/L), and a fluid pH reduced to levels less than 7.20. Additional studies of interest would be rheumatoid factor levels that are increased (≥1:320) to values at least as high as seen in serum, complement levels that are reduced, and a tendency to contain high quantities of cholesterol or cholesterol crystals.[62] Cytologic analysis of the pleural fluid may also suggest the diagnosis when distinct features are sought,[249] including the presence of a background necrotic material; round, giant, multinucleated macrophages; or multinucleated macrophages that are more slender or elongated. Closed pleural biopsies are generally not helpful, revealing only fibrosis or chronic inflammation in the majority of cases.

*Radiation Pleuritis:* External beam radiation therapy may cause direct injury to the pleural and subpleural capillaries as well as cause impaired lymphatic drainage of the pleural space and lung. The resulting increased permeability leads to small-to-moderate sized unilateral pleural effusions (nonspecific mononuclear exudate). Patients may be asymptomatic or present with pleuritic chest pain and/or dyspnea usually 2 to 6 months following irradiation.[250] The diagnosis is generally made presumptively, with an incidence of approximately 6% for breast cancer.[251] The incidence of pleuritis for other tumors treated with radiation therapy is unknown.

***Pneumothorax:*** Pneumothorax is defined as the accumulation of air or other gases in the pleural space. The predominant symptoms of a pneumothorax are chest pain (in 90% cases) and dyspnea (in 80% cases).[252] The chest pain is usually acute in onset, pleuritic in nature, and localized to the same side of the thorax as the pneumothorax. After a few hours pass, the patient's chest discomfort may take on more of a dull aching quality and, within 24 to 72 hours, some patients experience complete resolution of their symptoms despite continued roentgenographic evidence of 4rsistent pneumothorax.

Pneumothorax is just one form of extraalveolar air that also includes pulmonary interstitial emphysema, pneumomediastinum, pneumopericardium, subcutaneous emphysema, pneumoperitoneum, and systemic air embolism. Clinically, extraalveolar air may result from (1) direct generation of gas from gas-forming infectious microorganisms (occurs rarely); (2) introduced after traumatic penetration of cutaneous structures or disruption of mucosal (ie, tracheobronchial, alveolar) barriers; or (3) alveolar rupture due to generation of an excessive pressure gradient between the alveolus and the nearby interstitial space.[253]

**Primary spontaneous pneumothorax** occurs in generally healthy individuals who have no predisposing pulmonary disease. This is a relatively uncommon entity, with an incidence reported at 7.4 per 100,000 people per year for men and 1.2 per 100,000 people per year for women.[252,254−256] Peak incidence is in the third to fifth decades of life. Bilateral spontaneous pneumothorax does occur, but is even more rare.[256] Most of these patients are found to have small apical subpleural blebs whose developmental pathophysiology remains speculative. The majority of these patients are also cigarette smokers. Despite a popular misconception, only about 9% of spontaneous pneumothoraces occur during exercise or heavy exertion.[257,258]

**Secondary spontaneous pneumothorax** occurs in association with an underlying pulmonary disease. The incidence of this condition is surprisingly similar to that of primary spontaneous pneumothorax and has been reported at 6.3 per 100,000 people per year for men and 2.0 per 100,000 people per year for women.[252] Chronic obstructive pulmonary disease (COPD) is the most common of these associated causes.[254,255] Rupture of bullae through the visceral pleura causes spontaneous pneumothorax in patients with COPD. Catamenial pneumothorax is an uncommon idiopathic syndrome of recurring pneumothorax generally occurring within 24 to 72 hours of the onset of menses of women in their third to fourth decade of life.[259,260] Catamenial pneumothorax occurs predominantly on the right side (in approximately 88% of cases) and has been noted to occur bilaterally in 6% to 7% of cases.[260]

With the ever-increasing prevalence of AIDS, more cases of spontaneous pneumothorax in the setting of *Pneumocystis carinii* pneumonia have been noted (estimated at 2% to 6% of patients).[255,261] It has also been noted that the use of aerosolized pentamidine for the prophylactic treatment of *P carinii* infection appears to increase the risk of developing spontaneous pneumothorax.[261] At least one study[261] would also suggest that for AIDS patients who present with spontaneous pneumothorax, concurrent treatment for *P carinii* infection should administered.

Traumatic pneumothorax would include those cases due to blunt or penetrating thoracic trauma as well as those caused iatrogenically or associated with mechanical ventilation. Iatrogenic pneumothorax is a common procedure-related complication that is known to be a risk for numerous procedures, including central venous catheterization (in 3% to 6% of cases), thoracentesis (generally in less than 10%, but may in as many as 39% of cases), pleural biopsy, transthoracic (in up to 20% of cases) or transbronchial lung biopsy (in less than 10% of cases), tracheostomy, mediastinoscopy, liver biopsy, pericardiocentesis, and cardiopulmonary resuscitation.[256, 262–265] Chest roentgenograms should be obtained in all patients following these procedures to assess for the presence of pneumothorax. However, it should be remembered that a pneumothorax may not be evident immediately, and some take 24 hours or longer to develop.[262] Pneumothorax may complicate the course of 3% to 5% of patients undergoing positive-pressure mechanical ventilation.[254,266] A symmetric, sudden rise in peak and plateau inspiratory airway pressures occurs along with a fall in lung compliance and may be the only signs to warn of this complication.

Penetrating and blunt trauma to the chest wall may produce tension pneumothorax, massive hemothorax, and/or open pneumothorax (the so-called "sucking chest wound"), all of which are life-threatening emergencies.[255, 267–270] In the setting of blunt trauma, pneumothorax is the result of rib fractures or from sudden chest compression due to deceleration forces[262,271] and occurs in approximately 19% of trauma patients, approximately half of which will have no associated bony injuries. Less commonly, chest trauma may lead to pneumothorax due to tracheal or bronchial injuries (80% are within 2.5 cm of the carina), diaphragmatic injuries, or esophageal injuries [270,272,273].

*Physical Examination:* The patient's vital signs are generally normal in the setting of a pneumothorax, except for the presence of a moderate sinus tachycardia. Patients with heart rates greater than 140 bpm, diaphoresis, hypotension, cyanosis, or who appear in extremis should be suspected of having a tension pneumothorax.

Physical exam may reveal a decreased

respiratory excursion, enlargement of the hemithorax, decreased breath sounds, hyperresonance to percussion, and/or absence of tactile fremitus all on the side of the involved hemithorax. In the presence of a tension pneumothorax, distended neck veins and tracheal deviation away from the affected hemithorax may be noted. The exam in patients with underlying lung disease may not be as helpful, since many of these above-mentioned findings may be present in the absence of a pneumothorax. However, a high index of suspicion for the diagnosis of pneumothorax should be maintained in all patients with COPD who present with increasing dyspnea and/or unilateral chest pain.

*Diagnostic Testing:* Hypoxemia with an elevated alveolar-arterial (A-a) gradient may be seen on arterial blood gas measurements and is thought to result from shunting and areas of low ventilation-perfusion ratio ($\dot{V}/\dot{Q}$) matching in the partially or totally atelectatic lung.[252] Hypocarbia may also result from associated hyperventilation.

The ECG changes associated with pneumothorax, especially on the left, may be mistaken for those typically associated with a subendocardial MI. Electrical alternans has also been reported with left-sided pneumothorax,[274] as has a rightward deviation of the QRS axis, decreased R wave voltage in the precordial leads, and precordial T wave inversions.[252,254,255]

The classic roentgenographic finding in pneumothorax is the demonstration of a distinct visceral pleural line without lung markings peripheral to this line. Films taken in the erect position during end-expiration may help in visualizing this abnormality. This is especially important for the detection of pneumothorax in patients with COPD where even a small pneumothorax may produce severe symptoms. An important caveat when carefully examining these roentgenograms is not to confuse the pleural lines associated with cystic or bullous changes from underlying disease with the pleural line of pneumothorax. If this distinction cannot be made reliably based on routine chest roentgenography,

CT scanning of the chest may be helpful.[254,255] Roentgenograms in hospitalized patients frequently can only be obtained with the patient in the supine position, making the diagnostic signs of traumatic pneumothorax potentially difficult to recognize. In a supine or semierect film of the chest, collections of air may be seen to accumulate in one or more of the following regions: (1) anteromedial—the most common location on the supine film with noted lucent outlines of adjacent vascular structures, the lateral cardiac margin, or within the right minor fissure [275]; (2) subpulmonic—reported most commonly to occur in the left hemithorax and manifested as basilar hyperlucency, depression of the hemidiaphragm, distinct outlining of the cardiac apex, or as a lucency that extends deeply into the costophrenic sulcus (ie, deep sulcus sign) [275–277]; (3) apicolateral—generally seen only with large collections of air and after, or in conjunction with the previously mentioned locations [276,277]; and (4) posteromedial—generally seen with patients in the supine position and most commonly seen with lower lobe atelectasis.[275] These posteromedial signs of pneumothorax may be very subtle and have been reported to have been missed on initial review by radiologists in 30% of cases.[277]

**Pulmonary Embolism:** Studies have reported dyspnea (in 80% to 84%) and pleuritic chest pain (in 28% to 74%) as the most common symptoms in patients with ultimately confirmed PE.[278,279] The diagnosis should be considered in all patients with acute chest pain due to the frequency of pulmonary thromboembolism in the population and its prevalence as a cause of acute chest pain.

While more than 250,000 cases are diagnosed annually in the United States, it is estimated that the actual prevalence of venous thromboembolism is on the order of 600,000 cases per year,[280,281] and accounts for approximately 50,000 to 100,000 deaths per year in the United States, or between 5% to 10% of all hospital deaths.[282,283] When considering all patients who present to the emergency department with pleuritic chest pain, it has been shown that PE can be confirmed in about 21% of these cases.[217] Although common, PE is frequently underdiagnosed as a cause of acute chest pain. The literature suggests that major PE may go undiagnosed in up to 62% to 84% of cases.[281, 284–287] Unfortunately, clinical assessment is highly inaccurate in confirming or excluding PE with approximately one-half to two-thirds of cases of venous thromboembolism being "asymptomatic," and another one-half to two-thirds of patients with "classic" signs and symptoms for these diseases eventually shown not to actually have the disease.[286–289] Of note is the autopsy finding of multiple emboli and/or infarcts of different ages in at least 15% of cases,[290] further emphasizing the need of a high index of suspicion for these diagnoses since at least some of these deaths might have been preventable.

A number of **risk factors** have been convincingly shown to be associated with the development of venous thromboembolism (see Tables VIII and IX).[280,281] When there are no risk factors present, it is very unusual for a patient to develop venous thromboembolic disease. In fact, some evidence suggests that an individual's risk for disease increases directly as the number of risk factors present rises.[291,292] Up to 90% of all clinically important PE is known to arise from proximal leg (ie, iliac, femoral, popliteal veins) deep venous thrombosis (DVT).[293] Other less frequent potential sites of thrombosis formation include the pelvic veins following pregnancy or operations in the pelvic area; the superior vena cava and veins of the upper extremities, especially after intravenous catheterization; and the right atrium, particularly with atrial fibrillation.

It has previously been believed that hematologic abnormalities predisposing to PE (protein C and S deficiencies and the antiphospholipid antibody syndrome[294]) have been rare and account for only 5% to 10% of recurrent thromboembolism. This idea has recently been challenged by the discovery of a mutation in factor V. Individuals that are heterozygous carriers for a factor that destroys an activated protein

## Table VIII
### Risk Factors in Patients With a Diagnosis of Acute Deep Venous Thrombosis or Pulmonary Embolism

| Risk Factor | % (n = 1231) |
| --- | --- |
| Age ≥40 years | 88.5 |
| Obesity | 37.8 |
| History of venous thromboembolism | 26.0 |
| Cancer | 22.3 |
| Bed rest ≥5 days | 12.0 |
| Major surgery | 11.2 |
| Congestive heart failure | 8.2 |
| Varicose veins | 5.8 |
| Fracture (hip or leg) | 3.7 |
| Estrogen treatment | 2.0 |
| Stroke | 1.8 |
| Multiple trauma | 1.1 |
| Childbirth | 1.1 |
| Myocardial infarction | 0.7 |
| One or more risk factors | 96.3 |
| Two or more risk factors | 76.0 |
| Three or more risk factors | 39.0 |

Data from Anderson FA Jr, Wheeler HB. Physician practices in the management of venous thromboembolism: A community-wide survey. J Vasc Surg 1992;15: 707–714.

## Table IX
### Odds of Acute Proximal Deep Venous Thrombosis

| Patient Group | Odds |
| --- | --- |
| DVT signs or symptoms | 1:3 |
| Major abdominal surgery (no prophylaxis) | 1:20 |
| Major abdominal surgery (prophylaxis) | 1:50 |
| Hospital in-patients* | 1:100 |
| General United States population (per year) | 1:2000 |

* Approximately 1% of hospitalized patients are treated for an episode of acute DVT or PE. Two-thirds of these are recognized at admission. The remaining one-third develop symptoms of DVT or PE during hospitalization.[281]
DVT = deep venous thrombosis; PE = pulmonary embolism.
Adapted from Anderson FA Jr, Wheeler HB. Venous thromboembolism. Risk factors and prophylaxis. In: *Anonymous Clinics in Chest Medicine*. Philadelphia, Pa: WB Saunders Company, 1995;235–251.

C cleavage site (factor V Leiden) make up approximately 5% to 10% of the general population, but may account for up to 50% of the cases of recurrent venous thromboembolism. One study[295] has shown an eight-fold increase in risk of thrombosis for carriers of this mutation as compared with noncarriers, and a greater than 30-fold increased risk when combining this mutation with oral contraceptive use. Further research is required before screening recommendations can be formulated.

Pain in PE is due to the inflammation of the pleura adjacent to infarcted tissue, tissue with hemorrhagic consolidation, or due to the development of pulmonary hypertension. All may occur due to the abrupt changes in pulmonary circulation that result from embolization. However, due to the lung's dual blood supply (ie, pulmonary arteries and bronchial arteries) with extensive interconnections, ischemic damage to lung tissue from embolic obstruction of a pulmonary artery only rarely leads to infarction. In general, pulmonary infarction is unlikely to occur unless the patient has some pre-existing cardiovascular impairment. When infarcts do occur, they are situated in the peripheral lung parenchyma, especially involving the lower lobes. They tend to be cone- or wedge-shaped with the base along the edge of the pleura and the apex extending back towards the hilum.

*History:* The initial clinical suspicion for a PE diagnosis must be refined to allow prompt, accurate, and cost-effective diagnostic strategies. A highly sensitive strategy is warranted to initially identify all patients with this disorder. Classic teaching is that in patients with no preexisting cardiac or pulmonary disease, the presence of dyspnea, tachypnea, or chest pain (likelihood ratio of 5 to 6 if pleuritic) is present in 97% of patients with PE.[296,297] Classification schemes touted as being 95% sensitive[298] have identified three "typical" patterns of presentation: (1) pulmonary infarction, with the acute onset of dyspnea, pleuritic chest pain, hemoptysis, and pleural friction rubs; (2) acute cor pulmonale, with sudden onset dyspnea, hy-

potension, right ventricular failure, and cyanosis; and (3) unexplained dyspnea.[299] However, this high sensitivity is at the cost of evaluating many patients who will later be shown not to have PE, (the specificity of these clinical factors is low [only about 10%]). In addition, even common symptoms, such as dyspnea or pleuritic chest pain, may be absent in the elderly, as exemplified by the even lower rate of correct antemortem diagnosis of PE (approximately 30%) in older patients.[286] Other common symptoms include apprehension (63%), cough (39% to 50%), and diaphoresis (41%). Hemoptysis occurs in only 13% to 22% of cases.

*Physical Examination:* The most common physical signs observed in patients with a confirmed diagnosis of PE include tachypnea (59% to 92%), fever (54%, two-thirds of which will be $<38°C$), tachycardia (41%), and an increased $S_2$ (40%).[278,279] Neck vein distension (31%) and hypotension (24%) are other common signs. In patients with massive PE, neck vein distension may be present in 80% of cases.[300]

*Diagnostic Testing:* As of this writing, there exists no accurate, rapid, inexpensive blood test that reliably screens for the presence of DVT or PE. To date the most promising test may be the D-dimer assay, which is still undergoing clinical testing and refinement.

Similar to patient history and physical exam, there are generally no clearly helpful features on routine chest roentgenogram that diagnose or exclude PE.[301,302] The chest roentgenogram may be considered abnormal in 29% to 80% of cases, depending on the anatomic criteria used.[217,303] Frequently described signs include enlargement of the descending pulmonary artery in 66% of cases, elevation of the hemidiaphragm(s) in 74%, enlargement of the heart shadow in 56%, and small pleural effusions in 51%.[304,305] Westermark sign, a region of pulmonary parenchymal relative hyperlucency caused by diminished blood flow to that area, is considered typical for PE; however it only occurs in 13% to 15% of cases.[306]

Pulmonary densities suggestive of pulmonary infarction are not commonly seen but may appear as opacities in the costophrenic angles (ie, "Hampton's hump"), as rounded densities with indistinct margins above the diaphragm, or as the classic cone-shaped opacities described earlier.

Tachycardia and ST segment depression are the most common ECG findings in patients with confirmed PE.[307] Overall, the literature has associated more than 20 ECG patterns with PE.[307,308] The "classic" ECG sign for PE, the $S_1Q_3T_3$ pattern, occurs in only about 15% of the cases.[307] Abnormalities, such as T wave inversions in $V_1$ through $V_2$, a late R in lead aVR, and PR segment displacement, are significantly more frequent in subjects with PE and occur 23% to 36% of the time.[307,308] Additionally, the presence of ST segment depression and T wave inversion in leads $V_1$ through $V_2$ are associated with an increased severity of embolization.[307] Some of the identified ECG abnormalities may be the result of right ventricular ischemia.

The arterial blood gas pattern in patients with PE generally reveals hypoxemia with hypocapnia. Differential diagnosis based on these findings is problematic, however, due to the wide range of overlapping values between those subjects with confirmed PE versus those without PE. A "normal" $Pao_2$ (ie, >80 mm Hg) is not uncommon, especially in those with milder degrees of pulmonary vascular obstruction. The A-a $Po_2$ gradient is also unable to reliably exclude the diagnosis of acute PE [297,309]. While the $P(A-a)o_2$ gradient does exhibit a strong inverse linear correlation with the $Pao_2$ among patients with confirmed PE regardless of the presence of prior cardiopulmonary disease, approximately 12% to 23% of patients with confirmed acute PE may have "normal" $P(A-a)o_2$ gradients. A normal $P(A-a)o_2$ gradient, therefore, cannot be used to reliably exclude the diagnosis of acute PE.

Diagnostic specificity can be improved with the use of chest roentgenogram, ECG, and arterial blood gas analysis. However, this strategy raises the specificity to only 24% without sacrificing any

sensitivity.[296] Optimally, at this point, those patients with the highest probability of having PE should have therapy instituted empirically prior to proceeding with additional testing, providing no contraindications to systemic anticoagulation exist. The collective clinical assessment has been shown to further optimize risk stratification as well as the diagnostic value of potential lung scintigraphy.[310–312] Other clinical classification schemes using likelihood ratios, discriminant analysis, and multiple linear regression techniques[296,313] have been shown to be highly specific, at 90% to 92%, and with an overall diagnostic accuracy of 75% to 88%. Approximately one-third of those with clinically suspected PE will have the disease confirmed by further work-up[312,314] that includes evaluations for DVT, lung scanning, and pulmonary angiography.

Many diagnostic techniques are available for the evaluation of potential DVT. The "gold standard" test for DVT remains contrast venography. However, limitations due to patient discomfort, technical problems with performing or interpreting the test, and an 8% incidence of inducing a DVT have all served to establish noninvasive testing as the techniques of choice. The major noninvasive tests in use today for proximal vein thrombosis are impedance plethysmography (IPG) and compression ultrasonography. Both techniques are inexpensive, portable, have reported excellent accuracy, and have been studied extensively in clinical trials. These techniques also share the disadvantage of inaccuracy in the diagnosis of calf vein thrombosis. When performed according to protocol, IPG has a reported 91% sensitivity and a 96% specificity for detecting proximal vein thrombosis.[315] When a negative IPG result is used as a basis to withhold anticoagulant therapy in patients with suspected DVT, it is important to obtain serial studies over the ensuing 10 to 14 days since studies[316,317] have shown that up to 15% of proximal DVTs may be detected after an initial negative IPG. On the other hand, false-positive tests may result when testing patients with a history of previous venous disease, severe arterial disease, raised central venous pressure associated with congestive heart failure or pregnancy, and raised intrathoracic pressure from severe chronic obstructive lung disease.[318–320] These concerns, as well as reports of frequent technical difficulties with the test, have led to concern that IPG may not be as accurate a noninvasive diagnostic modality as previously believed.

In many institutions, the combination of duplex and compression ultrasonography has largely replaced the IPG as the primary screening examination for diagnosis of proximal vein thrombosis. This technique evaluates venous blood flow, the size (ie, dilation) of the veins, the presence of anechoic and/or echogenic thrombi, and the focal compressibility of the venous system (noncompressibility is the most reliable sonographic sign for DVT.). Representative results from multiple studies indicate a sensitivity of at least 95% and a specificity of at least 98% for the detection of DVT.[321–327] In a large, randomized, prospective study comparing IPG and compression ultrasonography directly, the false-negative rates of the tests were similarly low but compression ultrasonography had a noted superior positive predictive value of 94% as compared to 83% for IPGs.[328] Outcome analysis studies have also been performed on patients with symptomatic DVT and have shown that the risk of a false-negative ultrasound is less than the risk of contrast-induced DVT for patients having venography.[329] Similar to the case for IPGs, recent concern has arisen that compression ultrasonography is not as accurate as stated above for detection of DVT in asymptomatic patients who are at high risk for the development of thromboembolic disease.[119, 330–333] The thrombi that were missed primarily tended to be small, nonocclusive, and limited to the calf veins.

Perfusion and ventilation-perfusion lung scanning are important diagnostic tests in screening for the presence of PE. A normal or near-normal perfusion scan essentially rules out all clinically relevant PE and focuses the diagnostic evaluation on other possibilities. These patients do not need to be treated with anticoagulant therapy and do not require further testing for PE.[217,312,314,334] Unfortunately, normal or near-normal scans occur in only approximately 14% of patients being evaluated for PE. Abnormal scans are typically categorized as low, intermediate, high, and indeterminate probability for PE based on the size and number of perfusion defects and whether there are any corresponding ventilation defects. High-probability lung scans have a sensitivity of 41% to 57% with a specificity of 90% to 97% for PE.[312, 334–336] Unfortunately, this scan pattern occurs in less than half of the patients with PE and in only 13% of patients being evaluated for PE. Multiple studies have shown that the other abnormal scan patterns mentioned above have little diagnostic value.

Unless lung scanning reveals high probability or normal to near-normal scans or studies for DVT are positive, the clinician cannot reliably exclude or diagnose PE without the aid of pulmonary angiography. Pulmonary angiography is the most specific diagnostic examination available for establishing the diagnosis of PE, and as such is considered the "gold-standard" against which other techniques are compared. The procedure is generally safe, except for patients with contrast dye allergy or for patients with right ventricular end-diastolic pressures greater than 20 mm Hg,[337] In the hands of an experienced team, pulmonary angiography can be performed safely even in the presence of severe pulmonary hypertension and/or right ventricular failure.[338] With proper technique and the judicious use of nonionic contrast agents, the mortality rate for this underutilized procedure should not be in excess of 0.3%.[312,339] A practical limitation also exists in that approximately 10% to 15% of patients will have inadequate visualization of their pulmonary vasculature.[314] Pulmonary embolism cannot be excluded unless at least two different views reveal normal vasculature. The frequency of PE in patients who were suspected to have this disease but who had negative pulmonary angiograms is only 1.6% to 4.2% in follow-up studies.[340,341]

*Perspective:* The rationale described above has been studied prospectively in outpatients presenting with pleuritic chest pain.[217] When pulmonary angiography was used to confirm the diagnosis of PE in patients with non-high-probability abnormal lung scans, the sensitivity was 97% and the specificity was 100% for the diagnosis. This algorithm, however, required 43% of suspect patients to undergo angiography. The addition of noninvasive testing for DVT to those patients with nondiagnostic lung scans, followed by pulmonary angiography for only those patients with suspected venous thromboembolic disease who still had no confirmed disease, resulted in similar sensitivity (100%) and specificity (97%). This paradigm required only 26% of suspect patients to have angiography to establish a diagnosis. Because these results are expressed in terms of sensitivity and specificity, they are independent of disease prevalence and should thus remain the same for populations with greater or lesser frequencies of PE.

The above algorithms help establish the diagnosis of PE but do not necessarily diagnose the cause of chest pain. Since DVT does not cause chest pain, the presence of DVT does not clearly establish a cause of pain. A diagnosis of DVT permits definitive therapy with heparin to be started and thereby delays the urgency of evaluating the chest pain. Since most patients with DVT do not have PE, since DVT is relatively common, and since numerous other causes of chest pain may exist in patients with DVT, many patients require more definitive evidence of pulmonary embolism. The authors favor definitive proof of PE by arteriography or a high-probability ventilation-perfusion scan in patients with complicated or recurrent chest pain.

**Pulmonary Hypertension:** Pulmonary hypertension is a nonspecific term describing elevated pressures in the pulmonary artery. Although numerous diseases may result in pulmonary hypertension, the frequency of chest pain has only been reliably reported for primary pulmonary hypertension and recurrent PE. In the largest survey of patients with primary pulmonary hypertension, only 7% complained of chest pain.[342] Other smaller series report a higher rate of chest pain of approximately 75% in patients with primary pulmonary hypertension and recurrent thromboembolism.[343] Chest pain is usually described as precordial and is felt to arise from right ventricular ischemia, distention of the major pulmonary arteries, or both.[344,345] The pain sometimes radiates to the neck, but generally not into the arms. The natural history and clinical manifestations of patients with pulmonary hypertension will depend to a large extent on the underlying cause or causes of their disease which, to a great extent, is the main contributor to symptomatology. Patients with pulmonary hypertension most frequently complain of exertional dyspnea, syncope, exertional precordial chest pain, weakness, and later in the disease, dyspnea at rest. Palpitations also occur commonly and may be the result of ventricular tachyarrhythmias.

*Physical Examination:* Findings specific for pulmonary hypertension include large a waves in the jugular venous pulse; a carotid arterial pulse of normal upstroke, but of reduced volume; a left parasternal (right ventricular) heave; a closely split $S_2$ with a loud pulmonic component; and an $S_4$ originating from the right ventricle. Late in the course of the disease, right heart failure may result in hepatomegaly, ascites, and peripheral edema. Severe pulmonary hypertension may also lead to tricuspid regurgitation and prominent v waves in the jugular venous pulse tracing. Left-to-right shunts (eg, patent foramen ovale) may be transformed into right-to-left shunts with increasing pulmonary hypertension, leading to further decompensation and sometimes cyanosis.

*Diagnostic Testing:* Routine laboratory findings may be remarkable for arterial oxygen desaturation, a reactive polycythemia, or even elevated liver function tests as a result of right ventricular failure. The ECG findings of pulmonary hypertension may include right axis deviation and right atrial and right ventricular enlargement. A direct correlation has been shown between the amplitude of the R wave in $V_1$, the R/S ratio in $V_1$, and the level of pulmonary artery pressure.[346]

Roentgenographic findings will also vary depending on the underlying cause of the pulmonary hypertension. In patients with primary pulmonary hypertension (PPH), the main pulmonary arteries and their branches are enlarged with dramatic tapering of the more peripheral arteries.[347,348] It has been suggested that survival in PPH correlates inversely with the size of the main pulmonary artery.[348] The right atrium and ventricle may also be enlarged. Perfusion lung scans in patients with PPH are usually either normal or show small, nonspecific, subsegmental defects. Cardiac catheterization and/or pulmonary angiography can be used to help confirm the diagnosis of PPH. Both of these techniques carry an increased risk of complications in this population. Patients with PPH may tolerate diagnostic procedures poorly and have been known to experience sudden cardiovascular collapse and even death during diagnostic or therapeutic attempts.[349] Appropriate use of echocardiography, angiography, and cardiac catheterization can help exclude or narrow down the large differential diagnosis for causes of secondary pulmonary hypertension from PPH.

**Panic, Hyperventilation, and Anxiety Syndromes:** It is difficult to concisely define the hyperventilation syndrome, panic disorder, and anxiety syndromes. The definitions have varied over the past two decades, frequently overlap, and may employ phsyiologic or psychologic criteria or both. The formal definitions used in the Diagnostic and Statistical Manual, 4th edition (DSM-IV) have not been routinely used by the nonpsychiatric clinical community. Clinically, there is difficulty in determining when panic or anxiety reaches pathologic severity and whether hyperventilation during these episodes results in the symptom of chest pain. Although these syndromes are also discussed in the Chapter 2, Dyspnea, the

**Table X**
Criteria for the Diagnosis
of Panic Disorder

Dyspnea or Smothering Sensations
Choking or Smothering Sensations
Palpitations or Accelerated Heart Rate
Chest Pain or Discomfort
Sweating
Dizziness, Unsteady Feelings, or Lightheadedness
Flushes (hot flashes) or Chills
Trembling or Shaking
Fear of Dying
Fear of Going Crazy or Doing Something Uncontrolled
Nausea or Abdominal Distress
Depersonalization or Derealization
Numbness or Tingling Sensations

literature on dyspnea and chest pain is different.

*Definitions:* The DSM-IV establishes criteria for the diagnosis of panic disorder. Patients must have three attacks of intense fear or discomfort in 3 weeks accompanied by at least 4 of 13 symptoms (Tables X and XI) during an attack.

The diagnosis of the hyperventilation syndrome is less precise. Although Magarian has reported specific diagnostic criteria, clinical studies usually employ a definition of appropriate symptoms (eg, lightheadedness, respiratory rate above 16 breaths per minute at rest, end-tidal or arterial $P_{CO_2}$ below 36 mm Hg at rest, and thoracic breathing).[350]

The term anxiety syndrome is usually used to describe individuals who do not meet the criteria for panic disorder or hyperventilation syndrome, but appear anxious and have increased symptoms in situations with increased anxiety.

*Prevalence:* Due to the variety of definitions employed, the exact prevalence of these disorders has been difficult to estimate. The data describing the prevalence of panic disorder appear the most reproducible. Although only 1% to 2% of the general population has panic disorder,[351] up

## Table XI
### Sign and Symptoms of the Hyperventilation Syndrome

**General:** Chronic and easy fatigability, weakness, sleep disturbances, headache, excessive sweating, sensation of feeling cold, poor concentration, and performance of tasks.

**Neurologic:** numbness and tingling especially of distal extremities, giddiness, syncope, blurring or tunneling of vision, and impaired thinking.

**Respiratory:** sensation of breathlessness or inability to take a deep enough breath with sighing, yawning, and excessive use of upper chest and accessory muscles of respiration, nocturnal dyspnea superficially mimicking paroxysmal nocturnal dyspnea of cardiovascular origin, and nonproductive cough with frequent clearing of throat.

**Cardiovascular:** chest pains often mimicking angina, palpitations, and tachycardia.

**Gastrointestinal:** aerophagia resulting in full or bloated sensation, belching, flatus, esophageal reflux and heartburn, sharp lower chest pain, dry mouth, and sensation of lump in throat.

**Musculoskeletal:** myalgias, increased muscle tone with muscle tightness (stiffness), cramps with occasional carpopedal spasms and rarely a more generalized tetany.

**Psychiatric:** anxious, irritable, and tense though may superficially appear calm (suppression of emotional release), depersonalization or a feeling of being far away, phobias, and panic attacks.

to 13% of patients seeking care in a general family practice may have it.[352] Up to 60% of panic disorder patients complain of chest pain as a major symptom during an attack of panic.[353]

Panic disorder also occurs very commonly among patients with chest pain. Of patients in a coronary care unit for the evaluation of chest pain, 31% met criteria for a diagnosis of panic disorder, and 55% of those patients with noncardiac chest pain had a panic disorder.[354] Moreover, 34% to 43 % of patients referred for coronary angiography due to chest pain and who had normal coronary arteries met the criteria for panic disorder,[355] and up to 26% may have had a generalized anxiety

disorder.[356] Yingling et al.[357] reported that among consecutive patients seen in an emergency department for chest pain, 17.5% had panic disorder and 23% had depressive illness. In patients with acute coronary ischemia, 16.6% had a panic disorder, similar to the 19.4% rate of panic disorder in those without acute ischemia. Panic disorder patients were more likely to have visited the emergency department in the preceding year.

Physicians need to remember that panic patients may also have ischemic coronary disease.[354] Consequently, panic disorder as a sole cause of chest pain is typically a diagnosis of exclusion.

The diagnosis of panic disorder is more frequently dismissed in the elderly. The diagnosis of panic disorder as a cause of chest pain predominates in younger patients in part due to the lower prevalence of cardiac and GI disease in the younger age group. However, panic disorder may begin after 60 years of age and must not be dismissed in this age group.[358]

*Pathophysiology:* There is a familial tendency to panic disorder with chest pain.[359] In a study by Kushner et al., 16% of patients with both panic disorder and chest pain had a first-degree relative with panic disorder; only 4% of patients with cardiac chest pain alone had a first-degree relative with panic disorder.[359]

Most authors now believe that panic and anxiety produce chest pain as a consequence of hyperventilation. Hyperventilation causes thoracic sensations that are interpreted by a susceptible individual as pain. A triggering event starts the hyperventilation which produces the sensation and amplifies the trigger. Triggers may be emotional or physical, such as exercise. Hyperventilation also appears capable of inducing chest panic attacks with or without chest pain. This has been shown experimentally by inducing hyperventilation by the infusion of lactate or breathing higher concentration of carbon dioxide.[56,360]

While hyperventilation appears central to inducing chest pain, the pain threshold and response to the perception of pain in patients with panic disorder appear different from that in normal patients and are important in producing a chest pain syndrome. Bradley [361] demonstrated that patients with chronic, idiopathic, presumably psychogenic chest pain had lower pain thresholds to esophageal balloon distention and employed maladaptive coping strategies compared to normal patients, or patients with GI disease or coronary artery diseases. He postulated that the pain threshold and response to pain in these patients was behaviorally determined and could be treated with behavioral or cognitive strategies.

The personality trait of neuroticism appears to promote poor cognitive strategies in these patients. Neuroticism is felt to be a component of normal personality. Neurotic individuals tend to be negatively affective, more frequently experiencing negative distressing emotions and displaying fearfulness, irritability, low self-esteem, and poor inhibition of impulses.[362] Individuals with a high level of neuroticism tend to report higher rates of somatic complaints such as chest pain. As such, neuroticism appears to be a risk factor for chest pain and is usually negatively correlated with the presence of coronary artery disease. Neurotic chest pain appears more triggered by emotion than by exertion and is more frequently accompanied by sighing, breathlessness, and dizziness.

*History:* In order to establish that a hyperventilation or anxiety syndrome or panic disorder causes chest pain, one must first establish a diagnosis of anxiety, hyperventilation, or panic and then establish the relationship with the patient's chest pain. Epidemiologic studies have struggled with establishing that these syndromes are the exclusive cause of chest pain. In clinical practice, this distinction is probably unnecessary. Because these syndromes appear more commonly in the population of patients with chest pain, are associated with morbidity besides the chest pain, and are all treatable, one can argue that all chest pain patients should be screened for these disorders even if another cause of chest pain is apparent. It would be foolish to suggest that individuals with these common disorders require evaluation and treatment only if they have chest pain. If no other cause for the chest pain can be established in these anxiety/hyperventilation/panic patients, then the pain probably results from the syndrome. If another cause of pain can be established, patients probably still have an anxiety/hyperventilation/panic disorder that requires further evaluation and treatment.

The diagnosis of panic disorder can be established primarily by interview (Table X). The diagnosis of hyperventilation syndrome can be suggested by interview and evaluated by a provocative test (Table XII). Physicians typically do not ask chest pain patients about fear, panic, and anxiety and probably underdiagnose these disorders in chest pain patients. Wulsin et al.[363] assigned psychiatric diagnoses to patients presenting to the emergency department with chest pain based solely on responses to a standardized questionnaire. He found that 43% of patients met criteria for panic attack, 16% for panic disorder, and 39% for depression. However, only 2% were given a psychiatric diagnosis. Kushner et al.[364] attempted to determine which of 187 patients with noncardiac, atypical chest pain had panic disorder by using a structured clinical interview and several self-administered behavioral questionnaires [the Zung Self-rating Anxiety Scale (SAS), the Beck Depression Inventory, the Marks-Mathews Fear Questionnaire, and the Brief Symptom Inventory]. Only the SAS and the patient's age were predictive. The sensitivity of these two for correctly identifying patients with panic disorder was 71%, the specificity 76%, and the accuracy 74%. Seventy percent of cases could be correctly classified based on SAS score alone.

*Diagnostic Testing:* Provocative testing (Table XII) plays a very limited role in establishing a diagnosis [365]; it appears most helpful in ruling out hyperventilation and panic disorders. The carbon dioxide challenge test for the diagnosis of panic disorder has been reported to be highly sensitive but not specific.[360] Infusion of lactic acid will produce panic in up to 87% of

## Table XII
### Provocative Test for Hyperventilation Syndrome

1. Instruct patients that you are going to have them do a breathing test and that they are only to pay complete attention to how they feel during the test. The test should be done before you discuss hyperventilation with the patient so that they may more spontaneously recognize the association of their symptoms with hyperventilation. Others inform patients in advance that the test is being performed to provoke their symptoms.

2. Tell the patient to expect a very dry mouth and that it may be somewhat tiring, otherwise offer no suggestions of wht they may experience during the trial.

3. It is often of value to breathe with them initially to demonstrate the rate and depth you wish for them to breathe and show them using arm motions to increase the speed or depth of respirations if they slow down during the trial. A rate of 30 to 40 deep breathes per minute is generally used.

4. Patients should be encouraged to tell you whatever sensations they may feel as they hyperventilate. The test should be continued until 4 to 5 minutes of vigorous hyperventilation has occurred or until the patient complains of dizziness. If replication of at least some of the symptoms has not occurred by this time, an arterial blood gas should be obtained to document a respiratory alkalotic state. If respiratory alkalosis is not present, the test is inadequate.

5. For those with chest pain as a primary complaint, the test should be performed with electrocardiographic monitoring. If ischemic appearing changes occur, other diagnostic maneuvers will be necessary to distinguish whether this represents the "pseudoischemia" of hyperventilation or is reflective of true myocardial ischemia.

6. If symptoms are reproduced, it is desirable for the patient to make the connection spontaneously before asking them if they are feeling any of the symptoms they have been previously experiencing.

7. After the patient's recognition of the symptoms, bag rebreathing is used to demonstrate its ability to quickly relieve the symptoms and how patients can thereby regain control.

susceptible patients, but specificity data are not available. In practice, these tests may exacerbate cardiac chest pain, asthma, or COPD and cannot routinely be employed as first-line screening tests. Given this information, these tests should only be considered once other common causes of chest pain have been evaluated and probably need only be performed when the clinical suspicion of the diagnosis remains in doubt.

Identifying behavioral profiles are also more helpful in excluding the diagnosis than in establishing it. Low scores for neuroticism appear to make anxiety/hyperventilation/panic an unlikely cause of chest pain. Individuals who score highly for neuroticism, however, cannot be assumed to have a psychogenic cause of pain.[366,367]

Cardiopulmonary exercise testing (CPEX) with end-tidal or arterial blood gas $CO_2$ monitoring appears helpful in supporting the diagnosis. In a study of patients referred for an exercise testing due to chest pain,[368] hypocapnia at rest or during exercise was uncommon (14%) in patients with ischemic changes on ECG during exercise. Among patients without ischemic changes, hypocapnia occurred before or during exercise more frequently in patients with a clinical suspicion of hyperventilation syndrome than those without clinical suspicion of hyperventilation syndrome, (70% versus 40%, respectively).

### Gastrointestinal

**Esophageal Disease:** Esophageal disease is a common cause of chest pain. The esophageal abnormalities considered most likely to play a role in causing chest pain are gastroesophageal reflux disease (GERD) in 35% to 50%[369,370] and esophageal motility disorders (eg, "nutcracker" esophagus, nonspecific esophageal motility disorder, diffuse esophageal spasm, hypertensive lower esophageal sphincter, or achalasia) in 10% to 25%.[371-373] To confound the picture is the fact that GERD can provoke myocardial ischemia in patients with pre-existing stenotic coronary arteries.[374]

The mechanism of pain in the esophageal syndromes has not been clearly elucidated. Gastroesophageal reflux disease presumably creates chest pain via inflammation triggering vagal mucosal afferents. Dysmotility may give rise to pain via transient distention. At low-distending pressures, an esophageal balloon will frequently produce a sensation of retrosternal "fullness." This sensation will eventually evolve into frank pain as the distending pressure is increased. Although not clearly established, it is likely that distending pressures above 40 mm Hg or so will also be perceived as being painful in a majority of normal human subjects.[26] Vagal afferents preferentially innervate mucosal and muscle layers and encode for generated pressures in the 0 to 60 mm Hg range. Sympathetic afferents appear to preferentially innervate muscle and serosa, exhibiting lower firing rates than vagal afferents but encoding for pressures of up to 120 mm Hg or more.

Previously, investigators have focused on correlating the onset of chest pain symptoms with provocation tests that involved acid perfusion of the esophagus, distension of an intraluminal balloon, or challenge with the cholinergic stimulant, edrophonium sulfate. After extensive testing over the past few years with each of these stimuli, current thinking is that the exact stimulus that produces chest pain is not as important as the fact that this group of patients appears to have a lowered threshold for the experience of pain when compared to the "normal" population and that multiple different stimuli may result in the same type of chest pain.[370, 372, 375–377] The popular catchphrase in usage in the literature that encompassess all of these factors is "irritable esophagus." The criteria that ascribe chest pain to acid reflux events or abnormal esophageal motility both suffer from the fact that many episodes recorded are not associated with pain and at other times, painful events are not associated with any significant change from "normal" in the variable being studied.[375] It is difficult to reconcile cumulative data that report GERD to be a more common cause of chest pain than abnormal motility (71% versus 29%). When on provocation testing, the supposed "gold standard," motor-enhancing agents and acid perfusion are equally effective (28% versus 30%) in inducing chest pain.[375] The combined results of several studies[371–373, 378–382] involving 281 patients with noncardiac chest pain allowed categorization of 20% of the patients to have an acid-sensitive esophagus, 14% a mechano-sensitive esophagus, and 24% with an irritable esophagus.[375]

*History:* Approximately 10% of the patients with symptomatic esophageal disorders will manifest chest pain as their only symptom,[383] and this discomfort frequently mimics angina in location, character, radiation pattern, and factors that incite or alleviate the pain. An exertional component is frequently present and when pain is due to a motility disorder, it may be relieved by rest, nitroglycerin, or calcium channel blockers.[383–385] Fully 19% of patients with pain of esophageal origin will complain of pain that radiates into their neck, arms, and back.[386] While historic factors may add little to a clinician's ability to distinguish esophageal disorders from myocardial ischemia, heartburn and regurgitation, in general, are more suggestive of GERD,[54,387,388] and significantly more patients with esophageal disorders (82%) will complain of a dull background aching sensation that lasts for hours as compared to patients with angina (33%).[384] Although used for many years in evaluation of acute chest pain, the administration of oral antacid-topical anesthetic mixtures should **not** be relied upon for diagnostic purposes since the relief of symptoms does not adequately rule out coexisting coronary artery disease.[389] The role of specific diagnostic tests for esophageal disease is discussed later.

**Esophageal Rupture and Perforation/Incarcerated Diaphragmatic Hernias:** Transmural spontaneous esophageal rupture (ie, Boerhaave's syndrome) was first described more than 250 years ago, but remains an uncommon entity with a high mortality rate (reported up to 50%) due to delayed and/or missed diagnosis.[390,391] Only 21% to 50% of these patients are correctly diagnosed within the first 12 to 24 hours.[390,392] Most commonly, disruption of the integrity of the esophagus due to esophageal perforation is the result of instrumentation.[393] Historically, it has been reported that substantial alcohol and/or food intake with subsequent vomiting prior to the onset of symptoms is the "classic" presentation of rupture.[394,395] Further, a "classic" diagnostic triad of vomiting, chest pain, and subcutaneous emphysema has also been reported.[396] More recently, these descriptions have been challenged by a series of patients[390] who descriptively had infrequent food (50%) or alcohol (14%) consumption. The most common symptom of rupture was acute onset of severe pain (86%), with 21% describing only chest pain and another 29% chest and abdominal pain. Only 71% of patients vomited prior to the onset of pain and 29% exhibited subcutaneous emphysema. The primary chest roentgenographic abnormalities seen were pneumomediastinum (50%) and pleural effusion (36%).

Confirmation of the diagnosis can be made upon pleural fluid analysis, which typically shows a low pH and an elevated amylase level, and with Gastrografin swallow.

The most common congenital diaphragmatic hernia occurs in the posterolateral region of the diaphragm (ie, Bochdalek's hernia) 60% to 80% of the time on the left.[397] The overall prevalence of this hernia in the general adult population is around 6%,[397] with the majority being clinically silent.[398] Incarceration of abdominal contents resulting in chest pain or thoracoabdominal pain (67% of patients) has been reported in at least 100 cases in the English literature.[399,400] Abdominal contents most commonly herniated include small intestine, colon, and/or omentum,[401,402] with the stomach also being involved in 40% of cases.[403] Other symptoms may include dyspnea, cough, pleural effusion, or lower respiratory tract infection.[398,404] The diagnosis is generally made with chest roentgenogram or chest CT and the definitive diagnosis confirmed by upper and/or lower GI series. The clinical presentation may simulate that of Boerhaave's syndrome, and similarly, a favorable outcome depends on early diagnosis. Other diaphragmatic hernias associated with chest pain include the paraesophageal hiatus hernia and traumatic hernias. Athough most of these hernias remain asymptomatic for years or may cause mild recurrent pain, stomach, colon, pancreas, or small bowel may strangulate in these openings resulting in acute, catastrophic chest or epigastric pain.[405–408]

## Pancreatitis

Acute pancreatitis can prove to be a diagnostic challenge because it may present with an isolated chest pain syndrome that simulates MI, can cause transient ECG abnormalities similar to the changes seen with myocardial ischemia or MI, is frequently associated with a pleural effusion, and may also present with a pleuritic chest pain component that is the result of diaphragmatic irritation due to pseudocyst or abscess formation. Moreover, pancreatitis may also present in a patient with no obvious risk for the disease (eg, excessive alcohol use, cholelithiasis, hyperlipidemia, hyperparathyroidism, diuretic use); in up to 20% of cases the cause is idiopathic. Unless the diagnosis of pancreatitis is considered by the evaluating clinician, the diagnosis will be missed.

Patients with acute pancreatitis will generally complain of the gradual onset of epigastric and/or back pain (98%) that may become continuous and will sometimes exhibit diffuse abdominal tenderness and rebound on exam. The most common physical exam findings in acute pancreatitis are fever (80%), abnormal blood pressure (elevated in 40%, decreased in 25%), abdominal distension (60%), and pleural effusions (15%). These patients are generally anorectic or vomiting.

Elevated levels of serum amylase support the diagnosis; however, the limitations of the diagnostic utility of this test must be appreciated. It has a sensitivity between 55% to 80% acutely that decreases to 33% after 48 hours.[409] Serum levels may vary widely depending on the cause of pancreatitis—very sensitive for gallstone pancreatitis (90% to 100%) but poorly sensitive in alcoholic pancreatitis (perhaps 30%). The serum amylase test is also not a very specific test since a large number of organs (eg, intestines, kidney, and fallopian tubes) and disease conditions may contribute to elevated levels. Severe pancreatitis may be present in the setting of a "normal" serum amylase level. Pancreatic isoamylase levels and serum lipase levels are much more accurate markers for the presence of this disease but may not be routinely available at some institutions or may have a delayed turn-around time, thereby limiting their usefulness.

Plain abdominal x-rays will exhibit abnormalities in 40% to 50% of patients with acute pancreatitis (ie, colonic dilatation, small intestinal ileus, obscured psoas margins, apparent separation of the stomach from the colon, pleural effusions). Abdominal ultrasound is a reasonable initial diagnostic modality for the detection of acute pancreatitis (sensitivity 62% to 95%[409]), pseudocysts, abscesses, and presence of gallstones. If excessive bowel gas is present or if ultrasonography is suboptimal, CT is a potentially more useful diagnostic modality (sensitivity 92%, specificity 100%[409]), especially when used with rapid, dynamic contrast imaging to assess the degree of pancreatic vascularity.

## Biliary Tract Disease

This category of disease includes biliary colic, cholecystitis, and choledocholithiasis. One study has suggested that these conditions may be confused with angina 8% of the time.[3] One of the potential major confounding factors with these diseases is their ability to provoke true angina in those patients who may have coexisting coronary artery disease. Additionally, the pain of biliary tract disease may cause T wave inversions on an ECG regardless of the presence of any overt coronary disease.

Although pain probably arises from local inflammatory mediators within the biliary tree, careful studies regarding distention as the mechanism of pain have been published. Gallbladder distention in humans has been shown in numerous studies to cause pain in both experimental and pathological states when intraluminal pressures exceed 35 to 45 mm Hg.[26] The afferents that carry this pain are the sympathetic splanchnic nerves which have no ongoing basal activity and respond only to direct mechanical stimuli applied to certain sites within the gallbladder and its ducts.

Biliary colic characteristically is pain of acute onset (thought to result from the acute impaction of a gallstone into the proximal end of the cystic duct and possibly followed by spasm of the gallbladder) that rapidly reaches a plateau of moderate-to-severe intensity and lasts on the order of 30 minutes to 4 hours or more. Thereafter, there is dramatic relief of the severe pain (generally ascribed to dislocation of the offending calculus), and this is replaced with a lingering background discomfort for the next 12 to 24 hours. The pain is generally right subcostal or epigastric, but in some patients may extend into the low central anterior chest. Only rarely, however, is the pain confined to the chest and thereby possibly mimicks the pain of myocardial ischemia. The pain will frequently radiate into the back, especially to the inferior angle of the right scapula. Somewhat less frequently is the referral of pain to the right shoulder region. Neck, jaw, and upper extremity pain are distinctly unusual.

On physical examination fever is usually minimal or absent. The patient is uncomfortable but does not appear acutely ill, and jaundice is rare. Right upper quadrant/subcostal tenderness to palpation may be present, especially on deep inspiration (ie, Murphy's sign). Biliary colic is generally considered a predecessor of acute cholecystitis.

The pain of acute cholecystitis is generally similar to biliary colic except that it usually lasts for days rather than hours and is usually much more localized to the right upper quadrant. True chest pain is rare with this condition; however aggravation of the pain with respiration may be mistaken for pleurisy. Obstruction of the cystic duct is associated with calculus disease in more than 90% of patients.[410] The gallbladder wall subsequently becomes distended and inflamed and the retained bile may become infected over time. The diagnosis of cholecystitis is usually obvious in patients presenting with right upper quadrant or epigastric pain, fever, nausea, vomiting, and signs of a localized peritonitis.

On laboratory testing, these patients will generally exhibit a leukocytosis and at least a mild increase in the hepatic aminotransferases. Serum amylase may be elevated in some patients, and 10% to 15% of these patients may develop a mild hyperbilirubinemia.[410]

Ultrasonography of the right upper quadrant usually documents the presence of cholelithiasis with a distended, thick, and edematous gallbladder and occasionally pericholecystic fluid. The diagnostic sensitivity of this technique approaches 80%.[410] Another diagnostic modality available is radionuclide cholescintigraphy which confirms the diagnosis of cystic duct obstruction if the gallbladder is not visualized within 4 hours after the administration of radionuclide. Computed tomography may also be used in the evaluation of the "acute abdomen" and will show gallbladder distention, thickening of the wall of the gallbladder, and the presence of surrounding inflammatory fluid.[411]

Acute cholecystitis in the absence of gallbladder calculi (ie, acalculus cholecystitis) occurs 5% to 10% of the time. This disease generally occurs in the setting of critically ill patients.[412] This condition has also been recognized as a late complication of AIDS and is generally associated with cytomegalovirus or infection by *Cryptosporidium* species.[413] A functional obstruction of the cystic duct occurs by an unknown pathogenesis. The signs, symptoms, and diagnostic work-up of this disease are similar to that of calculus cholecystitis.

Choledocholithiasis is the result of stone impaction in the common bile duct that causes severe right upper quadrant pain. The pain typically fluctuates in intensity and may radiate to the inferior angle of the right scapula. Anterior chest pain occurs only very rarely.

## Peptic Ulcer

Uncommonly, a gastric ulcer may occur in the cardia of the stomach, and an ulcer in this location may frequently be the cause of chest pain, especially in the presence of a sliding hiatus hernia. The resulting chest pain is generally anterior, low, and central and may have associated lateral radiation. The diagnosis of peptic ulcer is made on the basis of upper GI contrast x-rays and/or endoscopy.

## Aerophagia/Gas Entrapment Syndromes

Air swallowing, ingestion of beer or carbonated beverages, or consumption of nondigestable sugars in beans or leafy green vegetables may lead to excess gas accumulation in the lumen of the GI system. Pain or discomfort resulting from gas entrapment syndromes depends on the location of the excess gas, the position of the patient, and any anatomical variations that may present a hindrance to the passage of gas (eg, cascade stomach, redundant splenic flexure). Pain results from the tension produced on the visceral peritoneum by focal or generalized distension of a hollow viscus. If the viscus lies adjacent to the diaphragm (eg, stomach, splenic flexure, hepatic flexure), chest pain, as well as referred pain to the left shoulder on occasion, may result (Figure 6). The discomfort is often dull and constant, worsening as the day progresses and at mealtime, since all swallowing causes some aerophagia. Early satiety and hiccoughs are common. The clinical presentation may be extremely variable, and occasionally, the patient may be a frequent visitor to the emergency department and/or be using potent

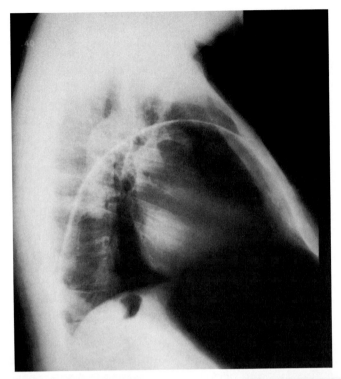

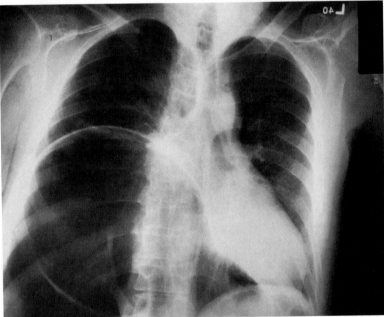

**Figure 6.** Posteroanterior and lateral chest roentgenogram of a patient with acute colonic pseudo-obstruction (Ogilvie's syndrome). Curvilinear densities seen in the right lower lung field represent stretched haustral markings. Chest pain probably results from distention of the colon and displacement of thoracic structures. (Reproduced with permission from American College of Chest Physicians. Critical Care Medicine. ACCP-SEEK, Test 1994; 4:40–41.)

analgesics. More typically, there is a prolonged history of abdominal bloating that is frequently associated with excess belching or flatus. Physical examination of these patients is usually normal. Although a tympanitic abdomen is sometimes present, distention of the abdomen may not be a striking finding, despite the history. Plain, upright, abdominal roentgenograms of the patient will usually reveal excess gas in a portion or in all of the GI tract. Pain relief occurs with passage of the excess gas. The presence of an anatomical gas entrapment syndrome signifies the need for further investigation and possible surgical intervention.

## Thoracic Muscles and Bones

### Pectoral Girdle Syndrome

Parasternal, submammary, lateral pectoral, axillary, cervical, and intercostal pain may result from overuse of or pressure trauma to the pectoral muscles[414] (Figure 7). Precipitants usually include

carrying weight in the hand, forearm, or on the shoulder or work involving unsupported use of the arms. Unsupported armwork, such as packing, machining with the arms raised, carrying heavy objects, sewing, and knitting, may cause pain in these cases. Of patients with the pectoral girdle syndrome, 50% have pain in the serratus anterior.[414] Prolonged forward flexion of the neck, such as during data entry or typing, may produce pain or tenderness. Elevated bra-strap pressure is a common cause of pain in these areas in women. Pressures greater than 0.5 to 1 kg may result in pain. Large-breasted women may experience left chest pain due to pectoral girdle strain.

### Fibromyalgia

Primary fibromyalgia or fibrositis/myofascial syndrome is a syndrome of diffuse chronic pain mediated by inflammation of muscles and may occur in up to 2% of the

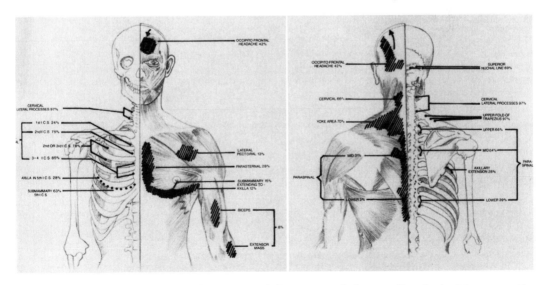

**Figure 7.** Diagrams indicate the location and frequency of chest-wall pain in 80 consecutive people with pain due to fatigue of the pectoral girdle muscles. The double-hatched areas on the muscle side of the diagrams indicate where the pain was most severe. The skeletal portions of the diagrams show areas tender to pressure and their frequency of occurrence. Common causes included repetitive activities due to one's occupation, heavy lifting, breastfeeding, and increased bra-strap pressure. I.C.S. = intercostal space (From Ryan, EL. Cervicothoracic pain due to fatigue of pectoral girdle masculature. MJA 1991; 155: 204–205. ©Copyright 1991 *The Medical Journal of Australia*—reproduced with permission)

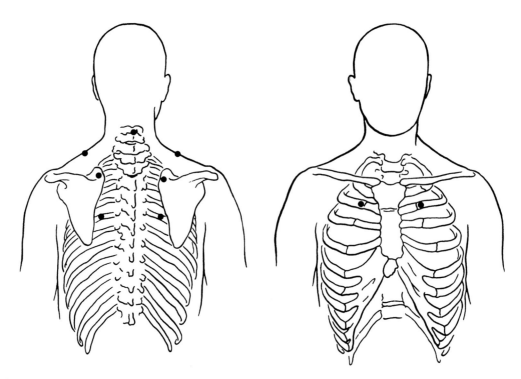

**Figure 8.** Dots indicate the most common thoracic location of trigger points in the fibrositis syndrome. (Reproduced with permission from Fam AG, Primary Care 1988;15:767.)

general population.[415] Fibromylagia may, in some patients, only involve the thorax and during the acute stage or exacerbations may present with puzzling chest pain. Diagnostic criteria include: (1) generalized aches and pains or prominent stiffness involving three or more sites for at least 3 months; (2) the presence of at least five typical, consistently tender or trigger points at characteristic sites (Figure 8) ; (3) the absence of systemic causes of pain confirmed by clinical examination, laboratory tests, and roentgenograms; and (4) at least three of the following: modulation of symptoms by anxiety, too little or too much physical activity, weather change, stress, poor sleep, general fatigue, chronic headaches, or irritable bowel syndrome.[416] Tender points are most common in the trapezius, the sternocleidomatoid, the costochondral junction, and distal to the lateral and medial epicondyles. Palpation of a trigger point may cause pain to radiate and parasthesias or autonomic

symptoms to appear.[417] Trigger points (Figure 8) occur commonly in the trapezius, deltoid, pectoralis, the muscles of the rotator cuff, and the posterior cervical muscles. Trigger points are best detected by pincer palpation and rolling the muscle fibers between the fingers to detect taut bands of muscle.[418] Although some authors have reported that trigger points show spontaneous electromyogram activity,[419] others have found no electromyogram abnormalities in these patients.[420]

### Benign Overuse

Overuse of the thoracic muscles may result in local inflammation of the involved muscle and chest pain. Typical overuse activities involve repetitive arm work such as raking, painting ceilings, or lifting. Cessation of the offending activities, rest of the involved muscles, and use of analgesics and nonsteroidal anti-inflammatory agents relieves the pain, providing diagnostically useful and reassuring information.

## Xyphoidynia, Xyphoidalgia

It is important to consider xyphoid pain as a cause of chest pain since it can be easily diagnosed and treated. Xyphoidynia or xyphoidalgia is probably frequently missed. The cause of xyphoid pain is felt to arise from perichondritis or apophysitis in the xiphisternal region. Inflammation is facilitated when the xyphoid is bifid with a fishtail deformity with projecting sharp spines, known as a tack-hammer deformity. Since the xyphoid attaches to the rectus abdominus, the internal and external oblique aponeuroses, and the diaphragm, pain results from lifting or aerobic activity[421,422] and is aggravated by deep breathing, coughing, leaning forward, walking, postprandial abdominal distention, or change in position.[423] Pain may be squeezing, achy, burning, or sharp and may radiate to the anterior chest, epigastrium, neck, shoulders, and back. Due to the pattern of radiation and aggravation by exertion many patients undergo exhaustive cardiac and GI evaluations before the diagnosis is established.[423] Reproduction of the pain by xyphoid and paraxyphoid pressure and subsequent relief with lidocaine injection establishes the diagnosis.

## Sternoclavicular Joint Disease

The sternoclavicular joint[424] is a diathrodial, synovial lined joint that articulates with the first rib, sternum, and clavicle. The joint is reinforced with anterior and posterior ligaments containing bursae. Shoulder abduction or flexion elevates the distal clavicle, causing rotation of the sternoclavicular joint. Inflammation of the joint causes edema of the surrounding tissues with warmth, erythema and tenderness, and occasionally crepitus. Therefore, pain may radiate to the shoulder and along the sternum.

Inflammation leading to chest pain may be due to a variety of diseases—infectious (eg, tuberculosis, leprosy, and syphilis), rheumatoid arthritis, ankylosing spondylitis, gout, degenerative arthritis due to overuse, Paget's disease, aseptic necrosis, and polymyalgia rheumatica. Sternocostoclavicular hyperostosis (ie, a process of osteosclerosis, ossifying periostitis, and hyperostosis) may lead to chest pain; it is a painful, chronic, slowly progressive swelling of the clavicles, sternum, and upper ribs. This region may also be involved with condensing osteitis, which presents with painful swelling of the medial clavicle and bony sclerosis, or trauma, which frequently results in dislocation. Anterior dislocation is more common than posterior.

## Precordial Catch

Precordial catch is a benign, self-limited chest pain most commonly found in children.[425–427] Although the pain is presumably musculoskeletal in origin, the pathophysiology remains poorly defined. Some speculate that pain results from tethering or pinching of pleuropericardial structures.[428] The pain is typically brief, lasting less than 3 minutes, occurring at rest, and centered in the left lower anterior chest; it can be well-localized to a small area, and does not radiate. The pain is increased with inspiration and may occur with a change in posture. As the pain is brief, most patients do not seek physician evaluation. Surveys have indicated that up to 1.4% of adolescents have had this type of pain.[428]

## Tietze's Syndrome and Costochondritis

Both Tietze's syndrome and costochondritis involve inflammation of the costochondral junction. Tietze's syndrome presents with pain in the anterior chest wall, is more common in people younger than 40, and in 70% of cases involves a single costochondral junction, usually the second or third.[429] Tenderness and swelling of the costochondral junction is usually obvious. Chest pain may be pleuritic and change with position. Although the syndrome may follow mild trauma or cough it is generally believed to be idiopathic and self-limited.

Costochondritis presents with pain in the anterior chest, is more common in people older than age 40, and in more than 90% of cases involves more than one costochondral junction. Swelling is unusual and the second through fifth junctions may be involved. Provocative maneuvers include the "crowing rooster" maneuver, extension of the cervical spine while applying posterior traction to the extended arms, and traction of an adducted arm with the head rotated to the same side.

### Ankylosing Spondylitis

Ankylosing spondylitis may cause chest pain via costosternal,[430] sternoclavicular,[431] or costovertebral pain[432] inflammation. Chest pain is usually more common in those patients with extensive, active disease. In one series of patients those with prolonged morning stiffness or with greater finger-to-floor distances on bending were more likely to have chest pain.[430] Ankylosing spondylitis patients have a chest expansion on inspiration usually less than 3 in and those affected with chest pain usually closer to 1 in.[430]

### Rib Pain

Trauma is usually an obvious cause of rib pain. Such patients will have point tenderness and swelling at the trauma site. In the absence of trauma, one must consider cough, even in otherwise healthy individuals (see the complications section of Chapter 1, Cough), primary bone diseases, and tumors. Paget's disease, osteoporosis, osteomalacia, and rheumatoid arthritis may result in rib fracture with minimal trauma, such as twisting. All of the more common types of adenocarcinoma metas-

tasize to the ribs, and the ribs may be involved in eosinophilic granuloma, multiple myeloma, and chondrosarcomas.

The slipping rib or rib tip syndrome, presents with intermittent, unilateral, sharp, or pressure-type pain in the anterior lower costal cartilages.[429,433] Pain is usually unilateral and occurs when an intercostal nerve is compressed by a mobile eighth to tenth rib rising up and touching the rib superior to it. Pain can be reproduced by hooking the fingers under the anterior costal margin and pulling anteriorly. A snap may be heard when the rib moves. Pain can be reduced by avoiding provocative movements or by using analgesics, nonsteroidal anti-inflammatory drugs, lidocaine infiltration, nerve block, and surgical resection of the involved cartilage.

### Spine

Chest pain may result from cervical or thoracic disk herniation or inflammatory processes affecting the vertebrae and exiting nerves. Osteomyelitis due to fungus, common bacteria or the organisms causing typhoid, tuberculosis, syphilis, and brucellosis may result in pain radiating to the chest. Although these patients may be otherwise asymptomatic they more typically present with fever and associated signs of infection. Spinal cord tumors may present with chest pain before there are obvious localizing neurologic signs.[434] Cervical spondylosis or herniation of cervical disks is a common problem that may infrequently causes chest pain.[435] Pain may arise in the C-5 to T-1 dermatomes ipsilateral to the pathology. Due to the sensory nerve distribution, pain may seem to center in the arm and radiate to the neck, shoulder, and chest or to center in the chest and radiate to the arm. Pain typically increases with maneuvers that increase nerve compression caused by the cervical spine disease (eg, neck hyperflexion or hyperextension, ipsilateral rotation of the neck, downward pressure applied to the head). Sneezing, coughing, straining at stool, or sighing may aggravate pain. Stiff neck, trapezius spasm, reduced arm reflexes, digital hypesthesia, and arm motor weakness all help to indicate the diagnosis. Cervical spine roentgenograms or magnetic resonance imaging and nerve conduction studies help to confirm the diagnosis.

## Shoulder

The clinician evaluating chest pain must possess a thorough understanding of shoulder disease because shoulder pain commonly radiates to both the anterior and posterior thorax and because many of the anterior chest pain syndromes radiate to the shoulder. Pain arising from the shoulder usually arises from the acromioclavicular joint or the rotator cuff.[436] Pain involves the C-4 and C-5 dermatomes and therefore radiates predominantly to the lateral upper arm, radial forearm, or deltoid region. Pain from the acromioclavicular joint radiates primarily to the C-4 dermatome. Pain also may be referred to the shoulder by numerous diseases in other locations. Inflammation of the pleura, Pancoast tumor, aortic arch disease, disease of the cervical spine or muscles at the C-5 through T-1 levels, gall bladder disease, pancreatic disease, or gastric disease may all be perceived in the shoulder or interscapular chest area. Evaluation of pain localized to the shoulder area should, therefore, always include a thorough evaluation of the remainder of the thorax, the abdomen, and neck.

The differential diagnosis of syndromes causing shoulder pain is limited and most problems can be diagnosed with a careful physical examination.[436] Figures 9A and 9B review the muscles, bones, and joints of the shoulder. The involvement of multiple joints suggests rheumatoid, gout, or systemic arthritis. Pain radiating to the forearm and wrist, marked reduction of mobility on abduction, and a duration of pain of 3 to 6 months suggests a frozen shoulder with involvement of the capsule and synovium. Involvement of the acromioclavicular joint can usually be detected by the presence of tenderness and deformity. Many pain syndromes result from injury of the rotator cuff. Four muscles that run from the scapula to the humerus form the rotator cuff and consist of the supraspinatus, infraspinatus, teres minor, and subscapularis. Pain usually follows exertion or trauma and increases over the 12 hours following injury. Pain results from tears, rupture, or avulsion. Pain from rotator cuff injuries is aggravated by downward pull on the relaxed arm and relieved by allowing the weight of the arm to fall away from the inflamed acromium. This can be accomplished by full-hip and trunk flexion and allowing the arm to hang limp. Tendinitis or bursitis of associated bursae frequently follows rotator cuff injury. Calcific tendinitis occurs more commonly in younger patients and occurs when 1- to 1.5-cm calcified masses on tendons develop an associated bursitis. Pain is typically acute, lasting less than 1 week. Examination reveals point tenderness in the rotator cuff group. A shoulder roentgenogram reveals calcific deposits. The humeral head may dislocate anteriorly or posteriorly. The diagnosis can usually be established by examination and confirmed by roentgenography.

## Thoracic Outlet Syndrome

The thoracic outlet syndrome is due to compression of the brachial plexus, subclavian artery, and subclavian vein at the root of the neck. Pain and parasthesias are most common in the C-8 through T-1 dermatomes. Advanced cases may demonstrate extremity weakness, muscle atrophy, or arm edema or pallor. Pain increases on downward traction of the resting arm and increases on abduction. Compression may be due to cervical ribs, the first rib, hypertrophy of the subclavius or scalene muscles, or compression following trauma.[437] Since pain usually predominates in the shoulder and arm, not the shoulder and chest, this syndrome is usually easily distinguished from other causes of chest pain. Diagnosis may be facilitated by Adson's maneuver or the costoclavicular maneuver. Both maneuvers consist of checking for decreased pulses or increased

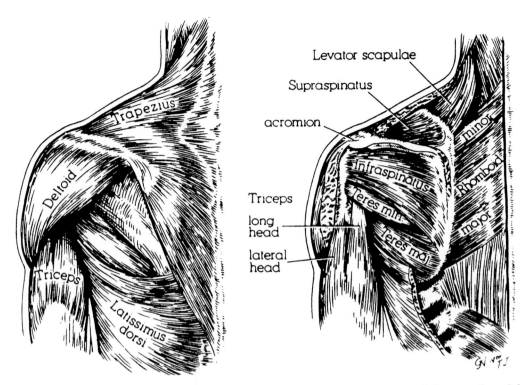

**Figure 9A.** This panel displays the surface muscles of the shoulder (left) and the muscles of the rotator cuff (right). maj = major. (Reproduced with permission from Bland JH, Merrit JA, Boushey DR. The painful shoulder. Semin Arthritis Rheum 1977; 7:21–47.[436])

symptoms while placing the patient in a position which narrows the thoracic outlet. Adson's maneuver involves extension of the patient's neck with the head turned to the opposite side with deep inspiration. During the costoclavicular maneuver, the patient stands in an "exaggerated military posture" with the shoulders back and down.

### Diaphragm

Isolated involvement of the diaphragm is an infrequent cause of chest pain. Overuse by exertion or recurrent hiccoughing may cause an ache in the area of the diaphragm (see Chapter 8, Singultus). More frequently the diaphragm is secondarily involved from inflammation in surrounding organs, and this may mislead the clinician by directing attention to the lower chest when the cause of pain may be upper thoracic or GI. This localization of pain may be due to the fact that the innervation of the diaphragm overlaps that of the peritoneum. Since the peripheral portions of the diaphragm are innervated by intercostal nerves and the intercostal nerves also contain the pain fibers for the parietal peritoneum, the referred pain area from the diaphragm may extend down over the abdomen and lumbar region as far as T-12. Any inflammatory myositis, such as polymyositis, or infectious myositis, such as trichinosis, may involve the diaphragm and cause chest pain. Isolated involvement of the diaphragm is rare in these diseases since most cases present with progressive systemic symptoms. Trichinosis occurs after eating infected meat, most commonly pork or game, and presents with myalgia, fever, facial edema, and diarrhea.[438–440] Eosinophilia is com-

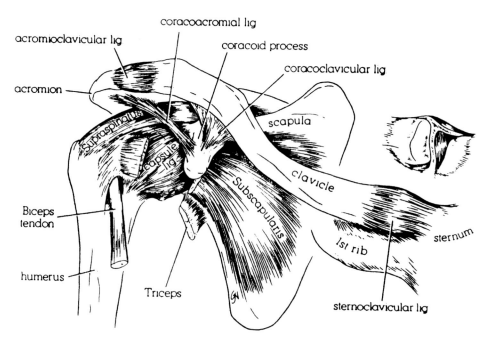

**Figure 9B.** This panel displays the bones and joints of the shoulder. lig. = ligament. (Reproduced with permission from Bland JH, Merrit JA, Boushey DR. The painful shoulder. Semin Arthritis Rheum 1977; 7:21–47.[436])

mon. The diagnosis of trichinosis can be confirmed by serology or muscle biopsy.[438,441]

## Neck

In addition to cervical spine disease, any structure in the neck that reaches a large enough size to compress or inflame adjacent tissues or nerves may cause pain. Pain may be localized to the neck or may be referred into the upper midchest. Pain may change with swallowing or respiration adding to the perception that the origin of the pain may be thoracic. Tumors, cysts and thyroid lesions, particularly pyogenic and subacute granulomatous thyroiditis, may all present with chest pain. Pain, however, is typically felt in the neck as well as in the chest. Pain also more typically radiates to the mandible, ear, or occiput. Inflammation of the cervical nerve roots or the phrenic or vagus nerves

as they transverse the neck may lead to referred pain at distant sites.

Pyogenic thyroiditis is rare, usually preceded by bacterial infection in another site, and usually presents with malaise, fever, and localized tenderness, erythema, and warmth. Subacute granulomatous thyroiditis usually follows an upper respiratory viral illness and may last months.[442,443] Since referred pain into the sternal area may dominate over local pain, the diagnosis may be easily missed. Examination usually reveals nodularity and tenderness of the thyroid typically with one side more involved than the other. Patients may develop clinically apparent thyrotoxicosis. Diagnosis can be confirmed by demonstrating a markedly elevated erythrocyte sedimentation rate and a symmetric, low radioactive iodine uptake.

## Skin

Chest pain may result from any irritating cutaneous thoracic lesion. Cutaneous pain may be confused with visceral pain because the skin involvement may not be obvious or may change with thoracic movement such as with respiration. Cutaneous pain may also be severe, prompting unnecessary evaluations for origins of life-threatening visceral pain syndromes if the skin examination is overlooked.

Cutaneous thoracic pain most commonly results from burns, inflammatory lesions, infiltrative diseases, and tumors. Burns may be easily diagnosed by their classic appearance and a history of contact with heat. Inflammatory lesions typically present with obvious tenderness, erythema, edema, pustules, or nodules. A diagnosis of bacterial cellulitis, impetigo, or excoriations may be easily established by inspection. The pain of herpes zoster virus may precede the appearance of viral lesions by several days, usually follows a dermatomal distribution, and may have associated hyperaesthesia of the involved skin. Pain that persists following resolution of the skin lesions is known as post-herpetic neuralgia. Cutaneous involvement of the skin with polyarteritis nodosa or dermatomyositis may cause pain, but rarely presents as isolated thoracic disease. Glomus tumors may present as areas of exquisite point tenderness with no visible skin lesion. Pain may result from touch or temperature change. Diagnosis can be established by suspicion and biopsy. Primary skin malignancies or metastases are infrequently painful but may produce a localized inflammation due to compression of adjacent structures or superinfection and necrosis.

## Breast

Chest pain due to breast involvement can occur with trauma, mastitis, fibrocystic disease, cancer, breast implants, and in gynecomastia.[444]

### Mastitis

Mastitis is an infection of the skin of the breast and the superficial galndular

ducts and surrounding structures. Infection is typically due to common skin flora, such as streptococcal or staphylococcal species, and is more common following trauma or with breastfeeding. The breast is usually erythematous, tender, and swollen. Granulomatous mastitis may also rarely occur and may mimic inflammatory carcinoma in its presentation.[445,446]

### Mammary Duct Ectasia

Elderly women with atrophic breasts may present with intermittent infra-areolar pain, bloody nipple discharge, and localized tenderness, erythema, and swelling. Pain results from mammary duct ectasia and inflammation due to lipid-rich material and cellular debris.[447]

### Fibrocystic Disease

Tenderness, nodularity, and engorgement may occur premenstrually due to cyclic hormonal change. The key to establishing fibrocystic disease as the cause of the pain lies in demonstrating the association with the menstrual cycle. The larger cysts in fibrocystic disease may mimic cancer on palpation and if they do not completely disappear during the cycle, they should be aspirated/ biopsed to rule out malignancy.[448,449]

### Breast Cancer

The presence of pain should not dissuade the clinician from evaluating the patient for cancer despite the increased likelihood that a painful lesion has an underlying inflammatory nonmalignant cause.[450] All types of breast cancer have been reported to present with painful lumps. Cancer classically appears as a hard, well-circumscribed, mass. Fixation of the mass, dimpling of the skin, edema of the skin, and nipple retraction make cancer more likely. Inflammatory breast cancer may involve a portion of or the entire breast and may present with diffuse erythema, induration, warmth, and tenderness.[451] Paget's disease of the breast presents as an eczematoid lesion of the areolar region and typically has a more itchy or burning character to the pain. All lesions suspicious for cancer should undergo an appropriate evaluation including biopsy. Benign breast tumors may also present with pain or tenderness.[450]

## Trauma to the Breast

Pain may occur at the time of trauma or may start at a later date due to the consequence of trauma. Fat necrosis may present several days afterwards with a painful lump which subsequently atrophies.[452] Mondor's syndrome, a subcutaneous phlebitis and thrombosis of the thoracoepigastric veins, may occur spontaneously or follow trauma. Tender cords may be palpable, are more common laterally, and extend to the axilla or abdomen.[453]

## Breast Implants

Silicone breast implants have been reported to result in a chest pain syndrome that may easily be confused with angina.[454] Pain may last from minutes to days, be pressing or stabbing in quality, and be accompanied by dyspnea, diaphoresis, nausea, and radiation to the jaw, shoulder, and arms. Pain may occur without rupture or leak of silicone. This pain has been believed to arise from neuroma formation or from major inflammation of the pectorals due to atrophy, myositis, or fasciitis. Pain typically resolves with removal of the implant.

## Gynecomastia

Hyperplasia of breast tissue in men may be extremely painful. When pain is present, it is localized to the periareolar area and glandular breast tissue is palpable. Physiologic gynecomastia may occur

at puberty. Pathologic gynecomastia results from decreased testosterone effect, increased estrogen, or drugs. The most widely used drugs that may cause gynecomastia include spironolactone, digitalis, $H_2$ blockers, isoniazid, benzodiazepines, and tricyclic antidepressants. Therapy for prostate cancer with antiandrogens, estrogens or castration also may result in gynecomastia.

## Mediastinum

Although mediastinitis and pneumomediastinum are the most commonly recognized causes of pain arising from the mediastinum, pain may also arise from compression or inflammation of all mediastinal structure and has been reported with enlarging masses of various types, such as traumatic hematoma, substernal thyroid, lipoma, metastatic or primary cancer or lymphoma, and dermoid cysts or hygromas. Epicardial pacing wires may migrate from the central vasculature and create chest pain with a foreign body reaction in the mediastinum.[455]

## Mediastinitis

Mediastinitis can occur due to rupture of thoracic structures or dissection of infection along tissue planes from the neck or abdomen. Pain presumably arises due to irritation of vagal afferants. Fever, pleural effusion, pneumomediastinum, or pneumothorax are frequently present. Infection may occur after thoracic or cardiac surgery and, more frequently, after a median sternotomy has been performed. Esophageal rupture due to trauma, tumor, or inflammation frequently results in mediastinitis. Any deep infection of the neck, pharynx, or abdomen may spread to the chest along the mediastinal tissue planes.[456]

## Pneumomediastinum

Spontaneous pneumomediastinum may arise with spontaneous pneumothorax or independently.[457] It also can occur in asthmatic patients, following root canal work with a high speed air drill, tracheostomy, mechanical ventilation, or during labor.[458] In one report, up to 1 in 368 admissions to the hospital in the 14- to 29-year-old age group of nonsurgical, nontrauma, nonobstetric patients had spontaneous pneumomediastinum. The prevalence has been estimated to occur at a ratio of 1:15 with spontaneous pneumothorax. More than 80% of cases occur in men. Physical examination detects the presence of subcutaneous emphysema in more than 90% of cases and Hamman's sign, a precordial adventitious sound auscultated over the sternum during systole, in more than 50% of cases.[458] Mediastinitis needs to always be evaluated and ruled out whenever air appears in the mediastinum or when a patient's complaint of chest pain occurs in association with subcutaneous emphysema.

## Nerves

Most pain arising from nerves involves a compression of the nerve root, as noted in the section on spine disease. Other less common nerve syndromes can also produce chest pain. Spinal subarachnoid hemorrhage can classically present with sudden posterior chest or neck pain known as "le coup de poignard" or "strike of the dagger."[459] Epilepsy has been reported to cause chest pain; it may result from uncontrolled muscle spasms but may also result directly from stimulation of the central nervous system.[460]

### Intercostal Nerve Injury Due to Internal Mammary Artery Grafting

Internal mammary artery (IMA) grafts are now widely used for coronary artery bypass grafting. Patients with IMA grafting may present with chest pain 4 months to 5 years postoperatively.[461] Intercostal nerve injury due to direct trauma and ischemia appears to be the cause of the pain. Pain

may occur after unilateral or bilateral procedures, is more frequently moderate-to-severe, typically constant, and may have a burning, dull, or pricking character. Distinguishing features include numbness to pinprick in the T-1 through T-6 dermatomes extending to or around the nipple line anteriorly, tenderness to palpation over the sternum or costosternal junctions from T-1 to T-6, and pain due to stimuli that do not normally cause pain (allodynia) such as clothes or light touch in the area of numbness. Bone scans show increased activity in the sternum in the delayed phase of the scan more than 1 year after surgery, suggesting poor sternal healing.

### Neuromas

Traumatic neuroma may arise from chest-wall injury or surgical section of nerves during thoracic surgery. Traumatic neuroma usually presents with point tenderness at the point-of-nerve injury or section. Pain may radiate along the course of the nerve.

### Sternal Wires

Sternal wire sutures applied post-median sternotomy have been reported to result in pain due to possible nickel hypersensitivity[462] and due to entrapment of sensory nerves.[463] Pain has been described as sharp, stabbing, or a deep ache, and patients have tenderness over the retained wires. Resected wires have demonstrated an intense fibrous reaction encasing the twisted portion of the wire and entrapment of sensory nerves. Pain has also occurred when wire fragments have migrated to the pleural space.[464] Pain resolves with removal of the sternal wires. The diagnosis is made clinically.

## Kidneys

Kidney pain typically results from inflammation and is directly sensed by visceral afferants. The vagus nerves innervate the kidneys; they are presumed to be the afferent nerve mediating the sensation of pain. Pyelonephritis, renal calculi, and renal infarct may all present with pain in the chest. Pain usually occurs in the flank, that is, the lateral posterior inferior portion of the chest overlying the affected kidney. Other renal conditions that result in renal inflammation, such as infected or hemorrhagic cysts, or intrarenal hemorrhage may also cause flank pain.

## Pyelonephritis

Pyelonephritis classically occurs acutely with fever, flank pain, pyuria, and leukocytosis.[465] The pain typically increases with percussion or firm palpation of the flank. Patients at increased risk for pyelonephritis include women, diabetics, pregnant women, patients after instrumentation of the urethra or ureters, patients with renal calculi, and individuals with impaired bladder function.[465,466] *Escherichia coli* accounts for 90% of cases of pyelonephritis.[467,468] The diagnosis frequently is obvious at presentation, and rarely mimics other causes of chest pain. Evaluation need only consist of considering the diagnostic possibility, identifying the patient as a member of a risk group, and obtaining a temperature, white blood cell count, and urinary dipstick for nitrites.[465] In complicated patients, a culture and sensitivity of a clean catch urine may be required. Pyelonephritis in men, children, pregnant women, immunocompromised patients, and patients suspected of having renal calculi merit additional evaluation with ultrasound or contrast CT. In children and in difficult diagnostic cases, renal scintigraphy with a dimercaptosuccinic acid scan (DMSA) has been shown to be 91% sensitive and 99% specific in establishing the diagnosis.[469–471]

## Renal Infarct

While small areas of the kidney may infarct without a sensation of pain, pain will result when a larger volume of the kidney acutely develops severe ischemia. Chronic ischemia typically produces a painless atrophy. Diseases that cause an abrupt severe ischemia may present with flank pain. This usually occurs due to abrupt, near-complete occlusion of the main renal artery due to trauma, or due to embolism in patients with atrial fibrillation, mitral stenosis, ventricular mural thrombi, endocarditis, or atherosclerosis. While pain may radiate to the posterior chest, it is usually abrupt, sharp and radiates to the abdomen and groin rather than to the chest. Fever, leukocytosis, and hematuria should occur almost universally when pain is present. When unclear, the diagnosis can be confirmed with angiography.

## Renal Calculi

While renal stones may be large and almost completely fill the collecting system without causing pain, stones that are associated with infection, enter the urethra, or obstruct with calyceal or ureteral dilatation may cause pain due to distention or, because ureteral passage is usually associated with hemorrhage, due to direct ureteral trauma from release of inflammatory mediators. Initially, pain is felt in the flank and is typically gradual in onset over 20 to 60 minutes. Pain may become severe, sharp, and necessitate analgesia. As the stone migrates downward, flank pain usually resolves and pain radiates to the lower abdomen, groin, and testicles. Patients at increased risk for renal calculi are those who have had prior calculi or gout, distal renal tubular acidosis, recurrent renal infections, hyperparathyroidism, and dehydration. Renal colic rarely mimics other causes of chest pain. The presence of hematuria or visualization of a distended ureter or stone by ultrasound or abdominal roentgenogram may confirm the diagnosis.

## Drugs

Numerous drugs have been reported to the Food and Drug Administration due to patients developing chest pain after their administration. Consequently, all patients with chest pain should be questioned as to their recent drug use: prescription, nonprescription, and illegal. While chest pain may result from the direct action of the drug (eg, cocaine), allergic reactions, nonallergic reactions, or non-drug-related substances are associated with administration. In most cases, the mechanism by which drugs potentially cause pain has not been studied, leaving the causative pathway speculative. When nine patients developed chest pain after the administration of alpha-1-proteinase inhibitor, the cause of chest pain was traced to impurities in the manufacturing process and appeared limited to specific lots of drug.[472]

In most cases, it is likely that drug-induced chest pain results from a direct action of the drug or a metabolite. The chemotherapeutic agents, 5 fluorouracil, bleomycin, and methotrexate have been reported to frequently cause chest pain. 5-fluorouracil cardiotoxicity[473,474] occurs in 1.6% to 18% of patients administered the drug, appears more frequent when delivered as a continuous intravenous infusion, and may be associated with profound, reversible left ventricular dysfunction or ECG changes of ischemia. Chest pain occurs several hours after the third intravenous bolus or on the third or fourth day of intravenous infusion. Up to 2.8% of patients receiving bleomycin[475] develop a substernal pressure or pleuritic chest pain which is sudden in onset and may last 4 to 72 hours. While pain in some cases is associated with pericarditis and/or pleural effusion, reactions are usually self-limited, do not stop with cessation of infusion, and do not typically recur on reinfusion. Methotrexate[476] when given in high doses of 8 g/m² or higher may cause a pleuritis in 8.5% of cases. Pain occurs usually after the third or fourth treatment, may be severe, and may last 3 to 5 days.

Drugs that have vasoactive properties may result in chest pain due to direct cardiac stimulation or changes in blood pressure. Shimp et al.[477] postulated that ranitidine caused acute severe chest pain by interaction with cardiac $H_2$ receptors. Corticotropin-releasing hormone delivered in a dose of 100 $\mu$g may cause chest pain due to coronary ischemia within 10 minutes of administration, presumably by hypotension resulting from mesenteric vascular dilatation.[478] Similarly, apraclonidine administered as a topical ophthalmic solution may rarely cause hypotension and chest pain.[479] Odansetron, a newer antiemetic, has been associated with exacerbating angina.[480]

Other drugs produce chest pain via well-described unique mechanisms. Mild, retrosternal pain, typically worse on inspiration, occurs almost universally after 17 hours of 100% oxygen administration and is felt to be due to tracheitis.[481] Vancomycin infusion may result in a histamine-mediated "pain and spasm syndrome."[482] The pain may be retrosternal and occur in individuals who have no evidence of coronary disease. Sertraline, a selective serotonin-reuptake inhibitor antidepressant, has been reported to cause chest pain due to possible coronary vasoconstriction or esophageal reactions.[483,484] Sumatriptan, a serotonin agonist prescribed for migraine, may cause chest pain possibly due to coronary ischemia or esophageal dysmotility.[485-487]

### Cocaine

Acute and chronic cocaine use frequently results in chest pain. In Hennepin County Hospital in Minneapolis, five cases of cocaine-induced chest pain were evaluated per month and accounted for 1.4% of coronary intensive care unit admissions.[488] Chest pain was described as pressure (46%), sharp (33%), dull (20%), and pleuritic (18%), and radiated to the neck, shoulders, and arms in 40% of cases.[488] Pain started during or within 1 hour of cocaine use in 27% to 55% of cases [367,488] and occurred more than 3 hours after cocaine use in only 13% of cases.

The cause of pain is multifactorial. Some believe that chest pain results from a local sensory response to acute airway irritation.[489] Although cocaine use has clearly resulted in MI, Gitter points out that only 65 cases of cocaine-related MI have been reported in the North American medical literature between 1982 and 1990,[488] despite admitted regular use of cocaine by 5 million North Americans. Pain by many is assumed to be anginal and due to coronary ischemia secondary to cocaine-mediated microangiopathy,[490] focal coronary vasospasm, thrombus formation, myocarditis, or increased coronary oxygen consumption due to the sympathomimetic effects of increased contractility, tachycardia, and hypertension.[490,491] The incidence of MI in cocaine users presenting to the emergency department with chest pain ranges from 0% to 6%. The low rate of infarction has led some to question whether the chest pain commonly seen with cocaine use might also relate to a toxic effect on thoracic skeletal muscle.[488] Cocaine use may rarely cause noncardiac, nonmuscular pain due to catastrophic events, such as aortic dissection.

Protocols for evaluating and treating patients with cocaine-induced chest pain remain in flux. Since the 0% to 6% infarction rate among cocaine users in not substantially different from the 4% rate of infarction rate among 25- to 39-year-olds presenting with chest pain,[367] identification of cocaine users is most important in that it helps guide further evaluation. A urine screen for recent cocaine use may be performed by assaying for benzoylecgonine. This should test positive within 5 minutes of intravenous injection or smoking and within 30 minutes of insufflation, and remain positive for 24 to 36 hours.[367] Patients with a positive urine screen who are ruled out for MI should require no further diagnostic evaluation since cocaine is the most likely cause of the chest pain episode. If the urine screen is negative, additional evaluation will be indicated even if MI is ruled out.

## References:

1. Kroenke K, Mangelsdorff D. Common symptoms in ambulatory care: incidence, evaluation, therapy, and outcome. Am J Med 1989; 86:262–266.
2. Gold M, Azevedo D. The content of adult primary care episodes. Public Health Reports 1982; 97:48–57.
3. Kemp HG, Vokonas PS, Cohn PF, et al. The anginal syndromes associated with normal coronary arteriograms: report of a six year experience. Am J Med 1973; 54: 735–742.
4. Marchandise B, Bourassa MG, Chaitman BR, et al. Angiographic evaluation of the natural history of normal coronary arteries and mild coronary atherosclerosis. Am J Cardiol 1978; 41:216–220.
5. Fineberg HV, Scadden D, Goldman L. Care of patients with a low probability of acute myocardial infarction. Cost effectiveness of alternatives to coronary care unit admission. N Engl J Med 1984; 310: 1301–1307.
6. Gibler WB. Chest pain evaluation in the ED: beyond triage. Am J Emerg Med 1994; 12:121–122.
7. Goldman L, Weinberg M, Weisberg M, et al. A computer-derived protocol to aid in the diagnosis of emergency room patients with acute chest pain. N Engl J Med 1982; 307:588–596.
8. Pozen MW, D'Agostino RB, Mitchell JB, et al. The usefulness of a predictive instrument to reduce innapropriate admissions to the coronary care unit. Ann Intern Med 1980; 92:238–242.
9. Pozen MW, D'Agostino RB, Selker HP, et al. A predictive instrument to improve coronary-care-unit admission practices in acute ischemic heart disease: a prospective multicenter clinical trial. N Engl J Med 1984; 310:1273–1278.
10. Bloom BS, Peterson OL. End results, cost and productivity of coronary-care units. N Engl J Med 1973; 288:72–78.
11. Eisenberg JM, Horowitz LN, Busch R, et al. Diagnosis of acute myocardial infarction in the emergency room: a prospective assessment of clinical decision making and the usefulness of immediate cardiac enzyme determination. J Community Health 1979; 4:190–198.
12. Fuchs R, Scheidt S. Improved criteria for admission to cardiac care units. JAMA 1981; 246:2037–2041.
13. Madias JE, Gorlin R. The myth of acute "mild" myocardial infarction. Ann Intern Med 1977; 86:347–352.
14. Tierney WM, Roth BJ, Psaty B, et al. Predictors of myocardial infarction in emer-

gency room patients. Crit Care Med 1985; 13:526–531.

15. Goldman L, Cook EF, Brand DA, et al. A computer protocol to predict myocardial infarction in emergency department patients with chest pain. N Engl J Med 1988; 318:797–803.

16. Melzack R. The McGill pain questionnaire: major properties and scoring methods. Pain 1975; 1:277–299.

17. Powley TL, Prechtl J, Fox E, et al. Fibers of the vagus nerve regulating gastrointestinal function. Dig Dis Sci 1989; 34:984.

18. Grant JCB. Grant's Atlas of Anatomy. Baltimore, Md: Williams & Wilkins Company; 1972.

19. Genereux GP, Howie JL. Normal mediastinal lymph node size and number: CT and 8anatomic study. AJR 1984; 142: 1095–1100.

20. Dockray GJ, Sharkey KA. Neurochemistry of visceral afferent neurons. In: Cervero F, Morrison JFB, eds. Progress in Brain Research. New York, NY: Elsevier Publishing Co; 1986:133–148.

21. Cunningham ET, Ravich WJ, Jones B, et al. Vagal reflexes referred from the upper aerodigestive tract: an infrequently recognized cause of common cardiorespiratory responses. Ann Intern Med 1992; 116: 575–582.

22. Ness TJ, Gebhart GF. Visceral pain: a review of experimental studies. Pain 1990; 41:167–234.

23. Cross SA. Pathophysiology of pain. Mayo Clin Proc 1994; 69:375–383.

24. Besson J, Chaouch A. Peripheral and spinal mechanisms of nociception. Physiol Rev 1987; 67:67–186.

25. Talbot JD, Marrett S, Evans AC, et al. Multiple representations of pain in human cerebral cortex. Science 1991; 251: 1355–1357.

26. McMahon SB. Mechanisms of cutaneous, deep and visceral pain. In: Wall PD, Melzack R, eds. Texbook of Pain.3rd ed. New York, NY: Churchill Livingstone; 1994: 129–150.

27. Nathan PW. Pain and the sympathetic system. J Auton Nerv Sys 1983; 7: 363–370.

28. Wheat MW, Jr. Acute dissecting aneurysms of the aorta: diagnosis and treatment 1979. Am Heart J 1980; 99:373–387.

29. Roberts WC. Aortic dissection: anatomy, consequences, and causes. Am Heart J 1981; 101:195–214.

30. Wheat MW. Pathogenesis of aortic dissec-

tion. In: Doroghazi RM, Slater EE, eds. Aortic Dissection. New York, NY: McGraw-Hill Book Company; 1983:55.

31. Daily PO, Trueblood HW, Stinson EB, et al. Management of acute aortic dissections. Ann Thorac Surg 1970;10:237–247.

32. Larson EW, Edwards WD. Risk factors for aortic dissection: a necropsy study of 161 cases. Am J Cardiol 1984;53:849–855.

33. Slater EE, DeSanctis RW. The clinical recognition of dissecting aortic aneurysm. Am J Med 1976;60:625–633.

34. Slater EE. Aortic dissection: presentation and diagnosis. In: Doroghazi RM, Slater EE, eds. Aortic Dissection. New York, NY: McGraw-Hill Book Company;1983:61.

35. Riley DJ, Liu RT, Saxanoff S. Aortic dissection: a rare cause of the superior vena cava syndrome. J Med Soc N J 1981;78: 187–189.

36. Roth JA, Parekh MA. Dissecting aneurysms perforating the esophagus. N Engl J Med 1978;299:776.

37. Erbel R, Engberding R, Daniel W, et al. Echocardiography in diagnosis of aortic dissection. Lancet 1989;i:457–461.

38. Adachi H, Kyo S, Takamoto S, et al. Early diagnosis and surgical intervention of acute aortic dissection by transesophageal color flow mapping. Circulation 1990; 82:19–23.

39. Eagle KA, DeSanctis RW. Diseases of the aorta. In: Braunwald E, ed. Heart Disease. A Textbook of Cardiovascular Medicine. 4th ed. Philadelphia, Pa: WB Saunders Company; 1992:1528–1557.

40. Collins JJ, Koster JK, Cohn LH, et al. Common aortic aneurysms: when to intervene. J Cardiovasc Med 1983;8:245–252.

41. Brundage BH, Rich S, Spigos D. Computed tomography of the heart and great vessels: present and future. Ann Intern Med 1984; 101:801–809.

42. Cigarroa JE, Isselbacher EM, DeSanctis RW, et al. Medical progress. Diagnostic imaging in the evaluation of suspected aortic dissection: old standards and new directions. AJR 1993; 161:485–493.

43. Seward JB, Khandheria BK, Oh JK, et al. Transesophageal echocardiography: technique, anatomic correlations, implementation, and clinical applications. Mayo Clin Proc 1988; 63:649–680.

44. Lupi-Herrera E, Sanchez-Torres G, Marcushamer J, et al. Takayasu's arteritis. Clinical study of 107 cases. Am Heart J 1977; 93:94–103.

45. Paulus HE, Pearson CM, Pitts W, Jr. Aortic

insufficiency in five patients with Reiter's syndrome. A detailed clinical and pathologic study. Am J Med 1972; 53:464–472.

46. Morgan SH, Asherson RA, Hughes GR. Distal aortitis complicating Reiter's syndrome. Br Heart J 1984; 52:115–116.

47. Gronemeyer PS, deMello DE. Takayasu's disease with aneurysm of right common iliac artery and iliocaval fistula in a young infant: case report and review of the literature. Pediatrics 1982; 69:626–631.

48. Morooka S, Saito Y, Nonaka Y, et al. Clinical features of aortitis syndrome in Japanese women older than 40 years. Am J Cardiol 1984; 53:859–861.

49. Ishikawa K. Diagnostic approach and proposed criteria for the clinical diagnosis of Takayasu's arteriopathy. J Am Coll Cardiol 1988; 12:964–972.

50. Salisbury RS, Hazleman BL. Successful treatment of dissecting aortic aneurysm due to giant cell arteritis. Ann Rheum Dis 1981;40:507–508.

51. National Center for Health Statistics. Utilization of short stay hospitals, United States, 1987. Vital Health Stat 1987;31:197.

52. Lee TH, Cook EF, Weisberg M, et al. Acute chest pain in the emergency room. Identification and examination of low-risk patients. Arch Intern Med 1985;145:65–69.

53. Castell DO. Chest pain of undetermined origin: overview of pathophysiology. Am J Med 1992; 92:2S-4S.

54. Davies HA. Anginal pain of esophageal origin: clinical presentation, prevalence, and prognosis. Am J Med 1992;92:5S-10S.

55. Lynn RB. Mechanisms of esophageal pain. Am J Med 1992; 92:11S-19S.

56. Beitman BD. Panic disorder in patients with angiographically normal coronary arteries. Am J Med 1992;92:33S-40S.

57. Benjamin SB. Microvascular angina and the sensitive heart: historical perspective. Am J Med 1992;92:52S-55S.

58. Kemp HG, Kronmal RA, Vliestra RE, et al. Seven year survival of patients with normal or near normal coronary arteriograms: A CASS registry study. J Am Coll Cardiol 1986;7:479–483.

59. Chambers J, Bass C. Chest pain with normal coronary anatomy: a review of natural history and possible etiologic factors. Prog Cardiovasc Dis 1990;33:161–184.

60. Ockene IS, Shay MJ, Alpert JS, et al. Unexplained chest pain in patients with normal coronary arteriograms. N Engl J Med 1980;303:1249–1252.

61. Ward BW, Wu WC, Richter JE, et al. Long-term follow-up of symptomatic status of patients with noncardiac chest pain: is diagnosis of esophageal etiology helpful? Am J Gastroenterol 1987;82:215–218.

62. Light RW. Pleural disease due to collagen vascular diseases. In: *Anonymous Pleural Diseases*. 3rd ed. Baltimore, Md: Williams & Wilkinsσ95:208–218.

63. Karlson BW, Herlitz J, Pettersson P, et al. Patients admitted to the emergency room with symptoms indicative of acute myocardial infarction. J Intern Med 1991;230:251–258.

64. Rouan GW, Lee TH, Cook EF, et al. Clinical characteristics and outcome of acute myocardial infarction in patients with initially normal or nonspecific electrocardiograms. A report from the multicenter chest pain study. Am J Cardiol 1989;64:1087–1092.

65. McCarthy BD, Wong JB, Selker HP. Detecting acute cardiac ischemia in the emergency department: a review of the literature. J Gen Int Med 1990;5:365–373.

66. Lee TH, Weisberg MC, Brand DA, et al. Candidates for thrombolysis among emergency room patients with acute chest pain-potential true- and false-positive rates. Ann Intern Med 1989;110:957–962.

67. Betriu A, Castaner A, Sanz GA,et al. Angiographic findings 1 month after myocardial infarction: a prospective study of 259 survivors. Circulation 1982;65:1099–1105.

68. Glover MU, Kuber MT, Warren SE, et al. Myocardial infarction before age 36: risk factor and arteriographic analysis. Am J Cardiol 1982;49:1600–1603.

69. Ciraulo DA, Bresnahan GF, Frankel PS, et al. Transmural myocardial infarction with normal coronary angiograms and with single vessel coronary obstruction. Clinical-angiographic features and 5-year follow-up. Chest 1983;83:196–202.

70. Pecora MJ, Roubin GS, Cobbs BW, Jr., et al. Presentation and late outcome of myocardial infarction in the absence of angiographically significant coronary artery disease. Am J Cardiol 1988;62:363–367.

71. Raymond R, Lynch J, Underwood D, et al. Myocardial infarction and normal coronary arteriography: a 10-year clinical and risk analysis of 74 patients. J Am Coll Cardiol 1988;11:471–477.

72. Tofler GH, Stone PH, Maclure M, et al. Analysis of possible triggers of acute myo-

cardial infarction (The MILIS Study). Am J Cardiol 1990;66:22–27.

73. Jenkins CD. Recent evidence supporting psychological and social risk factors for coronary disease. N Engl J Med 1976;294: 1033–1038.

74. Muller DW, Topol EJ, Califf RM, et al. Relationship between antecedent angina pectoris and short-term prognosis after thrombolytic therapy for acute myocardial infarction. Thrombolysis and Angioplasty in Myocardial Infarction (TAMI) Study Group. Am Heart J 1990;119: 224–231.

75. Muller JE, Stone PH, Turi ZG, et al. Circadian variation in the frequency of onset of acute myocardial infarction. N Engl J Med 1985;313:1315–1322.

76. Goldberg RJ, Brady P, Muller JE, et al. Time onset of symptoms of acute myocardial infarction. Am J Cardiol 1990;66: 140–144.

77. Muller JE, Ludmer PL, Willich SN, et al. Circadian variation in the frequency of sudden cardiac death. Circulation 1987; 75:131–138.

78. Tsementzis SA, Gill JS, Hitchcock ER, et al. Diurnal variation of and activity during the onset of stroke. Neurology 1985; 17:901–904.

79. Quyyumi AA, Mockus L, Wright C, et al. Morphology of ambulatory ST segment changes in patients with varying severity of coronary artery disease: investigation of the frequency of nocturnal ischemia and coronary spasm. Br Heart J 1985;53: 186–193.

80. Rocco MB, Barry J, Campbell S, et al. Circadian variation of transient myocardial ischemia in patients with coronary artery disease. Circulation 1987;75:395–400.

81. Ingram DA, Fulton RA, Portal RW, et al. Vomiting as a diagnostic aid in acute ischaemic cardiac pain. Br Med J 1980; 281:636–637.

82. Sigurdsson E, Thorgeirsson G, Sigvaldason H, et al. Unrecognized myocardial infarction: epidemiology, clinical characteristics, and the prognostic role of angina pectoris. The Reykjavik Study. Ann Intern Med 1995;122:96–102.

83. Margolis JR, Kannel WS, Feinleib M, et al. Clinical features of unrecognized myocardial infarction—silent and symptomatic. Eighteen year follow-up: The Framingham Study. Am J Cardiol 1973;32: 1–7.

84. Yano K, MacLean CJ. The incidence and prognosis of unrecognized myocardial infarction in the Honolulu, Hawaii, Heart Program. Arch Intern Med 1989;149: 1528–1532.

85. Webb SW, Adgey AA, Pantridge JF. Autonomic disturbance at onset of acute myocardial infarction. Br Med J 1972;3:89–92.

86. Shell WE, DeWood MA, Peter T, et al. Comparison of clinical signs and hemodynamic state in the early hours of transmural myocardial infarction. Am Heart J 1982;104:521–528.

87. Krainin FM, Flessas AP, Spodick DH. Infarction-associated pericarditis. Rarity of diagnostic electrocardiogram. N Engl J Med 1984;311:1211–1214.

88. Galve E, Garcia-Del-Castillo H, Evangelista A, et al. Pericardial effusion in the course of myocardial infarction: incidence, natural history, and clinical relevance. Circulation 1986;73:294–299.

89. Sobel BE, Shell WE. Serum enzyme determinations in the diagnosis and assessment of myocardial infarction. Circulation 1972;45:471–482.

90. Lee TH, Goldman L. Serum enzyme assays in the diagnosis of acute myocardial infarction. Recommendations based on quantitative analysis. Ann Intern Med 1986;105:221–233.

91. Hendricks GR, Amano J, Kenna T, et al. Creatine kinase release not associated with myocardial necrosis after short periods of coronary artery occlusion in conscious baboons. J Am Coll Cardiol 1985; 6:1299–1303.

92. Weidner N. Laboratory diagnosis of acute myocardial infarct. Usefulness of determination of lactate dehydrogenase (LDH)-1 level and the ratio of LDH-1 to total LDH. Arch Pathol Lab Med 1982;106: 375–377.

93. Vasudevan G, Mercer DW, Varat MA. Lactic dehydrogenase isoenzyme determination in the diagnosis of acute myocardial infarction. Circulation 1978;57: 1055–1057.

94. Graeber GM, Clagett P, Wolf RE, et al. Alterations in serum creatine kinase and lactate dehydrogenase. Chest 1990;97: 521–527.

95. Gerhardt W, Katus HA, Ravkilde J, et al. S-troponin T in suspected ischemic myocardial injury compared with mass and catalytic concentration of S-creatine kinase isoenzyme MB. Clin Chem 1991;37: 1405–1411.

96. Mach F, Lovis C, Chevrolet JC, et al. Rapid

bedside whole blood cardiospecific troponin T immunoassay for the diagnosis of
acute myocardial infarction. Am J Cardiol
1995;75:842–845.

97. Puelo PR, Meyer D, Wathen C, et al. Use
of a rapid assay of subforms of creatine
kinase MB to diagnose or rule out myocardial infarction. N Engl J Med 1994;331:
1405–1411.

98. Rude RE, Poole WK, Muller JE, et al.
Electrocardiographic and clinical criteria
for recognition of acute myocardial infarction based on analysis of 3,697 patients. Am J Cardiol 1983;52:936–942.

99. Fesmire FM, Percy RF, Wears RL, et al.
Initial ECG in Q-wave and non-Q-wave
myocardial infarction. Ann Emerg Med
1989;18:741–746.

100. Miller DH, Kligfield P, Schreiber TL, et
al. Relationship of prior myocardial infarction to false-positive electrocardiographic diagnosis of acute injury in patients with chest pain. Arch Intern Med
1987;147:257–261.

101. Zarling EJ, Sexton H, Milnor P Jr. Failure
to diagnose acute myocardial infarction—The clinicopathologic experience
at a large community hospital. JAMA
1983;250:1177–1181.

102. Behar S, Schor S, Kariv I, et al. Evaluation
of the electrocardiogram in the emergency
room as a decision-making tool. Chest
1977;71:486–491.

103. McGuiness JB, Begg TB, Semple T. First
electrocardiogram in recent myocardial
infarction. Br. Med J 1976; 2:449–451.

104. Gunraj DR, Rajapakse DA. Daily ECG confirmation in acute myocardial infarction.
Practitioner 1974;213:361–364.

105. The TIMI Study Group. The thrombolysis
in myocardial infarction (TIMI) trial.
Phase I findings. N Engl J Med 1985;312:
932–936.

106. Zaret BL, Wackers FJ, Soufer R. Nuclear
cardiology. In: Braunwald E, ed. *Heart
Disease. A Textbook of Cardiovascular
Medicine.* 4th ed. Philadelphia, Pa: WB
Saunders Company; 1992:276–311.

107. Skorton DJ, Schelbert HR, Wolf GL, et al.
Relative merits of imaging techniques. In:
Braunwald E, ed. *Heart Disease. A Text-
book of Cardiovascular Medicine.* 4th ed.
Philadelphia, Pa: WB Saunders Com-
pany; 1992:342–350.

108. Hilton TC, Thompson RC, Williams HJ, et
al. Technetium-99m sestamibi myocardial perfusion imaging in the emergency

room evaluation of chest pain. J Am Coll
Cardiol 1994;23:1016–1022.

109. Stratmann HG, Williams GA, Wittry MD,
et al. Exercise technetium-99m sestamibi
tomography for cardiac risk stratification
of patients with stable chest pain. Circulation 1994;89:615–622.

110. Haronian HL, Remetz MS, Sinusas AJ, et
al. Myocardial risk area defined by tech-
netium-99m sestamibi imaging during
percutaneous transluminal coronary angioplasty: comparison with coronary angiography. J Am Coll Cardiol 1993;22:
1033–1043.

111. Varetto T, Cantalupi D, Altieri A, et al.
Emergency room technetium-99m sestamibi imaging to rule out acute myocardial ischemic events in patients with nondiagnostic electrocardiograms. J Am Coll
Cardiol 1993;22:1804–1808.

112. Peels CH, Visser CA, Kupper AJ, et al.
Usefulness of two-dimensional echocardiography for immediate detection of
myocardial ischemia in the emergency
room. Am J Cardiol 1990; 65:687–691.

113. Mann DL, Gillam LD, Weyman AE. Cross-
sectional echocardiographic assessment
of regional left ventricular performance
and myocardial perfusion. Prog Cardiovasc Dis 1986;29:1–52.

114. Berning J, Steensgaard-Hansen F. Early
estimation of risk by echocardiographic
determination of wall motion index in an
unselected population with acute myocardial infarction. Am J Cardiol 1990;65:
567–576.

115. Chandraratna PA, Nanna M, McKay C, et
al. Determination of cardiac output by
transcutaneous continuous-wave ultra-
sonic Doppler computer. Am J Cardiol
1984;53:234–237.

116. Smyllie JH, Sutherland GR, Geuskens R,
et al. Doppler color flow mapping in the
diagnosis of ventricular septal rupture
and acute mitral regurgitation after myocardial infarction. J Am Coll Cardiol 1990;
15:1449–1455.

117. Miklozek CL, Crumpacker CS, Royal HD,
et al. Myocarditis presenting as acute
myocardial infarction. Am Heart J 1988;
115:768–776.

118. Abelmann WH. Myocarditis and dilated
cardiomyopathy. West J Med 1989;150:
458.

119. Davidson BL, Elliott CG, Lensing AW.
Low accuracy of color Doppler ultrasound in the detection of proximal leg
vein thrombosis in asymptomatic high-

risk patients. Ann Intern Med 1992;117: 735–738.

120. Heath D. Pathology of cardiac tumors. Am J Cardiol 1968;21:315–327.

121. Urba WJ, Longo DL. Primary solid tumors of the heart. In: Kapoor AS, ed. *Cancer of the Heart*. New York, NY: Springer-Verlag 1986:62.

122. Smith C. Tumors of the heart. Arch Pathol Lab Med 1986;110:371–374.

123. Cannon RO, Cunnion RE, Parrillo JE, et al. Dynamic limitation of coronary vasodilator reserve in patients with dilated cardiomyopathy and chest pain. J Am Coll Cardiol 1987;10:1190–1200.

124. Ferrans VJ. Pathologic anatomy of the dilated cardiomyopathies. Am J Cardiol 1989;64:9C-11C.

125. Maron BJ, Bonow RO, Cannon RO, et al. Hypertrophic cardiomyopathy: interrelations of clinical manifestations, pathophysiology, and therapy. N Engl J Med 1987;316:844–852.

126. Maron BJ, Wolfson JK, Epstein SE, et al. Intramural ("small vessel") coronary artery disease in hypertrophic cardiomyopathy. J Am Coll Cardiol 1986;8:545–557.

127. Wynne J, Braunwald E. The cardiomyopathies and myocarditides: toxic, chemical, and physical damage to the heart. In: Braunwald E, ed. *Heart Disease. A Textbook of Cardiovascular Medicine*. 4th ed. Philadelphia, Pa: WB Saunders Company; 1992:1394–1450.

128. Unterberg C, Buchwald A, Wiegand V. Traumatic thrombosis of the left main coronary artery and myocardial infarction caused by blunt chest trauma. Clin Cardiol 1989;12:672–674.

129. Miller FB, Richardson JD, Thomas HA, et al. Role of CT in diagnosis of major arterial injury after blunt thoracic trauma. Surgery 1989;106:596–602.

130. Matthews RV, French WJ, Criley JM. Chest trauma and subvalvular left ventricular aneurysms. Chest 1989;95:474–476.

131. Clifford RP, Gill KS. Traumatic rupture of the pericardium with dislocation of the heart. Injury 1984;16:123–125.

132. Tenzer ML. The spectrum of myocardial contusion: a review. J Trauma 1985;25: 620–627.

133. Sutherland GR, Cheung HW, Holliday RL, et al. Hemodynamic adaptation to acute myocardial contusion complicating blunt chest injury. Am J Cardiol 1986;57: 291–297.

134. Torres-Mirabal P, Gruenberg JC, Talbert JG, et al. Ventricular function in myocardial contusion: a preliminary study. Crit Care Med 1982;10:19–24.

135. Fox KM, Rowland E, Krikler DM, et al. Electrophysiological manifestations of nonpenetrating cardiac trauma. Br Heart J 1980;43:458–462.

136. Bognolo DA, Rabow FI, Vijayanagar RR, et al. Traumatic sinus node dysfunction. Ann Emerg Med 1982;11:319–321.

137. Evora PR, Ribeiro PJ, Brasil JC, et al. Late surgical repair of ventricular septal defect due to nonpenetrating chest trauma: review and report of two contrasting cases. J Trauma 1985;25:1007–1009.

138. Mattox KL, Limacher MC, Feliciano DV, et al. Cardiac evaluation following heart injury. J Trauma 1985;25:758–765.

139. Chapman JE, Jr., Rubin JW, Gross CM, et al. Congenital absence of pericardium: an unusual cause of atypical angina. Ann Thorac Surg 1988;45:91–93.

140. Warren MJ, Kay VJ. Pericardial cyst in a patient with acute chest pain. Clin Radiol 1991;44:212

141. Celers J, Celers P, Bertocchi A. Non-polio enterovirus in France from 1974 to 1985. Data collected from a system of 30 hospital virology laboratories. Pathol Biol 1988; 36:1221–1226.

142. Acierno LJ. Cardiac complications in acquired immune deficiency syndrome (AIDS): a review. J Am Coll Cardiol 1989; 13:1144–1154.

143. Kinney EL, Monsuez JJ, Kitzis M, et al. Treatment of AIDS-associated heart disease. Angiology 1989;40:970–976.

144. Spodick DH. Pericardial rub: prospective, multiple observer investigation of pericardial friction rub in 100 patients. Am J Cardiol 1975;35:357–362.

145. Spodick DH. Diagnostic electrocardiographic sequences in acute pericarditis: significance of PR segment and PR vector changes. Circulation 1973;48:575–580.

146. Bruce MA, Spodick DH. Atypical electrocardiogram in acute pericarditis: characteristics and prevalence. J Electrocardiol 1980;13:61–66.

147. Wanner WR, Schaal SF, Bashore TM, et al. Repolarization variant vs. acute pericarditis. A prospective electrocardiographic and echocardiographic evaluation. Chest 1983;83:180–184.

148. Ginzton LE, Laks MM. The differential diagnosis of acute pericarditis from the normal variant: new electrocardiographic criteria. Circulation 1982;65:1004–1009.

149. Dressler N. Sinus tachycardia complicating and outlasting pericarditis. Am Heart J 1966;72:422–425.

150. Weiss JM, Spodick DH. Association of left pleural effusion with pericardial disease. N Engl J Med 1983;308:696–697.

151. Karjalainen J, Heikkila J. "Acute pericarditis": myocardial enzyme release as evidence for myocarditis. Am Heart J 1986; 111:546–552.

152. Permanyer-Miralda G, Sagrista-Sauleda J, Soler-Soler J. Primary acute pericardial disease: a prospective series of 231 consecutive patients. Am J Cardiol 1985;56: 623–630.

153. Usher BW, Popp RL. Electrical alternans: mechanism in pericardial effusion. Am Heart J 1972;83:459–463.

154. Singh S, Wann LS, Klopfenstein HS, et al. Usefulness of right ventricular diastolic collapse in diagnosing cardiac tamponade and comparison to pulsus paradoxus. Am J Cardiol 1986;57:652–656.

155. Engle MA, Ito T. The postpericardiotomy syndrome. Am J Cardiol 1961;7:73–84.

156. Engle MA, Gay WA Jr., Zabriskie JB, et al. The postpericardiotomy syndrome: 25 years' experience. J Cardiovasc Med 1984; 4:321–330.

157. Kaminsky ME, Rodan BA, Osborne DR, et al. Postpericardiotomy syndrome. AJR 1982;138:503–508.

158. Kassanoff AH, Martirossian MG. Postpericardiotomy and postmyocardial infarction syndrome presenting as noncardiac pulmonary edema. Chest 1991;99: 1410–1414.

159. Ofori-Krakye SK, Tyberg TI, Geha AS, et al. Late cardiac tamponade after open heart surgery: incidence, role of anticoagulants in its pathogenesis and its relationship to the postpericardiotomy syndrome. Circulation 1981;63:1323–1328.

160. Lorell BH, Braunwald E. Pericardial disease. In: Braunwald E, Ed. *Heart Disease. A Textbook of Cardiovascular Medicine.* 4th ed. Philadelphia, Pa: WB Saunders Company; 1992:1465–1516.

161. Mukai K, Shinkai T, Tominaga K, et al. The incidence of secondary tumors of the heart and pericardium: A ten-year study. Jpn J Clin Oncol 1988;18:195–201.

162. Press OW, Livingston R. Management of malignant pericardial effusion and tamponade. JAMA 1987;257:1088–1092.

163. Posner MR, Cohen GI, Skarin AT. Pericardial disease in patients with cancer. The differentiation of malignant from idiopathic and radiation-induced pericarditis. Am J Med 1981;71:407–413.

164. Yazdi HM, Hajdu SI, Melamed MR. Cytopathology of pericardial effusions. Acta Cytologica 1980;24:401–412.

165. Dressler W. The post-myocardial infarction syndrome. A report of forty-four cases. Arch Intern Med 1959;103:28–42.

166. Van der Geld H. Anti-heart antibodies in the post-pericardiotomy and the post-myocardial infarction syndrome. Lancet 1964;ii:617–618.

167. Dressler W. A postmyocardial infarction syndrome. Preliminary report of a complication resembling idiopathic recurrent benign pericarditis. JAMA 1956;160: 1379–1382.

168. Holloway JD. Post-myocardial infarction pericarditis. Chronic symptoms in a middle-aged man. Postgrad Med 1989;85: 57–60.

169. Roberts WC. Valvular, subvalvular, and supravalvular aortic stenosis. Morphologic features. Cardiovasc Clin 1973;5: 97–126.

170. Panidis IP, Segal BL. Aortic valve disease in the elderly. In: Frankl WS, Brest AN, eds. *Cardiovascular Clinics. Valvular Heart Disease: Comprehensive Evaluation and Management.* Philadelphia, Pa: FA Davis; 1986:289–312.

171. Levinson GE. Aortic stenosis. In: Dalen JE, Alpert JS, eds. *Valvular Heart Disease.* 2nd ed. Boston, Ma: Little Brown and Company; 1987:197–282.

172. Smucker ML, Tedesco CL, Manning SB, et al. Demonstration of an imbalance between coronary perfusion and excessive load as a mechanism of ischemia during stress in patients with aortic stenosis. Circulation 1988;78:573–582.

173. Matsuo S, Tsuruta M, Hayano M, et al. Phasic coronary artery flow velocity determined by Doppler flowmeter catheter in aortic stenosis and aortic regurgitation. Am J Cardiol 1988;62:917–922.

174. Kennedy KD, Nishimura RA, Holmes DR, Jr., et al. Natural history of moderate aortic stenosis. J Am Coll Cardiol 1991;17: 313–319.

175. Frank S, Johnson A, Ross J Jr. Natural history of valvular aortic stenosis. Br Heart J 1973;35:41–46.

176. Kelly TA, Rothbart RM, Cooper CM, et al. Comparison of outcome of asymptomatic to symptomatic patients older than 20 years of age with valvular aortic stenosis. Am J Cardiol 1988;61:123–130.

177. Fowler NO. Aortic stenosis. In: *Anonymous Diagnosis of Heart Disease.* New York, NY: Springer-Verlag; 1991: 134–145.

178. Abrams J. Aortic stenosis. In: *Anonymous Essentials of Cardiac Physical Diagnosis.* Philadelphia, Pa: Lea & Febiger; 1987: 205–224.

179. Caulfield WH, deLeon AC, Jr., Perloff JK, et al. The clinical significance of the fourth heart sound in aortic stenosis. Am J Cardiol 1971;28:179–182.

180. Forsell G, Jonasson R, Orinius E. Identifying severe aortic valvular stenosis by bedside examination. Acta Med Scand 1985; 218:397–400.

181. Gooch AS, Calatayud JB, Rogers PA, et al. Analysis of the P wave in severe aortic stenosis. Dis Chest 1966;49:459–463.

182. Nair CK, Aronow WS, Stokke K, et al. Cardiac conduction defects in patients older than 60 years with aortic stenosis with and without mitral annular calcium. Am J Cardiol 1984;53:169–172.

183. Galan A, Zoghbi WA, Quinones MA. Determination of severity of valvular aortic stenosis by Doppler echocardiography and relation of findings to clinical outcome and agreement with hemodynamic measurements determined at cardiac catheterization. Am J Cardiol 1991;67: 1007–1012.

184. Yeager M, Yock PG, Popp RL. Comparison of Doppler-derived pressure gradient to that determined at cardiac catheterization in adults with aortic valve stenosis: implications for management. Am J Cardiol 1986;57:644–648.

185. Reichek N, Shelburne JC, Perloff JK. Clinical aspects of rheumatic valvular disease. Prog Cardiovasc Dis 1973;15:491–537.

186. Kinare SG, Kulkarni HL. Quantitative study of the mitral valve in chronic rheumatic heart disease. Int J Cardiol 1987;16: 271–284.

187. Olson LJ, Subramanian R, Ackermann DM, et al. Surgical pathology of the mitral valve: a study of 712 cases spanning 21 years. Mayo Clin Proc 1987;62:22–34.

188. Bell MH, Mintz GS. Mitral valve disease in the elderly. In: Frankl WS, Brest AN, eds. *Cardiovascular Clinics. Valvular Heart Disease: Comprehensive Evaluation and Management.* Philadelphia, Pa: FA Davis; 1986:313–324.

189. Chopra P, Tandon HD, Raizada V, et al. Comparative studies in mitral valves in rheumatic heart disease. Arch Intern Med 1983;143:661–666.

190. Reis RN, Roberts WC. Amounts of coronary arterial narrowing by atherosclerotic plaques in clinically isolated mitral valve stenosis: analysis of 76 necropsy patients older than 30 years. Am J Cardiol 1986; 57:1117–1123.

191. Chun PK, Gertz E, Davia JE, et al. Coronary atherosclerosis in mitral stenosis. Chest 1982;81:36–41.

192. Baxter RH, Reid JM, McGuiness JB, et al. Relation of angina to coronary artery disease in mitral and aortic valve disease. Br Heart J 1978;40:918–922.

193. Barrington WW, Boudoulas H, Bashore T, et al. Mitral stenosis: mitral dome excursion and MI and the mitral opening snap—the concept of reciprocal heart sounds. Am Heart J 1988;115:1280–1290.

194. Amplatz K. The roentgenographic diagnosis of mitral and aortic valvular disease. Am Heart J 1962;64:556–561.

195. Melhem RE, Dunbar JD, Booth RW. "B" lines of Kerley and left atrial size in mitral valve disease: their correlation with mean left atrial pressure as measured by left atrial puncture. Radiology 1961;76: 65–68.

196. Walston A, Harley A, Pipberger HV. Computer analysis of the orthogonal electrocardiogram and vectorcardiogram in mitral stenosis. Circulation 1974;50: 472–478.

197. Cueto J, Toshima H, Armijo G, et al. Vectorcardiographic studies in acquired valvular disease with reference to the diagnosis of right ventricular hypertrophy. Circulation 1966;33:588–598.

198. Zoghbi WA, Farmer KL, Soto JG, et al. Accurate noninvasive quantification of stenotic aortic valve area by Doppler echocardiography. Circulation 1986;73: 452–459.

199. Savage DD, Garrison RJ, Deveroux RB, et al. Mitral valve prolapse in the general population. I. Epidemiologic features: The Framingham Study. Am Heart J 1983; 106:571–576.

200. Procacci PM, Savran SV, Schreiter SL, et al. Prevalence of clinical mitral valve prolapse in 1,169 young women. N Engl J Med 1976;294:1086–1088.

201. Guy FC, MacDonald RP, Fraser DB, et al. Mitral valve prolapse as a cause of hemodynamically important mitral regurgitation. Can J Surg 1980;23:166–170.

202. Gaffney FA, Bastian BC, Lane LB, et al.

Abnormal cardiovascular regulation in the mitral valve prolapse syndrome. Am J Cardiol 1983; 52:316–320.

203. Puddu PE, Pasternac A, Tubau JF, et al. QT interval prolongation and increased plasma catecholamine levels in patients with mitral valve prolapse. Am Heart J 1983;105:422–428.

204. Tomaru T, Uchida Y, Mohri N, et al. Post-inflammatory mitral and aortic valve prolapse: a clinical and pathological study. Circulation 1987;76:68–76.

205. Boudoulas H, Kolibash AJ Jr., Baker P, et al. Mitral valve prolapse and the mitral valve prolapse syndrome: a diagnostic classification and pathogenesis of symptoms. Am Heart J 1989;118:796–818.

206. Panidis IP, McAllister M, Ross J, et al. Prevalence and severity of mitral regurgitation in the mitral valve prolapse syndrome: a Doppler echocardiographic study of 80 patients. J Am Coll Cardiol 1986;7:975–981.

207. Lembo NJ, Dell'Italia LJ, Crawford MH, et al. Bedside diagnosis of systolic murmurs. N Engl J Med 1988;318:1572–1578.

208. Pocock WA. Mitral leaflet billowing and prolapse. In: Barlow JB, ed. *Perspectives on the Mitral Valve*. Philadelphia, Pa: FA Davis; 1987:45–112.

209. Campbell RW, Godman MG, Fiddler GI, et al. Ventricular arrhythmias in syndrome of balloon deformity of mitral valve. Definition of possible high risk group. Br Heart J 1976;38:1053–1057.

210. Pocock WA, Bosman CK, Chesler E, et al. Sudden death in primary mitral valve prolapse. Am Heart J 1984;107:378–382.

211. Chesler E, King RA, Edwards JE. The myxomatous mitral valve and sudden death. Circulation 1983;67:632–639.

212. Hershman WY, Moskowitz MA, Marton KI, et al. Utility of echocardiography in patients with suspected mitral valve prolapse. Am J Med 1989;87:371–376.

213. MacMahon SW, Hickey AJ, Wilcken DE, et al. Risk of infective endocarditis in mitral valve prolapse with and without precordial systolic murmurs. Am J Cardiol 1987;59:105–108.

214. Danchin N, Voiriot P, Briancon S, et al. Mitral valve prolapse as a risk factor for infective endocarditis. Lancet 1989;i: 743–745.

215. Barletta GA, Gagliardi R, Benvenuti L, et al. Cerebral ischemic attacks as a complication of aortic and mitral valve prolapse. Stroke 1985;16:219–223.

216. Makino H, Al-Sadir J. Myocardial infarction in patients with mitral valve prolapse and normal coronary arteries. J Am Coll Cardiol 1983;1:661.

217. Hull RD, Raskob GE, Carter CJ, et al. Pulmonary embolism in outpatients with pleuritic chest pain. Arch Intern Med 1988;148:838–844.

218. Branch WT, Jr., McNeil BJ. Analysis of the differential diagnosis and assessment of pleuritic chest pain in young adults. Am J Med 1983;75:671–679.

219. Fine NL, Smith LR, Sheedy PF. Frequency of pleural effusions in mycoplasma and viral pneumonias. N Engl J Med 1970;283:790–793.

220. Michon P, Niviere J, Larcan A. Les epanchements pleuraux d'origine virale: a propos de 45 observations. Bull Soc Med Hosp Paris 1959;75:33–42.

221. Lau RC. Coxsackie B virus infections in New Zealand patients with cardiac and noncardiac diseases. J Med Virology 1983;11:131–137.

222. Archard LC, Richardson PJ, Olsen EG, et al. The role of Coxsackie B viruses in the pathogenesis of myocarditis, dilated cardiomyopathy, and inflammatory muscle disease. Biochem Soc Symp 1988;53: 51–62.

223. Helin M, Savola J, Lapinleimu K. Cardiac manifestations during a Coxsackie B5 epidemic. Br Med J 1968;3:97–99.

224. Lau RC. Coxsackie B virus-specific IgM responses in coronary care unit patients. J Med Virology 1986;18:193–198.

225. Chong AY, Lee LH, Wong HB. Epidemic pleurodynia (Bornholm Disease) outbreak in Singapore. A clinical and virological study. Trop Geogr Med 1975;27: 151–159.

226. Artenstein MS, Cadigan FC, Jr., Buescher EL. Clinical and epidemiological features of Coxsackie group B virus infections. Ann Intern Med 1965;63:597–603.

227. Taryle DA, Potts DE, Sahn SA. The incidence and clinical correlates of parapneumonic effusions in pneumococcal pneumonia. Chest 1978;71:666–668.

228. Light RW, Girard WM, Jenkinson SG. Para-pneumonic effusions. Am J Med 1980;69:507–512.

229. Batungwanayo J, Taelman H, Allen S, et al. Pleural effusion, tuberculosis and HIV-1 infection in Kigali, Rwanda. AIDS 1993; 7:73–79.

230. Mehta JB, Dutt A, Harvill L, et al. Epide-

miology of extrapulmonary tuberculosis. Chest 1991;99:1134–1138.

231. Seibert AF, Haynes J Jr., Middleton R, et al. Tuberculous pleural effusion: twenty-year experience. Chest 1991;99:883–886.

232. Moudgil H, Sridhar G, Leitch AG. Reactivation disease: the commonest form of tuberculous pleural effusion in Edinburgh, 1980–1991. Respir Med 1994;88:301–304.

233. Chan CH, Arnold M, Chan CY, et al. Clinical and pathological features of tuberculous pleural effusion and its long-term consequences. Respiration 1991;58:171–175.

234. Berger HW, Mejia E. Tuberculous pleurisy. Chest 1973;63:88–92.

235. Ocana I, Martinez-Vazquez JM, Segura R. Adenosine deaminase in pleural fluids: test for diagnosis of tuberculous pleural effusion. Chest 1983;84:51–53.

236. Valdes L, San Jose E, Alvarez D, et al. Diagnosis of tuberculous pleurisy using the biologic parameters adeonosine deaminase, lysozyme, and interferon gamma. Chest 1993;103:458–465.

237. Scharer L, McClement JH. Isolation of tubercle bacilli from needle biopsy specimens of parietal pleura. Am Rev Respir Dis 1968;97:466–468.

238. Levine H, Metzger W, Lacera D, et al. Diagnosis of tuberculous pleurisy by culture of pleural biopsy specimen. Arch Intern Med 1970;126:269–271.

239. Harvey AM, Shulman LE, Tumulty PA. Systemic lupus erythematosus: review of the literature and clinical analysis of 138 cases. Medicine 1954;33:291–437.

240. Blomgren SE, Condemi JJ, Vaughan JH. Procainamide-induced lupus erythematosus. Am J Med 1972;52:338–348.

241. Halla JT, Schronhehloher RE, Volanakis JE. Immune complexes and other laboratory features of pleural effusions. Ann Intern Med 1980;92:748–752.

242. Winslow WA, Ploss LN, Loitman B. Pleuritis in systemic lupus erythematosus: its importance as an early manifestation in diagnosis. Ann Intern Med 1958;49:70–88.

243. Good JT Jr., King TE, Antony VB, et al. Lupus pleuritis. Clinical features and pleural fluid characteristics with special reference to pleural fluid antibodies. Chest 1983;84:714–718.

244. Khare V, Baethge B, Lang S, et al. Antinuclear antibodies in pleural fluid. Chest 1994;106:866–871.

245. Walker WC, Wright V. Rheumatoid pleuritis. Ann Rheum Dis 1967;26:467–474.

246. Joseph J, Sahn SA. Connective tissue diseases and the pleura. Chest 1993;104:262–270.

247. Horler AR, Thompson M. The pleural and pulmonary complications of rheumatoid arthritis. Ann Intern Med 1959;51:1179–1203.

248. Lillington GA, Carr DT, Mayne JG. Rheumatoid pleurisy with effusion. Arch Intern Med 1971;128:764–768.

249. Naylor B. The pathognomonic cytologic picture of rheumatoid pleuritis. Acta Cytol 1990;34:465–473.

250. Light RW. Pleural effusion due to miscellaneous diseases. In: *Anonymous Pleural Diseases*. 3rd ed. Baltimore, Md: Williams & Wilkins; 1995:224–241.

251. Bachman AL, Macken K. Pleural effusions following supervoltage radiation for breast carcinoma. Radiology 1959;72:699–709.

252. O'Neill S. Spontaneous pneumothorax: aetiology, management and complications. Ir Med J 1987;80:306–311.

253. Maunder RJ, Pierson DJ, Hudson LD. Subcutaneous and mediastinal emphysema: pathophysiology, diagnosis and management. Arch Intern Med 1984;144:1447–1453.

254. Jenkinson SG. Pneumothorax. Clin Chest Med 1985;6:153–161.

255. Kirby TJ, Ginsberg RJ. Management of pneumothorax and barotrauma. Clin Chest Med 1992;13:97–112.

256. Vukich DJ. Diseases of the pleural space. Emerg Med Clin North Am 1989;7:309–324.

257. O'Hara VS. Spontaneous pneumothorax. Milit Med 1978;143:32–35.

258. Serementis MG. The management of spontaneous pneumothorax. Chest 1970;78:65–68.

259. Carter EJ, Ettensohn DB. Catamenial pneumothorax. Chest 1990;98:713–716.

260. Shiraishi T. Catamenial pneumothorax: report of a case and review of the Japanese and non-Japanese literature. Thorac Cardiovasc Surg 1991;39:304–307.

261. Sepkowitz KA, Telzak EE, Gold JW. Pneumothorax in AIDS. Ann Intern Med 1991;114:455–459.

262. Light RW. Pneumothorax. In: Murray JJ, Nadel JA, eds. *Textbook of Respiratory Medicine*. Philadelphia, Pa: WB Saunders Company; 1988:1745–1759.

263. Hillman K, Albin M. Pulmonary barotrauma during cardiopulmonary resuscitation. Crit Care Med 1986;14:606–609.

264. Raptopoulos V, Davis LM, Lee G, et al. Factors affecting the development of pneumothorax associated with thoracentesis. Am J Roentgenol 1991;156:917–920.

265. Grogan DR, Irwin RS. Thoracentesis. In: Rippe JM, Irwin RS, Fink MP, Cerra FB, Curley FJ, Heard SO, eds. *Procedures and Techniques in Intensive Care Medicine*. Boston, Ma: Little Brown and Company; 1995:156–164.

266. Pierson DJ. Complications of mechanical ventilation. In: *Anonymous Current Pulmonology*. Chicago, Ill: Year Book Medical Publishers; 1990:19–46.

267. Beaver BL, Laschinger JC. Pediatric thoracic trauma. Semin Thorac Cardiovasc Surg 1992;4:255–262.

268. Pate JW. Chest wall injuries. Surg Clin North Am 1989;69:59–70.

269. Pepe JW. Acute post-traumatic respiratory physiology and insufficiency. Surg Clin North Am 1989;69:157–173.

270. Symbas PN. Cardiothoracic Trauma. Curr Probl Surg 1991;28:741–797.

271. Shorr RM, Crittenden M, Indeck M. Blunt thoracic trauma: analysis of 515 patients. Ann Surg 1987;206:200–205.

272. Millham RH, Rajii-Khorasani A, Birkett DF. Carinal injury: diagnosis and treatment—case report. J Trauma 1991;31:1420–1422.

273. Spencer JA, Rogers CE, Westaby S. Clinico-radiological correlates in rupture of the major airways. Clin Radiol 1991;43:371–376.

274. Kounis NG, Zavras GM, Kitrou MP. Unusual electrocardiographic manifestations in conditions with increased intrathoracic pressure. Acta Cardiol 1988;43:653–661.

275. Buckner CB, Harmon BH, Plallin JS. The radiology of abnormal intrathoracic air. Curr Probl Diagn Radiol 1988;17:37–71.

276. Tocino IM. Pneumothorax in the supine patient: radiographic anatomy. Radiographics 1985;5:557–586.

277. Tocino IM, Miller MH, Fairfax WR. Distribution of pneumothorax in the supine and semierect critically ill adult. AJR 1985;144:901–905.

278. Stein PD, Willis PW, DeMets DL. History and physical examination in acute pulmonary embolism in patients without preexisting cardiac or pulmonary disease. Am J Cardiol 1981;47:218–223.

279. Anonymous. The Urokinase Pulmonary Embolism Trial. A national cooperative study. Circulation 1973;47:86–90.

280. Anderson FA, Jr., Wheeler HB. Venous thromboembolism. Risk factors and prophylaxis. In: *Anonymous Clinics in Chest Medicine*. Philadelphia, Pa: WB Saunders Company; 1995:235–251.

281. Anderson FA Jr., Wheeler HB, Goldberg RJ. A population-based perspective of the hospital incidence and case-fatality rates of deep vein thrombosis and pulmonary embolism: The Worcester DVT Study. Arch Intern Med 1991;151:933–938.

282. Dismuke SE, Wagner EH. Pulmonary embolism as a cause of death: the changing mortality in hospitalized patients. JAMA 1986;255:2039–2042.

283. Salzman EW, Hirsh J. The epidemiology, pathogenesis and natural history of venous thromboembolism. In: Colman RW, Hirsh J, Marder VJ, Salzman EW, eds. *Hemostasis and Thrombosis*. Philadelphia, Pa: Lippincott; 1994:1275–1296.

284. Dalen JE, Alpert JS. Natural history of pulmonary embolism. Prog Cardiovasc Dis 1975;17:257–270.

285. Lilienfeld DE, Chan E, Ehland J. Mortality from pulmonary embolism in the United States: 1962 to 1984. Chest 1990;98:1067–1072.

286. Goldhaber SZ, Hennekens CH, Evand DA. Factors associated with an antemortem diagnosis of major pulmonary embolism. Am J Med 1982;73:822–826.

287. Bergqvist D, Lindblad B. A 30-year survey of pulmonary embolism verified at autopsy: An analysis of 1274 surgical patients. Br J Surg 1985 72:105–108.

288. Cranley JJ, Canos AJ, Sull WJ. The diagnosis of deep vein thrombosis: fallibility of clinical symptoms and signs. Arch Surg 1976;1:497–498.

289. Haeger K. Problems of acute deep venous thrombosis: 1. The interpretation of signs and symptoms. Angiology 1969;20:219–223.

290. Morpurgo M, Schmid C. Clinico-pathological correlations in pulmonary embolism: a posteriori evaluation. Prog Respir Res 1980;13:8–15.

291. Nicolaides AN, Irving D. Clinical factors and the risk of deep venous thrombosis. In: Nicholaides AN, ed. *Thromboembolism Etiology, Advances in Prevention*

*and Management.* Baltimore, Md: University Park Press; 1975: 193–204.

292. Wheeler HB, Anderson FA Jr., Cardullo PA. Suspected deep vein thrombosis: management by impedance plethysmography. Arch Surg 1982;117:1206–1209.

293. Browse NL, Thomas MD. Source of nonlethal pulmonary emboli. Lancet 1974;i: 258–259.

294. Khamashta MA, Cuadrado MJ, Mujic F, et al. The management of thrombosis in the antiphospholipid antibody syndrome. N Engl J Med 1995;332:993–997.

295. Vandenbroucke JP, Koster T, Briet E. Increased risk of venous thrombosis in oral-contraceptive users who are carriers of factor V Leiden mutation. Lancet 1994; 344:1453–1457.

296. Palla A, Petruzzelli S, Donnamaria V, et al. The role of suspicion in the diagnosis of pulmonary embolism. Chest 1995;107: 21S-24S.

297. Stein PD, Terrin ML, Hales CA, et al. Clinical, laboratory, roentgenographic, and electrocardiographic findings in patients with acute pulmonary embolism and no pre-existing cardiac or pulmonary disease. Chest 1991;100:598–603.

298. Dalen JE. Clinical diagnosis of acute pulmonary embolism. When should a V̇/Q̇ scan be ordered? Chest 1991;100: 1185–1186.

299. Sharma GVRK, Sasahara AA. Diagnosis and treatment of pulmonary embolism. Med Clin N Am 1979;63:239–250.

300. Sutton GC, Honey M, Gibson RV. Clinical diagnosis of acute massive pulmonary embolism. Lancet 1969;i:271–273.

301. Hildner FJ, Ormond RS. Accuracy of the clinical diagnosis of pulmonary embolism. JAMA 1967;202:567–570.

302. Greenspan RH, Ravin CE, Polansky SM. Accuracy of the chest radiograph in diagnosis of pulmonary embolism. AJR 1982; 141:513–517.

303. Manganelli D, Palla A, Donnamaria V, Giuntini C. Clinical features of pulmonary embolism: doubts and certainties. Chest 1995;107:25S-32S.

304. Palla A, Donnamaria V, Petruzzelli S. Enlargement of the right descending pulmonary artery in pulmonary embolism. AJR 1983;141:513–517.

305. Donnamaria V, Palla A, Petruzzelli S. Early and late follow-up of pulmonary embolism. Respiration 1993;60:15–20.

306. Palla A, Bronzini R, Petruzzelli S. Ruolo della radiografia del torace nel formulare il sospetto di embolia polmonare. Ital J Chest Dis 1990;44:309–313.

307. Petruzzelli S, Palla A, Pieraccini F. Routine electrocardiography in screening for pulmonary embolism. Respiration 1986; 50:233–243.

308. Petruzzelli S, Palla A, Donnamaria V. Diagnosi di embolia polmonare: ruolo delle tecniche non invasive. G Ital Cardiol 1991;21:675–682.

309. Stein PD, Goldhaber SZ, Henry JW. Alveolar-arterial oxygen gradient in the assessment of acute pulmonary embolism. Chest 1995;107:139–143.

310. Stein PD, Gottschalk A, Henry JW. Stratification of patients according to prior cardiopulmonary disease and probability assessment based on the number of mismatched segmental equivalent perfusion defects: approaches to strengthen the diagnostic value of ventilation/perfusion lung scans in acute pulmonary embolism. Chest 1993;104:1461–1467.

311. Stein PD, Henry JW, Gottschalk A. The addition of clinical assessment to stratification according to prior cardiopulmonary disease further optimizes the interpretation of ventilation/perfusion lung scans in pulmonary embolism. Chest 1993;104:1472–1476.

312. PIOPED INVESTIGATORS. Value of ventilation/perfusion scan in acute pulmonary embolism. JAMA 1990;263: 2753–2759.

313. Celi A, Palla A, Petruzzelli S. Prospective study of a standardized questionnaire to improve clinical estimate of pulmonary embolism. Chest 1988;95:332–337.

314. Hull RD, Hirsh J, Carter CJ, et al. Diagnostic value of ventilation-perfusion lung scanning in patients with suspected pulmonary embolism. Chest 1985;88: 819–828.

315. Hull RD, Taylor DW, Hirsh J, et al. Impedance plethysmography: the relationship between venous filling and sensitivity and specificity for proximal vein thrombosis. Circulation 1978;58:898–902.

316. Hull RD, Hirsh J, Carter CJ, et al. Diagnostic efficacy of impedance plethysmography for clinically suspected deep-vein thrombosis: a randomized trial. Ann Intern Med 1985;102:21–28.

317. Huisman MV, Buller HR, Ten Cate JW, et al. Serial impedance plethysmography for suspected deep-vein thrombosis in outpatients. N Engl J Med 1986;314:823–828.

318. D'Amico A. Imaging for deep venous

thrombosis. Emerg Med Clin North Am 1992;10:121–132.

319. Glew D, Cooper T, Mitchelmore AE. Impedance plethysmography and thrombo-embolic disease. Br J Radiol 1992;65:306–308.

320. Patterson RB, Fowl RJ, Keller JD. The limitations of impedance plethysmography in the diagnosis of acute deep venous thrombosis. J Vasc Surg 1989;9:725–730.

321. Lensing AW, Prandoni P, Brandjes D. Detection of deep vein thrombosis by real-time B-mode ultrasonography. N Engl J Med 1989;320:342–345.

322. Montefusco-von Kleist CM, Bakal C, et al. Comparison of duplex ultrasonography and ascending contrast venography in the diagnosis of venous thrombosis. Angiology 1993;44:169–175.

323. Dauzat MM, Laroche JP, Charras C. Real-time B-mode ultrasonography for better specificity in the noninvasive diagnosis of deep venous thrombosis. J Ultrasound Med 1986;5:625–631.

324. Appleman PT, DeJong TE, Lampmann LE. Deep venous thrombosis of the leg: US findings. Radiology 1987;163:743–746.

325. Cronan JJ, Dorfman GS, Grusmark J. Lower-extremity deep venous thrombosis: further experience with and refinements of US assessment. Radiology 1988; 168:101–107.

326. Rose SC, Zwiebel WJ, Nelson BD. Symptomatic lower extremity deep venous thrombosis: accuracy, limitations, and role of color duplex flow imaging in diagnosis. Radiology 1990; 175:639–644.

327. Hull RD, Feldstein W, Pineo GF, et al. Cost effectiveness of diagnosis of deep venous thrombosis in symptomatic patients. Thrombosis and Haemostasis 1995; 74:189–196.

328. Heijboer H, Buller HR, Lensing AWA, et al. A comparison of realtime compression ultrasonography with impedance plethysmography for the diagnosis of deep vein thrombosis in symptomatic outpatients. N Engl J Med 1993;329:1365–1369.

329. Vaccaro JP, Cronan JJ, Dorfman GS. Outcome analysis of patients with normal compression US examinations. Radiology 1990;175:645–649.

330. Ginsberg JS, Caco CC, Brill-Edwards PA. Venous thrombosis in patients who have undergone major hip or knee surgery: detection with compression US and impedance plethysmography. Radiology 1991; 181:651–654.

331. Mattos MA, Londrey GL, Leutz DW. Color-flow duplex scanning for the surveillance and diagnosis of acute deep venous thrombosis. J Vasc Surg 1992;15: 366–375.

332. Barnes CL, Nelson CL, Nix ML. Duplex scanning versus venography as a screening examination in total hip arthroplasty patients. Clin Orthop 1991;271:180–189.

333. Agnelli G, Volpato R, Radicchia S. Detection of asymptomatic deep vein thrombosis by real-time B-mode ultrasonography in hip surgery patients. Thromb Haemost 1992;68:257–260.

334. Hull RD, Raskob GE, Coates G, et al. Clinical validity of a normal perfusion lung scan in patients with suspected pulmonary embolism. Chest 1990;97:23–26.

335. Biello DR, Mattar AG, McKnight RC, et al. Ventilation-perfusion studies in suspected pulmonary embolism. AJR 1979; 133:1033–1037.

336. McNeil BJ. Ventilation-perfusion studies and the diagnosis of pulmonary embolism: concise communication. J Nucl Med 1980;21:319–323.

337. Perlmutt LM, Braun SD, Newman GE, et al. Pulmonary arteriography in the high-risk patient. Radiology 1987;162: 187–189.

338. Nicod P, Peterson K, Levine M, et al. Pulmonary angiography in severe chronic pulmonary hypertension. Ann Intern Med 1987;107:565–568.

339. Kramer FL, Teitelbaum G, Merli GJ. Panvenography and pulmonary angiography in the diagnosis of deep vein thrombosis and pulmonary thromboembolism. Radiol Clin North Am 1986;24:397–418.

340. Henry JW, Relyea B, Stein PD. Continuing risk of thromboemboli among patients with normal pulmonary angiograms. Chest 1995;107:1375–1378.

341. Hull RD, Raskob GE, Ginsberg JS. A noninvasive strategy for the treatment of patients with suspected pulmonary embolism. Arch Intern Med 1994;154:289–297.

342. D'Alonzo GE, Bower JS, Dantzker DR. Differentiation of patients with primary and thromboembolic pulmonary hypertension. Chest 1984;85:457–461.

343. Rich S, Dantzker DR, Ayres SM, et al. Primary pulmonary hypertension: a national prospective study. Ann Intern Med 1987; 107:216–223.

344. Ross RS. Right ventricular hypertension as a cause of precordial pain. Am Heart J 1961;61:134.

345. Viar WN, Harrison TR. Chest pain in association with pulmonary hypertension; its similarity to the pain of coronary disease. Circulation 1952;5:1–6.

346. Kanemoto N. Electrocardiographic and hemodynamic correlations in primary pulmonary hypertension. Angiology 1988;39:781–787.

347. Kanemoto N, Furuya H, Etoh T, et al. Chest roentgenograms in primary pulmonary hypertension. Chest 1979;76:45–49.

348. Anderson G, Reid L, Simon G. The radiographic appearances in primary and in thromboembolic pulmonary hypertension. Clin Radiol 1973;24:113–120.

349. Child JS, Wolfe JD, Tashkin D, et al. Fatal lung scan in a case of pulmonary hypertension due to obliterative pulmonary vascular disease. Chest 1975;67:308–310.

350. DeGuire S, Gevirtz R, Kawahara Y, et al. Hyperventilation syndrome and the assessment of treatment for functional cardiac symptoms. Am J Cardiol 1992;70:673–677.

351. Markowitz MM, Merikangas KR. The epidemiology of anxiety and panic disorders: an update. J Clin Psychiatry 1986;47(suppl):11–17.

352. Katon W, Vitaliano PP, Russo J. Panic disorder: epidemiology in primary care. J Fam Pract 1986;23:233–239.

353. Ballenger J. Pharmacotherapy for panic disorder. J Clin Psychiatry 1986;47:27–32.

354. Carter C, Maddock R, Amsterdam E, et al. Panic disorder and chest pain in the coronary care unit. Psychosomatics 1992;33:302–309.

355. Beitman BD, Mukerji V, Lamberti JW, et al. Panic disorder in patients with chest pain and angiographically normal coronary arteries. Am J Cardiol 1989;63:1399–1403.

356. Kane FJ, Jr., Wittels E, Harper RG. Chest pain and anxiety disorder. Texas Medicine 1990;86:104–110.

357. Yingling KW, Wulsin LR, Arnold LM, et al. Estimated prevalences of panic disorder and depression among consecutive patients seen in an emergency department with acute chest pain. J Gen Int Med 1993;8:231–235.

358. Beitman BD, Kushner M, Grossberg GT. Late onset panic disorder: evidence from a study of patients with chest pain and normal cardiac evaluations. Int J Psych Med 1991;21:29–35.

359. Kushner MG, Thomas AM, Bartels KM, et al. Panic disorder history in the families of patients with angiographically normal coronary arteries. Am J Psych 1992;149:1563–1567.

360. Beitman BD, Mukerji V, Kushner M, et al. Validating studies for panic disorder in patients with angiographically normal coronary arteries. Med Clin North Am 1991;75:1143–1155.

361. Bradley LA, Richter JE, Scarinci IC, et al. Psychosocial and psychophysical assessments of patients with unexplained chest pain. Am J Med 1992;92:65S-73S.

362. Costa PT Jr. Influence of the normal personality dimension of neuroticism on chest pain symptoms and coronary artery disease. Am J Cardiol 1987;60:20J-26J.

363. Wulsin LR, Hillard JR, Geier P, et al. Screening emergency room patients with atypical chest pain for depression and panic disorder. Int J Psych Med 1988;18:315–323.

364. Kushner MG, Beitman BD, Beck NC. Factors predictive of panic disorder in cardiology patients with chest pain and no evidence of coronary artery disease: a cross-validation. J Psychosomatic Res 1989;33:207–215.

365. Roll M, Zetterquist S. Acute chest pain without obvious organic cause before the age of 40 years: response to forced hyperventilation. J Int Med 1990;228:223–227.

366. McCroskery JH, Schell RE, Sprafkin RP, et al. Differentiating anginal patients with coronary artery disease from those with normal coronary arteries using psychological measures. Am J Cardiol 1991;67:645–646.

367. Zimmerman JL, Dellinger RP, Majid PA. Cocaine-associated chest pain. Ann Emerg Med 1991;20:611–615.

368. Chambers JB, Kiff PJ, Gardner WN, et al. Value of measuring end tidal partial pressure of carbon dioxide as an adjunct to treadmill exercise testing. Br Med J Clin Res Ed 1988;296:1281–1285.

369. Richter JE, Bradley LA. Chest pain with normal coronary arteries. Another perspective. Dig Dis Sci 1990;35:1441–1444.

370. Vantrappen G, Janssens J. What is irritable esophagus? Another point of view. Gastroenterology 1988;94:1092–1094.

371. Soffer EE, Scalabrini P, Wingate DL. Spontaneous noncardiac chest pain: value of ambulatory esophageal pH and motility monitoring. Dig Dis Sci 1989;34:1651–1655.

372. Peters L, Maas L, Petty D, et al. Sponta-

neous noncardiac chest pain. Evaluation by 24-hour ambulatory esophageal motility and pH monitoring. Gastroenterology 1988;94:878–886.

373. Janssens J, Vantrappen G, Ghillebert G. 24-hour recording of esophageal pressure and pH in patients with noncardiac chest pain. Gastroenterology 1986;90:1978–1984.

374. Anonymous. Angina and oesophageal disease. Lancet 1986;i:191–192.

375. Janssens JP, Vantrappen G. Irritable esophagus. Am J Med 1992;92:27S–32S.

376. Richter JE, Barish CF, Castell DO. Abnormal sensory perception in patients with esophageal chest pain. Gastroenterology 1986;91:845–852.

377. Vantrappen G, Janssens J, Ghillebert G. The irritable oesophagus: a frequent cause of angina-like chest pain. Lancet 1987;i:1232–1234.

378. Humeau B, Cloarec D, Simon J. Douleurs pseudo-angineuses d'origine oesophagienne: resultats de l'exploration fonctionnelle et interet du test de distention mecanique par ballonnet. Gastroenterol Clin Biol 1990;14:334–341.

379. Hewson EG, Dalton CB, Richter JE. Comparison of esophageal manometry, provocative testing, and ambulatory monitoring in patients with unexplained chest pain. Dig Dis Sci 1990;35:302–309.

380. Ghillebert G, Janssens J, Vantrappen G, et al. Ambulatory 24-hour intraesophageal pH and pressure recordings vs. provacative tests in the diagnosis of chest pain of oesophageal origin. Gut 1990; 31: 738–744.

381. Kaufmann HJ. Chest pain and esophageal motility: what is the role of manometry? J Clin Gastroenterol 1982;4:466–467.

382. Nevens F, Janssens J, Piessens J, Ghillebert G, De Geest H, Vantrappen G. Prospective study on prevalence of esophageal chest pain in patients referred on an elective basis to a cardiac unit for suspected myocardial ischemia. Dig Dis Sci 1991;36:229–235.

383. Richter JE, Bradley LA, Castell DO. Esophageal chest pain: current controversies in pathogenesis, diagnosis, and therapy. Ann Intern Med 1989;110:66–78.

384. Davies HA, Jones DB, Rhodes J. 'Esophageal angina' as the cause of chest pain. JAMA 1982;248:2274–2278.

385. Levine HJ. Difficult problems in the diagnosis of chest pain. Am Heart J 1980;100:108–118.

386. Bernstein JM, Fruinn RC, Pacini R. Differentiation of esophageal pain from angina pectoris: role of the esophageal acid perfusion test. Medicine 1962;41:143–148.

387. Price S, Castell DO. Esophageal mythology. JAMA 1978;240:44–46.

388. Henderson RD, Marryatt G. Characteristics of esophageal pain. Acta Med Scand 1980;644:49–51.

389. Howell JM, Hedges JR. Differential diagnosis of chest discomfort and general approach to myocardial ischemia decision making. Am J Emerg Med 1991;9:571–579.

390. Walker WS, Cameron EWJ, Walbaum PR. Diagnosis and management of spontaneous transmural rupture of the oesophagus (Boerhaave's syndrome). Br J Surg 1985;72:204–207.

391. Bradley SL, Pairolero PC, Spencer Payne W, et al. Spontaneous rupture of the esophagus. Arch Surg 1981;116:755–758.

392. Abbott OA, Mansour KA, Dogan WD Jr., et al. Atraumatic so-called 'spontaneous' rupture of the esophagus. J Thorac Cardiovasc Surg 1970;59:67–83.

393. Michel L, Grillo HC, Malt RA. Esophageal perforation. Ann Thorac Surg 1982;33:203–210.

394. Samson PC. Post emetic rupture of the esophagus. Surg Gynecol Obstet 1951;93:221–229.

395. Derrick JR, Harrison WH, Howard JM. Factors predisposing to spontaneous perforation of the esophagus. Surgery 1958;43:486–489.

396. Mackler SA. Spontaneous rupture of the esophagus: an experimental and clinical study. Surg Gynecol Obstet 1952;95:345–356.

397. Gale ME. Bochdalek hernia: prevalence and CT characteristics. Radiology 1985;156:449–452.

398. Osebold WR, Soper RT. Congenital posterolateral diaphragmatic hernia past infancy. Am J Surg 1976;131:748–754.

399. Powers RC, Sejdinaj I, Oberschneider PB. Strangulated foramen of Bochdalek hernia in the adult. Am J Surg 1966;111:749–751.

400. Karanikas ID, Dendrinos SS, Liakakos TD, et al. Complications of congenital posterolateral diaphragmatic hernia in the adult: report of two cases and literature review. J Cardiovasc Surg 1994;35:555–558.

401. Ahrend TR, Thompson BW. Hernia of the

foramen of Bochdalek in the adult. Am J Surg 1971;122:612–615.

402. Sugg WL, Roper CL, Carlsson E. Incarcerated Bochdalek hernias in the adult. Ann Surg 1964;160:847–851.

403. Heaton ND, Adam G, Howard ER. The late presentation of posterolateral congenital diaphragmatic hernias. Postgrad Med J 1992;68:445–448.

404. Perhoniemi V, Helminen J, Luosto R. Posterolateral diaphragmatic hernia in adults. Acute symptoms, diagnosis and treatment. Scand J Cardiovasc Surg 1992; 26:225–227.

405. Kafka NJ, Leitman IM, Tromba J. Acute pancreatitis secondary to incarcerated paraesophageal hernia. Surgery 1994;115: 653–655.

406. Oddsdottir M, Franco AL, Laycock WS, et al. Laparoscopic repair of paraesophageal hernia. New access, old technique. Surg Endoscopy 1995;9:164–168.

407. Allen B, Tompkins RK, Mulder DG. Repair of large paraesophageal hernia with complete intrathoracic stomach. Am Surgeon 1991;57:642–647.

408. Farrell B, Gerard PS, Bryk D. Paraesophageal hernia causing colonic obstruction. J Clin Gastroenterol 1991;13:188–190.

409. Gumaste VV. Diagnostic tests for acute pancreatitis. The Gastroenterologist 1994; 2:119–130.

410. Cohen SA, Siegel JH. Biliary tract emergencies: endoscopic and medical management. In: Fisher RL, ed. Critical Care Clinics. Philadelphia, Pa: WB Saunders Company; 1995:273–294.

411. Kane RA, Costello P, Duszlak E. Computed tomography in acute cholecystitis. AJR 1983;141:697–701.

412. Howard RJ. Acute acalculus cholecystitis. Am J Surg 1981;141:194–198.

413. Cohen SA, Siegel JH. Biliary disorders in AIDS. Practical Gastroenterology 1993; 17:10–19.

414. Ryan EL. Cervicothoracic pain due to fatigue of pectoral girdle musculature. MJA 1991;155:204–205.

415. Davies AH, Walton J, Stuart E, et al. Surgical management of the thoracic outlet compression syndrome. Br J Surg 1991; 78:1193–1195.

416. Yunus M, Masi AT, Calabro JJ, et al. Primary fibromyalgia (fibrositis): clinical study of 50 patients with matched normal controls. Semin Arthitis Rheum 1981;11: 151–171.

417. Pellegrino MJ. Atypical chest pain as an initial presentation of primary fibromyalgia. Arch Physical Med Rehab 1990;71: 526–528.

418. Simons DG. Trigger point origin of musculoskeletal chest pain. South Med J 1990;83:262–263.

419. Hubbard DR, Berkoff GM. Myofascial trigger points show spontaneous needle EMG activity. Spine 1993;18:1803–1807.

420. Durette MR, Rodriquez AA, Agre JC, et al. Needle electromyographic evaluation of patients with myofascial or fibromyalgic pain. Am J Phys Med Rehabil 1991;70: 154–156.

421. Howell JM. Xiphoidynia: a report of three cases. J Emerg Med 1992;10:435–438.

422. Howell J. Xiphoidynia: an uncommon cause of exertional chest pain. Am J Emer Med 1990;8:176.

423. Sklaroff HJ. Xiphoidynia-another cause of atypical chest pain: six case reports. Mount Sinai J Med 1979;46:546–548.

424. Yood RA, Goldenberg DL. Sternoclavicular joint arthritis. Arthritis Rheum 1980; 23:232–239.

425. Pickering D. Precordial catch syndrome. Arch Dis Child 1981;56:401–403.

426. Sparrow MJ, Bird EL. "Precordial catch": a benign syndrome of chest pain in young persons. New Zealand Med J 1978;88: 325–326.

427. Reynolds JL. Precordial catch syndrome in children. South Med J 1989;82: 1228–1230.

428. Anonymous. Texidor's twinge (editorial). Lancet 1979;ii:133

429. Fam AG. Approach to musculoskeletal chest wall pain. Primary Care Clin Office Pract 1988;15:767–782.

430. Dawes PT, Sheeran TP, Hothersall TE. Chest pain—a common feature of ankylosing spondylitis. Postgrad Med 1988;64: 27–29.

431. Reuler JB, Girard DE, Nardone DA. Sternoclavicular joint involvement in ankylosing spondylitis. South Med J 1978;71: 1480–1481.

432. Arroyo JF, Jolliet P, Junod AF. Costovertebral joint dysfunction: another misdiagnosed cause of atypical chest pain. Postgrad Med 1992;68:655–659.

433. Taubman B, Vetter VL. Slipping rib syndrome as a cause of chest pain in children. Clin Pediatr 1996;35:403–405.

434. Akiyama H, Tamura K, Takatsuka K, et al. Spinal cord tumor appearing as unusual pain. Spine 1994;19:1410–1412.

435. Yeung MC, Hagen NA. Cervical disc her-

niation presenting with chest wall pain. Can J Neurol Sci 1993;20:59–61.

436. Bland JH, Merrit JA, Boushey DR. The painful shoulder. Semin Arthritis Rheum 1977;7:21–47.

437. Razi DM, Wassel HD. Traffic accident induced thoracic outlet syndrome: decompression without rib resection, correction of associated recurrent thoracic aneurysm. Int Surg 1993;78:25–27.

438. Stack PS. Trichinosis. Still a public health threat. Postgrad Med 1995;97: 137–144.

439. Limsuwan S, Siriprasert V. A clinical study on trichinosis in Changwat Phayao, Thailand. Southeast Asian J Trop Med Public Health 1994;25:305–308.

440. Santos Duran-Ortiz J, Garcia-de la Torre I, Orozco-Barocio G, et al. Trichinosis with severe myopathic involvement mimicking polymyositis. Report of a family outbreak. J Rheumatol 1992;19:310–312.

441. Mahannop P, Setasuban P, Morakote N, et al. Immunodiagnosis of human trichinellosis and identification of specific antigen for Trichinella spiralis. Int J Parasitol 1995;25:87–94.

442. Singer PA. Thyroiditis. Acute, subacute, and chronic. Med Clin North Am 1991; 75:61–77.

443. Sakiyama R. Thyroiditis: a clinical review. Am Fam Physician 1993;48: 615–621.

444. BeLieu RM. Mastodynia. Obstet Gynecol Clin North Am 1994;21:461–477.

445. Donn W, Rebbeck P, Wilson C, et al. Idiopathic granulomatous mastitis. a report of three cases and review of the literature. Arch Pathol Lab Med 1994;118:822–825.

446. Jorgensen MB, Nielsen DM. Diagnosis and treatment of granulomatous mastitis. Am J Med 1992;93:97–101.

447. Hughes LE. Non-lactational inflammation and duct ectasia. Br Med Bull 1991;47: 272–283.

448. Fiorica JV. Fibrocystic changes. Obstet Gynecol Clin North Am 1994;21: 445–452.

449. Dixon JM. Cystic disease and fibroadenoma of the breast: natural history and relation to breast cancer risk. Br Med Bull 1991;47:258–271.

450. Isaacs JH. Benign tumors of the breast. Obstet Gynecol Clin North Am 1994;21: 487–497.

451. Mogavero GT, Fishman EK, Kuhlman JE. Inflammatory breast cancer: CT evaluation. Clin Imaging 1992;16:183–186.

452. Van Gelderen WF. Atypical fat necrosis of the breast: the 'mycetoma' appearance. Aust Radiol 1994;38:76–77.

453. Fiorica JV. Special problems. Mondor's disease, macrocysts, trauma, squamous metaplasia, miscellaneous disorders of the nipple. Obstet Gynecol Clin North Am 1994;21:479–485.

454. Lu LB, Shoaib BO, Patten BM. Atypical chest pain syndrome in patients with breast implants. South Med J 1994;87: 978–984.

455. Gentry WH, Hassan AA. Complications of retained epicardial pacing wires: an unusual bronchial foreign body. Ann Thorac Surg 1993;56:1391–1393.

456. Jacobs TE, Irwin RS, Raptopoulos V. Severe upper airway infections. In: Rippe JM, Irwin RS, Alpert JS, Fink MP, eds. *Intensive Care Medicine.* 2nd ed. Boston, Ma: Little Brown and Company; 1991: 695–713.

457. Yellin A, Gapany-Gapanavicius M, Lieberman Y. Spontaneous pneumomediastinum: is it a rare cause of chest pain? Thorax 1983;38:383–385.

458. Dattwyler RJ, Goldman MA, Bloch KJ. Pneumomediastinum as a complication of asthma in teenage and young adult patients. J Allergy Clin Immunol 1979;63: 412–416.

459. Barton CW. Subarachnoid hemorrhage presenting as acute chest pain: a variant of le coup de poignard. Ann Emerg Med 1988;17:977–978.

460. Richardson DE. Does epileptic pain really exist? Appl Neurophysiol 1987;50: 365–368.

461. Mailis A, Chan J, Basinski A, et al. Chest wall pain after aortocoronary bypass surgery using internal mammary artery graft: a new pain syndrome? Heart Lung 1989; 18:553–558.

462. Fine PG, Karwande SV. Sternal wire-induced persistent chest pain: a possible hypersensitivity reaction. Ann Thorac Surg 1990;49:135–136.

463. Eastridge CE, Mahfood SS, Walker WA, et al. Delayed chest wall pain due to sternal wire sutures. Ann Thorac Surg 1991;51: 56–59.

464. McWilliams R, Hooper T, Lawson R. A late complication of pectus excavatum repair. Postgrad Med 1992;68:473–474.

465. Tenner SM, Yadven MW, Kimmel PL. Acute pyelonephritis. Preventing complications through prompt diagnosis and

proper therapy. Postgrad Med 1992;91: 261–268.

466. Plattner MS. Pyelonephritis in pregnancy. J Perinatal Neonatal Nurs 1994;8: 20–27.

467. Meyrier A, Guibert J. Diagnosis and drug treatment of acute pyelonephritis. Drugs 1992;44:356–367.

468. Roberts JA. Etiology and pathophysiology of pyelonephritis. Am J Kidney Dis 1991; 17:1–9.

469. Eggli DF, Tulchinsky M. Scintigraphic evaluation of pediatric urinary tract infection. Semin Nuc Med 1993;23:199–218.

470. Rushton HG, Majd M. Dimercaptosuccinic acid renal scintigraphy for the evaluation of pyelonephritis and scarring: a review of experimental and clinical studies. J Urol 1992;148:1726–1732.

471. Majd M, Rushton HG. Renal cortical scintigraphy in the diagnosis of acute pyelonephritis. Semin Nuc Med 1992;22: 98–111.

472. Clark JA, Gross TP. Pain and cyanosis associated with alpha 1-proteinase inhibitor. Am J Med 1992;92:621–626.

473. Eskilsson J, Albertsson M. Failure of preventing 5-fluorouracil cardiotoxicity by prophylactic treatment with verapamil. Acta Oncologica 1990;29:1001–1003.

474. Eskilsson J, Albertsson M, Mercke C. Adverse cardiac effects during induction chemotherapy treatment with cis-platin and 5-fluorouracil. Radiotherapy & Oncology 1988;13:41–46.

475. White DA, Schwartzberg LS, Kris MG, et al. Acute chest pain syndrome during bleomycin infusions. Cancer 1987;59: 1582–1585.

476. Urban C, Nirenberg A, Caparros B, et al. Chemical pleuritis as the cause of acute chest pain following high-dose methotrexate treatment. Cancer 1983;51:34–37.

477. Shimp LA, Smith MA, Wahr DW. Ranitidine-induced chest pain. DICP 1989;23: 224–226.

478. Paloma VC, Montse MD, Gomez Eliseo P,

et al. Chest pain after intravenous corticotropin-releasing hormone. Lancet 1989;i: 222

479. King MH, Richards DW. Near syncope and chest tightness after administration of apraclonidine before argon laser iridotomy. Am J Ophthalmol 1990;110: 308–309.

480. Ballard HS, Bottino G, Bottino J. Ondansetron and chest pain. Lancet 1992; 340:1107

481. Montgomery AB, Luce JM, Murray JF. Retrosternal pain is an early indicator of oxygen toxicity. Am Rev Respir Dis 1989; 139:1548–1550.

482. Miralles R, Pedro-Botet J, Rubies-Prat J. Chest pain—another adverse reaction to vancomycin. Chest 1990;97:1504

483. Iruela LM. Sudden chest pain with sertraline. Lancet 1994;343:1106

484. Berti CA, Doogan DP. Sudden chest pain with sertraline. Lancet 1994;343: 1510–1511.

485. Houghton LA, Foster JM, Whorwell PJ, et al. Is chest pain after sumatriptan oesophageal in origin? Lancet 1994;344: 985–986.

486. Hillis WS, Macintyre PD. Sumatriptan and chest pain. Lancet 1993;341: 1564–1565.

487. Hillis WS, Macintyre PD. Sumatriptan and chest pain. Lancet 1993;342:683

488. Gitter MJ, Goldsmith SR, Dunbar DN, et al. Cocaine and chest pain: clinical features and outcome of patients hospitalized to rule out myocardial infarction. Ann Intern Med 1991;115:277–282.

489. Haim DY, Lippman ML, Goldberg SK, et al. The pulmonary complications of crack cocaine; a comprehensive review. Chest 1995;107:233–240.

490. Majid PA, Patel B, Kim HS, et al. An angiographic and histologic study of cocaine-induced chest pain. Am J Cardiol 1990;65:812–814.

491. Olshaker JS. Cocaine chest pain. Emerg Med Clin North Am 1994;12:391–396.

# 6

# Chest Pain:
## Diagnostic Strategies and Treatment

Mark M. Wilson, M.D.
Frederick J. Curley, M.D.

## Diagnostic Strategy

The previous chapter reviewed in detail the pathophysiology of chest pain and the classic presentation of each of the major chest pain syndromes. However, many patients do not present with a pathognomonic history and physical examination. This chapter presents strategies for discriminating among the major causes of chest pain when the presentation is not classic. Through the use of a systematic evaluation the cause of chest pain should not only be identified but be identified in a cost-effective manner. Once the cause is known, the physician can prescribe therapy specific for the underlying disease. At the end of this chapter we discuss both specific and nonspecific therapies for chest pain.

Diagnostic algorithms are presented at the end of this section for the evaluation of acute and chronic chest pain in the adult. The evaluation of chest pain in the pediatric population is also discussed. The algorithms are intended for use when the cause of chest pain remains unclear after history and physical examination.

Abnormalities identified on history and physical examination strongly suggesting a cause of chest pain should be evaluated as outlined in the diagnostic sections describing individual diseases above. Since up to one third of patients with chest pain will have more than one cause of pain,[1] patients should be re-evaluated and new studies should be considered when specific therapy for the identified cause of pain fails to completely eliminate pain.

Any attempt to design a strategy for evaluating chest pain will be controversial in that the data necessary to resolve crucial questions frequently do not exist. This section will review the available data that support our algorithms with an emphasis on the role of history, physical examination, and the major diagnostic tests for screening patients with chest pain.

Most published work is biased toward accurately diagnosing cardiac chest pain in patients presenting either to the emergency department or for cardiology consultation. However, large series of patients with chest pain suggest that only 30% to 40% of patients will have a cardiac cause. Only one third of patients referred to a car-

From Irwin RS, Curley FJ, Grossman RF (eds): Diagnosis and Treatment of Symptoms of the Respiratory Tract. Armonk, New York, Futura Publishing Company, Inc., © 1997.

diologist will have a definite cardiac cause of chest pain[2] and up to one third of patients undergoing cardiac angiography will have *normal* coronary anatomy.[3,4] Overall, only 15% to 20% of those patients who present to the emergency department will be found to have an acute myocardial infarction (MI). Patients subsequently released from the emergency department after an unrevealing evaluation for MI and coronary ischemia will later prove to only have a 2% to 5% incidence of acute MI after all.[5-7]

Our diagnostic strategies have been developed to deal with the two thirds of cases that are noncardiac in origin as well as those cases arising from cardiac causes. It can be anticipated that approximately 11% of these patients with noncardiac causes of chest pain will have an easily recognizable musculoskeletal cause,[8] approximately 20% to 30%[9] will have an anxiety/hyperventilation syndrome, and at least 30% will have esophageal abnormalities that could explain pain.[10,11] Based on our clinical experience, we would suspect that at least another 10% of patients should have an extremely obvious cause of chest pain, such as herpes zoster, aortic dissection, trauma or traumatic pneumothorax, breast, or kidney disease. When these data are considered, it is surprising that 30% to 50% of patients in whom cardiac disease has been ruled out actually are reported to have idiopathic pain.

## History

Many studies have attempted to address the role of history in separating patients with cardiac disease from those with noncardiac disease. Screening questionnaires have been designed to evaluate the yield of history alone in determining the cause of central chest pain. In one series from Sweden, the questionnaire had a sensitivity of 83%, specificity of 48%, and predictive accuracy of 82% for ischemic coronary disease and a sensitivity of 34%, specificity of 93% and predictive accuracy of 82% for detecting esophageal disease.

When comparing patients with MI with those without MI, the frequency of the symptoms of palpitations was 10 times more frequent and that of dizziness/limpness or tingling in the fingers five times more likely in the non-MI group.[12] Additionally, pain that radiates into the left shoulder, neck, or left arm occurs twice as often in patients subsequently proven to have acute MI compared with those that do not.[13-16] No questionnaire has attained a diagnostic accuracy high enough to exclude cardiac chest pain without further objective evaluation.

Chest pain that is central or left-sided but does not clearly match the definition of classic angina has been referred to over the years as "atypical chest pain." Those pain characteristics that have most often been described as representing a cause other than angina include pleuritic pain (sharp or knifelike pain brought on by respiration or coughing), pain that can be precisely localized with one finger, pain that is reproducible with movement or palpation of the chest wall or arms, pain that is constant or lasts for days, and pain that is exceptionally brief lasting a few seconds or less. While it is true that these descriptions are more apt to be found in clinical entities other than coronary ischemia, it must be remembered that these characteristics by no means rule out myocardial ischemia. Lee et al.[17] showed that patients with proven coronary artery atherosclerosis resulting in ischemia will present with "atypical pain" in up to 20% of cases overall. More specifically, it was shown that coronary ischemia can be present in 23% of those presenting with "burning or indigestion," 22% of those with "sharp" or "stabbing" pains, 13% of those with pleuritic pain, 7% of those with pain that is reproducible with palpation, and 24% of those with "other" atypical pain descriptions.

History should be extremely sensitive in diagnosing possible hyperventilation/anxiety syndromes; musculoskeletal disorders such as benign overuse, trauma, or pectoral girdle syndromes; fibrocystic breast disease; and renal disease. In most of these cases, the primary criterion for establishing the diagnosis is the history. Conversely, without a specific history these diagnoses will not be established.

## Physical Examination

A complete physical examination for patients with chest pain of unknown causes is summarized in Table I. Physical examination will most often be helpful in the following conditions: herpes zoster, trauma, breast disease, shoulder disease, cervicothoracic disc disease, and most musculoskeletal problems.

Since 10% or more of chest pain results from musculoskeletal disease,[8] a thorough musculoskeletal exam should always be performed and should include the provocative maneuvers depicted in figure 1.[8,18] Particular emphasis should be placed on examination of the shoulder because many shoulder syndromes radiate to the left chest and angina radiates to the left arm and shoulder. All major muscle groups, the costochondral junctions, the spine, and the xiphoid process should be palpated. Studies estimate that, with practice, a thorough screening musculoskeletal examination adds only 5 minutes to the total examination time.[8]

In order to be considered a cause of the patient's chest pain, palpation or a provocative maneuver must reproduce the patient's pain. In one study of patients undergoing cardiac catheterization,[8] 78% of patients had some thoracic tenderness. In 11% of patients, when palpation reproduced pain, a definitive diagnosis of a noncardiac cause could be established. However, tenderness that did not reproduce pain was not helpful and occurred in 78% of those with coronary ischemia and 56% of those without coronary ischemia (Figures 2A and 2B).

The specificity of physical examination for determining acute central chest pain to be due to ischemic coronary disease has been estimated at from 71% to 80%.[19] Examination is most helpful when patients have femoral or carotid bruits or clear-cut abnormalities on cardiac auscultation.

## Diagnostic Testing

### Electrocardiography

The initial electrocardiogram (ECG) findings in patients who are evaluated during an acute episode of chest pain can be very valuable. Diagnostic changes on the initial ECG that are suggestive of an acute MI occur in 18% to 65% of those who are subsequently shown to have had a MI. This incidence increases to 83% to 93% for ECG tracings followed serially over ensuing hours to days.[20,21] In the setting of new ST segment elevations in two or more contiguous leads and the presence of new pathologic Q waves, the incidence of MI is 82% to 100%.[21] With only ST segment elevations present, the incidence of MI decreases to around 40% to 60% and this same pattern can also be seen in 12% to 25% of patients with unstable angina.[22,23] When the initial ECG in symptomatic patients shows generalized or focal ST segment depressions, the incidence of MI has been reported at 46% to 56% and may also be seen in 5% to 7% of patients with unstable angina.[21] In the presence of isolated T wave inversions, the incidence of MI is only 23% and the incidence of unstable angina with these same findings is around 3% to 16%.[24,25] A "normal" pattern on the initial ECG can be seen in 6% to 20% of the overall patient population presenting with acute chest pain. While a normal ECG is reassuring, the clinician should not be lulled into a false sense of security since 1% to 10% of these patients will go on to have an acute MI and another 4% of this group will have unstable angina.[17,26,27]

The clinician in the emergency department, then, can expect to find an ECG strongly suggestive of MI in only approximately one half of those patients with ischemia/infarct. Despite its poor sensitivity for diagnosing myocardial infarction, patient selection for thrombolytic or revascularization therapies is based on the ECG. The clinical implications of the rate of true- and false-positive ECG tracings in the emergency department evaluation of acute chest pain have been studied

**Table I**
Physical Examination in Chest Pain Patients

**Vital Signs**
  Blood Pressure (both arms)
  Pulsus Paradoxus
  Temperature
  Pulse
  Respiratory Rate
**Inspection**
  Scoliosis
  Kyphosis
  Pectus Excavatum
  Trauma
  Skin Rash
  Deformity of Acromioclavicular Joints
  Deformity of Costochondral Joints
  Horner's Syndrome
  Tracheal Deviation
  Jugular Venous Distention
  Ankle Edema
  Nail Bed Cyanosis
  Obesity
**Palpation**
  Neck
    Goiter
    Thyroid Tenderness
    Cyst
    Mass
    Adenopathy
  Muscles
    Sternocleidomastoid
    Trapezius
    Rotator Cuff
    Deltoids
    Biceps
    Paraspinal
    Trigger Points
  Bones
    Acromioclavicular Joint
    Xiphoid
    Ribs
    Cervicothoracic Spine
    Sternum
    Costochondral Junctions
    Scapula
  Heart
    Second Intercostal Space Thrill
    Heaves
  Abdomen
    Splenomegaly
    Right Upper Quadrant Tenderness
    Epigastric Tenderness
    Mass
    Gravid Uterus

  Breasts
    Cysts
    Masses
    Superficial Thromboses
    Nipple Discharge
    Implants
    Gynecomastia
  Kidneys
    Flank Pain
  Blood Vessels
    Equality of Pulses
    Parvus et Tardus Carotid Artery Pulse
  Lymph Nodes
**Maneuvers**
  Spurling's
  Crowing Rooster
  Adson's
  Rib Hooking
  Horizontal Arm Flexion
  Cervical Compression
  Range of Motion of Shoulder
  Range of Motion of Cervical Spine
**Auscultation**
  Neck
    Carotid Bruit
  Heart
    Murmurs
    Rub
    Gallop
    Opening Snap
    Midsystolic Click
    Loud P2
  Lungs
    Rub
    Crackle
    Wheeze
    Unilateral Decrease in Breath Sounds
    Bilateral Decrease in Breath Sounds
  Abdomen
    Absent Bowel Sounds
    Renal Bruit
  Groin
    Femoral Bruit
**Percussion**
  Lungs
    Basilar Dullness of Pleural Effusion
    Hyperresonance of Pneumothorax

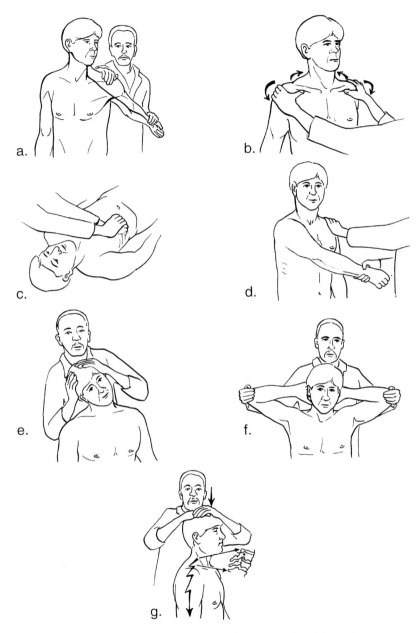

**Figure 1.** These figures illustrate the maneuvers that are helpful in eliciting musculoskeletal causes of chest pain. (a) Adson's maneuver and (b) the costoclavicular maneuver (position of attention) help identify thoracic outlet syndrome by increasing symptoms or palpating a diminishing pulse. (c) Rib hooking seeks to identify a slipping rib. (d) Horizontal arm flexion helps identify shoulder lesions. (e) Spurling's maneuver and (f) the crowing rooster maneuver identify costochondral inflammation. (g) Cervical compression narrows the neural foramina and may identify cervical sources of pain referred to the chest.

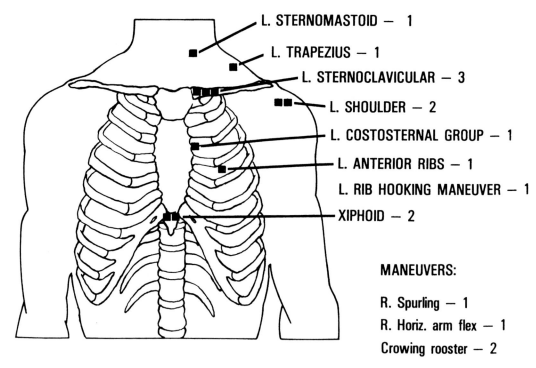

**Figure 2A.** This figure indicates the locations of tenderness that reproduced the patients' pain in 7 patients during a thorough musculoskeletal examination. The study examined 62 patients with chest pain who underwent coronary arteriography. Reprinted with permission from Levine PR, Mascette AM, Southern Medical Journal (82;580:1989).[8]

by at least one group[28] who documented a sensitivity of 43% and a positive predictive value of 76% for the ECG. This amounts to less than half of the appropriate patients being evaluated for possible maximal therapy, and for every eight patients correctly chosen for thrombolytic therapy, two inappropriate patients were also selected.

### Chest Roentgenograms

The value of chest radiography in patients with chest pain has been examined in several studies.[29–31] Data suggest that when chest roentgenograms are conventionally ordered in patients with acute chest pain, 56% are normal but 23% reveal information likely to influence clinical management. In 82% of cases where roentgenograms were helpful, the abnormalities were primarily related to acute or chronic pulmonary inflammation (35%), congestive heart failure-cardiomegaly-pleural effusion-pulmonary edema (34%), or pneumothorax (3%). Clinicians should not forget to evaluate the shoulders on chest roentgenograms. Although no studies have been performed evaluating the yield of chest roentgenograms when administered to all patients with chest pain, it appears likely that these roentgenograms will be most helpful when there is a suspected cardiac or pulmonary cause of chest pain. No studies have evaluated the role of roentgenograms in chronic chest pain.

### Cardiac Enzymes

Currently available measurements of cardiac enzymes are still not quite sensi-

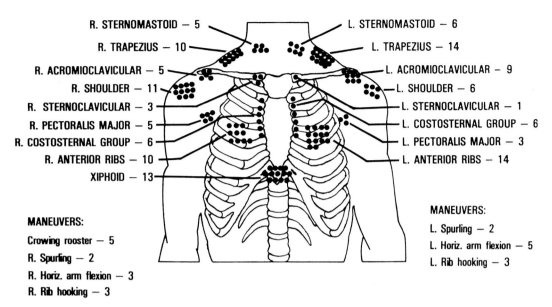

R. STERNOMASTOID — 5
R. TRAPEZIUS — 10
R. ACROMIOCLAVICULAR — 5
R. SHOULDER — 11
R. STERNOCLAVICULAR — 3
R. PECTORALIS MAJOR — 5
R. COSTOSTERNAL GROUP — 6
R. ANTERIOR RIBS — 10
XIPHOID — 13

L. STERNOMASTOID — 6
L. TRAPEZIUS — 14
L. ACROMIOCLAVICULAR — 9
L. SHOULDER — 6
L. STERNOCLAVICULAR — 1
L. COSTOSTERNAL GROUP — 6
L. PECTORALIS MAJOR — 3
L. ANTERIOR RIBS — 14

MANEUVERS:
Crowing rooster — 5
R. Spurling — 2
R. Horiz. arm flexion — 3
R. Rib hooking — 3

MANEUVERS:
L. Spurling — 2
L. Horiz. arm flexion — 5
L. Rib hooking — 3

**Figure 2B.** This figure indicates the locations of tenderness in 43 patients that did not reproduce the patients' pain during a thorough musculoskeletal examination. The study examined 62 patients with chest pain who underwent coronary arteriography. Sites of tenderness that did not reproduce pain were symmetrically distributed and very common. Reprinted with permission from Levine PR, Mascette AM, Southern Medical Journal (82;580:1989).[8]

tive enough to be used reliably as urgent screening tests for MI, particularly for those patients presenting within 4 hours or so of the onset of chest pain. Cardiac creatine phosphokinase (CPK) is composed of 85% MM isoenzyme and 15% MB isoenzyme. The newer immunochemical detection methods have greatly improved the usefulness of measuring CPK levels for the emergency department detection of MI, as compared to the older electrophoretic methods.[32–34] The sensitivity of CPK-MB analysis on specimens obtained upon patient arrival to the emergency department is approximately 50% to 62% (previously averaged around 35% with electrophoresis).[33] Repeat measurements 3 hours after arrival showed a 92% to 97% sensitivity and a specificity of 83% to 96% (improved from previous sensitivity of 77% with a specificity of 99%). Other markers of myocyte necrosis (eg, CPK-MB isoforms, myoglobin, troponin T) are currently being evaluated for use in the early detection of infarction.

## Exercise Testing

Treadmill exercise testing may be performed on individuals suspected of having true angina pectoris when their resting ECG is normal. The final assessment as to the significance of any ECG changes with exercise depends on both the type and degree of any ST segment abnormality as well as the pretest likelihood of disease (see "Mathematically Based Diagnostic Aids" section below). Individuals who develop ST segment depressions of greater than 1 mm on exertion that are associated with anginalike chest pain have a high likelihood of coronary artery stenosis (83% to 97% for men and 42% to 95% for women, depending on their age profiles [35]). Patients with significant ST segment depressions at low levels of exertion are suspect for possible multivessel disease or left main coronary artery disease.[36] Difficulties with interpreting these tests come about when an intermediate probability for the existence of disease results. This will tend to occur in patients with a low pretest likelihood of disease who have an abnormal ST segment response to exercise (potential false-positive) or for patients with substantial risk factors for the presence of coronary artery disease who do not exhibit any exertional ST segment abnormalities (potential false-negative). Overall, the sensitivity of routine exercise treadmill testing is approximately 60% to 70% and the specificity approaches 80%.[36]

### Diagnostic Cardiac Imaging

A potential role in the emergency department detection of MI has been suggested for such diverse modalities as echocardiography, thallium[201] scintigraphy, technetium[99m] pyrophosphate scanning, as well as [99m]sestamibi SPECT scanning. None of these imaging techniques has been adequately evaluated prospectively, however, and despite high anticipated sensitivities for the detection of acute MI, all of these modalities would be expected to be limited by their inability to distinguish old versus new abnormalities. In the absence of ongoing chest pain, these tests would also be expected to have low sensitivity for unstable angina. Additional factors, such as limited availability at many hospitals, logistic problems for rapid diagnosis of emergency department patients, the subjective nature of test interpretation, and the high cost of these exams, would seem to limit their general applicability in the near future.

### Gastrointestinal Provocative Tests

Separating gastrointestinal from cardiac causes of chest pain remains a diagnostic challenge. In some cases, it is impossible or nearly impossible to separate out these entities since both may coexist in the same patient. For example, since up to 50% of patients with coronary artery disease will also have an associated esophageal disorder,[37] it is generally agreed that an esophageal origin for chest pain should be considered after cardiac disease has been reliably excluded.

When all patients who present to the emergency department for evaluation of acute chest pain are evaluated and followed until a final diagnosis is established, esophageal abnormalities may be found in up to 12% to 20% of cases.[38,39] Using this same cohort of patients, once those with evidence of ischemic heart disease have been excluded, esophageal problems can be seen in 29% to 60% of the remaining patients.[38,39] This makes patients with esophageal problems the largest single diagnostic group among those with chest pain of uncertain origin. The difficulty with this finding relates to the fact that although esophageal abnormalities are common, they may not be causing the patient's symptoms. Therefore, definitive diagnosis frequently requires invasive testing.

A variety of esophageal provocative tests are available. Unfortunately there are no "gold standard" reference tests to compare these tests with, and the overall diagnostic yield appears to be relatively low.[10] Prolonged ambulatory esophageal pH and pressure-monitoring is well suited for determining if a patient's infrequent complaints of chest pain are related to gastroesophageal reflux disease (GERD), abnormal esophageal motility, or both. Ambulatory monitoring of both pH and manometry can now be performed with a simple, single nasoesophageal catheter positioned without fluoroscopic guidance. The sensors on the catheter store data to a small disk worn on the patient's belt. Data can then be analyzed after transfer to a computer. With these tests, acid reflux disease has been shown to be associated with chest pain on the order of two to three times more commonly than motility abnormalities.[10] What is troubling about this finding is that nearly 50% of the chest pain in patients with abnormal esophageal episodes has no identifiable esophageal cause. It is unclear if this is due to the coexistence of another disease responsible for the chest pain syndrome, or if our understanding of the pathophysiology of pain is inadequate to explain this occurrence, or both. The concept of the "irritable esophagus" was introduced earlier to explain how in many patients, noncardiac chest pain of esophageal origin may be induced by more than one type of stimulus. Thus, patients with no abnormalities on a 24-hour esophageal pH manometry study are unlikely to have an irritable esophagus or an esophageal cause of chest pain. Patients with an abnormal study may have an esophageal cause of chest pain.

The available literature would suggest that the cumulative diagnostic yields for the esophageal provocative tests would favor ambulatory esophageal pH and pressure-monitoring as a first assessment.[10,40–42] This test is much more sensitive and specific than the esophageal acid perfusion test (ie, Bernstein test) and appears to better predict clinical outcome.[42] Cholinergic stimulation using edrophonium allows a small increase in the diagnostic yield, but may be associated with significant side effects. Balloon distention of the esophagus offers a more physiologic stimulus for chest pain and is capable of identifying most if not all of those patients who have positive cholinergic or acid infusion provocation tests. The role of esophagoscopy in the evaluation of esophageal disease is controversial.[43] We recommend ambulatory esophageal pH and pressure-monitoring as the best single test and balloon provocation as the next best test in patients with unexplained chest pain.

## Mathematically Based Diagnostic Aids—Assessment of Cardiac Risk

Diagnostic and/or therapeutic algorithms have attempted to translate clinical acumen into probability by employing mathematical models based on the results of large groups of subjects with the aid of numerous statistical methods: logistic regression, recursive partition analysis, Bayesian inference, or artificial intelligence. The remainder of this subsection will address what additional aids are available to help the clinician predict the risk for acute MI or the presence of ischemic cardiac disease.

Table II lists several predictive instruments that have been developed and tested prospectively in the emergency department for the detection of patients most likely to have acute MI.[13,44–49] In general, none of these aids are any better than clinical judgement when considering patients that can clearly be classified into acute MI versus no MI categories (ie, all share similar sensitivities for the diagnosis of MI). Any real benefit from these models is in their improved specificity for the diagnosis of MI when compared to clinicians' judgement in those patients with an "intermediate" probability of MI. This important ability has been used to decrease the admission rate to the cardiac intensive care unit by approximately one third in those patients who in actuality do not have an acute MI.[45,46] While still far from perfect, in 1988[44] it was estimated that use of one of these algorithms to guide coronary care unit admissions had the potential to save $85 million per year in the United States. This is not intended to imply that we feel any one of these instruments is clearly better than another. However, from purely numerical and performance standpoints, it would appear that the Acute Ischemic Heart Disease Predictive Instrument[46] or the Decision Tree for the Classification of Patients with Acute Chest Pain[44] might be highly useful in decision support. The major caveat to remember when considering more wide-scale application of these predictive instruments is that the patient population these protocols were derived from may be entirely different from the patient population that frequents other emergency departments.

A similar approach has been used to address the issue of estimating the probability of coronary artery disease in patient subgroups. This reasoning will have an influence on those patients who do not present with acute MI but in whom possible ischemia may still be a consideration. Since any noninvasive testing is imperfect, its reliability for screening patients for the presence of disease is critically affected by the likelihood that the disease exists in the first place (ie, the prevalence of the disease in that population).[50] No

**Table II**
Predictive Instruments for the Detection of Myocardial Infarction
in the Emergency Department

| Study | Study Technique | Prospective Validation | N* | Sensitivity | Specificity | + Predictive Value | Overall Accuracy |
|---|---|---|---|---|---|---|---|
| 1) Goldman et al. 1982[13] | Recursive Partitioning Analysis | Y | 482 (468) | 88% | 77% | 42% | 79% |
| 2) Goldman et al. 1988[44] | Recursive Partitioning Analysis | Y | 1379 (4770) | 88% | 74% | 32% | 76% |
| 3) Pozen et al. 1980[45] | Logistic Regression | Y | 925 (856) | 86% | 92% | — | 91% |
| 4) Pozen et al. 1984[46] | Logistic Regression | Y | 2801 (2320) | 95% | 78% | — | 83% |
| 5) Tierney et al. 1985[47] | Logistic Regression | Y | 284 (256) | 81% | 86% | 43% | 88% |
| 6) Jonsbu et al. 1991[48] | Statistical Pattern Recognition | Y | 200 (1574) | 89%–95% | 63%–69% | 59%–78% | 74%–80% |
| 7) Lee et al. 1991[49] | Bayesian Inference | Y | 976 (2684) | 79% | 56% | 71% | — |

* The first number indicates the size of the population used to develop the model. The second parenthesized number indicates the size of the population used to validate the model; Y = yes.

matter how sensitive or specific any individual test may be, the possibility of a false-negative and a false-positive test result must be factored in when applying those results to that patient at hand. Thus, in a patient population with a high prevalence rate of disease (eg, an elderly male smoker with hypertension, diabetes, hypercholesterolemia, and typical angina), a negative test is of little diagnostic accuracy since it is more than likely to have a false-negative result. On the other hand, in a population with a low prevalence rate (eg, a teenage female without risk factors and asymptomatic), the result is likely to be a true-negative result. The establishment of a patient's pretest likelihood of coronary artery disease, then, is a valuable aid in the clinical assessment of chest pain presentations.

Reliable data have been gathered to provide strong predictors of a patient's pretest clinical likelihood of coronary artery disease. Estimates exist for risk based on age, sex, characteristics of chest pain, and disease prevalence in the population. A review of the medical literature reveals that the prevalence of coronary artery disease in persons with typical angina is around 90% overall, whereas it is only 50% in those with atypical angina and 16% overall for those with a nonanginal type pain.[35] Asymptomatic adults also have a low risk of coronary artery disease, which is estimated at around 4%.[35] Further refinement in these estimates is possible when accounting for sex differences and subdividing into age groups. Table III summarizes the prevalence of atherosclerotic disease in the adult population in the United States and is based on autopsy data and angiographically confirmed evidence of coronary artery disease in symptomatic patients. There is a wide range of pretest likelihoods for each combination of age, sex, and symptoms. Further refinement in these estimates can be achieved by consideration of additional risk factors for the

**Table III**
Pretest Likelihood of Coronary Artery Disease According to Age and Sex*

| Age (years) | Typical Angina | | Atypical Angina | | Nonanginal Chest Pain | | Asymptomatic | |
|---|---|---|---|---|---|---|---|---|
| | Men | Women | Men | Women | Men | Women | Men | Women |
| 30–39 | 69.7 ± 3.2 | 25.8 ± 6.6 | 21.8 ± 2.4 | 4.2 ± 1.3 | 5.2 ± 0.8 | 0.8 ± 0.3 | 1.9 ± 0.3 | 0.3 ± 0.1 |
| 40–49 | 87.3 ± 1.0 | 55.2 ± 6.5 | 46.1 ± 1.8 | 13.3 ± 2.9 | 14.1 ± 1.3 | 2.8 ± 0.7 | 5.5 ± 0.3 | 1.0 ± 0.2 |
| 50–59 | 92.0 ± 0.6 | 79.4 ± 2.4 | 58.9 ± 1.5 | 32.4 ± 3.0 | 21.5 ± 1.7 | 8.4 ± 1.2 | 9.7 ± 0.4 | 3.2 ± 0.4 |
| 60–69 | 94.3 ± 0.4 | 90.6 ± 1.0 | 67.1 ± 1.3 | 54.4 ± 2.4 | 28.1 ± 1.9 | 18.6 ± 1.9 | 12.3 ± 0.5 | 7.5 ± 0.6 |

* Each value represents the percent ± 1 standard error of the percent.
Modified from: Diamond GA, Forrester JS. N Engl J Med 1979;300:1350–1358.[35]

presence of disease other than age and sex. Using a slightly different patient population, Pryor et al.[51] developed nomograms for estimating the likelihood of significant coronary artery disease that incorporate age, sex, smoking, hyperlipidemia, symptoms, ECG findings, and clinical history. A representative nomogram is shown as Figure 3.

Using a nomogram or equation to assign a probability of disease to the patients with chest pain, the clinician can more wisely order and interpret cardiac tests. With disease probabilities less than 10% or greater than 90%, further testing is unnecessary since the presence of coronary artery disease has been satisfactorily dismissed or confirmed, respectively.[52] Patients with intermediate levels of probability will require further testing. By using the sensitivities and specificities for each noninvasive test for coronary artery disease, a quantitative post-test likelihood of disease can be determined,[35,50,53] according to Bayes' theorem of conditional probability. Serial use of independent tests may be required to attain the necessary risk estimates and diagnostic endpoints.

Applying these techniques to data from published series, it has been estimated that technetium-imaging of the blood pool of the left ventricle during rest and with exercise has the highest predictive value in establishing risk for those patients with intermediate pretest levels of disease.[50] Thallium perfusion imaging would have the next best predictive value, followed by analysis of ST segment changes with exercise. Our diagnostic algorithms are faithful to the data that address the cardiac work-up of chest pain.

Implementation of diagnostic testing algorithms will necessarily depend on availability of these tests and on development of more sensitive and specific tests in the future. With the emphasis placed on rapid diagnosis of cardiac ischemia and infarction and the additional emphasis on cost-effectiveness, we expect that numerous diagnostic tests will be evaluated in the emergency department setting in the future. Currently, in the United States, many institutions have opted to have separate "chest pain treatment centers" where patients will be evaluated expeditiously and the diagnosis of MI or ischemia will be established within the first 12 hours of stay. Their success or failure will determine the diagnostic algorithms of the future and will require continual re-evaluation as newer and improved techniques become available.

## Psychologic Considerations

Studies suggest that the performance of laboratory tests in patients with chest pain, even when of no diagnostic value, affect the outcome of care. Patients who have undergone ECG and CPK testing versus those who did not, have experienced less short-term disability and improved satisfaction with care.[54] These data would strongly suggest that reassurance in the absence of testing is inadequate for many patients. While we cannot advocate "useless" diagnostic testing, we recognize that

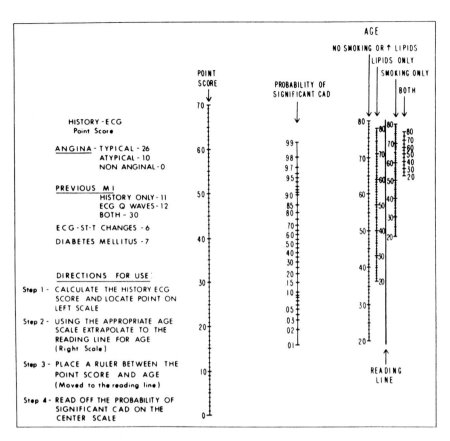

**Figure 3.** The figure shows a typical nomogram used for estimating the risk of significant coronary artery disease. This nomogram displayed is for women and determines risk on the basis of symptoms, age, history, lipid profile, and ECG. Reprinted by permission of the publisher from (Pryor DB et al. Estimating the likelihood of significant coronary artery disease.) Am J Med, 75, 771–780. Copyright 1983 by Excerpta Medical Inc. [51]

testing at times may be necessary to prevent needless re-evaluation of concerned, dissatisfied patients.

## Acute Pain in the Adult

Table IV lists the most common causes of acute chest pain in the adult. Figure 4 displays a suggested algorithm for evaluation. Any algorithm for evaluating acute chest pain should detect the most common diseases and should not miss the less common but potentially fatal causes of acute chest pain (Table V). Initial history and physical examination should detect patients with classic presentations of

disease, identify those at high risk for the anxiety/hyperventilation syndrome, and accurately diagnose musculoskeletal, skin, trauma, breast, and neurologic causes of pain. The algorithm is designed for those cases when the cause of pain remains unclear.

Due to the high prevalence of cardiac causes of pain in the population, we recommend that all patients in whom a diagnosis remains unclear after history and physical examination be screened by electrocardiography and chest roentgenography. This should identify many patients with atypical MI, angina, pneumothorax, aortic disease, tamponade, pneumonia, pleurisy, and pericarditis. All patients at

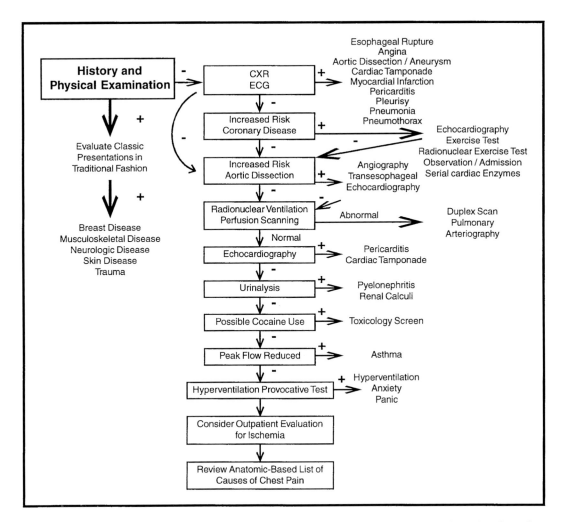

**Figure 4.** Algorithm for evaluating acute chest pain of unclear etiology in adults. The algorithm is intended for use when a thorough history and physical examination fail to suggest likely causes. CXR = chest roentgenogram; ECG = electrocardiogram; + = abnormal or diagnostic;— = normal or not diagnostic.

increased risk for cardiac disease (Table III) should undergo a more definitive cardiac evaluation to include exercise testing, radioisotope exercise testing, or echocardiography. If definitive testing is not available, patients who have an intermediate or higher risk for coronary disease may require evaluation or re-evaluation over 12 to 24 hours and serial cardiac enzyme determinations. Those with risk factors for aortic dissection and a compatible history should have a more definitive evaluation with transesophageal echocardiography or angiography. Due to the relatively high frequency of pulmonary embolism (PE) in the population, all remaining patients should undergo ventilation-perfusion scanning. All patients with other than a normal scan require a more definitive evaluation for PE. The remainder of the algorithm is based upon our perception of the frequency of disease, the accuracy of screening tests, and the potential for death from the causative diseases. Patients with no di-

## Table IV
### Common Causes of Acute Chest Pain in the Adult

Angina
Benign Overuse Syndrome
Cardiac Trauma
Cocaine
Costosternal Syndrome
Gall Bladder Disease
Gastroesophageal Reflux Disease
Gastroesophageal Dysmotility
Herpes Zoster
Hyperventilation/Anxiety
Myocardial Infarction
Pectoral Girdle Syndrome
Pericarditis
Pleurisy
Pneumonia
Renal Calculi
Rib Trauma

## Table VI
### Common Causes of Chronic Chest Pain in Adults

Angina
Aortic Stenosis
Asthma
Benign Overuse Syndrome
Breast Cancer
Cardiomyopathy
Drugs
Fibrocystic Breast Disease
Gastroesophageal Reflux Disease
Gastroesophageal Dysmotility
Hyperventilation/Anxiety Syndrome
Mitral Valve Prolapse
Mitral Stenosis
Pectoral Girdle Syndrome

agnosis at the end of the algorithm should be considered for further outpatient evaluation directed to cardiac and gastrointestinal causes and the hyperventilation/anxiety syndrome.

## Chronic Pain in the Adult

Table VI lists the common causes of chronic chest pain in adults, and Figure 5 displays an algorithm for the evaluation of chronic pain. The evaluation of chronic chest pain differs from acute chest pain in that diseases causing chronic chest pain by definition are less likely to be acutely

## Table V
### Less Common But Potentially Fatal Causes of Acute Chest Pain in the Adult

Aortic Dissection
Aortic Aneurysm
Cardiac Tamponade
Esophageal Rupture
Pneumothorax

fatal. History and physical examination should be performed thoroughly. As with acute chest pain we suspect that the majority of patients will have an obvious cause of pain identified after a history and physical examination have been performed. This should identify classic presentations of disease (eg, a classic aortic stenosis murmur, history of angina, or frequent regurgitation of food) which can then be evaluated in a traditional manner. Other diseases such as skin, breast, neurologic, and musculoskeletal diseases should be apparent without further testing or with simple confirmatory tests specific for these diseases.

In patients in whom the cause of disease remains unapparent, the algorithm suggests that the evaluative tests be ordered in a sequence reflecting the prevalence of the suspected diseases and accuracy of the screening tests. Asthma occurs in at least 5% of the population, typically presents with chest pain or tightness, and is frequently underdiagnosed. Most patients with aortic stenosis should have easily heard murmurs when symptomatic. Mitral stenosis and cardiomyopathy may only be apparent on echocardiography. Echocardiography should detect those individuals with valvular disease or cardio-

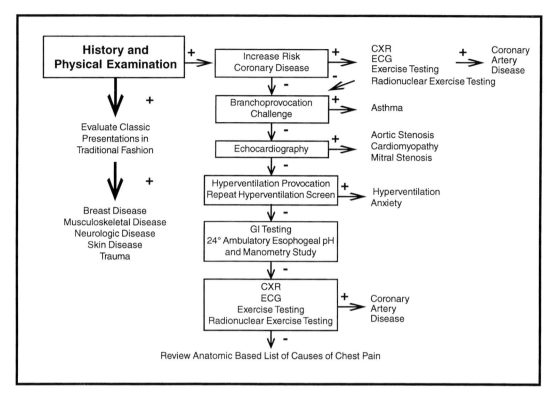

**Figure 5.** Algorithm for evaluating chronic chest pain of unclear etiology in adults. The algorithm is intended for use when a thorough history and physical examination fail to suggest a likely cause. CXR = chest roentgenogram; ECG = electrocardiogram; + = abnormal or diagnostic;— = normal or not diagnostic.

myopathy with normal cardiac examinations.

## Pediatric and Adolescent Chest Pain

The spectrum of causes and morbidity of chest pain in the pediatric age group is significantly different from that of adults and requires a different strategy for diagnostic evaluation. Most authors agree that, in this age group, history and physical examination constitute the best initial screen and can separate potentially serious problems from benign ones without other extensive testing.

### Prevalence of Causes of Pediatric Chest Pain

Table VII summarizes the frequencies of the causes of pediatric chest pain found in five major reported studies. Results differ depending on whether the study site was an outpatient clinic, emergency department, or inner city care center, or whether patients were admitted to the hospital. Evaluation of 100 adolescents seen in an outpatient clinic for the evaluation of chest pain revealed the following causes: 31% musculoskeletal, 20% hyperventilation, 5% breast-related, and 39% idiopathic.[55] Selbst et al.[56] systematically evaluated 407 children presenting with chest pain to a Philadelphia emergency department. The most common causes of chest pain were musculoskeletal (due to cough, costochondritis, and trauma) 39%, idiopathic 21%, psychogenic 9%, and asthma 7%. In a study of 43 children evaluated in an outpatient clinic in an urban pediatric hospital, Driscoll et al.[57] found 45% of cases to be idiopathic, 33% were musculo-

**Table VII**
Causes of Chest Pain in the Pediatric Age Group
(Percent of Total for Each Diagnosis in Five Major Studies)

| | Driscoll et al. 1976[57] N = 43 | Pantell and Goodman 1983[55] N = 100 | Selbst et al. 1988[56] N = 407 | Kaden et al. 1991[385] N = 42 | Zavaras-Angelidou et al. 1992[58] N = 134 |
|---|---|---|---|---|---|
| Idiopathic | 45 | 39 | 21 | 52 | 20 |
| Musculoskeletal | 33 | 31 | 29 | 8 | 16 |
| Cardiac | | 1 | 4 | 22 | 19 |
| Respiratory | 13 | 2 | 21 | 4 | 10 |
| Psychiatric | | 20 | 9 | 8 | 6 |
| Gastrointestinal | | 2 | 4 | | 10 |
| Sickle Cell | | | 2 | | 7 |
| Viral | | | | | 4 |
| Miscellaneous | 10 | 5 | 9 | 6 | 11 |

skeletal, 10% were due to cough, and 10% due to miscellaneous causes. A study from a Milwaukee emergency department found the following spectrum among 134 pediatric patients: idiopathic 20%, cardiac 19%, musculoskeletal 16%, respiratory 10%, gastrointestinal 7%, sickle cell 7%, viral 6%, and psychogenic 6%, cocaine 2%, and miscellaneous 6%. Although precordial catch is mentioned in case reports as commonly occurring in the pediatric age group, the diagnosis infrequently appears in large series.

The initial evaluation of chest pain in an urgent care setting appears to identify accurately patients with a serious problem. One Scottish study reports that 22% of patients of age younger than 35 years who presented to an emergency department due to chest pain required hospital admission. The admission rates in the adolescent and pediatric age group are probably comparable, with one center reporting a 27% admission rate.[58] In children sick enough to require admission approximately half had a cardiac problem, most commonly arrhythmia, pericarditis, or dilated cardiomyopathy. Asthma, spontaneous pneumothorax, pneumonia, sickle cell crisis, and cocaine use account for most of the other causes for admission. Case reports document chest pain due to

seizure,[59] myocarditis,[60] and anomalous coronary vasculature.[61]

Age does appear to influence the likelihood of diagnosis.[56] Children younger than 12 years were twice as likely to have a cardiorespiratory cause of chest pain. Children older than 12 years were 2.5 times more likely to have a psychogenic cause.

Long-term follow-up of pediatric patients with chest pain confirms that the chest pain in patients judged not to require hospital admission is usually benign and extensive evaluation unnecessary. Follow-up of Selbst's patients[62] indicated that chest pain persisted in 43% of children. Serious organic disease not suspected at initial evaluation was not detected over the course of follow-up. Similarly, Rowland and Richards[63] report that chest pain resolved in 81% of pediatric patients followed over 3 years and that initially unsuspected organic diseases were rarely detected on follow-up.

## Diagnostic Testing

Routine laboratory evaluation with ECG, chest roentgenography, pulmonary function tests, or esophageal studies in the absence of abnormalities appears unhelpful. In Selbst's original series, ECG established a new diagnosis in only one patient. Physical examination was abnormal in 40% of patients. Although 27% of chest roentgenograms were abnormal, chest roentgenogram was helpful only when pneumonia or pneumothorax was suspected. The prevalence of exercise-induced asthma in the testing population probably greatly influences the value of an exercise test with prespirometric, postspirometric, or peak flow measurements. Wiens et al.[64] report that 72% of 88 children undergoing exercise testing for the evaluation of chest pain had spirometric evidence of exercise-induced asthma. However, Nudel evaluated 180 patients with exertional pain and found only 9.5% had exercise-induced asthma. Although the study by Glassman et al.[65] suggests that pediatric patients with chest pain should undergo esophogogastroscopy and esophageal manometry, these data do not support such a strong statement. In 83 patients referred due to a suspicion of gastrointestinal etiologies of chest pain 57% were normal, 18% had esophagitis, 16% dysmotility, and 10% dysmotility and esophagitis. The prevalence of abnormalities would likely be lower if these studies were performed in a screening fashion on an unselected population. Since only those with esophagitis were responsive to therapy, a trial of $H_2$ blockers may be more cost-effective than routine testing.

When the cause of chest pain is not apparent after history and physical examination and the child appears nontoxic, no further evaluation apart from routine follow-up appears indicated. Screening for asthma with serial peak flows or bronchoprovocation challenge may be helpful when chest pain persists. When the child appears toxic and the cause is not apparent, ECG, chest roentgenogram, an echocardiogram, and a spirometric evaluation should reveal most potentially serious problems.[58,66,67]

Physicians should always inquire about recent stress in the child's life, such as active illnesses in other family members. Psychogenic chest pain in the pediatric and adolescent age groups appears to be frequently triggered by an identifiable stressful emotional event.[55,68] In 47% of cases another family member has similar symptoms or vague somatic complaints. In the presence of a normal physical examination and an otherwise nondiagnostic history, one can make a presumptive diagnosis of psychogenic chest pain.

## Treatment

Treatment for chest pain may be either specific or nonspecific. Specific therapy is therapy that is directed at reversing the causative pathophysiologic mechanism of the pain. Nonspecific therapy, such as analgesics, is therapy directed at the pain rather than the underlying disease. In attributing a cause of chest pain based upon a favorable response to specific therapy, clinicians should be cautious since specific therapy for one illness can also be specific therapy for another. Nitroglycerin when administered to patients with known coronary artery disease may also treat esophageal spasm and can relieve some muscular pains due to changes in muscle perfusion.[37,69–72] Ingestion of antacids has been helpful in some cases of cardiac pain.[1,73,74] We recommend the use of specific therapy whenever available because specific therapy may resolve the underlying disease and nonspecific pharmacologic therapy is typically associated with significant long-term side effects.

### Specific Therapy

#### *Cardiovascular*

***Aortic Dissection:*** Without treatment, aortic dissection has a high fatality rate—greater than 25% within 24 hours, greater than 50% at 1 week, greater than 75% after 1 month, and more than 90% within 1 year.[75] The goals of initial (ie, medical) therapy are to prevent further propagation of the dissection by reducing the systolic blood pressure and reducing the aortic wall stress from the ejection of the left ventricular stroke volume.

All patients should be admitted to a highly monitored setting for pain relief and reducing the systolic arterial blood pressure to approximately 100 to 120 mm Hg (mean arterial pressure of 60 to 75 mm Hg). Potent vasodilators, such as sodium nitroprusside, are effective for acute reduction of blood pressure. Starting doses of 25 to 50 $\mu$g/min intravenously are used and the infusion can then be titrated to blood pressure response while maintaining adequate vital organ perfusion. When used for more than 48 hours continuously, cyanide or thiocyanate toxicity may occur. In addition, when used alone for blood pressure control, this agent may inadvertently cause an increase in aortic wall stress levels and serve to extend the dissection.[76] Therefore, it is recommended that adequate beta adrenergic blockade be used simultaneously with this drug.[77]

Several different beta-blocking agents have been shown to be efficacious in the management of aortic dissection. Satisfactory therapy is generally that which reduces the heart rate to 60 to 80 bpm acutely. Intravenous propranolol has had the longest use and can be given as a 0.5-mg test dose followed by incremental doses of 1.0 mg every 5 minutes until the heart rate goal is achieved or a total dose of 0.15 mg/kg has been reached. Subsequent dosing is generally in the 2- to 6-mg range every 4 to 6 hours. Atenolol and metoprolol are more cardioselective agents that may occasionally be preferable to propranolol for specific patients (eg, asthmatics) when given in equivalent doses. The alpha and beta adrenergic blocker, labetalol, is effective for blood pressure reduction and reducing wall stresses when used as a single agent.[78] This agent is initially given as 5 to 20 mg intravenously, followed by 20 to 40 mg every 10 to 15 minutes until the target blood pressure is reached or a total of 300 mg has been given.

Use of the intravenous angiotensin-converting enzyme inhibitor enalapril maleate (1 to 2 mg every 4 to 6 hours) may be quite effective in cases with refractory hypertension due to renal artery occlusion. Calcium channel antagonists have also had favorable effects in the management of acute hypertensive crises.

Medical therapy offers a relative advantage over surgery in the management of most cases of uncomplicated distal dissections and in stabilizing patients with proximal dissection prior to proceeding with surgical repair.[79,80] This difference in therapy is based on the fact that any progression of a proximal dissection may have catastrophic results and that, in general, patients with distal dissections will have more advanced atherosclerosis and pose a higher surgical risk. Medical therapy has been shown to have an equivalent outcome to surgical treatment of uncomplicated distal dissections.[81] Hospital survival is 80% to 90% for those patients with proximal dissections treated surgically and approximately 80% for patients with distal dissections treated medically.[81,82] Initially successful medical or surgical therapy is usually sustained over the course of long-term follow-up. Long-term medical therapy with antihypertensives and agents to reduce aortic wall stress is generally indicated for all patients after an aortic dissection, regardless of whether they have received surgical or medical therapy.

***Aortic Aneurysm:*** Historically, patients with untreated symptomatic thoracic aneurysms have a 27% 5-year survival.[83] Surgical excision is the treatment of choice when feasible. The details of the procedure itself must be tailored to each specific aneurysm; however, total cardiopulmonary bypass is generally required for all ascending aortic aneurysm resections. Most major centers now report an approximately 90% operative and 66% 5-year survival rate for elective resection of ascending or descending aneurysms.[84,85] Although the risk of technical complications is not negligible despite extensive precautions (eg, a 5% incidence of spinal cord injury [84,86,87]), the major complications encountered in these patients are directly due to the massive physiologic stress of surgery in the setting of multisystem involvement with arteriosclerosis.

***Myocardial Infarction:*** Improvements in therapy for acute MI have resulted in a decrease in early mortality from greater than 20% to less than 10% over the last decade.[88] However, since most deaths related to acute MI are still due to ventricular fibrillation and occur in the first hour of onset,[89] public education remains a prime concern to encourage patients to seek immediate medical attention when they experience chest pain. This is true not only to prevent potentially treatable dysrhythmias but also to improve the chances of salvaging myocardium at risk. The rapid triage of patients is essential as it has been estimated that for every hour of delay in initiating therapy, a reduction in survival benefit is noted on the order of two lives per 1000 treated patients.[90]

Because ongoing ischemia is responsible for the pain associated with MI, interventions to improve the balance of myocardial oxygen supply and demand should decrease or relieve that pain. It is an accepted common practice to treat all patients suspected of having acute MI with oxygen based on the frequent occurrence of hypoxemia in this setting[91,92] and the belief that oxygen supply may be augmented. Experimental data suggest that, if the goal of oxygen administration is to limit infarct size, high-inspired concentrations may be needed.[93,94] Some authors advise that 40% oxygen be administered by mask for 4 to 5 days after infarction.[95] Patients with severe pulmonary edema may require endotracheal intubation and institution of mechanical ventilation.

*Nitrates:* Nitrates are generally first-line agents for anti-ischemic effects as long as patients do not exhibit hypotension (defined as a systolic blood pressure <100 mm Hg or a drop of >25 mm Hg from that patient's baseline). In the acute MI setting, intravenous nitroglycerin lowers left ventricular filling pressure, improves cardiac output, and improves regional ischemia.[88,96,97] From a hemodynamic standpoint, the most beneficial effects of this therapy will be seen in those patients with the most severe left ventricular failure. Careful monitoring of vital signs is

warranted and if symptoms are severe or occur for prolonged periods of time with a waxing/waning quality, consideration should be given to intravenous nitroglycerin. Nitrates should be used judiciously in patients with inferior wall MI because of the propensity for acute hypotension and bradycardia in this setting. Likewise, nitrates might be considered to be relatively contraindicated in the setting of right ventricular MI due to the well-documented preload dependence of these patients.[98] Invariably, tachyphylaxis to nitrate therapy will occur after 24 hours of continuous administration, regardless of the route of delivery. This diminution in effectiveness can be prevented by providing at least a 10- to 12-hour nitrate-free interval per day. When using intravenous nitroglycerin, it may be more appropriate to overcome tachyphylaxis by progressively increasing the dose every 12 to 24 hours as determined by the patients' blood pressure response and headache tolerance.

*Narcotic Agents:* Narcotic agents, especially morphine, have been used extensively to treat the pain associated with MI. Intravenous morphine sulfate (2 to 8 mg) can be given every 5 to 15 minutes until the pain is controlled or toxicity occurs (eg, hypotension, severe vomiting, depression of respiratory drive). Among the numerous beneficial effects of this medication are reduction of anxiety (and therefore metabolic demand), peripheral arterial and venous dilation, reduction of the work of breathing, and decreased sympathetic tone in conjunction with augmented vagal tone.

*Beta adrenergic Blocking Agents:* Beta adrenergic blocking agents are especially useful in the setting of acute MI to reduce ischemia and limit the size of any resulting infarct. Especially suited are those patients with hypertension and sinus tachycardia. Metoprolol is a popular and safe agent and can be given as 50 to 100 mg orally, bid. If needed, an extremely short-acting agent, such as esmolol can be used intravenously or as a means of determining relative hemodynamic stability prior to starting more long-acting agents. A reduced ejection fraction is **not** an absolute contraindication to beta blockade and, in fact, these patients may actually derive the most benefit from these agents. Either metoprolol (5 mg intravenously every 2 to 5 minutes for three doses) or atenolol (10 to 20 mg intravenously) can be used as routinely recommended adjunctive agents for patients with acute MI who are treated within 4 to 6 hours of symptom onset. These agents have been convincingly shown to reduce both infarct size and associated hospital mortality, especially in those patients with elevated systolic blood pressures, sinus tachycardia, or both.[99,100] Moreover, the use of intravenous beta-blocking agents is recommended as part of routine care for acute MI, regardless of concomitant use of thrombolytic agents.

Unlike beta blockers, calcium channel antagonists are of little value in the setting of acute MI.[101,102]

*Limitation of Physical Activity:* Limitation of physical activity has long been a mainstay of acute MI therapy. Unless there is evidence of hemodynamic instability or other complications coexist, patients need not be confined to bed for more than 24 to 36 hours. Progression of activity level should then be individualized with a clear goal towards early ambulation given its potent psychologic and physical benefits without any clearly increased medical risks.[103,104]

*Thrombolytic Therapy:* Close to 90% of patients in the early stages of an acute MI will have an intracoronary arterial thrombus documented by angiography.[105] This finding has led to several large randomized trials comparing the effectiveness of a variety of intravenous thrombolytic agents since the early 1980's. Compared to placebo these initial trials[106,107] documented significant reductions in the mortality rates (ranging from 18% to 48%) for patients receiving streptokinase, anisoylated plasminogen streptokinase activator complex (APSAC), or recombinant human tissue-type plasminogen activator (rt-PA). Based on these studies and subsequent work,[108,109] the current consensus for the

use of these agents is that any patient, regardless of age, presenting with a symptom complex suggestive of an acute MI, with at least 1 mm of ST segment elevation in two or more contiguous ECG leads and presenting within 12 hours of the onset of symptoms should be considered for thrombolytic therapy. Such patients next should have a careful individualized assessment of the risk-to-benefit ratio prior to using these agents. Important contraindications to the use of thrombolytic agents include a history of cerebral vascular accident; known intracranial malignancy; known arteriovenous malformation or aneurysm; history of a bleeding diathesis; recent (within 2 months) spinal, intracranial, or major surgery at a noncompressible site; significant surgery within 2 weeks; pericarditis; aortic dissection; uncontrolled hypertension; or any active bleeding.[88] Once it has been determined that there is no contraindication to thrombolytic therapy, it should be given promptly. An absolute reduction in mortality of approximately 30 lives per 1000 patients is achieved when treatment is begun within 6 hours of symptom onset. Thrombolytic therapy begun 7 to 12 hours after the onset of symptoms results in an estimated mortality reduction of 20 lives per 1000 patients.[90] Because recent evidence[110] suggests no advantage for the use of thrombolytic therapy in patients with non—Q wave MI or unstable angina, these agents are not indicated in these settings. Although a small (14%, at least half due to earlier reperfusion), but significant survival advantage has been shown for rt-PA,[111–113] currently no single thrombolytic protocol is considered to be ideal.[114,115]

Thrombolytic therapy in the setting of acute MI has clearly not turned out to be the originally hoped for panacea. Failure to reperfuse coronary stenoses/occlusions occurs in 20% to 30% of patients treated with these agents.[111,116] An additional 10% to 25% of patients who were initially successfully thrombolysed, will experience reocclusion.[113,117] Of increasing importance then, given these failure rates for thrombolytic agents, is the development of adjunctive therapies whose goals would include the following: (1) maintaining coronary artery patency; (2) preventing ventricular dilation; (3) minimizing myocardial ischemia by improving "supply" (coronary artery blood flow), decreasing "demand" (myocardial oxygen needs), or both; and (4) reducing infarct size.[118] Current recommendations to achieve these goals are outlined in several recent review articles[88,118] and are summarized below.

*Antiplatelet Agents:* Aspirin therapy, 160 to 325 mg daily, should begin immediately in patients with known or suspected acute MI, regardless of whether thrombolytic agents are also used. The use of aspirin alone has been shown to result in a 23% reduction in mortality and a 49% reduction in the reinfarction rate when compared with placebo.[119] When aspirin has been used with streptokinase, there has been a 42% reduction in mortality from acute MI as compared with placebo. For secondary prophylaxis against recurrent MI in acute MI survivors, meta-analysis of aspirin therapy trials showed a 13% reduction in mortality and a 31% reduction in long-term reinfarction rate.[120] When patients are placed on warfarin, the use of aspirin should be postponed. The combination of aspirin and warfarin should be strictly avoided due to the increased risks for bleeding complications and the unproven benefit of the combined agents compared with the use of either agent alone. Unfortunately, despite the proven efficacy, simplicity, and low cost of aspirin therapy, the benefits of aspirin apparently remain a well-kept secret since only 72% of MI patients in the United States receive aspirin.[121]

*Thrombin Inhibitors:* Intravenous heparin (5000 intravenous units (IU) bolus followed by continuous infusion at 1000 IU/h and then titrated to maintain the activated prothrombin time at 1.5 to 2.0 times control values for 5 to 7 days) is routinely recommended in all patients with acute MI who are treated with a thrombolytic agent.[122] This is especially true for rt-PA since it has a fibrin-specific site of action

and has a short duration of action, thereby increasing the chance for rethrombosis.[123,124] This therapy is also generally recommended for those treated with streptokinase. As the risk for coronary rethrombosis is highest in the first 24 hours after an acute MI, it is generally advisable to not decrease the infusion rate of heparin below 1000 IU/h, even if the activated prothrombin time increases to greater than two times baseline levels. The optimal duration of heparin therapy has not been clearly established in the literature. Since heparin has also been shown to prevent the progression of unstable angina,[125] it is reasonable to give it for unstable angina and non–Q wave infarction.[126] Even though warfarin has similar beneficial effects (approximately 25% reduction in mortality and a 34% to 55% reduction in reinfarction rate[127,128]) to aspirin, aspirin is much more widely used than warfarin at the present time.

The results of TIMI 5[129] indicate that the selective thrombin-inhibiting agent, hirudin, is effective for the prevention of coronary artery reocclusion after thrombolysis without increasing the occurrence of spontaneous bleeding. While this agent is both a more selective and more potent inhibitor of thrombin than heparin, it has only been evaluated in pilot studies to date and is not a recommended agent at this time. The role of this agent as an adjunct to thrombolysis in acute MI will likely be determined by the results of the TIMI 9 trial. Another promising class of agents under investigation as potential successors to aspirin and heparin are the platelet fibrinogen receptor antagonists (the IIb/IIIa inhibitors). These compounds block the final common pathway of platelet aggregation and have looked promising in pilot studies.[130,131] Phase III trials are now underway.

*Coronary Angioplasty:* Routine use of coronary angioplasty after successful thrombolysis is not recommended for all patients with acute MI.[132,133] This is also true for those patients who fail to reperfuse after thrombolytic therapy, so-called "rescue" coronary angioplasty.[133] It may be considered an acceptable alternative therapy, however, in those patients with a contraindication to thrombolytic therapy, persistent ischemia, or cardiogenic shock despite optimal medical management in whom coronary artery bypass surgery might carry a very high risk of morbidity. Primary percutaneous transluminal coronary angioplasty (without antecedent thrombolysis) may also be considered in this last patient population. Some believe that coronary angioplasty may produce higher coronary artery patency rates and less residual stenosis than thrombolytic agents, and also reduce mortality, recurrent ischemia/infarction, and hemorrhagic strokes.[134–136]

*Other Agents:* Clinical trials of the use of magnesium to reduce acute MI mortality[137–139] and trials with angiotensin-converting enzyme inhibitors to prevent postinfarction left ventricular dilatation [140,141] have shown disparate results; therefore, at present these agents are not recommended for routine use in the acute MI setting. Recently completed large studies[139,142] suggest a possible modest survival benefit to patients with acute MI treated with captopril early on.

*Immediate Cardiac Surgery:* Immediate cardiac surgery and/or coronary revascularization can be a lifesaving procedure when necessary due to severe mechanical complications from MI, such as acute severe mitral regurgitation due to papillary muscle rupture, ventricular septal defect, or myocardial rupture with tamponade. Evidence of a reduction in mortality also exists in patients treated with early surgery in the setting of cardiogenic shock, left-main disease, three-vessel coronary artery disease, and recurrent ischemia.[143]

**Myocarditis:** Treatment is often not sought out in the subclinical presentations and is primarily supportive in the case of more prominent manifestations. In general, patients with myocarditis should be followed closely for any evidence of involvement of the conduction system. Animal studies suggest that the damage from in-

flammation can be intensified with exercise, therefore adequate rest is felt to be important.[144] Congestive heart failure responds to routine therapy (eg, diuretics, cardiac glycosides). Beta blockers are usually avoided due to concern over their negative inotropic effects. The use of corticosteroids in this condition remains controversial.[144,145] Cyclosporine, indomethacin, salicylates, and ibuprofen are contraindicated in the first 2 weeks of viral myocarditis because these agents have been shown to increase the extent of myocardial damage.[146,147] In the late phase of myocarditis, however, nonsteroidal anti-inflammatory agents appear to be safe.[146,148] Appropriate antibiotics are beneficial when therapy can be focused to a specific organism .

**Cardiac and Pericardial Tumors:** The treatment of choice for the majority of benign tumors of the heart—approximately 75% of all cardiac tumors are benign—is operative resection and results in a complete cure in most cases.[149,150] The bulk of intracavitary and intramural lesions will require excision under direct visualization in order to minimize the risk of embolic phenomena. The recurrence rate for cardiac myxomas is approximately 1% to 5%,[151] with a much higher recurrence rate reported for patients with a genetic (familial) predisposition. Operative management for the great majority of malignant cardiac tumors is not generally effective for anything other than to confirm a diagnosis. The natural history for these malignancies may be altered for the better in some patients receiving chemotherapy and/or radiation therapy.

The mean survival for patients with neoplastic pericarditis treated for cardiac tamponade is about 4 months; with only 25% surviving 1 year.[152,153] The outcome for patients with breast cancer is strikingly better than for those with lung cancer or other metastatic disease. In general, the choice of management techniques used will depend on the underlying condition of the patient, with less invasive means (eg, catheter pericardiocentesis, subxiphoid pericardiotomy) used to palliate symptoms in the severely ill, to more aggressive options for those with a generally better prognosis (eg, partial [window] pericardiectomy, chemotherapy, external beam radiation therapy).

***Cardiomyopathy:*** Therapy for cardiomyopathy varies depending on whether the myopathy is of the dilated or hypertrophic type. Since dyspnea and debility are the most common symptoms arising from cardiomyopathy, most treatment regimens have aimed to reduce these symptoms. Little data exist on treatment of the chest pain associated with cardiomyopathy. Treatment is discussed briefly in Chapter 2, "Dyspnea."

***Pericardial and Myocardial Trauma:*** As a general rule, uncomplicated pericarditis due to thoracic trauma is self-limited. The postpericardiotomy syndrome may occur in a small portion of these patients and generally responds well to nonsteroidal anti-inflammatory agents. Constrictive pericarditis occurs rarely and may be seen in those with or without recurrent pericardial effusions. Cardiac tamponade requires emergent treatment and is described elsewhere in this chapter.

With respect to myocardial contusion, several investigators have concluded that routine intensive care unit monitoring and routine imaging studies of trauma patients in stable condition are not warranted.[154,155] Moreover, anticoagulant and thrombolytic therapies are contraindicated for cardiac contusion as intrapericardial and/or intramyocardial hemorrhage may be precipitated or worsened. Nitroglycerin and related drugs generally have little effect for pain relief for these patients; instead, chest pain is best treated with narcotic agents (eg, morphine). Aneurysmal complications generally require surgical resection only if the patient develops heart failure. On the other hand, pseudoaneurysms require immediate repair. Prognosis for partial and complete recovery after cardiac contusion is generally excellent with careful follow-up to monitor for the development of late complications, such as left ventricular failure.

***Pericarditis:*** Specific therapy is based on confirmation of the underlying causes (See Chapter 5, "Chest Pain: Pathophysiology and Differential Diagnosis," Table VI).[156] Nonspecific therapy consists of bed rest and a period of observation to exclude the possibilities of a pyogenic process, associated MI, or the development of cardiac tamponade. Acute pericarditis due to viral, idiopathic, post-MI, or post-pericardiotomy causes are generally self-limited with resolution of inflammation over 2 to 6 weeks. Nonsteroidal anti-inflammatory agents (aspirin 650 mg orally, every 3 to 4 hours or indomethacin 25 to 50 mg orally, every 6 hours) generally work well in relief of chest pain. When severe pain does not respond to the above agents within 48 hours, consideration should be given to a trial of corticosteroids (prednisone 60 to 80 mg (or its equivalent) orally, everyday for 5 to 7 days and then tapered to zero over 1 to 2 weeks). Regardless of the cause, avoidance of oral anticoagulant therapy will minimize the likelihood of a tension hemopericardium. If anticoagulation is required for a patient, such as for a prosthetic heart valve, intravenous heparin can be used and its effects rapidly reversed with protamine if need be. The most troublesome complication, experienced by 20% to 28% of patients,[157,158] is recurrent episodes of pericardial inflammation leading to fever with disabling chest pain at intervals of weeks to months, and perhaps over a period of years, after the initial episode. In this setting, pericardiectomy is not always followed by pain relief.[159] Hemodynamic complications due to cardiac compression are uncommon but may be life-threatening and include cardiac tamponade (discussed later), constrictive pericarditis due to the development of fibrosis and/or calcification of the pericardium, and a combination of effusive and constrictive disease.

***Cardiac Tamponade:*** The specific cause of tamponade should be vigorously sought and treated. Because tamponade physiology is developing, it can be halted or delayed by aggressive intravascular volume expansion; this will delay the appearance of right ventricular diastolic collapse. Inotropic support may also be of value, but the use of vasodilators, diuretics or positive-pressure mechanical ventilation are all best avoided if possible given their effects on blood pressure, intravascular volume, and cardiac output. Hemodynamic instability is best treated with removal of pericardial fluid by percutaneous pericardiocentesis or a surgical approach. The major risks from pericardiocentesis include lacerations to the coronary arteries, heart, or lung. Prior to the 1970's, when this procedure was performed without any form of central hemodynamic monitoring, the risk of death or of a life-threatening complication was as high as 20%.[160] Now, using fluoroscopic guidance with central hemodynamic monitoring, continuous electrocardiography, and an experienced operator, the risk of death or a life-threatening complication has decreased to 0% to 5%.[161,162] Surgical drainage is generally preferred in cases of purulent or tuberculous pericarditis. The technique for performing pericardiocentesis is presented in detail elsewhere.[163]

**Postpericardiotomy Syndrome:** This syndrome is generally self-limited but may also be prolonged and disabling. Nonsteroidal anti-inflammatory agents are the medications of choice for fever and chest discomfort. If these symptoms persist after 48 hours, a trial of corticosteroids should be considered.

**Postinfarction Pericarditis (Dressler's Syndrome):** As in other patients with acute pericarditis, severe fever and chest pain generally respond to bed rest and nonsteroidal anti-inflammatory agents. Severe cases of pericarditis warrant hospital admission for observation for the development of cardiac tamponade. All anticoagulants should be avoided if possible due to the risk of pericardial hemorrhage. Episodes of Dressler's syndrome are usually self-limited, but do have a tendency to recur. Recurrent episodes of this syndrome will occasionally require systemic corticosteroids and/or pericardiectomy.

**Aortic Stenosis:** Because of the tendency for the left ventricular obstruction of aortic stenosis to progress slowly over time, asymptomatic patients should be followed carefully and re-evaluated regularly for evidence of progression. Endocarditis prophylaxis[164] should be fully explained and given for invasive procedures. Therapeutic interventions that reduce preload (ie, diuretics) or depress myocardial function (ie, beta blockers) should be used only with extreme caution, if at all. Given the potential adverse hemodynamic effects that would result from loss of the atrial "kick," preventive therapy for atrial fibrillation should be considered if premature atrial contractions become frequent. This arrhythmia requires prompt treatment when it occurs, and the possibility of mitral valvular disease also should be considered. If any symptoms develop, all adults with severe aortic stenosis should have catheterization of the left ventricle to evaluate for possible surgical treatment.

In the majority of adults with calcific aortic stenosis, valvular function cannot be restored adequately with anything less than total valve replacement. Valve replacement is the treatment of choice for those patients with severe aortic stenosis who are symptomatic. It may also be recommended for asymptomatic patients with evidence of progressive left ventricular dysfunction. Operative mortality for those without overt left ventricular failure is in the range of 2% to 8% at most centers.[165] In this setting, hemodynamic and symptomatic improvements are striking with almost every patient obtaining a normal ventricular performance, relief of symptoms of myocardial ischemia, and relief of symptoms associated with elevated left atrial pressures.[166] Operative mortality in the order of 10% to 25% occurs when valve replacement is attempted on patients with reduced ejection fractions or frank left ventricular failure.[167]

Valves[168] may be replaced with prosthetic mechanical or tissue valves. Mechanical valves have excellent durability records while the major limitation of porcine tissue valves is a 20% failure rate by 10 years and a 50% to 55% failure rate by

15 years. Both types of valves in either the aortic or mitral position require anticoagulation. For mechanical prostheses, the risk of thromboembolism is greatest in the first postoperative year. Anticoagulation decreases this incidence three- to six-fold. Anticoagulation with warfarin begins 2 days postoperatively and continues for the patient's lifetime. The prothrombin time should be maintained 1.5 to 2 times control values. The incidence of fatal thromboembolic complications remains 0.2 per 100 patient years; the incidence of nonfatal complications, 1 to 2 per 100 patient years, despite anticoagulation. The complications of warfarin therapy occur at approximately similar rates. The incidence of thromboembolic complications is slightly higher for mechanical valves in the mitral rather than in the aortic position. Tissue valves require anticoagulation for the first 3 months postoperatively while the sewing ring endothelializes. Thereafter, porcine aortic valves or mitral valves in patients with normal sinus rhythm do not require anticoagulation. The rate of thromboembolism in these situations without anticoagulation is approximately 1 to 2 per 100 patient years. One third of the patients who undergo mitral valve replacement with porcine prostheses remain in atrial fibrillation and due to a three-fold increased risk of thromboembolism require lifelong anticoagulation.

Patients felt to be at too high an operative risk for valve replacement can be considered for balloon valvuloplasty, which results in an average 60% improvement in initial valve area, a 50% reduction in the mean valve gradient, and an improved ejection fraction.[169,170] Of these patients, 50% or more will experience restenosis within 6 months, and the 1-year mortality is approximately 25%. In critically ill patients, the procedure-related mortality is 3% to 7%, with an additional 6% developing serious complications. In the adult population, aortic balloon valvuloplasty should not be considered a substitute for surgery when feasible (as mitral balloon valvuloplasty might sometimes be).

**Mitral Stenosis:** All patients, with or without symptoms, with a history of rheumatic heart disease are candidates for antibiotic prophylaxis to prevent endocarditis in the setting of procedures or events recognized as being potential bacterial portals of entry.[164] Symptomatic patients may show substantial improvement with diuretic therapy and minimizing sodium intake. Beta blockers may be of benefit to improve exercise performance by slowing the heart rate of these patients. While digitalis glycosides are not of any benefit for patients in normal sinus rhythm, they can be very useful in decreasing the ventricular rate of patients with atrial fibrillation. Anticoagulant therapy is helpful in these patients with heart failure and/or atrial fibrillation to prevent thromboembolic complications. Immediate treatment after the onset of atrial fibrillation is aimed at reducing the resulting rapid ventricular rate to 60 to 65 bpm with digitalis and/or beta blockade, and at re-establishing sinus rhythm, if possible, with pharmacologic therapy and/or electrical cardioversion. The risk of systemic embolization following electrical or pharmacologic cardioversion is at least 1% to 2% in patients with mitral stenosis.[160]

The natural history of untreated mitral stenosis in temperate zones is one of a prolonged asymptomatic period of 20 to 25 years followed by the rapid progression from mild disability to severe disability over the next 5 years or so. Patients in more tropical environments show a more accelerated course. Medically treated patients show improved survival rates; however, once severe stenosis develops the disease will progress rapidly unless surgical intervention occurs. There is no evidence to suggest any improvement in prognosis with surgical therapy for those patients with slight or no functional impairments. Asymptomatic patients with a history of systemic embolism, however, should be considered for surgical treatment because of the high rate of recurrence.

There are three basic operative techniques available for the treatment of mitral stenosis [171,172]: (1) closed mitral valvulotomy; (2) mitral commissurotomy, generally an open-chest procedure with the aid of cardiopulmonary bypass; and (3) mitral valve replacement. (See the discussion above in the section on aortic valve replacement) Striking reduction in pulmonary artery pressures and right-sided heart failure is characteristic with the effective relief of mitral valvular obstruction.[173,174] The mortality rate after commissurotomy is from 1 to 3% and carries an actuarial 10 year survival rate of 95% [175,176]. This procedure is a palliative rather then a curative operation and these patients are subject to restenosis[177]; approximately 10% of patients will require a repeat operation within 5 years and 60% by 10 years.[178,179] Adequate reconstruction of the valve is frequently not possible at the time of reoperation and valve replacement is often necessary. Mitral valve replacement is also the procedure of choice for those patients with combined mitral stenosis and mitral regurgitation or who exhibit extensive calcification of the commissures. The operative mortality for this more definitive surgery ranges from 3% to 8% in most hospitals. The long-term effects of lifelong anticoagulant therapy and the fate of prosthetic valves is not well studied as yet.

An alternative to surgical intervention for patients unsuitable for surgery because of high operative risks is the technique of balloon valvuloplasty. In this procedure, a transseptal puncture of the interatrial septum allows passage of a balloon flotation catheter across the orifice of the mitral valve. Subsequent balloon inflation causes commissural separation resulting in an average 20% improvement in cardiac output and a 50% to 100% expansion of the calculated valve area. The reported mortality ranges from 0% to 4%, with the associated risks of thromboembolic events, cardiac perforation, and development of severe mitral regurgitation. The restenosis rate is approximately 10% over 1 to 2 years of follow-up. The most impressive results for this relatively new technique have been in younger patients without significant valvular calcification or thickening.[180]

### Mitral Valve Prolapse (Barlow's Syndrome):
Asymptomatic mitral valve prolapse (MVP) patients with no evidence of paroxysmal arrhythmias, normal ECG findings, and no evidence of serious mitral regurgitation have an excellent prognosis and require only limited long-term follow-up. Prophylaxis for infective endocarditis is advisable for all those with a systolic murmur. Patients with symptoms suggestive of diminished cardiac reserve (eg, lightheadedness, dizziness, syncope), ventricular arrhythmias, or prolonged QT intervals should be considered for therapy with beta blockers. Nitrates should be used cautiously as they may exaggerate the prolapse by diminishing venous return. Patients with symptoms attributable to mitral regurgitation should receive treatment like other patients with severe mitral regurgitation and may require reconstructive surgery or valve replacement. Those patients with exertional angina or ischemic changes on ECG or during other noninvasive cardiac testing should have further work-up and management for myocardial ischemia. Any patients with evidence of systemic thromboembolization without any other apparent cause should be considered for anticoagulant therapy and/or aspirin.

### Pulmonary

**Pleurisy:** The treatment of pleurisy varies depending on the causative agents. Virtually all cases benefit from symptomatic relief with analgesics, such as nonsteroidal anti-inflammatories. Pleurisy resulting from bacterial pneumonia resolves with appropriate antibiotic treatment of the pneumonia. Complicated effusions and empyema require drainage of the pleural space. Treatment of **neoplastic pleurisy**[181] should always be directed at the underlying malignancy, whenever effective therapy is available. Radiation of the chest wall and pleura may reduce pain. In cases where chemotherapy is ineffective, tube thoracoscopy and sclerosis may help reduce pain. **Benign asbestos pleurisy** resolves spontaneously and should be treated symptomatically.[182] Localized mesothelioma requires resection for cure and relief of pain. Diffuse mesothelioma may be treated with combination protocols of chemotherapy and resection. With modern protocols of treatment in the 20% of patients eligible for surgery, cure rates for mesothelioma have been reported to be as high as 40% at 2 years and 10% at 5 years.[183,184]

Most cases of **tuberculous pleuritis** will resolve spontaneously without any specific therapy over the course of 2 to 4 months, but 43%[185] to 65%[186] of these patients will subsequently develop active tuberculosis at a later date if left untreated. The current American Thoracic Society recommendations[187] would be for a 6-month regimen of isoniazid and rifampin, with the addition of pyrazinamide for the first 2 months of therapy along with ethambutol hydrochloride until the results of drug susceptibility studies are known. Given the usually small bacterial burden in these patients, it has been suggested that administration of 6 months of isoniazid and rifampin is sufficient in these patients to prevent subsequent development of active tuberculosis, provided the patient does not have resistant organisms.[188] Use of corticosteroids has been shown to decrease the duration of fever and the time required for complete resorption of the pleural fluid in these patients,[189,190] however, corticosteroids do not influence the development of residual pleural thickening (incidence 50% after 6 to 12 months of therapy).[191] Rarely, these patients may require decortication if a significant fibrothorax results. Pain usually resolves within a few weeks of starting therapy.

*Lupus pleuritis* has shown a definitely beneficial response (clearance of pleural effusions in 80% to 90%) to administration of systemic corticosteroids,[192,193] in contrast to the case seen in rheumatoid arthritis. Doses on the order of of 80 mg of prednisone given every other day and then with rapid tapering once symptoms are controlled have been recommended.[194] In those situations, when the pleural effusion is large and/or does not respond to corticosteroid therapy, consideration should be given to chemical pleurodesis and possibly a pleuroperitoneal shunt.[194]

**Rheumatoid pleuritis** exhibits a variable natural history with the primary goal of therapy being to prevent the progression to pleural fibrosis.[195,196] In one series,[195] just over 75% of patients experienced a spontaneous recovery within 3 months of the onset of the effusion. The literature is somewhat sparse and contradictory, however, it appears that some patients may respond favorably to systemic corticosteroids.[195] Despite the lack of efficacy data or controlled studies, it is recommended that nonsteroidal anti-inflammatory drugs (NSAIDs), such as aspirin or ibuprofen, be used in the initial 2 to 3 months. For effusions that persist after this time despite therapy, consideration should be given to therapeutic thoracentesis and possibly intrapleural injection of corticosteroids.[194] In patients who are symptomatic with dyspnea and have evidence of a thickened pleura, a decortication procedure should be considered.[196]

The effusions and pain due to **radiation pleuritis** may persist from months to years and the addition of steroids to their management may relieve symptoms and hasten resolution.[197,198]

*Pneumothorax:* The presence of extra-alveolar air does not necessitate specific treatment in and of itself. Patients with mild symptoms and pneumothorax (PTX) volumes less than 10% to 15% of a hemithorax may be considered for observation alone.[199,200] The body will reabsorb the air in the pleural space at a rate of about 1.25% of the volume of the hemithorax per day. This reabsorption rate can be hastened 4-fold to 6-fold by administering supplemental oxygen, due to the gradient between the partial pressure of nitrogen of the air in the pleural space and the partial pressure of nitrogen in the blood being enhanced. Concentrations of inspired oxygen higher than 40% are probably unnecessary.[201] Patients who are symptomatic, have more than a 15% PTX, or have a progressively increasing PTX can be treated with simple aspiration of the air or with tube thoracostomy.[199,200] The success rates for simple catheter aspiration in primary spontaneous PTX range from 45% to

83%.[200,202,203] Aspiration is not recommended for initial treatment of secondary spontaneous PTX or for recurrent primary PTX.[199,204] If the patient fails to re-expand the lung or if there is recurrent PTX after simple aspiration, tube thoracostomy is indicated. Most patients can be managed successfully with small-bore (ie, 7.0 F to 9.4 F) chest tubes. Chest tubes are generally left in place until at least 24 hours after the lung has totally re-expanded and there is no indication of an air leak.

Given PTX recurrence rates of 36% to 52% for either primary or secondary spontaneous PTX, followed by a 62% chance of recurrence after a second PTX, and an 83% chance after a third PTX, some authors advocate pleurodesis to decrease the risk of recurrence after treatment of the initial episode. Others favor chemical or operative pleurodesis only after a recurrence, unless the patient lives in a remote area or has an occupational risk (eg, pilot, diver). Many different materials have been used as sclerosing agents, including quinacrine, talc, olive oil, tetracycline, and bleomycin. Since quinacrine and tetracycline are no longer commercially available, doxycycline, aerosolized talc, and bleomycin appear to have become the more favored agents in use. Open thoracotomy with scarification of the pleura is an alternative to chemical pleurodesis; it is generally favored in patients with persistent air leaks or partially expanded lungs after 5 to 7 days of tube thoracostomy.

The occurrence of a tension PTX is a true medical emergency. When a patient is in respiratory distress and physical examination suggests the presence of a PTX, specific therapy should not be delayed for roentgenographic confirmation of the diagnosis.[204–206] These patients should receive high-concentration supplemental oxygen to treat and/or prevent severe hypoxemia and a large-bore needle or angiocath should be inserted into the pleural space through the second intercostal space at the midclavicular line of the presumably affected side. Escape of air from the needle with a rapid improvement in the patient's condition confirms the diagnosis; the procedure is followed up by definitive tube thoracostomy as soon as possible.[204,207]

***Pulmonary Embolism and Infarction:*** Unfractionated heparin is the drug of choice for both prophylaxis[208,209] against the development of PE and/or deep venous thrombosis (DVT), as well as for short-term treatment of these conditions once established.[210–212] Warfarin sodium is used for the prevention of venous thromboembolic disease in high-risk patients and in the long-term (ie, at least 3 months) treatment of DVT or PE.

The currently accepted short-term standard prophylactic regimen for venous thromboembolism is to give low, fixed subcutaneous doses (5000 U every 8 to 12 hours) of unfractionated heparin. This regimen is comparable in effectiveness to intermittent pneumatic compression of the calf in reducing the incidence of DVT. Only low-dose heparin, however, has been shown to reduce the incidence of fatal PE (a 60% to 70% reduction) and total mortality.[213–215] Since these methods are relatively ineffective for patients undergoing orthopedic procedures or major urologic surgery, an adjusted-dose heparin regimen should be used, starting with 3500 U subcutaneously, tid, and adjusted as needed to maintain the midinterval activated partial thromboplastin time at the upper limits of the normal range. Low molecular weight heparins do not share this inconvenience and are as effective, but further randomized trials are needed to document the safety and efficacy profile of this agent prior to its routine use. Oral warfarin can also be used for prophylaxis of venous thromboembolism with benefit noted for regimens begun on or before the first postoperative day targeted at achieving an international normalized ratio (INR) of 2.0 to 3.0.[216]

The treatment of calf-vein thrombosis remains somewhat controversial. The likelihood of proximal extension of clot within 1 to 2 weeks in patients who do not receive anticoagulant therapy is approximately 20%. Currently, these patients should either receive heparin and warfarin in the "usual" fashion for the treatment of established DVT (see below), or are followed serially with noninvasive testing while anticoagulants are withheld.[217]

Heparin is currently the standard initial treatment for the majority of patients with venous thromboembolic disease, and has been shown recently[218] to be required for the prevention of extension of DVT or occurrence of PE when compared with oral anticoagulants alone. Heparin may be administered by subcutaneous injection or by intravenous infusion. Continuous infusion is preferred over intermittent injections because the incidence of hemorrhagic complications are less frequent.[219] Failure to achieve adequate anticoagulation in a timely fashion is responsible for early recurrences and/or extensions.[218,220–223] Recent evidence suggests that the use of weight-based nomograms for intravenous heparin results in significantly better early anticoagulation (97% of subjects with therapeutic levels within 24 hours) and fewer recurrences.[221] Beginning with a bolus infusion of 80 U/kg and a continuous drip at 18 U/kg per hour, the dose is strictly adjusted according to a standard regimen to maintain the activated partial thromboplastin time in the range of 1.5 to 2.3 times control value.

Conventionally, the duration of treatment with heparin for DVT or PE has been 7 to 10 days, followed by oral anticoagulation for 3 to 6 months.[224,225] More recently, studies have shown that a 5-day regimen of heparin is safe provided that oral anticoagulation is begun at approximately the same time and that the prothrombin time is in the therapeutic range for at least 24 hours prior to discontinuing the heparin.[226,227] The frequency of bleeding complications was 9% to 12% for these regimens, and this is similar to previously reported bleeding rates.[212,220,226]

The optimal duration of longer-term secondary prevention anticoagulant therapy remains unclear. Most authorities recommend at least 3 to 6 months of oral anticoagulation for proximal DVT or PE. Patients with persistent risk factors for venous thromboembolic disease or with recurrent DVT and/or PE should receive warfarin therapy for greater than 3 months.[210] Furthermore, those with more than two episodes of DVT and/or PE, those with uncontrolled cancer, and those patients with inherited abnormalities of the clotting cascade should be indefinitely treated with warfarin . The optimal intensity of oral anticoagulation is generally recommended at doses that provide an INR of 2.0 to 3.0.[225,228] However, in the case of the antiphospholipid antibody thrombosis syndrome, the INR should be maintained at 3.0 or greater.[229] These levels of long-term anticoagulation are efficacious in preventing recurrent thromboembolism and are associated with a less than 5% risk of bleeding complications. While higher intensity warfarin therapy (ie, INR of 3.0 to 4.5) has been shown to increase the risk of bleeding to around 20%,[230,231] this has not been the case in the antiphospholipid antibody thrombosis syndrome.[229]

The use of low-molecular-weight heparins, selective thrombin inhibitors (eg, hirudin), and factor Xa inhibitors have just recently begun to be studied in clinical efficacy trials in humans and it is too soon to tell what their roles will become. Low-molecular-weight heparins have received the most study to date and are currently FDA approved for the treatment of DVT.

A subgroup of patients with venous thromboembolic disease will develop severe bleeding complications from anticoagulant use, develop recurrent DVT and/or PE while on therapeutic concentrations of anticoagulant agents, or initially have an absolute contraindication to the use of these medications. In this group of patients, interruption of the inferior vena cava either surgically or with the use of intraluminal mechanical devices (ie, "filters"), may be an effective alternative to anticoagulation.[232] Pulmonary embolism after placement of inferior vena cave filters occurs in up to 2.4% of cases, but fatal events occur in fewer than 1%.

Thrombolysis has a somewhat controversial role in the management of PE. In the past, this modality had been relegated to the role of being a "heroic measure" used only in situations of impending death from acute right heart failure. As more and more physicians have gained experience with thrombolytic agents, now used almost routinely in the therapy of acute MI, proponents have argued for more expanded indications for thrombolysis in PE. Current estimates are that no more than about 10% of patients with PE receive thrombolytics in the United States.[233] As the major long-term morbidity of PE is chronic pulmonary hypertension, complete dissolution of the thrombus is now seen by some as being just as imperative as accelerated clot lysis is for the emergent reversal of cardiogenic shock. For those patients with PE who are treated with heparin alone, the risk for recurrent PE or death within 14 days of initial diagnosis is at least 10%.[233,234] While PIOPED hinted at an improved long-term outcome for those patients treated with thrombolysis, to date there have been no convincing studies that support a reduction in the fatality rate from PE treated with thrombolytic agents. Streptokinase, urokinase, and rt-PA have all received FDA approval for use in PE (Table VIII) and these agents have been shown in prospective trials in comparison to heparin therapy alone to cause more rapid and complete clot dissolution, improved right ventricular function, improved pulmonary perfusion, and improved exercise tolerance and quality of life.[235–237] Until further supportive data are available, we would not recommend the routine use of thrombolytics.

***Pulmonary Hypertension:*** Secondary pulmonary hypertension accounts for the majority of those patients with pulmonary hypertension and often responds well to therapy, but even when poorly responsive to therapy, the prognosis is generally not as grim as it is for those with primary pulmonary hypertension. Treatment is most successful when an underlying cause can be identified and eliminated prior to the onset of irreversible damage to the pulmonary vasculature. For those patients in whom removal of an inciting cause is not possible, therapy is aimed at decreasing pulmonary resistance and improving compensatory mechanisms to manage right ventricular pressure overload.

When specific causes of secondary pulmonary hypertension exist (eg, those that cause left ventricular failure), decreased resistance to pulmonary blood flow can be accomplished by lowering left atrial and/or ventricular diastolic pressures. Only when there is significant active vasoconstriction of the small muscular arteries or arterioles will pulmonary vasodilators be potentially effective. Various vasodilating agents have been used for acute and/or chronic management of pulmonary hypertension, including oxygen, hydralazine hydrochloride, phentolamine, isoproterenol, diazoxide, nifedipine, prostacyclin, tolazoline hydrochloride, verapamil, nitroglycerin, and captopril. These agents have met with variable, and sometimes conflicting, efficacy. Evidence exists that favorable hemodynamic findings during acute drug testing trials predicts the long-term results of treatment for patients with primary pulmonary hypertension.[238,239]

Both single-lung and heart-lung transplantation have been performed on patients with advanced, otherwise untreatable, pulmonary vascular disease.[240,241] With current surgical techniques and immunosuppressive therapy, survival at 3 years is approximately 65%.[241]

Chronic anticoagulation is clearly indicated in those with pulmonary hypertension on the basis of recurrent pulmonary emboli. Its role in other forms of secondary pulmonary hypertension is not of proven benefit. Clinical evidence does suggest, however, that anticoagulants may

---

**Table VIII**
FDA-Approved Thrombolytic Regimens for Pulmonary Embolism

**Streptokinase:** 250,000 IU as a loading dose over 30 minutes, followed by 100,000 IU/hr for 24 hours—approved in 1977

**Urokinase:** 4400 IU/kg as a loading dose over 10 minutes, followed by 4400 IU/kg/h for 12 to 24 hours—approved in 1978

**rt-PA:** 100 mg as a continuous peripheral infusion administered over 2 hours—approved in 1990 improve the prognosis in at least some patients with severe primary pulmonary hypertension.[242,243]

Stellate ganglion blocks have been successfully used in relieving chest pain associated with pulmonary hypertension.[244]

## Panic, Hyperventilation, and Anxiety

Failure to diagnose and treat anxiety/hyperventilation syndrome/panic disorder is been expensive. Although panic disorder and hyperventilation syndrome are a common cause of chest pain, up to 79% of these patients receive no specific therapy.[245] These patients, on average, visit physicians or emergency departments 2.2 times per month and are hospitalized almost once a year due to chest pain. The average cost of evaluating these patients has been estimated to be $3500 per year.[37] Up to 50% may fail to return to work or resume normal physical activity. All patients with unexplained chest pain should be screened for panic/anxiety/hyperventilation syndromes and, when the diagnosis is likely, be referred to a qualified practitioner for therapy.

Although numerous therapies have been reported to be effective for panic disorder and hyperventilation syndrome, few studies have evaluated the efficacy of treatment on the symptom of chest pain. Most reports of efficacy in the treatment of chest pain due to these disorders have come from case reports or small, frequently uncontrolled studies. Since controlled studies have indicated a 30% response to placebo,[246] initial therapy should be conservative and only those patients with persistent or severe disease should receive formal therapy. Therapy typically involves cognitive-behavioral therapy, pharmacotherapy, and breathing/relaxation retraining.

Cognitive-behavioral therapy[247] aims to educate the patient that anxiety, panic, and associated symptoms, such as chest pain, result from the misinterpretation of sensations produced in the chest as a result of hyperventilation. Identification of the problem as a misattribution of sensations seeks to reassure the patient that the symptoms are not a sign of danger thereby reducing anxiety and subsequent autonomic arousal. This allows the patient to understand the symptoms and not catastrophize about them. Voluntary hyperventilation may produce symptoms demonstrating to patients the benign nature of the problem and indicating that voluntary hypoventilation at the time of increased symptoms may result in resolution of the symptoms. This cognitive approach allows patients to understand how symptoms arise and how they may be controlled. All patients are typically counselled to avoid alcohol, caffeine, and psychoactive substances, such as cocaine and marijuana, since the consumption of or withdrawal from these substances may trigger an attack.

When cognitive-behavioral therapy fails or is not available for panic disorder or hyperventilation syndrome, pharmacotherapy may be effective. While beta blockade has been helpful in some patients, overall results have been conflicting. Imipramine or desipramine hydrochloride starting at a dose of 10 mg/day and increasing if necessary to more than 150 mg/day has been effective in some patients.[246] Although fluoxetine hydrochloride (Prozac) and sertraline hydrochloride (Zoloft) also have been helpful in patients with panic attacks who have failed behavioral therapy, there are no studies published on their efficacy in reducing chest pain. Beitman et al.[248] evaluated the role of alprazolam in treating patients with chest pain and panic disorder and reported a 50% or greater reduction in the frequency of panic attacks and complete elimination of the symptoms of chest pain during attacks in 57% of responders. The effective drug dose ranged from 1.25 to 6 mg/day. In a study of 15 patients with panic disorder and chest pain, the frequency of chest pain decreased (p = 0.06) after 8 weeks of treatment.[249] Uncontrolled studies of clonazepam and other benzodiazepines have claimed efficacy in treating panic disorder.

Behavioral therapy aimed at modifying the breathing pattern has also been successful. Evans and Lum[250] reported that 50 patients with hyperventilation-induced chest pain were taught diaphragmatic breathing and control strategies for an average of 10 sessions and instructed to avoid both acute and chronic hyperventilation. After 6 months, 53% were symptom-free and 47% improved. Hegel et al.[251] reported significant decreases in chest pain in three women with hyperventilation syndrome and chest pain who were instructed in diaphragmatic breathing and progressive muscle relaxation training. DeGuire et al.[252] compared the effects of three methods: (1) guided breathing retraining, (2) guided breathing retraining with thoracoabdominal movement and temperature monitoring, and (3) guided breathing retraining with thoracoabdominal movement and temperature monitoring and end-tidal $CO_2$ monitoring. Compared to untreated controls, all three strategies were equally effective in reducing respiratory rate, increasing end-tidal $CO_2$ and decreasing the frequency of hyperventilation episodes. However, the frequency of chest pain or the mean severity of symptoms during an attack did not change. Other controlled studies suggest that breathing retraining is effective.[253] In 640 patients treated with the above general strategy, Lum reported that 70% were rendered asymptomatic, 20% to 25% improved, and 5% to 10% failed to respond.[254] One third of patients can be completely treated in two to three visits.[255]

## Gastrointestinal

**Esophageal Diseases:** The structural integrity of the lower esophageal sphincter is the primary determinant of esophageal injury in GERD. Other important pathogenic factors in the degree of reflux-induced injury include the volume of the gastric refluxate, the potency (eg, pH, presence of pepsin and/or other digestive enzymes) of the refluxate, the efficiency of gastroesophageal clearance, and the tissue resistance and repair capabilities of the esophageal mucosa. The pathogenesis of GERD

and management and treatment options are discussed more fully in Chapter 1, "Cough." The basis of therapy for GERD is similar when considering treatment of GERD-induced chronic cough or GERD-induced chest pain and will be discussed only briefly here.

Conservative therapy to alleviate symptoms of GERD includes dietary/behavioral interventions, mechanical measures, and antacids . More aggressive medical therapy includes the use of $H_2$ receptor antagonists, proton pump inhibitors, prokinetic agents, sucralfate, and combinations of these.

Data on the efficacy of medical therapy for GERD-induced chest pain are unfortunately limited. At least one study[256] has shown symptomatic relief of heartburn (34%), acid regurgitation (67%), and chest pain (67%) in patients treated with sucralfate. It would also appear from this study that endoscopic healing of the esophageal mucosa is not required for the relief of chest pain symptoms. Preliminary data also indicate that omeprazole and ranitidine may be helpful.[228,257]

Overall it is clear that many questions remain unanswered with respect to treatment of GERD and symptomatic relief from chest pain. Additional studies are underway in an effort to resolve some of these issues. In the meantime, some authorities would recommend considering empiric therapy for GERD in patients with unexplained chest pain. Duration of therapy and the endpoints of interest would have to be defined on an individual basis and it is unclear if this approach has any clear advantages over initially performing direct testing.

The medical therapy for painful esophageal motility disorders is principally aimed at reducing smooth muscle spasm.[258] Nitrate preparations have been studied given the finding that the smooth muscle of the esophagus relaxes in a similar manner to vascular smooth muscle.[258] Unfortunately, these studies have shown conflicting results and are further limited due to small numbers of patients studied and lack of randomized, placebo-controlled investigations. Several studies have documented the ability of anticholinergic agents to decrease the amplitude of esophageal pressures during peristalsis and to lower the pressure in the lower esophageal sphincter.[259,260] While these agents might be potentially useful in the treatment of hypercontractile esophageal motility disorders, there are no published clinical trials that assess their use in the treatment of patients with unexplained chest pain. A high incidence of psychiatric disorders has been reported in patients with esophageal motility disorders.[261] While it is unclear if these agents (trazodone, alprazolam) actually improve the manometric abnormalities under investigation, they have been reported to be associated with a significantly greater global improvement in symptoms and panic scores[248,262] in these patients. Calcium channel antagonists interfere with the entry of calcium into smooth muscle cells and therefore would be expected to produce a decrease in the amplitude of esophageal contraction and a decrease in lower esophageal sphincter pressures. Both nifedipine (10 to 40 mg, tid) and diltiazem (60 to 90 mg, qid.) have demonstrated this effect in conjunction with improvement in chest pain,[263–265] however, long-term (12-week) studies of nifedipine have not shown sustained benefit for symptom control. Verapamil has not been studied in this regard.

### Esophageal Rupture and Perforation/Incarcerated Diagphramatic Hernias: The importance of an early diagnosis of esophageal rupture is borne out by surgical mortality data—simple repair performed within 24 hours carries a 20% mortality[266] whereas a mortality of 29% to 50% is associated with repairs performed later than 24 hours (due to breakdown of suture lines). In contrast, "conservative therapy" (eg, "nothing by mouth" (*nil per os*, NPO) instructions, nasogastric suction, drainage of pleural fluid, antibiotics, supplemental nutrition) may yield mortality rates down to approximately 9%.[266] Currently most authorities[267–269] recommend immediate thoracotomy and esophageal repair for those patients presenting within 24 to 48 hours.

Once beyond this time frame, a more conservative approach is advocated with emphasis placed on maintaining adequate pleural drainage (thoracoscopy with irrigation, broad spectrum antibiotics, and reduction of acid reflux with the use of $H_2$ blockers.

Patients presenting in extremis due to gastrointestinal viscera incarcerated in a diaphragmatic hernia (up to 46% of presentations[270]) have at least a 32% mortality. Definitive therapy involves surgical exploration and possible resection of any strangulated viscera. Most authors recommend resection of paraesophageal hernias even when asymptomatic to prevent possible gastric volvulus and strangulation of herniated viscera.[271–273] Successful laparoscopic reduction of paraesophageal hernias has now been reported.[272,274,275]

### Pancreatitis: The majority of patients with acute pancreatitis will recover without suffering any major sequelae. Overall the mortality in acute pancreatitis is about 10%[276,277]; however, if complications develop (eg, pancreatic necrosis, phlegmon, pseudocyst, infection, hypovolemic shock, renal failure, acute respiratory distress syndrome) mortality may increase to more than 50%.[278,279] Death within the first week is generally the result of one of the systemic complications while death occurring after the first week can generally be attributed to a local complication.[280] Overall, about 25% of patients will develop a complication, and this is the group that suffers the greatest mortality. Multiple prognostic systems that can be used in an attempt to estimate the severity of acute pancreatitis exist,[278,281,282] but each suffers from a substantial rate of falsely high and falsely low estimates of severity.[283] The appearance of the pancreas on computed tomography may also be used as a marker of severity in acute pancreatitis with the lack of vascular enhancement suggesting the presence of pancreatic necrosis.[284,285] Computed tomography of the pancreas shares a prognostic capability similar to the other grading systems.

Initial medical therapy is aimed at general supportive measures (eg, aggressive intravenous hydration, parenteral analgesics, enforcing NPO instructions, and managing any potential metabolic derangements) with the goals of minimizing the ongoing pancreatic injury and directing specific therapies at any complications that may occur. Clinical trials testing various agents that may reduce pancreatic secretion[286,287] or inhibit pancreatic proteases[288–290] have been unable to show any convincing therapeutic effects. Likewise, total parenteral nutrition[291,292] and peritoneal lavage[293,294] have also been evaluated and generally failed to show any significant benefits.

In patients at high risk of developing infection, especially those with 30% or more pancreatic necrosis seen on dynamic computed tomography scanning, imipenem or the quinolones are both acceptable for the majority of organisms that may be responsible.[295,296]

The primary therapy for large or complicated pseudocysts is generally surgical, although catheter drainage may also be attempted in those collections that do not contain areas of necrosis or multiple septations that would serve to prevent complete drainage of the pseudocyst.[297] The tried and true method of waiting 6 to 8 weeks before surgical intervention remains a valid concept, allowing time for the wall of the pseudocyst to mature.

**Biliary Disease:** The definitive treatment of cholecystitis is primarily surgical. Medical management involves intravenous hydration, analgesic agents, antibiotic therapy, and nasogastric tube decompression if a significant ileus coexists. Surgery is generally performed after a few days of medical treatment unless there is a clinical suspicion of complications (perforation or empyema) or if the patient's status deteriorates. Laparoscopic surgery is an option in some of these patients but as many as 50% may require conversion to open cholecystectomy in the setting of intense inflammation.[298,299] Percutaneous or endoscopic drainage of the gallbladder are alternate therapies for patients too ill or debilitated to undergo cholecystectomy. Most patients with biliary colic will require treatment with potent analgesic agents, either opiates or intramuscular diclofenac sodium.[300]

**Gastric Disease:** Treatment regimens for peptic ulcer disease have changed dramatically in the last few years with the appreciation of the importance of *Helicobacter pylori* in the natural history of chronic gastritis, duodenal ulcers, and most gastric ulcers. Patients treated with antisecretory agents alone frequently recur (35% to 55%[301,302]) when these agents are discontinued.[303] Epidemiologic studies have shown, however, that eradication of *H pylori* virtually abolishes relapses. The current debate is ongoing regarding the optimal therapy for these patients and in whom attempts at eradication are warranted.

At present the most effective drug regimen for eradication of *H pylori* is a 2-week course of triple therapy comprised of colloidal bismuth subcitrate (120 mg, qid) plus metronidazole (400 mg, tid) plus tetracycline (500 mg, qid).[303] The single most important factor for success with this regimen is ensuring patient compliance, which may be particularly difficult given the frequency of dosing and common onset of side effects (nausea, vomiting, diarrhea, taste disturbance). When at least 60% of the regimen is administered, successful eradication occurs in more than 90% of patients.[304,305] Amoxicillin (500 mg, qid) may be substituted for tetracycline, however, more patients are reportedly intolerant to this drug.[303]

An alternative regimen that is nearly as effective as triple therapy is the combination of omeprazole (20 mg, bid) with amoxicillin (1 g, bid) for a total of 14 days. This combination has an efficacy in the vicinity of 80%, has fewer side effects than triple therapy, and is generally easier for patients to comply with.[303]

In cases where the initial attempt at eradication of *H pylori* is unsuccessful, consideration should be given to a trial with the alternate combination (ie, substitute dual therapy for triple therapy and vice versa). Ultimately, maintenance on $H_2$ receptor antagonists may be necessary in some cases when attempts at eradication fail.

For a patient whose course is complicated with perforation or active bleeding, surgical intervention is frequently required.[306] This is especially common in elderly females with gastric ulcers who have been taking corticosteroids or NSAIDs.

**Aerophagia:** Perhaps the most important therapeutic modality for aerophagia is its prevention by avoidance of those food substrates known to be associated with excess gas production. Medications such as simethicone can help to absorb some of the gas burden and may also prove helpful. In cases of massive gastric or colonic distension, decompression with nasogastric and/or rectal tubes may be indicated. In situations where hollow viscera are distended to the point of ischemia or impending/documented perforation, surgical intervention may be lifesaving. Therapy should be individualized for each patient with consideration also given to the chronicity or acuteness of the presentation to help guide therapy.

## Thoracic Muscles and Bones

**Pectoral Girdle Syndrome:** In most cases, acute pectoral girdle syndrome resolves with muscle rest and anti-inflamatories or analgesics. Long-term therapy should concentrate on altering work ergonomics. In cases where bra-strap pressure has resulted in pain, effective treatment includes not wearing a bra,[307] wearing a wider bra strap, and reduction mammoplasty.[308]

**Fibrositis:** Treatment usually consists of xylocaine injection of trigger points, stretching, flexibility, heat or ice to affected areas, avoidance of provocative factors, and aerobic conditioning. No studies have thoroughly evaluated this "conventional" regimen. Provocative factors have been reported to include keyboard activities, prolonged standing or walking, heavy lifting or bending, or repetitive move-

ments.[309] Active exercise does not trigger exacerbations[310] and results in an increased quality of life and self-efficacy.[311]

Low-dose antidepressant medications administered at bedtime appear helpful. Double-blind, placebo-controlled trials have demonstrated short-term efficacy of amitriptyline hydrochloride (25 to 75 mg/day),[312,313] or cyclobenzaprine hydrochloride (10 mg/day), or a combination of ibuprofen and alprazolam.[314] The addition of ibuprofen to cyclobenzaprine reduces morning stiffness.[315] Fluoxetine,[316] chlormezanone,[317] and the more catecholaminergic antidepressants (eg, bupropion)[318] are ineffective. A randomized, double-blinded trial of electroacupuncture has also been used to reduce pain.[319]

**Benign Overuse:** Effective treatment includes rest of affected muscles, analgesics or anti-inflammatory drugs, and future avoidance of overuse.

**Xiphodynia, Xiphoidalgia:** While pain is frequently self-limited and may resolve without treatment,[320] injection with 5 to 15 cc of 1% xylocaine with a 22- to 25-gauge needle effectively relieves persistent symptoms.[321–323] Anti-inflammatories and steroid injections are also helpful.[322] The xiphoid may be difficult to palpate and care must be taken to avoid perforation of underlying viscera. Tack hammer xiphoid may require surgical resection.

**Sternoclavicular Joint Disease:** Treatment usually involves analgesics, anti-inflammatories, rest, and therapy directed at the underlying disease. Infection is usually treated with intravenous antibiotics. Gout and rheumatoid arthritis are treated in the conventional fashion. Traumatic disruption of the joint may require evaluation by an orthopedic surgeon.

**Precordial Catch:** Precordial catch is self-limited and requires no treatment.

**Tietze's Syndrome and Costochondritis:** Treatment for Tietze's syndrome and costochondritis consists of heat, nonsteroidal anti-inflammatories, and analge-

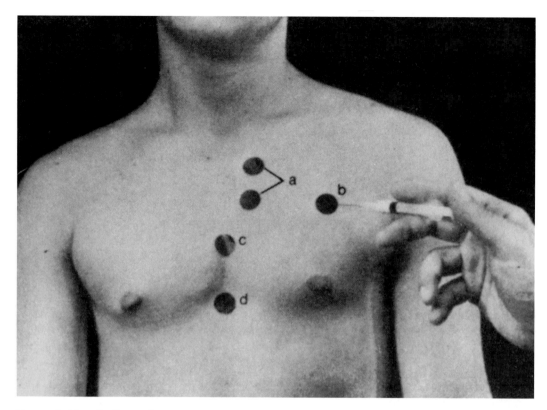

**Figure 6.** Dots indicate the most common sites requiring injection in the anterior chest wall: (a) the 2nd and 3rd costochondral junctions, (b) the pectoralis major muscle, (c) sternalis muscle, and (d) xiphoid. Reproduced by permission from the Southern Medical Journal (1988;81:64).

sics. Injection (similar to that for xiphodynia) with lidocaine-corticosteroid solution is also helpful (Figure 6).[320]

***Ankylosing Spondylitis:*** The treatment for ankylosing spondylitis resulting in chest pain is no different than that for ankylosing spondylitis in general. Patients improve with physiotherapy and conditioning rehabilitation,[324] anti-inflammatory medications, and avoidance of activities prone to inflame the sites of pain.

***Rib Pain:*** Rib pain usually resolves with rest and mild analgesics. In severe cases, nerve block may be useful.

***Cervical and Thoracic Disks and Spine Disease:*** Treatment remains controversial. Patients not responding to analgesics, non-

steroidal anti-inflammatories, muscle relaxants, and decreased mobilization may require surgical correction. Osteomyelitis should be treated with antibiotics appropriate to the infecting organism.

***Thoracic Outlet Syndrome:*** The pain from thoracic outlet syndrome may resolve with use of an orthosis,[325] a short-term graduated exercise program,[326] or an occupational change that eliminates exposure to the inciting injury. The role of surgery remains controversial and surgery should only be considered when the diagnosis is firmly established, the anatomy is well defined preoperatively, and severe symptoms persists despite failure of conservative therapy. The efficacy of surgery appears to vary depending on the operation performed and the cause of the nerve compression. Transaxillary first rib resection alone is successful in only 52% of cases.[327] When first rib resection is combined with scalenectomy success rates have been reported as 54% excellent, 28% good, 10% fair, and 8% had recurrent symptoms.[328] Others have reported a 72% success rate and argued that there is no difference in outcome whether the first rib is resected or not.[329] Most authors agree that cervical ribs, when present, should be resected. When symptoms follow trauma surgery appears to be more effective. With supraclavicular neurolysis and scalenectomy, 90% of patients report a good or excellent outcome.[330]

**Diaphragm:** When pain arises from irritation of the peritoneal surface of the diaphragm, pain resolves with appropriate treatment of the underlying abdominal process. Polymyositis is treated with high-dose steroids. Trichinosis is treated with rest, analgesics, antipyretics, and antihelminthics.[331]

## Neck: Thyroiditis

Bacterial pyogenic thyroiditis is treated with antibiotics and drainage if local abscess occurs. Antibiotic therapy should be guided by needle aspiration cultures. Subacute granulomatous thyroiditis, when mild, may be managed with analgesics such as aspirin. More severe cases respond to prednisone (20 to 30 mg per day) tapered over a few weeks. If hyperthyroidism develops, beta blockers are effective until normal thyroid function returns.

## Skin

The pain of varicella-zoster (ie, shingles) may be shortened in duration by the use of acyclovir (Zovirax) (800 mg orally, five times a day for 7 to 10 days) or famciclovir (500 to 750 mg, tid for 7 days).[332] An intravenous preparation of acyclovir is available for patients unable to take oral medication. Pain decreases markedly over approximately 8 days.[333,334] Preliminary

data indicate that alpha-2-interferon is also effective but probably has more side effects than acyclovir therapy.[335,336] Intralesional or intramuscular injection of hyperimmune anti–varicella-zoster immunoglobulins (Uman-VZIG) has been reported to shorten the duration of acute pain to approximately 5 days.[334] Post herpetic neuralgia, pain persisting weeks after the skin lesions have resolved, can be difficult to treat and several treatment regimens have been recommended. Famciclovir when started soon after the rash appeared had a two-fold faster resolution of postherpetic neuralgia, reducing the median duration of postherpetic neuralgia to 2 months.[332] Sympathetic blocks appear helpful if performed within the first 2 months of symptoms.[337] Studies performed prior to the release of acyclovir and famciclovir concluded that the best therapy is amitriptyline, topical capsaicin, and transcutaneous electrical stimulation.[333] Steroids are not recommended due to inadequate data supporting their value and the availability of less toxic, more effective therapy.

## Breasts

**Mastitis:** Mastitis usually responds well to a penicillinase-resistant synthetic penicillin, a first generation cephalosporin, or vancomycin hydrochloride. Some prescribe bromocriptine mesylate for lactating women to decrease lactation.[338]

**Mammary Duct Ectasia:** The treatment for mammary duct ectasia remains controversial. Analgesics, excisional surgery, and antibiotics have been effective in individual cases.[339]

**Fibrocystic Disease:** Therapy for fibrocystic mastalgia remains nonstandardized and frequently unsuccessful. Initial therapy usually consists of reassurance, mild analgesics, a decrease in dietary fat, cessation of oral contraceptives and hormone supplements, and wearing a well-fitting bra. Patients who have persistent life-altering pain may be prescribed primrose oil supplements, bromocriptine, tamoxifen citrate, or GnRH analogues.[338] The five most common treatments in Great Britain include danazol, analgesics, diuretics, local excision, and bromocriptine. Less than 50% of patients note an obvious improvement with treatment. In those noting improvement, noncyclic pain usually resolves within 2 years and cyclic pain responded more favorably to hormonal manipulation.[338]

**Breast Cancer:** Patients with breast cancer require definitive staging and then appropriate radiation, chemotherapy, or surgery.

**Trauma:** Pain from trauma responds to analgesics and resolves within a few weeks. Mondor's disease requires anticoagulation, anti-inflammatory drugs, and analgesia.[340]

**Breast Implants:** Pain typically resolves with removal of the implant.

**Gynecomastia:** Therapy consists of eliminating the offending drugs, treating any underlying endocrinologic disorder, and prescribing analgesics.

## Mediastinum

Spontaneous pneumomediastinum typically resolves without specific treatment.[341] Mediastinitis due to rupture of an airway or the esophagus requires surgical exploration and drainage, repair of the perforation, and prolonged antibiotic therapy. When infection extends from the neck or below the diaphragm, antibiotics coverage must include anaerobic coverage with high-dose clindamycin and metronidazole being the preferred choices of antibiotics. Surgical drainage may also be necessary. Mass lesions compressing adjacent mediastinal structures may require excision for relief of pain.

## Nerves

**Intercostal Nerve Injury due to Internal Mammary Artery Grafting:** Pain has been effectively treated with transcutaneous electrical nerve stimulator (TENS), amitriptyline, and desensitization.[342]

**Sternal Wires:** Pain due to sternal wires resolves with removal of the sternal wires.

**Neuromas:** No study addresses treatment of thoracic neuromas. One would assume that, like other neuromas, these would be treated by section and reimplantation of the proximal nerve with or without excision of the neuroma itself. External neurolysis does not appear to be effective.[343]

## Kidneys

**Pyelonephritis:** Uncomplicated pyelonephritis in nonpregnant women is typically treated on an outpatient basis with 3 weeks of antibiotics primarily directed at *Escherichia coli*.[344] Pregnant women, men, diabetics, elderly patients, immunocompromised patients, and patients with renal calculi require further diagnostic evaluation and inpatient parenteral antibiotic therapy until clinically improving.[345–347] Treatment in most cases is highly successful and surgical intervention is rarely required.

**Renal Infarct:** Since most cases of renal infarction result from embolization, all patients with no obvious source of emboli should be evaluated by echocardiography and blood cultures. Identification of endocarditis or an intracardiac thrombus necessitates treatment of the underlying disease with antibiotics, anticoagulation, anti-arrhythmic medications, cardioversion, or valvular surgery depending on the patient. Pain from the renal infarct is treated symptomatically with analgesics. Angiography to assess the potential for surgical revascularization should be considered. Cases that demonstrate collateral perfusion of the renal vascular tree on angiography may benefit from revascularization in that nutrient but not functional levels of perfusion may have preserved the renal cortex.

***Renal Calculi:*** Pain should be controlled with analgesics, and narcotics may be necessary for adequate relief. Pain resolves with stone passage and may be promoted by hydration. Although most stones pass spontaneously, surgical removal, lithotripsy, and retrograde basket retrieval may all be indicated in selected patients.

***Drugs:*** When a drug has resulted in chest pain, withdrawal of the causative agent constitutes effective therapy.

Chest pain due to cocaine may be complicated by MI and requires additional therapy. Patients who develop infarction usually have a typical ECG pattern of injury with a creatine kinase rise maximal 12 to 16 hours after the onset of pain. In 101 consecutive patients with cocaine-associated chest pain who did not infarct,[348] ECG abnormalities and creatine kinase elevations were also common. Of these patients, 43% had ST segment elevations that met criteria for thrombolytic therapy and 47% had elevations in creatine kinase. Contrary to those experiencing an MI, creatine kinase concentrations fell after admission. Young patients with resolved pain and normal ECG do not infarct and do not require admission due to chest pain. Patients with coronary risk factors, especially smoking, and an abnormal ECG require admission but can safely be discharged if evaluation is negative at 12 hours.[349] Treatment for cocaine-induced MI does not substantially differ from that of any given MI.

## Nonspecific Treatment of Chest Pain Syndromes

While these therapies theoretically apply to virtually all causes of chest pain, they are at times the only therapy available. Of patients with noncardiac chest pain, 50% continue to experience pain and at least 30% suffer significant disability at up to 4 years after catheterization.[350]

The available literature describes many potential treatments, although mostly on the basis of case reports or small series of patients. As might be expected there is a paucity of prospective, double-blind, placebo-controlled human studies on this topic, and one must be cautious in generalizing the results from one group of patients to another. Clinicians must try to avoid treating patients presenting with **acute chest pain syndromes** with nonspecific therapies, since nonspecific treatment may only confuse or interfere with specific treatments once a cause is established, and may actually cause additional morbidity or mortality due to delay in diagnosis and institution of definitive therapy when available. The potential role for nonspecific treatments is limited to those patients exhibiting **chronic chest pain syndromes**, especially those who remain without a specific diagnosis for their pain after appropriate evaluation has ruled out the existence of life-threatening disease or when specific therapy has failed. Various drug therapies, physiotherapy, hypnotherapy, acupuncture, behavioral/relaxation techniques, nerve stimulation/ablation procedures, and surgical alternatives have been studied. These modalities are usually somewhat controversial owing to a lack of agreement concerning their indications for use and a lack of consistency in any reported efficacy.

### Analgesics

Systemic analgesic administration is usually the clinician's first choice of therapy, with NSAIDs and narcotic agents most frequently employed. Unlike narcotics, physical dependence or tolerance does not develop with the use of aspirin, acetaminophen, or NSAIDs; however, a ceiling effect is present whereby further increases in dosage beyond a certain point do not provide any additional analgesia.

Opioids are conveniently classified in terms of receptor subtype affinities (ie, mu, delta, kappa). Most of the clinically useful opioids are mu agonists. While there is a clear consensus on the use of morphine and other strong opiods in treatment of severe pain from cancer, their chronic use for the nonmalignant pain remains more controversial.[351-353] Opioids exhibit variable effectiveness in the short-term, and it is noteworthy that not all pain is responsive to narcotic administration.

The various potential side effects or toxicities that may occur with these nonspecific therapies must be considered. They may include asthma exacerbations, bleeding diathesis, tinnitus, gastrointestinal irritation (bleeding, ulcers, perforation), renal failure, leukopenia, bone marrow suppression for NSAIDs; and hypoventilation, sedation, alteration in mood, confusion, nausea and vomiting, postural hypotension, ileus, tolerance to opiates, and urinary retention for narcotics. Readers interested in additional details regarding these agents and their use are referred to recent, more comprehensive sources.[351,352,354]

## Psychotropic Drugs

When systemic analgesic therapy is not entirely successful for the relief of chronic or intractable pain, the next most frequent management alternatives or adjuncts include psychotropic agents. Since a sizeable number of patients with chronic pain are clinically depressed, tricyclic antidepressants, such as amitriptyline, imipramine, or desipramine, and monoamine oxidase inhibitors, such as phenelzine sulfate, have been studied extensively in a number of chronic pain syndromes.[355] These agents likely have separate analgesic and antidepressant actions as a result of alterations in central neurotransmitter functions in the brain, thalamus, and spinal cord. While there is little evidence to support the use of any one tricyclic antidepressant agent over any other, the relative side effect profiles can be used in an attempt to minimize any adverse effects. Physicians should be aware that relapse or lack of any noted response may be due to inadequate regimens and/or poor patient compliance.

Neuroleptic agents, anticonvulsants (especially carbamazepine, clonazepam, valproic acid, or diphenylhydantoin) and antianxiety-sedative drugs (benzodiazepines) have also been effectively used, alone and in combination with other medications, in the treatment of chronic pain syndromes. A review of the numerous clinical trials involving these agents is beyond the scope of this discussion; further details of dosing, effectiveness, and treatment descriptions can be found elsewhere.[355]

## Cognitive-behavioral Strategies

Since the desire to seek care for chest pain has been shown to be related to the personality traits of neuroticism, type A behavior, and "vital exhaustion," behavioral interventions directed toward these traits may reduce utilization of health care resources or the patient's perception of morbidity even if symptoms are not reduced.[356] This demonstrates that learned behaviors (eg, avoidance, escape) and cognitive responses (helplessness, fear of harm) can be altered independently of perceived chest pain and that a patient's overall functional improvement is **not** dependent solely on reducing the frequency of chest pain symptoms.[357]

Behavioral interventions have been demonstrated to improve functional morbidity in patients in with persistent noncardiac chest pain even when symptom severity or frequency is not reduced.[357] This type of therapy typically emphasizes: (1) that physicians and patients agree on the diagnosis, good prognosis, and absence of need for further evaluation; (2) increased physical fitness; (3) the development of self-efficacy cognitions; and (4) a shift in attribution away from harmful diseases and toward fitness. The best improvement in disability is seen with individual or group interdisciplinary cognitive-behavioral education sessions. Others have reported that this form of therapy, when compared to controls, has increased the number of pain-free days, decreased the number of pain episodes, reduced disability, and improved mental state.[358] Since these behavioral studies did not screen patients for anxiety/hyperventilation syndrome and the successful outcome may have been due to the presence of patients with this syndrome, one must be cautious about the general applicability of such therapy.

This section has highlighted the necessity of interdisciplinary approaches in the management of chronic pain syndromes. The various psychotherapeutic approaches to the management of chronic chest pain are beyond the scope of this chapter. Excellent discussions of topics such as the placebo effect, the behavior of pain and illness, relaxation and biofeedback techniques, hypnotic analgesia, behavior therapy, other cognitive-behavioral approaches to chronic pain management, and compensation issues[359,360] are available.

## Neural Blockade

Pain associated with peripheral nerve injury (ie, neuropathic pain) often paradoxically produces an area of increased pain with an associated loss of sensory function. This pain may be amenable to neural blockade. Local infiltration of analgesics to produce a thoracic intercostal nerve block in the posterior axillary line may be useful for the relief of pain caused by processes involving the ribs or anterior chest wall, but does not relieve pain caused by diseases of the thoracic or upper abdominal viscera. Conversely, sympathetic chain nerve blocks can be useful for pain relief due to disease involving the viscera. Neural blockade, then, can be used for diagnostic, prophylactic, therapeutic, and/or prognostic applications. The prerequisites for optimal results involve an extensive knowledge of pain syndromes in general; the pharmacology of the agents being used; an appreciation of the indications, limitations, and complications of these procedures; and a thorough evaluation of the patient in question. A detailed discussion of the techniques of paravertebral block of the thoracic spinal nerves; posterior, lateral, anterior, and continuous intercostal blocks; and sympathetic nerve blocks can be found elsewhere.[361,362]

Open surgery involving the cervical and thoracic spinal cord with the intent to transect the anterolateral quadrants of the spinal cord (cordotomy) that contains the pain and temperature pathways has been a successful technique for the relief of intractable pain since the early 1900's.[363] More recently, a percutaneous approach has been developed. Neither of these techniques is in wide usage given that the number of patients with intractable pain has decreased and that nondestructive neurosurgical alternatives (ie, chronic epidural narcotic administration, electrical stimulation of the posterior columns of the spinal cord) have been successful in treating many of these patients. Similarly, surgical techniques aimed at sectioning dorsal spinal roots (rhizotomy) are no longer considered primary therapeutic approaches given the availability of other, less traumatic and potentially equally successful options. Stereotactic brain surgery can also be performed for the relief of chronic pain and has involved such procedures as medullary tractotomy, mesencephalic tractotomy, pontine tractotomy, thalamotomy, pulvinarotomy, hypothalamotomy, and cingulotomy.[364] Patient selection for any of these surgical procedures is based on individual case histories, repeated failure of other less invasive therapies, and an "acceptable" chance of success while the risk of complications are minimized.

## Afferent Nerve Stimulation: TENS and Acupuncture

The selective activation of afferent nerve fibers by vibration, implanted electrodes, or TENS can diminish acute pain in 60% of all patients and can control chronic intractable pain for prolonged periods in up to 30% of patients who have been refractory to other conventional treatment modalities [365]. The analgesic effects of electrical stimulation have been well known since the time of the Romans, when the shock from an electrogenic fish was used to treat the pains of gout, arthritis, and headache.[366,367] The rationale behind peripheral nerve stimulation is to activate local inhibitory circuits within the dorsal horn of the spinal cord to generate non-painful paresthesias in the region of the body where the pain is located. For practical purposes, this needs to be accomplished without also causing muscle contractions, dysesthesias, or local tissue injury.

The most effective site for the applied stimulation can sometimes be difficult to establish and "adequate" trials (at least 1 hour in length) are necessary to determine the appropriate position, frequency, pulse-width, and current amplitude. For TENS, the majority of patients prefer 0.1 to 0.5 millisecond pulse-widths with frequencies in the range of 40 to 70 Hz.[368,369] The induction time for analgesia with TENS varies from instantaneous to several hours (average time approximately 20 minutes).[365] In cases of chronic pain, often a cumulative analgesic effect that slowly builds up over the course of weeks is produced by continuous TENS stimulation. Transcutaneous electrical nerve stimulator therapy is particularly suited for the treatment of neurogenic pain from disorders such as intercostal neuritis, postherpetic neuralgia, peripheral nerve injury, radiculopathies, nerve compression syndromes, and causalgia.[370,371] In 1986, Mannheimer et. al.[372] reported on the use of TENS for the treatment of angina pectoris and showed an increased exercise tolerance and diminished ST segment depression. Some patients will require treatment periods of up to 9 hours per day in order to control their pain syndrome.

In the early stages of therapy, TENS appears to provide substantial relief in chronic pain patients, with some of this benefit being attributable to placebo effect. While any placebo effect will tend to fall off rapidly, tolerance to the analgesic effect develops and the therapeutic effectiveness of TENS decreases at a slower rate, finally settling in at an overall long-term success rate of 20% to 30%.

The use of TENS has been remarkably free of adverse effects, except for mild skin irritation in one third of the patients. Allergic reactions and electrical skin burns are uncommon. The only contraindications to the use of TENS are noncompliant patients, avoid stimulating over the anterior neck since laryngospasm and/or vasovagal reflexes may result, avoid stimulation over a pregnant uterus, and avoid use in patients with coexisting pacemakers or other implanted electrical devices. If an adequate supervised trial of TENS yields only partial or ineffective pain relief from severe, unremitting, and intractable chronic pain, consideration may be given to the use of implanted electrodes. Several thousand of these devices have been implanted, but these procedures remain somewhat controversial due to lack of agreement over precise indications, lack of consistency in reported efficacy, and a lack of understanding concerning the mechanism of action of analgesia.[365,373–375]

As reported in a recent consensus conference on the neurosurgical management of chronic pain,[374] stimulation of deep brain structures has reverted to investigational status in the United States under a ruling by the Food and Drug Administration.

The intense sensory input produced from a TENS unit is but one example of the many techniques available to produce "hyperstimulation analgesia." In fact, the idea of causing brief, moderate pain in an attempt to relieve another more prolonged and severe pain is an ancient form of pain treatment that has existed in every culture known to man.[376] The so-called rediscovery of the ancient Chinese practice of acupuncture is but one of the recent changes in the way the Western world has come to view "folk medicine." The basic procedure of acupuncture involves the insertion of fine needles through specifically defined points in the skin. The needles are then twirled slowly for some time and then left in place for additional periods of varying length. An induction time of around 20 minutes may be required for full analgesic effect to occur. The duration of analgesia is frequently at least several hours, and may occasionally last for days or even weeks.[377] Traditional acupuncture charts are exceptionally complex, but in general the points used in the treatment of a pain-

## Shoulder Joint

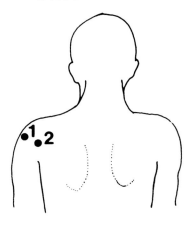

## Shoulder-Back

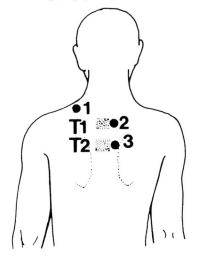

**Figure 7A.** Traditional acupuncture points (represented by dots) for the treatment of shoulder joint (top) and shoulder-back (bottom) pain. Modified with permission from *Textbook of Pain*. 3rd ed. Wall PD, Melzack R, eds. Edinburgh: Churchill Livingstone; 1994:1209–1217.[376]

## Chest or Rib

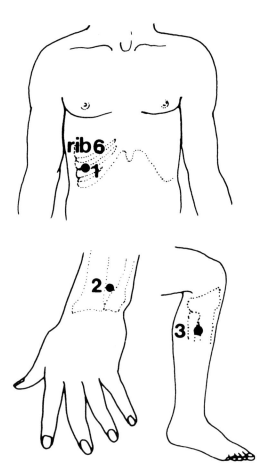

**Figure 7B.** Traditional acupuncture points (dots 1–3) for the treatment of chest or rib pain. Modified with permission from *Textbook of Pain*. 3rd ed. Wall PD, Melzack R, eds. Edinburgh: Churchill Livingstone; 1994:1209–1217.[376]

ful malady are usually clustered at or near the site of pain, with only a few points being located more distantly.

A number of carefully controlled studies have shown impressive results and served to place this technique on firmer scientific ground.[378,379] Research has shown that effective sites of stimulation are not necessarily the precise points on the skin indicated by the acupuncture charts of old, but rather that larger areas can provide equally efficacious pain relief.[380,381] More important than the precise site of stimulation is the intensity of the stimulation. Interestingly, the distribution of every trigger point reported in the Western medical literature and the deep, aching feeling experienced when these sites are stimulated with pressure, corresponds very closely (at least 71%) with the location of established acupuncture sites for therapy of specific pain syndromes.[382–386] Figures 7A-C illustrate some of the acupuncture points associated with the treatment of shoulder, back, and chest pain.

## Chest or Rib (Accessory Points)

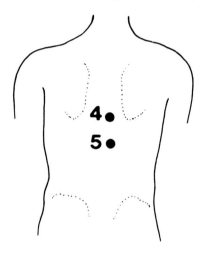

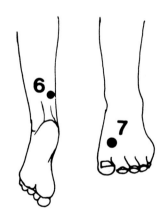

**Figure 7C.** Traditional acupuncture accessory points (dots 4–7) for the treatment of chest or rib pain. Modified with permission from *Textbook of Pain*. 3rd ed. Wall PD, Melzack R, eds. Edinburgh: Churchill Livingstone; 1994: 1209–1217.[376]

### References

1. Davies HA, Jones DB, Rhodes J, et al. Angina-like esophageal pain: differentiation from cardiac pain by history. J Clin Gastroenterol 1985;7:477–481.
2. Mayou R. Invited review: atypical chest pain. J Psychosomatic Res 1989;33: 393–406.
3. Kemp HG, Vokonas PS, Cohn PF, et al. The anginal syndromes associated with normal coronary arteriograms: report of a six year experience. Am J Med 1973;54: 735–742.
4. Marchandise B, Bourassa MG, Chaitman BR, et al. Angiographic evaluation of the natural history of normal coronary arteries and mild coronary atherosclerosis. Am J Cardiol 1978;41:216–220.
5. Lee TH, Rouan GW, Weisberg MC, et al. Clinical characteristics and natural history of patients with acute myocardial infarction sent home from the emergency room. Am J Cardiol 1987;60:219–224.
6. Behar S, Schor S, Kariv I, et al. Evaluation of the electrocardiogram in the emergency room as a decision-making tool. Chest 1977;71:486–491.
7. Hedges JR, Rouan GW, Toltzis R. Use of cardiac enzymes identifies patients with acute myocardial infarction otherwise unrecognized in the emergency department. Ann Emerg Med 1987;16:248–252.
8. Levine PR, Mascette AM. Musculoskeletal chest pain in patients with "angina": a prospective study. South Med J 1959; 82:580–585.
9. Higgins GL, 3d, Lambrew CT, Hunt E, et al. Expediting the early hospital care of the adult patient with nontraumatic chest pain: impact of a modified ED triage protocol. Am J Emerg Med 1993;11:576–582.
10. Richter JE. Overview of diagnostic testing for chest pain of unknown origin. Am J Med 1992;92:41S-45S.

11. Richter JE. Gastroesophogeal reflux disease as a cause of chest pain. Med Clin North Am 1991;75:1065–1080.
12. Beunderman R, Duyvis DJ. Myocardial infarction patients during the prodromal and acute phase: a comparison with patients with a diagnosis of 'noncardiac chest pain. Psychotherapy & Psychosomatics 1983;40:129–136.
13. Goldman L, Weinberg M, Weisberg M, et al. A computer-derived protocol to aid in the diagnosis of emergency room patients with acute chest pain. N Engl J Med 1982; 307:588–596.
14. Levene DL. Chest pain—prophet of doom or nagging neurosis. Acta Med Scand 1981;644:11–13.
15. Sawe U. Pain in acute myocardial infarction. A study of 137 patients in a coronary care unit. Acta Med Scand 1971;190: 79–81.
16. Sievers J. Myocardial infarction. Clinical features and outcome in three thousand thirty-six cases. Acta Med Scand 1964; 406:1–120.
17. Lee TH, Cook EF, Weisberg M, et al. Acute chest pain in the emergency room. Identification and examination of low-risk patients. Arch Intern Med 1985;145:65–69.
18. Hoppenfield S. Physical Examination of the Spine and Extremities. Norwalk: Appleton & Lange, 1976.
19. Dilger J, Pietsch-Breitfeld B, Stein W, et al. Simple computer-assisted diagnosis of acute myocardial infarction in patients with acute thoracic pain. Meth Inform Med 1992;31:263–267.
20. Zarling EJ, Sexton H, Milnor P Jr. Failure to diagnose acute myocardial infarction-The clinicopathologic experience at a large community hospital. JAMA 1983; 250:1177–1181.
21. Rude RE, Poole WK, Muller JE, et al. Electrocardiographic and clinical criteria for recognition of acute myocardial infarction based on analysis of 3,697 patients. Am J Cardiol 1983;52:936–942.
22. Huey BL, Gheorghiade M, Crampton RS, et al. Acute non-Q wave myocardial infarction associated with early ST segment elevation: evidence for spontaneous coronary reperfusion and implications for thrombolytic trials. J Am Coll Cardiol 1987;9:18–25.
23. Willich SN, Stone PH, Muller JE, et al. High-risk subgroup of patients with non-Q wave myocardial infarction based on

24. Granborg J, Grande P, Pedersen A. Diagnostic and prognostic implications of transient isolated negative T waves in suspected acute myocardial infarction. Am J Cardiol 1986;57:203–207.
25. Varat MA. Non-transmural infarction: clinical distinction between patients with ST depression and those with T wave inversion. J Electrocardiol 1985;18:15–20.
26. Slater DK, Hlatky MA, Mark DB, et al. Outcome in suspected acute myocardial infarction with normal or minimally abnormal admission electrocardiographic findings. Am J Cardiol 1987;60:766–770.
27. Karlson BW, Herlitz J, Wiklund O, et al. Early prediction of acute myocardial infarction from clinical history, examination and electrocardiogram in the emergency room. Am J Cardiol 1991;68: 171–175.
28. Lee TH, Weisberg MC, Brand DA, et al. Candidates for thrombolysis among emergency room patients with acute chest pain-potential true- and false-positive rates. Ann Intern Med 1989;110:957–962.
29. Templeton PA, McCallion WA, McKinney LA, et al. Chest pain in the accident and emergency department: is chest radiography worthwhile? Arch Emerg Med 1991;8:97–101.
30. Buenger RE. Five thousand acute care/ emergency department chest radiographs: comparison of requisitions with radiographic findings. J Emerg Med 1988; 6:197–202.
31. Russel NJ, Pantin CFA, Emerson PA, et al. The role of chest radiography in patients presenting with anterior chest pain to the accident and emergency department. J Royal Soc Med 1988;81:626–628.
32. Gibler WB, Young GP, Hedges JR, et al. Acute myocardial infarction in chest pain patients with nondiagnostic ECGs: serial CK-MB sampling in the emergency department. The Emergency Medicine Cardiac Research Group. Ann Emerg Med 1992;21:504–512.
33. Gibler WB, Lewis LM, Erb RE, et al. Early detection of acute myocardial infarction in patients presenting with chest pain and nondiagnostic ECGs: serial CK-MB sampling in the emergency department. Ann Emerg Med 1990;19:1359–1366.
34. Mair J, Artner-Dworzak E, Dienstl A, et.al. Early detection of acute myocardial infarction by measurement of mass concen-

tration of creatine kinase-MB. Am J Cardiol 1991;68:1545–1550.

35. Diamond GA, Forrester JS. Analysis of probability as an aid in the clinical diagnosis of coronary-artery disease. N Engl J Med 1979;300:1350–1358.

36. Hackshaw BT. Excluding heart disease in the patient with chest pain. Am J Med 1992;92:46S-51S.

37. Richter JE, Bradley LA, Castell DO. Esophageal chest pain: current controversies in pathogenesis, diagnosis, and therapy. Ann Intern Med 1989;110:66–78.

38. Bennett JR, Atkinson M. The differentiation between esophageal and cardiac pain. Lancet 1966;ii:1123–1127.

39. Alban Davies H, Lewis M, Rhodes J. "Esophageal angina" as a cause of chest pain. JAMA 1982;248:2274–2278.

40. Janssens JP, Vantrappen G. Irritable esophagus. Am J Med 1992;92:27S-32S.

41. Smout AJ, Lam HG, Breumelhof R. Ambulatory esophageal monitoring in noncardiac chest pain. Am J Med 1992;92:74S-80S.

42. Nostrant TT. Provocation testing in noncardiac chest pain. Am J Med 1992;92:56S-64S.

43. Hsia PC, Maher KA, Lewis JH, et al. Utility of upper endoscopy in the evaluation of noncardiac chest pain. Gastrointestinal Endoscopy 1991;37:22–26.

44. Goldman L, Cook EF, Brand DA, et al. A computer protocol to predict myocardial infarction in emergency department patients with chest pain. N Engl J Med 1988;318:797–803.

45. Pozen MW, D'Agostino RB, Mitchell JB, et al. The usefulness of a predictive instrument to reduce inappropriate admissions to the coronary care unit. Ann Int Med 1980;92:238–242.

46. Pozen MW, D'Agostino RB, Selker HP, et al. A predictive instrument to improve coronary-care-unit admission practices in acute ischemic heart disease: a prospective multicenter clinical trial. N Engl J Med 1984;310:1273–1278.

47. Tierney WM, Roth BJ, Psaty B, et al. Predictors of myocardial infarction in emergency room patients. Crit Care Med 1985;13:526–531.

48. Jonsbu J, Rollag A, Lippestad CT, et al. Rapid and correct diagnosis of myocardial infarction: standardized case history and clinical examination provide important information for correct referral to monitored beds. J Intern Med 1991;229:143–149.

49. Lee TH, Juarez G, Cook EF, et al. Ruling out acute myocardial infarction. A prospective multicenter validation of a 12-hour strategy for patients at low risk. N Engl J Med 1991;324:1239–1246.

50. Epstein SE. Implications of probability analysis on the strategy used for noninvasive detection of coronary artery disease: role of single or combined use of exercise electrocardiographic testing, radionuclide cineangiography and myocardial perfusion imaging. Am J Cardiol 1980;46:491–499.

51. Pryor DB, Harrell FE, Jr., Lee KL, et al. Estimating the likelihood of significant coronary artery disease. Am J Med 1983;75:771–780.

52. Diamond GA, Forrester JS, Hirsch M, et al. Application of conditional probability analysis to the clinical diagnosis of coronary artery disease. J Clin Invest 1980;65:1210–1221.

53. Henderson RD, Marryatt G. Characteristics of esophageal pain. Acta Med Scand 1980;644:49–51.

54. Sox HC, Jr., Margulies I, Sox CH. Psychologically mediated effects of diagnostic tests. Ann Intern Med 1981;95:680–685.

55. Pantell RH, Goodman BW, Jr. Adolescent chest pain: a prospective study. Pediatrics 1983;71:881–887.

56. Selbst SM, Ruddy RM, Clark BJ, et al. Pediatric chest pain: a prospective study. Pediatrics 1988;82:319–323.

57. Driscoll DJ, Glicklich LB, Gallen WJ. Chest pain in children: a prospective study. Pediatrics 1976;57:648–651.

58. Zavaras-Angelidou KA, Weinhouse E, Nelson DB. Review of 180 episodes of chest pain in 134 children. Ped Emerg Care 1992;8:189–193.

59. Gulati S, Kumar L. 'Chest epilepsy' in a child. Postgrad Med J 1992;68:369–370.

60. Hallagan LF, Dawson PA, Eljaiek LF, Jr. Pediatric chest pain: case report of a malignant cause. Am J Emerg Med 1992;10:43–45.

61. Click RL, Spittell JA, Jr., Puga FJ. Chest pain in a young woman. Mayo Clin Proc 1988;63:368–372.

62. Selbst SM, Ruddy R, Clark BJ. Chest pain in children. Follow-up of patients previously reported. Clin Ped 1990;29:374–377.

63. Rowland TW, Richards MM. The natural history of idiopathic chest pain in chil-

dren. A follow-up study. Clin Ped 1986; 25:612–614.

64. Wiens L, Sabath R, Ewing L, et al. Chest pain in otherwise healthy children and adolescents is frequently caused by exercise-induced asthma. Pediatrics 1992;90: 350–353.

65. Glassman MS, Medow MS, Berezin S, et al. Spectrum of esophageal disorders in children with chest pain. Dig Dis Sci 1992;37:663–666.

66. Selbst SM. Evaluation of chest pain in children. Ped Rev 1986;8:56–62.

67. Selbst SM. Chest pain in children. Am Fam Physician 1990;41:179–186.

68. Asnes RS, Santulli R, Bemporad JR. Psychogenic chest pain in children. Clin Ped 1981;20:788–791.

69. Swamy N. Esophageal spasm: clinical and manometric response to nitroglycerine and long acting nitrates. Gastroenterology 1977;72:23–27.

70. Donat WE. Chest pain: cardiac and noncardiac causes. Clin Chest Med 1987;8: 241–252.

71. Davies HA, Jones DB, Rhodes J. 'Esophageal angina' as the cause of chest pain. JAMA 1982;248:2274–2278.

72. Levine HJ. Difficult problems in the diagnosis of chest pain. Am Heart J 1980;100: 108–118.

73. Demeester TR, O'Sullivan GC, Bermudez G, et al. Esophageal function in patients with angina-type chest pain and normal coronary angiograms. Ann Surg 1982;196: 488–497.

74. Howell JM, Hedges JR. Differential diagnosis of chest discomfort and general approach to myocardial ischemia decision making. Am J Emerg Med 1991;9: 571–579.

75. Anagnostopoulos CE, Prabhakar MJ, Kittle CF. Aortic dissections and dissecting aneurysms. Am J Cardiol 1972;30: 263–273.

76. Palmer RF, Lasseter KC. Nitroprusside and dissecting aortic aneurysm. N Engl J Med 1976;294:1403.

77. Wheat MW. Intensive drug therapy. In: Doroghazi RM, Slater EE, eds. *Aortic Dissection.* New York, NY: McGraw-Hill Book Company; 1983:165.

78. Grubb BP, Sirio C, Zelis R. Intravenous labetalol in acute aortic dissection. JAMA 1987;258:78–79.

79. Doroghazi RM, Slater EE, DeSanctis RW, et al. Long-term survival of patients with treated aortic dissection. J Am Coll Cardiol 1984;3:1026–1034.

80. Miller DC, Mitchell RC, Oyer PE, et al. Independent determinants of operative mortality for patients with aortic dissections. Circulation 1984;70:153–164.

81. Glower DD, Fann JI, Speier RH, et al. Comparison of medical and surgical therapy for uncomplicated descending aortic dissection. Circulation 1994;82:39–46.

82. Crawford ES, Svensson LG, Coselli JS, et al. Aortic dissection and dissecting aortic aneurysms. Ann Surg 1988;208:254–273.

83. Joyce JW, Fairbairn JF, Kincaid OW, et al. Aneurysms of the thoracic aorta—a clinical study with special reference to prognosis. Circulation 1964;29:176–180.

84. Cabrol C, Pavie A, Mesnildrey P, et al. Long-term results with total replacement of the ascending aorta and reimplantation of the coronary arteries. J Thorac Cardiovasc Surg 1986;91:17–25.

85. Crawford ES, Svensson LG, Coselli JS, et al. Surgical treatment of aneurysm and/or dissection of the ascending aorta, transverse aortic arch, and ascending aorta and transverse aortic arch: factors influencing survival in 717 patients. J Thorac Cardiovasc Surg 1989;98:659–673.

86. Pressler V, McNamara JJ. Aneurysms of the thoracic aorta. Review of 260 cases. J Thorac Cardiovasc Surg 1985;89:50–54.

87. Crawford ES, Mizrahi EM, Hess KR, et al. The impact of distal aortic perfusion and somatosensory evoked potential monitoring on prevention of paraplegia after aortic aneurysm operation. J Thorac Cardiovasc Surg 1988;95:357–367.

88. Simmons J, Willens HJ, Kessler KM. Acute myocardial infarction: then and now. Chest 1995;107:1731–1743.

89. Gibler WB, Kereiakes DJ, Dean EN, et al. Prehospital diagnosis and treatment of acute myocardial infarction: a North-South perspective. The Cincinnati Heart Project and the Nashville Prehospital TPA Trial. Am Heart J 1991;121:1–11.

90. Fibrinolytic Therapy Trialists' (FTT) Collaborative Group. Indications for fibrinolytic therapy in suspected acute myocardial infarction: Collaborative overview of early mortality and major morbidity results from all randomized trials of more than 1,000 patients. Lancet 1994;343: 311–322.

91. Fillmore SJ, Shapiro M, Killip T. Arterial oxygen tension in acute myocardial infarction. Serial analysis of clinical state

and blood gas changes. Am Heart J 1970; 79:620–629.

92. Madias JE, Hood WB, Jr. Reduction of precordial ST-segment elevation in patients with anterior myocardial infarction by oxygen breathing. Circulation 1976;53: 198–200.

93. Maroko PR, Radvany P, Braunwald E. Reduction of infarct size by oxygen inhalation following acute coronary occlusion. Circulation 1975;52:360–368.

94. Madias JE, Madias NE, Hood WB. Precordial ST-segment mapping. 2. Effects of oxygen inhalation on ischemic injury in patients with acute myocardial infarction. Circulation 1976;53:411–417.

95. Irwin RS, French CL, Mike RW. Respiratory adjunct therapy. In: Rippe JM, Irwin RS, Alpert JS, Fink MP, eds. *Intensive Care Medicine.* 2nd ed. Boston, Ma: Little Brown and Company; 1991:585–595.

96. Flaherty J. Role of nitrates in acute myocardial infarction. Am J Cardiol 1992;70: 73B-81B.

97. Judgett B. Role of nitrates after acute myocardial infarction. Am J Cardiol 1992;70: 82B-87B.

98. Ferguson JJ, Diver DJ, Boldt M, et al. Significance of nitroglycerin-induced hypotension with acute myocardial infarction. Am J Cardiol 1989;64:311–314.

99. Hjalmarson A, Herlitz J, Holmberg S. The Goteborg Metoprolol Trial-effects on mortality and morbidity in acute myocardial infarction. Circulation 1983;67(suppl 1): 126–132.

100. The TIMI Study Group. Comparison of invasive and conservative strategies after treatment with intravenous tissue plasminogen activator in acute myocardial infarction. N Engl J Med 1989;320:618–627.

101. Goldbourt V, Behar S, Reicher-Reiss J. Early administration of nifedipine in suspected acute myocardial infarction: Secondary Prevention Reinfarction Israel Nifedipine Trial 2 Study. Arch Intern Med 1993;153:345–353.

102. Gibson R, Boden WE, Theroux P. Diltiazem and reinfarction in patients with non-Q wave myocardial infarction. N Engl J Med 1986;315:423–429.

103. Miller RR, Lies JE, Carretta RF. Prevention of lower extremity venous thrombosis by early mobilization: confirmation in patients with acute myocardial infarction by I125 fibrinogen uptake and venography. Ann Intern Med 1976;84:700–703.

104. Rowe MH, Jelinek MV, Liddell N. Effect of rapid mobilization on ejection fractions and ventricular volumes after myocardial infarction. Am J Cardiol 1989;63:1037–1041.

105. DeWood MA, Spores J, Notske R. Prevalence of total coronary occlusion during the early hours of transmural myocardial infarction. N Engl J Med 1980;303: 897–902.

106. Gruppo Italiano per lo Studio della Streptochinasi nell'Infarto Miocardico (GISSI). Effectiveness of intravenous thrombolytic treatment in acute myocardial infarction. Lancet 1986;1:397–402.

107. Wilcox RG, Olsson CG, Skene AM. Trial of tissue plasminogen activator for mortality reduction in acute myocardial infarction:anglo-scandinavian study of early thrombolysis (ASSETT). Lancet 1988;2:525–530.

108. Grines CL, DeMaria AN. Optimal utilization of thrombolytic therapy for acute myocardial infarction: Concepts and controversies. J Am Coll Cardiol 1990;16: 223–231.

109. EMERAS (Estudio Multicentrico Estreptoquinasa Republicas de America del Sur) Collaborative Group. Randomized trial of late thrombolysis in patients with suspected acute myocardial infarction. Lancet 1993;342:767–772.

110. The TIMI III B Investigators. Effects of tissue-plasminogen activator and a comparison of early invasive and conservative strategies in unstable angina and non-Q-wave myocardial infarction: results of the TIMI III B trial. Circulation 1994;89: 1545–1556.

111. The GUSTO Investigators. An international randomized trial comparing four thrombolytic strategies for acute myocardial infarction. N Engl J Med 1993;329: 673–682.

112. Neuhaus KL, Von Essen R, Tebbe U. Improved thrombolysis in acute myocardial infarction with front-loaded administration of alteplase: results of the rt PA-APSAC patency study(TAPS). J Am Coll Cardiol 1992;19:885–891.

113. The GUSTO Angiographic Investigators. The effects of tissue plasminogen activator, streptokinase, or both on coronary artery patency, ventricular function, and survival after acute myocardial infarction. N Engl J Med 1993;329:1615–1622.

114. Fuster V. Coronary thrombolysis-a perspective for the practicing physician. N Engl J Med 1993;329:723–725.

115. Ridker PM, O'Donnell C, Marder VJ. Large-scale trials of thrombolytic therapy for acute myocardial infarction: GISSI-2, ISIS-3,and GUSTO. Ann Intern Med 1993; 119:530–532.

116. Neuhaus KL, Feuerer W, Jeep-Tebbe S. Improved thrombolysis with a modified dose regimen of recombinant tissue-type plasminogen activator. J Am Coll Cardiol 1989;14:1566–1569.

117. Becker RC. Thrombin antagonists and antiplatelet agents. Am J Cardiol 1992;69: 39A-51A.

118. Habib GB. Current status of thrombolysis in acute myocardial infarction Part III. optimalization of adjunctive therapy after thrombolytic therapy. Chest 1995;107: 809–816.

119. ISIS-2 (Second International Study of Infarct Survival) Collaborative Group. Randomized trial of intravenous streptokinase,oral aspirin, both, or neither among 17,187 cases of suspected acute myocardial infarction. Lancet 1988;2:349–360.

120. Antiplatelet Trialists' Collaboration. Secondary prevention of vascular disease by prolonged antiplatelet treatment. BMJ (Clin Res Ed) 1988;296:316–330.

121. Hennekens CH, Jonas MA, Buring JE. The benefits of aspirin in acute myocardial infarction: still a well-kept secret in the United States. Arch Intern Med 1994;154: 37–39.

122. Gunnar RM, Bourdillon PD, Dixon DW. Guidelines for the early management of patients with acute myocardial infarction: a report of the American College of Cardiology/American Heart Association Task Force on Assessment of Diagnostic and Therapeutic Cardiovascular Procedures (Subcommittee to Develop Guidelines for the Early Management of Patients with Acute Myocardial Infarction). J Am Coll Cardiol 1990;16:249–292.

123. Bleich SD, Nichols TC, Schumacher RR. Effect of heparin on coronary arterial patency after thrombolysis with tissue plasminogen activator in acute myocardial infarction. Am J Cardiol 1990;66: 1412–1417.

124. de Bono DP, Simoons ML, Tijssen J. Effect of early intravenous heparin on coronary patency, infarct size, and bleeding complications after alteplase thrombolysis: results of a randomized double blind European Cooperative Study Group trial. Br Heart J 1992;67:122–128.

125. Theroux P, Ouimet H, McCans J. Aspirin, heparin or both to treat acute unstable angina. N Engl J Med 1988;319:1105–1111.

126. The RISC Group. Risk of myocardial infarction and death during treatment with low dose aspirin and intravenous heparin in men with unstable coronary artery disease. Lancet 1990;336:827–830.

127. Chalmer TC, Matta RJ, Smith JJ. Evidence favoring the use of anticoagulants in the hospital phase of acute myocardial infarction. N Engl J Med 1977;297:1091–1096.

128. The EPSIM Research Group. A controlled comparison of aspirin and oral anticoagulants in prevention of deaths after myocardial infarction. N Engl J Med 1982;307: 701–708.

129. Cannon CP, McCabe CH, Henry TD. A pilot trial of recombinant desulfatohirudin compared with heparin in conjunction with tissue-type plasminogen activator and aspirin for acute myocardial infarction: results of the thrombolysis in myocardial infarction (TIMI) 5 trial. Am J Coll Cardiol 1994;23:993–1003.

130. Schulman SP, Goldschmidt-Clermont PJ, Navetta RI. Integrelin in unstable angina: a double-blind, randomized trial. Circulation 1993;88:608.

131. Simoons ML, deBoer MF, van den Brand MJ. Randomized trial of a PG IIb/IIIa platelet receptor blocker in refractory unstable angina. Circulation 1994;89: 596–603.

132. Simoons ML, Betriu A, Col J. Thrombolysis with tissue plasminogen activator in acute myocardial infarction: no additional benefit from immediate percutaneous coronary angioplasty. Lancet 1988;1: 197–202.

133. TIMI Study Group. Comparison of invasive and conservative strategies after treatment with intravenous tissue plasminogen activator in acute myocardial infarction: results of the Thrombolysis in Myocardial Ischemia (TIMI) II Trial. N Engl J Med 1989;320:618–627.

134. Grines CL, Browne KF, Marco J. A comparison of immediate angioplasty with thrombolytic therapy for acute myocardial infarction. N Engl J Med 1993;328: 673–679.

135. Zilstra F, deBoer MJ, Hoorntje JCA. A comparison of immediate coronary angioplasty with intravenous streptokinase in acute myocardial infarction. N Engl J Med 1993;328:680–684.

136. Simari RD, Berger PB, Bell MR, et al. Coronary angioplasty in acute myocardial in-

farction: primary, immediate adjunctive, rescue, or deferred adjunctive approach? Mayo Clin Proc 1994;69:346–358.

137. Horner SM. Efficacy of intravenous magnesium in acute myocardial infarction in reducing arrhythmias and mortality: meta-analysis of magnesium in acute myocardial infarction. Circulation 1992; 86:774–779.

138. Woods K, Fletcher S, Roffe C. Intravenous magnesium sulphate in suspected acute myocardial infarction: results of the second Leicester Intravenous Magnesium Intervention Trial (LIMIT-2). Lancet 1992; 339:1553–1558.

139. ISIS-4 (Fourth International Study of Infarct Survival) Collaborative Group. A randomized factorial trial assessing early oral captopril, oral mononitrate, and intravenous magnesium sulphate in 58,050 patients with suspected acute myocardial infarction. Lancet 1995;345:669–685.

140. Pfeffer M, Lamas G, Vaughn D. Effect of captopril on progressive ventricular dilatation after anterior myocardial infarction. N Engl J Med 1988;319:80–86.

141. Gruppo Italiano per lo Studio della Sopravivenza nell'Infarcto Miocardico G. Effects of lisinopril and transdermal trinitrate singly and together on 6 week mortality and ventricular function after acute myocardial infarction. Lancet 1994;343: 1115–1122.

142. Chinese Cardiac Study Collaborative Group. Oral captopril versus placebo among 13,634 patients with suspected acute myocardial infarction: interim report from the Chinese Cardiac Study (CCS-1). Lancet 1995;345:686–687.

143. International Society and Federation of Cardiology and World Health Organization Task Force on Myocardial Reperfusion. Reperfusion in acute myocardial infarction. Circulation 1994;90:2091–2102.

144. Marboe CC, Fenoglio JJ, Jr. Pathology and natural history of human myocarditis. Pathol Immunopathol Res 1988;7:226–239.

145. Chan KY, Iwahara M, Benson LN, et al. Immunosuppressive therapy in the management of acute myocarditis in children: A clinical trial. J Am Coll Cardiol 1991; 17:458–460.

146. Rezkalla SH, Kloner RA. Management strategies in viral myocarditis. Am Heart J 1989;117:706–708.

147. Kishimoto C, Abelmann WH. Absence of effects of cyclosporine on myocardial lymphocyte subsets in Coxsackievirus B3

myocarditis in the aviremic stage. Circ Res 1989;65:934–945.

148. Rezkalla S, Khatib R, Khatib G, et al. Effect of indomethacin in the late phase of Coxsackievirus myocarditis in a murine model. J Lab Clin Med 1988;112:118–121.

149. Becker RC, Loeffler JS, Leopold KA, et al. Primary tumors of the heart: a review with emphasis on diagnosis and potential treatment modalities. Semin Surg Onc 1985;1:161–170.

150. Dapper F, Gorlach G, Hoffmann C, et al. Primary cardiac tumors- clinical experiences and late results in 48 patients. Thorac Cardiovasc Surg 1988;36:80–85.

151. McCarthy PM, Piehler JM, Schaff HV, et al. The significance of multiple, recurrent, and "complex" cardiac myxomas. J Thorac Cardiovasc Surg 1986;91: 389–396.

152. Piehler JM, Pluth JR, Schaff HV, et al. Surgical management of effusive pericardial disease. Influence of extent of pericardial resection on clinical course. J Thorac Cardiovasc Surg 1985;90:506–516.

153. Posner MR, Cohen GI, Skarin AT. Pericardial disease in patients with cancer. The differentiation of malignant from idiopathic and radiation-induced pericarditis. Am J Med 1981;71:407–413.

154. Dubrow TJ, Mihalka J, Eisenhauer DM, et al. Myocardial contusion in the stable patient: what level of care is appropriate? Surgery 1989;106:267–273.

155. Hossack KF, Moreno CA, Vanway CW, et al. Frequency of cardiac contusion in nonpenetrating chest injury. Am J Cardiol 1988;61:391–394.

156. Lorell BH, Braunwald E. Pericardial disease. In: Braunwald E, Ed. Heart Disease. A Textbook of Cardiovascular Medicine. 4th ed. Philadelphia, Pa: WB Saunders Company; 1992:1469

157. Torija Martinez RN, Gonzalez Hermosillo JA. Acute nonspecific pericarditis. Arch Inst Cardiol Mex 1987;57:307–312.

158. Sagrista-Sauleda J, Permanyer-Miralda G, Candell-Riera J, et al. Transient cardiac constriction: an unrecognized pattern of evolution in effusive acute idiopathic pericarditis. Am J Cardiol 1987;59: 961–966.

159. Fowler NO, Harbin AD. Recurrent acute pericarditis: follow-up study of 31 patients. J Am Coll Cardiol 1986;7:300–305.

160. Kilpatrick ZM, Chapman CB. On pericardiocentesis. Am J Cardiol 1965;16: 722–728.

161. Levine MJ, Lorell BH, Diver DJ, et al. Implications of echocardiographically assisted diagnosis of pericardial tamponade in contemporary medical patients: detection before hemodynamic embarrassment. J Am Coll Cardiol 1991;17:59–65.

162. Morgan CD, Marshall SA, Ross JR. Catheter drainage of the pericardium: its safety and efficacy. Can J Surg 1989;32:331–334.

163. Focht G, Becker RC. Pericardiocentesis. In: Rippe JM, Irwin RS, Fink MP, Cerra FB, Curley FJ, Heard SO, eds. *Procedures and Techniques in Intensive Care Medicine*. Boston, Ma: Little Brown and Company; 1995:111–116.

164. Dajani AS, Bisno AL, Chung KJ, et al. Prevention of bacterial endocarditis. JAMA 1990;264:2919–2922.

165. Kirklin JW, Barratt-Boyes BG. *Aortic Valve Disease*. New York, NY: John Wiley and Sons; 1986.

166. Pantely G, Morton M, Rahimtoola SH. Effects of successful, uncomplicated valve replacement on ventricular hypertrophy, volume and performance in aortic stenosis and aortic incompetence. J Thorac Cardiovasc Surg 1978;75:383–391.

167. O'Toole JD, Geiser EA, Reddy PS, et al. Effect of preoperative ejection fraction on survival and hemodynamic improvement following aortic valve replacement. Circulation 1978;58:1175–1184.

168. Braunwald E. Valvular heart disease. In: Braunwald E, ed. *Heart Disease. A Textbook of Cardiovascular Medicine*. 4th ed. Philadelphia, Pa: WB Saunders Company; 1992:1007–1077.

169. Kuntz RE, Tosteson AN, Berman AD, et al. Predictors of event-free survival after balloon aortic valvuloplasty. N Engl J Med 1991;325:17–23.

170. Nishimura RA, Holmes DR, Jr., Michela MA. Follow-up of patients with low output, low gradient hemodynamics after percutaneous balloon aortic valvuloplasty: The Mansfield Scientific Aortic Valvuloplasty Registry. J Am Coll Cardiol 1991;17:828–833.

171. John S, Bashi VV, Jairaj PS, et al. Closed mitral valvotomy: early results and long-term follow-up of 3724 consecutive patients. Circulation 1983;68:891–896.

172. Gautam PC, Coulshed N, Epstein EJ, et al. Preoperative clinical predictors of long-term survival in mitral stenosis: analysis of 200 cases followed up for 27 years after closed mitral valvotomy. Thorax 1986;41:401–406.

173. Ward C, Hancock BW. Extreme pulmonary hypertension caused by mitral valve disease. Natural history and results of surgery. Br Heart J 1975;37:74–78.

174. Dalen JE, Matloff JM, Evans GL, et al. Early reduction of pulmonary vascular resistance after mitral valve replacement. N Engl J Med 1967;277:387–394.

175. Ben Farhat M, Boussadia H, Gandjbakhch I, et al. Closed versus open mitral commissurotomy in pure noncalcific mitral stenosis: hemodynamic studies before and after operation. J Thorac Cardiovasc Surg 1990;99:639–644.

176. Cohn LH, Allred EN, Cohn LA, et al. Long-term results of open mitral valve reconstruction for mitral stenosis. Am J Cardiol 1985;55:731–734.

177. Heger JJ, Wann LS, Weyman AE, et al. Long-term changes in mitral valve area after successful mitral commissurotomy. Circulation 1979;59:443–448.

178. Aora R, Khalillullah M, Gupta MP, et al: Mitral restenosis: Incidence and epidemiology. Indian Heart J 1978;30:265.

179. John S, Bashi VV, Jaira PS, et al: Closed mitral valvotomy; Early results and long-term follow-up of 3724 consecutive patients. Circulation 1983;68:891–896.

180. Kirklin JW. Percutaneous balloon versus surgical closed commissurotomy for mitral stenosis. Circulation 1991;83: 1450–1451.

181. Light RW. Malignant pleural effusions. In: *Anonymous Pleural Diseases*. 3rd ed. Baltimore, Md: Williams & Wilkins; 1995: 94–116.

182. Light RW. Pleural effusion due to miscellaneous diseases. In: *Anonymous Pleural Diseases*. 3rd ed. Baltimore, Md: Williams & Wilkins; 1995:224–241.

183. Sugarbaker DJ, Strauss GM, Lynch TJ. Node status has prognostic significance in the multimodality therapy of diffuse, malignant mesothelioma. J Clin Oncol 1993; 11:1172–1178.

184. Vogelzang NJ. Malignant mesothelioma: diagnostic and management strategies for 1992. Semin Oncol 1992;19:64–71.

185. Patiala J. Initial tuberculous pleuritis in the Finnish Armed Forces in 1939–1945 with special reference to eventual post pleuritic tuberculosis. Acta Tuberc Scand 1954;36:1–57.

186. Roper WH, Waring JJ. Primary serofibrinous pleural effusion in military personnel. Am Rev Respir Dis 1955;71:616–634.

187. Bass JB, Jr., Farer LS, Hopewell PC, et al.

Treatment of tuberculosis and tuberculosis infection in adults and children. Am J Respir Crit Care Med 1994;149: 1359–1374.

188. Light RW. Tuberculous pleural effusions. In: *Anonymous Pleural Diseases.* 3rd ed. Baltimore, Md: Williams & Wilkins; 1995: 154–166.

189. Tani P, Poppius H, Makipaja J. Cortisone therapy for exudative tuberculous pleurisy in the light of the follow-up study. Acta Tuberc Scand 1964;44:303–309.

190. Lee CH, Wang WJ, Lan RS. Corticosteroids in the treatment of tuberculous pleurisy: a double-blind, placebo-controlled, randomized study. Chest 1988;94: 1256–1259.

191. Barbas CSV, Cukier A, de Varvalho CRR, et al. The relationship between pleural fluid findings and the development of pleural thickening in patients with pleural tuberculosis. Chest 1991;100: 1264–1267.

192. Winslow WA, Ploss LN, Loitman B. Pleuritis in systemic lupus erythematosus: its importance as an early manifestation in diagnosis. Ann Intern Med 1958; 49:70–88.

193. Hunder GG, McDuffie FC, Hepper NGG. Pleural fluid complement in systemic lupus erythematosus and rheumatoid arthritis. Ann Intern Med 1972;76:357–362.

194. Light RW. Pleural disease due to collagen vascular diseases. In: *Anonymous Pleural Diseases.* 3rd ed. Baltimore, Md: Williams & Wilkins; 1995:208–218.

195. Walker WC, Wright V. Rheumatoid pleuritis. Ann Rheum Dis 1967;26: 467–474.

196. Yarbrough JW, Sealy WC, Miller JA. Thoracic surgical problems associated with rheumatoid arthritis. J Thorac Cardiovasc Surg 1975;68:347–354.

197. Gross NJ. Pulmonary effects of radiation therapy. Ann Intern Med 1977;86:81–92.

198. Libshitz HI, Southard ME. Complications of radiation therapy: the thorax. Semin Roentgen 1974;9:41–49.

199. Kirby TJ, Ginsberg RJ. Management of pneumothorax and barotrauma. Clin Chest Med 1992;13:97–112.

200. O'Neill S. Spontaneous pneumothorax: aetiology, management and complications. Ir Med J 1987;80:306–311.

201. Jantz MA, Pierson DJ. Pneumothorax and barotrauma. In: *Anonymous Clinics in Chest Medicine.* Philadelphia, Pa: WB Saunders Company; 1994:75–91.

202. Delius RE, Obeid FN, Horst M. Catheter aspiration for simple pneumothorax. Arch Surg 1989;124:833–836.

203. Talbot-Stern J. Catheter aspiration for simple pneumothorax. J Emerg Med 1986; 4:437–442.

204. Light RW. Pneumothorax. In: Murray JJ, Nadel JA, eds. *Textbook of Respiratory Medicine.* Philadelphia, Pa: WB Saunders Company; 1988:1745–1759.

205. Jenkinson SG. Pneumothorax. Clin Chest Med 1985;6:153–161.

206. Vukich DJ. Diseases of the pleural space. Emerg Med Clin North Am 1989;7: 309–324.

207. Symbas PN. Cardiothoracic Trauma. Curr Probl Surg 1991;28:741–797.

208. Clagett GP, Anderson FA, Jr., Levine MN. Prevention of venous thromboembolism. Chest 1992;102:391S-407S.

209. Nicolaides AN. Prevention of venous thromboembolism. Int Angio 1992;11: 151–159.

210. Hyers TM, Hull RD, Weg J. Antithrombotic therapy for venous thromboembolic disease. Chest 1992;102:408S-425S.

211. Moser KM. Venous thromboembolism. Am Rev Respir Dis 1990;141:235–249.

212. Salzman EW, Deykin D, Shapiro RM. Management of heparin therapy: controlled prospective trial. N Engl J Med 1976;292:1046–1050.

213. Collins R, Scrimgeour A, Yusuf S. Reduction in fatal pulmonary embolism and venous thrombosis by perioperative administration of subcutaneous heparin. N Engl J Med 1988;318:1162–1170.

214. Anonymous. Prevention of fatal postoperative pulmonary embolism by low doses of heparin: an international multicenter trial. Lancet 1975;1:45–51.

215. Sagar S, Massey J, Sanderson JM. Low-dose heparin prophylaxis against fatal pulmonary embolism. Br Med J 1975;4: 257–259.

216. Francis CW, Marder VJ, Evarts CM. Two-step warfarin therapy: prevention of postoperative venous thrombosis without excessive bleeding. JAMA 1983;249: 374–378.

217. Hull RD, Pineo GF. Current concepts of anticoagulation therapy. In: *Anonymous Clinics in Chest Medicine.* Philadelphia, Pa: WB Saunders Company; 1995: 269–280.

218. Brandjes DP, Hejiboer H, Butler HR. Acenocoumarol and heparin compared with acenocoumarol alone in the initial

treatment of proximal-vein thrombosis. N Engl J Med 1992;327:1485–1489.

219. Glazier RL, Crowell EB. Randomized prospective trial of continuous vs intermittent heparin therapy. JAMA 1976;236:1365–1367.

220. Hull RD, Raskob GE, Hirsh J. Continuous intravenous heparin compared with intermittent subcutaneous heparin in the initial treatment of proximal vein thrombosis. N Engl J Med 1986;315:1109–1114.

221. Raschke RA, Reilly BM, Guidry JR. The weight-based heparin dosing nomogram compared with a "standard care" nomogram. Ann Intern Med 1993;119:874–881.

222. Wheeler AP, Jaquiss RD, Newman JH. Physician practices in the treatment of pulmonary embolism and deep-venous thrombosis. Arch Intern Med 1988;148:1321–1325.

223. Hull RD, Raskob GE, Rosenbloom DR. Optimal therapeutic level of heparin therapy in patients with venous thrombosis. Arch Intern Med 1992;152:1589–1595.

224. Hull RD, Delmore T, Genton E. Warfarin sodium versus low-dose heparin in the long-term treatment of venous thrombosis. N Engl J Med 1979;301:855–859.

225. Hull RD, Hirsh J, Jay R. Different intensities of oral anticoagulant therapy in the treatment of proximal vein thrombosis. N Engl J Med 1982;307:1676–1681.

226. Gallus A, Jackaman J, Tillett J. Safety and efficacy of warfarin started early after submassive venous thrombosis or pulmonary embolism. Lancet 1986;2:1293–1296.

227. Hull RD, Raskob GE, Rosenbloom D. Heparin for 5 days as compared with 10 days in the initial treatment of proximal venous thrombosis. N Engl J Med 1990;322:1260–1264.

228. Richter JE, Schan C, Burgard S, et al. Placebo controlled trial of omeprazole in the treatment of acid-related non-cardiac chest pain (NCCP). Am J Gastroenterol 1992;87:1255

229. Khamashta MA, Cuadrado MJ, Mujic F, et al. The management of thrombosis in the antiphospholipid antibody syndrome. N Engl J Med 1995;332:993–997.

230. Petitti DB, Strom BL, Melmon KL. Duration of warfarin anticoagulant therapy and the probabilities of recurrent thromboembolism and hemorrhage. Am J Med 1986;81:255–259.

231. Schulman S, Lockner D, Juhlin-Dannfelt A. The duration of oral anticoagulants after deep-vein thrombosis: a randomized

study. Acta Med Scand 1985;217:547–552.

232. Becker DM, Philbrick JT, Selby JB. Inferior vena cava filters, indications, safety, effectiveness. Arch Intern Med 1992;152:1985–1994.

233. Agnelli G. Anticoagulation in the prevention and treatment of pulmonary embolism. Chest 1995;107:39S-44S.

234. PIOPED Investigators. Value of ventilation/perfusion scan in acute pulmonary embolism. JAMA 1990;263:2753–2759.

235. Come PC, Kim D, Parker JA. Early reversal of right ventricular dysfunction in patients with acute pulmonary embolism after treatment with intravenous tissue plasminogen activator. J Am Coll Cardiol 1987;10:971–978.

236. Wolfe MW, Lee RT, Fedlstein ML. Prognostic significance of right ventricular hypokinesis and perfusion lung scan defects in pulmonary embolism. Am Heart J 1994;127:1371–1375.

237. Goldhaber SZ, Vaughan DE, Markis JE. Acute pulmonary embolism treated with tissue plasminogen activator. Lancet 1986;2:886–889.

238. Rich S, Brundage BH. High-dose calcium channel-blocking therapy for primary pulmonary hypertension: evidence of long-term reduction in pulmonary arterial pressure and regression of right ventricular hypertrophy. Circulation 1987;76:135–141.

239. Ruskin JN, Hutter AM. Primary pulmonary hypertension treated with oral phentolamine. Ann Intern Med 1979;90:772

240. Jamieson SW, Stinson EB, Oyer PE. Heart and lung transplantation for pulmonary hypertension. Am J Surg 1984;147:740–742.

241. McCarthy PM, Starnes VA, Theodore J. Improved survival after heart-lung transplantation. J Thorac Cardiovasc Surg 1990;99:54–59.

242. Cohen M, Edwards WD, Fuster V. Regression in thromboembolic type of primary pulmonary hypertension during 2 1/2 years of antithrombotic therapy. J Am Coll Cardiol 1986;7:172–175.

243. Fuster V, Steele PM, Edwards WD, et al. Primary pulmonary hypertension: natural history and the importance of thrombosis. Circulation 1984;70:580–587.

244. Parris WC, Lin S, Frist W Jr. Use of stellate ganglion blocks for chronic chest pain associated with primary pulmonary hypertension. Anesth Analg 1988;67:993–995.

245. Kane FJ Jr., Wittels E, Harper RG. Chest pain and anxiety disorder. Texas Medicine 1990;86:104–110.

246. Beitman BD. Panic disorder in patients with angiographically normal coronary arteries. Am J Med 1992;92:33S-40S.

247. Salkovskis PM. Psychological treatment of noncardiac chest pain: the cognitive approach. Am J Med 1992;92:114S-121S.

248. Beitman BD, Basha IM, Trombka LH, et al. Alprazolam in the treatment of cardiology patients with atypical chest pain and panic disorder. J Clin Psychopharmacol 1988;8:127–130.

249. Beitman BD, Basha IM, Trombka LH, et al. Pharmacotherapeutic treatment of panic disorder in patients presenting with chest pain. J Fam Practice 1989;28:177–180.

250. Evans DW, Lum LC. Hyperventilation: an important cause of pseudoangina. Lancet 1977;1:155–157.

251. Hegel MT, Abel GG, Etscheidt M, et al. Behavioral treatment of angina-like chest pain in patients with hyperventilation syndrome. J Behavior Ther Exp Psychiatry 1989;20:31–39.

252. DeGuire S, Gevirtz R, Kawahara Y, et al. Hyperventilation syndrome and the assessment of treatment for functional cardiac symptoms. Am J Cardiol 1992;70:673–677.

253. Grossman P, DeSwart CG, Defares PB. A controlled study of a breathing therapy for treatment of hyperventilation syndrome. J Psychosomatic Res 1985;29:49–58.

254. Lum LC. The syndrome of chronic habitual hyperventilation. In: Hill OW, ed. *Modern Trends in Psychosomatic Medicine*. London, England: Butterworth; 1976:196.

255. Magarian GJ. Hyperventilation syndromes: infrequently recognized common expressions of anxiety and stress. Medicine 1982;61:219–236.

256. Bremner CG, Marks IN, Segal I, et al. Reflux esophagitis therapy: sucralfate versus ranitidine in a double-blind multicenter trial. Am J Med 1991;91:119S-122S.

257. Stahl WG, Beton RR, Johnson CS, et al. High-dose ranitidine in the treatment of patients with non-cardiac chest pain and evidence of gastroesophageal reflux. Gastroenterology 1992;102:A168

258. Achem SR, Kolts BE. Current medical therapy for esophageal motility disorders. Am J Med 1992;92:98S-105S.

259. Dodds WJ, Dent J, Hogan WJ, et al. Effect of atropine on esophageal motor function in humans. Am J Physiol 1981;240:290–296.

260. Allen M, Mellow M, Robinson MG, et al. Comparison of calcium channel blocking agents and an anticholinergic agent on esophageal function. Aliment Pharmacol Therapeut 1987;1:153–159.

261. Clouse RE, Lustman PJ, Reidel WL. Correlation of esophageal motility abnormalities with neuropsychiatric status in diabetics. Gastroenterology 1986;90:1146–1154.

262. Clouse RE, Lustman PJ, Eckert TC. Low-dose trazodone for symptomatic patients with esophageal contraction abnormalities: a double-blind, placebo-controlled trial. Gastroenterology 1987;92:1027–1036.

263. Thomas E, Witt P, Willis M, et al. Nifedipine therapy for diffuse esophageal spasm. Southern Med J 1986;79:847–849.

264. Cattau EL, Jr., Castell DO, Johnson DA, et al. Diltiazem therapy for symptoms associated with nutcracker esophagus. Am J Gastroenterol 1991;86:272–276.

265. Richter JE, Dalton CB, Bradley LA, et al. Oral nifedipine in the treatment of noncardiac chest pain in patients with the nutcracker esophagus. Gastroenterology 1987;93:21–28.

266. Lyons WS, Seremetis MG, de Guzman VC, et al. Ruptures and perforation of the esophagus: the case for conservative supportive management. Ann Thorac Surg 1978;25:346–350.

267. Walker WS, Cameron EWJ, Walbaum PR. Diagnosis and management of spontaneous transmural rupture of the oesophagus (Boerhaave's syndrome). Br J Surg 1985;72:204–207.

268. Hutter JA, Fenn A, Braimbridge MV. The management of spontaneous oesophageal perforation by thoracoscopy and irrigation. Br J Surg 1985;72:208–209.

269. Campbell TC, Andrews JL, Neptune WB. Spontaneous rupture of the esophagus (Boerhaave's syndrome): necessity of early diagnosis and treatment. JAMA 1976;235:526–528.

270. Fingerhut A, Baillet P, Oberlin PH, et al. More on congenital diaphragmatic hernia in the adult. Int Surg 1984;69:182–183.

271. Kafka NJ, Leitman IM, Tromba J. Acute pancreatitis secondary to incarcerated paraesophageal hernia. Surgery 1994;115:653–655.

272. Oddsdottir M, Franco AL, Laycock WS, et

al. Laparoscopic repair of paraesophageal hernia. New access, old technique. Surg Endoscopy 1995;9:164–168.

273. Landreneau RJ, Johnson JA, Marshall JB, et al. Clinical spectrum of paraesophageal herniation. Dig Dis Sci 1992;37:537–544.

274. Cloyd DW. Laparoscopic repair of incarcerated paraesophageal hernias. Surgical Endoscopy 1994;8:893–897.

275. Allen B, Tompkins RK, Mulder DG. Repair of large paraesophageal hernia with complete intrathoracic stomach. Am Surgeon 1991;57:642–647.

276. Imrie CW, Whyte AS. A prospective study of acute pancreatitis. Br J Surg 1975;62:490–494.

277. Wilson C, Imrie CW, Carter DC. Fatal acute pancreatitis. Gut 1988;29:782–788.

278. Ranson JHC, Rifkind KM, Turner JW. Prognostic signs and nonoperative peritoneal lavage in acute pancreatitis. Surg Gynecol Obstet 1976;143:209–219.

279. Williamson RCN. Early assessment of severity in acute pancreatitis. Gut 1984;25:1331–1339.

280. Renner IG, Savage WT, Pantoja JL. Death due to acute pancreatitis: a retrospective analysis of 405 autopsy cases. Dig Dis Sci 1985;30:1005–1018.

281. Rabeneck L, Feinstein AR, Horwitz RI. A new clinical prognostic staging system for acute pancreatitis. Am J Med 1993;95:61–70.

282. Agarwal N, Pitchumoni CS. Assessment of severity in acute pancreatitis. Am J Gastroenterol 1991;86:1385–1391.

283. Forsmark CE, Toskes PP. Acute pancreatitis: medical management. In: Fisher RL, editor. *Gastrointestinal Emergencies.* Philadelphia: WB Saunders Company, 1995:295–309.

284. Balthazar EJ. CT diagnosis and staging of acute pancreatitis. Radiol Clin North Am 1989;27:19–37.

285. Bradley EL, Murphy F, Ferguson C. Prediction of pancreatic necrosis by dynamic pancreatography. Ann Surg 1989;210:495–504.

286. Beechy-Newman N. Controlled trial of high-dose octreotide in treatment of acute pancreatitis: evidence of improvement in disease severity. Dig Dis Sci 1993;38:644–647.

287. Saario IA. 5-Fluorouracil in the treatment of acute pancreatitis. Am J Surg 1983;145:349–352.

288. Valderrama R, Perez-Mateo M, Navarro S. Multicenter double-blind trial of gabexate mesylate (FOY) in unselected patients with acute pancreatitis. Digestion 1992;51:65–70.

289. Buchler M, Malfertheiner P, Uhl W. Gabexate mesilate in human acute pancreatitis. Gastroenterology 1993;104:1165–1170.

290. Larvin M, Wilson C, Heath D. A prospective, multi-center randomized trial of intra-peritoneal anti-protease therapy for acute pancreatitis. Gastroenterology 1992;102:A274

291. Sax HC, Warner BW, Talamini MA. Early total parenteral nutrition in acute pancreatitis: lack of beneficial effects. Am J Surg 1987;153:117–124.

292. Kalfarentzos FE, Karavia D, Karatzas T. Total parenteral nutrition in severe acute pancreatitis. J Am Coll Nutr 1991;10:156–162.

293. Ihse I, Evander A, Holmberg JT. Influence of peritoneal lavage on objective prognostic signs in acute pancreatitis. Ann Surg 1986;204:122–127.

294. Ranson JHC, Berman RS. Long peritoneal lavage decreases pancreatic sepsis in acute pancreatitis. Ann Surg 1990;211:708–718.

295. Pederzolli P, Bassi C, Vesentini S. A randomized multicenter clinical trial of antibiotic prophylaxis of septic complications in acute necrotizing pancreatitis with imipenem. Surg Gynecol Obstet 1993;176:480–483.

296. Buchler M, Malfertheiner P, Friel H. Human pancreatic tissue concentration of bactericidal antibiotics. Gastroenterology 1992;103:1902–1908.

297. Baker CC, Huynh T. Acute pancreatitis: surgical management. In: Fisher RL, ed. *Gastrointestinal Emergencies.* Philadelphia, Pa: WB Saunders Company; 1995:311–322.

298. Cooperman AM. *Laparoscopic Cholecystectomy: Difficult Cases and Creative Solutions.* St. Louis: Quality Medical, 1992.

299. Meyers WC, and the Southern Surgeons Club. A prospective analysis of 1518 laparoscopic cholecystectomies. N Engl J Med 1991;324:1073–1078.

300. Goldman G, Kahn PJ, Alon R, et al. Biliary colic treatment and acute cholecystitis prevention by prostaglandin inhibitor. Dig Dis Sci 1989;34:809–811.

301. Banks L, Wright JP, Lucke W, et al. Peptic ulcer: a follow-up study. J Clin Gastroenterol 1986;8:381–384.

302. Jorde R, Bostad L, Burhal BC. Asymptom-

atic gastric ulcer: a follow-up study on patients with previous gastric ulcer disease. Lancet 1986;1:119–121.

303. Katelaris P. Treatment of Helicobacter pylori infection. Biomed & Pharmacother 1995;49:5–10.

304. Chiba N, Rao BV, Rademaker JW, et al. Meta analysis of the efficacy of antibiotic therapy in eradicating Helicobacter pylori. Am J Gastroenterol 1992;87:1716–1727.

305. Graham DY, Lew GM, Malaty HM. Factors influencing the eradication of Helicobacter pylori with triple therapy. Gastroenterology 1993;102:493–496.

306. Henry DA, Johnson A, Dobson A, et al. Fatal peptic ulcer complications and the use of non-steroidal anti-inflammatory drugs, aspirin and corticosteroids. Br Med J 1987;295:1225–1227.

307. Ryan EL. Cervicothoracic pain due to fatigue of pectoral girdle musculature. Med J Aust 1991;155:204–205.

308. Pellegrino MJ. Atypical chest pain as an initial presentation of primary fibromyalgia. Arch Physical Med Rehab 1990;71:526–528.

309. Waylonis GW, Ronan PG, Gordon C. A profile of fibromyalgia in occupational environments. Am J Phys Med Rehab 1994;73:112–115.

310. Mengshoel AM, Komnaes HB, Forre O. The effects of 20 weeks of physical fitness training in female patients with fibromyalgia. Clin Exp Rheum 1992;10:345–349.

311. Burckhardt CS, Mannerkorpi K, Hedenberg L, et al. A randomized, controlled clinical trial of education and physical training for women with fibromyalgia. J Rheumatol 1994;21:714–720.

312. Carette S, Bell MJ, Reynolds WJ, et al. Comparison of amitriptyline, cyclobenzaprine, and placebo in the treatment of fibromyalgia. A randomized, double-blind clinical trial. Arthritis Rheum 1994;37:32–40.

313. Goodnick PJ, Sandoval R. Psychotropic treatment of chronic fatigue syndrome and related disorders. J Clin Psychiatry 1993;54:13–20.

314. Russell IJ, Fletcher EM, Michalek JE, et al. Treatment of primary fibrositis/fibromyalgia syndrome with ibuprofen and alprazolam. A double-blind, placebo-controlled study. Arthritis Rheum 1991;34:552–560.

315. Fossaluzza V, De Vita S. Combined therapy with cyclobenzaprine and ibuprofen in primary fibromyalgia syndrome. Int J Clin Pharm Res 1992;12:99–102.

316. Wolfe F, Cathey MA, Hawley DJ. A double-blind placebo controlled trial of fluoxetine in fibromyalgia. Scand J Rheum 1994;23:255–259.

317. Pattrick M, Swannell A, Doherty M. Chlormezanone in primary fibromyalgia syndrome: a double blind placebo controlled study. Br J Rheum 1993;32:55–58.

318. Goodnick PJ, Sandoval R: Psychotropic treatment of chronic fatigue syndrome and related disorders. J Clin Psychiatry 1993;54:13–20.

319. Deluze C, Bosia L, Zirbs A, et al. Electroacupuncture in fibromyalgia: results of a controlled trial. Br Med J 1992;305:1249–1252.

320. Kaufmann HJ. Chest pain and esophageal motility: what is the role of manometry? J Clin Gastroenterol 1982;4:466–467.

321. Howell JM. Xiphoidynia: a report of three cases. J Emerg Med 1992;10:435–438.

322. Howell J. Xiphoidynia: an uncommon cause of exertional chest pain. Am J Emerg Med 1990;8:176

323. Sklaroff HJ. Xiphoidynia-another cause of atypical chest pain: six case reports. Mount Sinai J Med 1979;46:546–548.

324. Viitanen JV, Suni J, Kautiainen H, et al. Effect of physiotherapy on spinal mobility in ankylosing spondylitis. Scand J Rheum 1992;21:38–41.

325. Nakatsuchi Y, Saitoh S, Hosaka M, et al. Conservative treatment of thoracic outlet syndrome using an orthosis. J Hand Surg 1995;20:34–39.

326. Kenny RA, Traynor GB, Withington D, et al. Thoracic outlet syndrome: a useful exercise treatment option. Am J Surg 1993;165:282–284.

327. Cuypers PW, Bollen EC, van Houtte HP. Transaxillary first rib resection for thoracic outlet syndrome. Acta Chir Belgica 1995;95:119–122.

328. Cina C, Whiteacre L, Edwards R, et al. Treatment of thoracic outlet syndrome with combined scalenectomy and transaxillary first rib resection. Cardiovasc Surg 1994;2:514–518.

329. Davies AH, Walton J, Stuart E, et al. Surgical management of the thoracic outlet compression syndrome. Br J Surg 1991;78:1193–1195.

330. Dellon AL. The results of supraclavicular brachial plexus neurolysis (without first rib resection) in management of post-trau-

matic "thoracic outlet syndrome". J Reconstruct Microsurg 1993;9:11–17.

331. Stack PS. Trichinosis. Still a public health threat. Postgrad Med 1995;97:137–144.

332. Tyring S, Barbarsh RA, Nahlik JE, et al. Famciclovir for the treatment of acute herpes zoster: effects on acute disease and postherpetic neuralgia, a randomized, double-blind, placebo-controlled study. Ann Intern Med 1995;123:89–96.

333. Carmichael JK. Treatment of herpes zoster and postherpetic neuralgia. Am Fam Physician 1991;44:203–210.

334. Agostini G, Agostini S. Immunoglobulins in the treatment of herpes zoster. Clin Therapeutica 1992;141:11–16.

335. Rossi S, Whitfield M, Berger TG. The treatment of acyclovir-resistant herpes zoster with trifluorothymidine and interferon alfa. Arch Derm 1995;131:24–26.

336. Yu B. Treatment of Herpes Zoster: recombinant alpha-2a-interferon versus acyclovir (ACV) and vitamin therapy. Clinical study group on interferon. Chinese Med Sci J 1993;8:38–40.

337. Winnie AP, Hartwell PW. Relationship between the time of treatment of acute herpes zoster with sympathetic blockade and prevention of post-herpetic neuralgia: clinical support for a new theory of the mechanism by which sympathetic blockade provides therapeutic benefit. Reg Anesth 1993;18:277–282.

338. BeLieu RM. Mastodynia. Obstet Gynecol Clin North Am 1994;21:461–477.

339. Petersen L, Graversen HP, Andersen JA, et al. The duct ectasia syndrome—an overlooked disease entity. Ugeskrift for Laeger 1993;155:1540–1545.

340. Fiorica JV. Special problems. Mondor's disease, macrocysts, trauma, squamous metaplasia, miscellaneous disorders of the nipple. Obstet Gynecol Clin North Am 1994;21:479–485.

341. Yellin A, Gapany-Gapanavicius M, Lieberman Y. Spontaneous pneumomediastinum: is it a rare cause of chest pain? Thorax 1983;38:383–385.

342. Mailis A, Chan J, Basinski A, et al. Chest wall pain after aortocoronary bypass surgery using internal mammary artery graft: a new pain syndrome? Heart Lung 1989;18:553–558.

343. Barbera J, Albert-Pamplo R. Centrocentral anastomosis of the proximal nerve stump in the treatment of painful amputation neuromas of major nerves. J Neurosurg 1993;79:331–334.

344. Meyrier A, Guibert J. Diagnosis and drug treatment of acute pyelonephritis. Drugs 1992;44:356–367.

345. Plattner MS. Pyelonephritis in pregnancy. J Perinatal Neonatal Nurs 1994;8:20–27.

346. Rushton HG, Majd M. Dimercaptosuccinic acid renal scintigraphy for the evaluation of pyelonephritis and scarring: a review of experimental and clinical studies. J Urol 1992;148:1726–1732.

347. Tenner SM, Yadven MW, Kimmel PL. Acute pyelonephritis. Preventing complications through prompt diagnosis and proper therapy. Postgrad Med 1992;91:261–268.

348. Gitter MJ, Goldsmith SR, Dunbar DN, et al. Cocaine and chest pain: clinical features and outcome of patients hospitalized to rule out myocardial infarction. Ann Intern Med 1991;115:277–282.

349. Olshaker JS. Cocaine chest pain. Emerg Med Clin North Am 1994;12:391–396.

350. Van Dorpe A, Piessens J, Willems JL, et al. Unexplained chest pain with normal coronary arteriograms. A follow-up study. Cardiology 1987;74:436–443.

351. McMahon SB. Mechanisms of cutaneous, deep and visceral pain. In: Wall PD, Melzack R, eds. *Textbook of Pain*. 3rd ed. Edinburgh: Churchill Livingstone; 1994:129–150.

352. Twycross RG. Opioids. In: Wall PD, Melzack R, eds. *Textbook of Pain*. 3rd ed. Edinburgh: Churchill Livingstone; 1994:943–962.

353. Gourlay GK, Cherry DA. Response to controversy corner: Can opioids be successfully used to treat severe pain in nonmalignant conditions? Clin J Pain 1991;7:347–349.

354. Sunshine A, Olson NZ. Nonnarcotic analgesics. In: Wall PD, Melzack R, eds. *Textbook of Pain*. 3rd ed. Edinburgh: Churchill Livingstone; 1994:923–942.

355. Monks R. Psychotropic drugs. In: Wall PD, Melzack R, eds. *Textbook of Pain*. 3rd ed. Edinburgh: Churchill Livingstone; 1994:963–989.

356. Roll M, Theorell T. Acute chest pain without obvious organic cause before age 40—personality and recent life events. J Psychosomatic Res 1987;31:215–221.

357. Cott A, McCully J, Goldberg WM, et al. Interdisciplinary treatment of morbidity

in benign chest pain. Angiology 1992;43: 195–202.

358. Klimes I, Mayou RA, Pearce MJ, et al. Psychological treatment for atypical non-cardiac chest pain: a controlled evaluation. Psychol Med 1990;20:605–611.

359. Wall PD. The placebo and the placebo response. In: Wall PD, Melzack R, eds. Textbook of Pain. 3rd ed. Edinburgh: Churchill Livingstone; 1994:1297–1308.

360. Mendelson G. Chronic pain and compensation issues. In: Wall PD, Melzack R, eds. Textbook of Pain. 3rd ed. Edinburgh: Churchill Livingstone; 1994:1387–1400.

361. Bonica JJ, Butler SH. Local anaesthesia and regional blocks. In: Wall PD, Melzack R, eds. Textbook of Pain. 3rd ed. Edinburgh: Churchill Livingstone; 1994: 997–1023.

362. Hannington-Kiff JG. Sympathetic nerve blocks in painful limb disorders.In: Wall PD, Melzack R, eds. Textbook of Pain. 3rd ed. Edinburgh: Churchill Livingstone; 1994:1035–1052.

363. Sweet WH, Poletti CE, Gybels JM. Operations in the brainstem and spinal canal, with an appendix on the relationship of open to percutaneous cordotomy. In: Wall PD, Melzack R, eds. Textbook of Pain. 3rd ed. Edinburgh: Churchill Livingstone; 1994:1113–1135.

364. Tasker RR. Stereotactic surgery. In: Wall PD, Melzack R, eds. Textbook of Pain. 3rd ed. Edinburgh: Churchill Livingstone; 1994:1137–1157.

365. Woolf CJ, Thompson JW. Stimulation-induced analgesia: transcutaneous electrical nerve stimulation (TENS) and vibration. In: Wall PD, Melzack R, eds. Textbook of Pain. 3rd ed. Edinburgh: Churchill Livingstone; 1994:1191–1208.

366. Kellaway P. The part played by electric fish in the early history of bioelectricity and electrotherapy. Bull Hist Med 1946; 20:112–137.

367. Kane K, Taub A. A history of local electrical analgesia. Pain 1975;1:125–138.

368. Linzer M, Long DM. Transcutaneous neural stimulation for relief of pain. IEEE Trans Biomed Eng 1976;23:341–345.

369. Ledergerber CP. Postoperative electro-analgesia. Obstet Gynaecol 1978;151: 334–338.

370. Wall PD, Sweet WH. Temporary abolition of pain in man. Science 1967;155: 108–109.

371. Bates JA, Nathan PW. Transcutaneous electrical nerve stimulation for chronic pain. Anaesthesia 1980;35:817–822.

372. Mannheimer C, Carlsson CA, Vedin A, et al. Transcutaneous electrical nerve stimulation (TENS) in angina pectoris. Pain 1986;26:291–300.

373. Simpson BA. Spinal cord stimulation in 60 cases of intractable pain. J Neurol Neurosurg Psych 1991;54:196–199.

374. North RB, Levy RM. Consensus conference on the neurosurgical management of pain. Neurol 1994;34:756–761.

375. Shimoji K, Hokari T, Kano T, et al. Management of intractable pain with percutaneous epidural spinal cord stimulation: differences in pain-relieving effects among diseases and sites of pain. Anesth Analg 1993;77:110–116.

376. Melzack R. Folk medicine and the sensory modulation of pain. In: Wall PD, Melzack R, eds. Textbook of Pain. 3rd ed. Edinburgh: Churchill Livingstone; 1994: 1209–1217.

377. Melzack R. Prolonged relief of pain by brief, intense transcutaneous somatic stimulation. Pain 1975;1:357–373

378. Reichmanis M, Becker RO. Relief of experimentally induced pain by stimulation at acupuncture loci. Comparative Medicine East and West 1977;5:281–288.

379. Gaw AC, Chang LW, Shaw LC. Efficacy of acupuncture on osteoarthritic pain. N Engl J Med 1975;293:375–378.

380. Taub HA, Beard MC, Eisenberg L, et al. Studies of acupuncture for operative dentistry. J Am Dental Assoc 1977;95: 555–561.

381. Lewit K. The needle effect in the relief of myofascial pain. Pain 1979;6:83–90.

382. Travell J, Rinzler SH. The myofascial genesis of pain. Postgrad Med 1952;11: 425–434.

383. Melzack R, Stillwell DM, Fox EJ. Trigger points and acupuncture points for pain: correlations and implications. Pain 1977; 3:3–23.

384. Liu YK, Varela M, Oswald R. The correspondence between some motor points and acupuncture loci. Am J Chinese Med 1975;3:347–358.

385. Kaden GG, Shenker IR, Gootman N. Chest pain in adolescents. J Adolescent Health 1991;12:251–255.

386. Kao. Acupuncture Therapeutics. New Haven: Eastern Press, 1973.

# 7

# Snoring

Stephen E. Lapinsky, M.D.
David R. Goldfarb, M.D.
Ronald F. Grossman, M.D.

## Introduction

### Definition and Classification

Snoring is an inspiratory noise produced during sleep by vibration of the oropharyngeal walls.[1] It is a symptom of an underlying abnormality of the upper airway and presents with various ranges of severity. In its mildest form, it may occur only intermittently often in the supine position, while severe snoring usually occurs every night and may be associated with obstructive apneas.[1] The diagnosis of snoring is usually subjective, and based on the impression of noise during sleep by a bed partner, family member, or sleep technologist. Similar imprecise diagnostic criteria are used in the majority of epidemiological studies of the prevalence and health risk of snoring, and often no definition has been given.[2]

For the purposes of research studies, a more objective assessment of snoring has been achieved using acoustic recordings during polysomnography. By measuring spikes in sound intensity greater than that produced by normal breathing, a uniform objective grading of snoring frequency and severity can be established.[3,4] However, sound intensity monitoring alone does not distinguish between snoring and other respiratory noises, and more complex techniques, such as spectral analysis, may be necessary.[5] Distinctive acoustic features may provide information about the pathogenic mechanisms, possibly allowing the differentiation of pathologic and simple snoring.[5,6]

The most important aspect in the classification of snoring is the presence or absence of obstructive sleep apnea (OSA). Nonapneic snorers appear to be at a lower risk of cardiovascular complications than apneic snorers.[7,8] The role of polysomnography in the diagnosis of OSA is discussed later in this chapter. Other techniques, such as nasal airflow recording and lateral pharyngeal cineradiography, have been used to differentiate subgroups of snorers.[9] Use of an electroencephalogram (EEG) arousal index may be of value to determine the degree of sleep fragmentation and identify snorers at risk of hypersomnolence.[10] Respiratory-related arousal may occur in the absence of obstructive sleep apnea, and appears to be related to increases in ventilatory effort.[11-13]

While a practical definition and clas-

From Irwin RS, Curley FJ, Grossman RF (eds): Diagnosis and Treatment of Symptoms of the Respiratory Tract. Armonk, New York, Futura Publishing Company, Inc., © 1997.

sification of snoring does not currently exist, the importance of this common affliction is gaining recognition. Once more objective diagnostic criteria have been established, further research will be necessary to distinguish pathologic from non-pathologic snoring.

## Epidemiology

Snoring is a common phenomenon, with a reported prevalence varying from 15% to 60% of the adult population. One of the earliest epidemiological surveys, a study of nearly 6000 people in the Republic of San Marino (northern Italy), determined that 40% of men and 28% of women reported snoring, with an increasing prevalence up to the seventh decade.[14] In this study, more than 60% of men and 40% of women older than 60 years reported snoring.[14] Other studies suggest that a slight decrease in prevalence occurs with increasing age over 60.[15,16] A study of middle-aged women demonstrated a prevalence of snoring of 23% in the younger age group (40 to 44 years) increasing to 40% at ages 50 to 59 years.[17] Comparable results have been reported from other epidemiological studies. Snorers represent 30% of men and 15% to 20% of women in a self-reported study of 7500 Finnish adults between the ages of 40 and 69 years.[18,19] The prevalence of self-reported snoring occurring "every or most nights" was 17% in a North American survey of more than 2000 adults, with men aged 40 to 64 years having the highest frequency at 30%.[20]

A significant bias may occur in these epidemiological studies, since snoring is generally self-reported. A higher prevalence of snoring has been noted when reporting was by the spouse, where 71% of husbands and 51% of wives were reported to snore.[15] A study comparing self-reporting with spouse-reporting demonstrated that self-reporting underestimates the prevalence of snoring. In this study, the prevalence in men increased from 34% (self-reported) to 43% (spouse reported).[21] Also, a significant bias occurs in all of these surveys due to the subjective nature of the assessment of snoring. A significant percentage (6% to 37%) of subjects in these surveys do not know whether they snore.[19,20] With no clear definition or standard objective measurement, these studies resort to the use of arbitrary descriptions such as "habitual snorers," "frequent snorers," or "snores most nights." The true incidence and spectrum of severity of snoring is thus difficult to determine.

The objective diagnosis of OSA, a clinically important complication of snoring, allows a more accurate estimation of the public health risk of snoring. A study of a random sample of 30- to 60-year-old state employees in Wisconsin revealed the prevalence of sleep disordered breathing (defined as an abnormal sleep study with apnea-hypopnea index greater than 5) to be 24% in men and 9% in women.[22] Subjects with symptomatic sleep-disordered breathing were estimated to account for 4% of men and 2% of women.[22]

## Clinical Significance

Snoring has traditionally been considered more of a social nuisance than a significant health problem, but it is apparent that this common affliction may pose a health risk. Epidemiological studies have demonstrated a correlation between snoring and hypertension, ischemic heart disease, and stroke.[14,15,17–19,23] However, this association may be largely due to concomitant obesity or sleep apnea and prospective studies have not confirmed an association when corrected for these parameters.[7,8] Heavy snoring is, nevertheless, an important marker of OSA, which appears to be an independent cardiovascular risk factor.[8,23–27] A common complaint of snorers is the occurrence of excessive daytime somnolence, which may occur even in the absence of OSA. Recent studies suggest that snoring may independently cause symptoms of daytime sleepiness and fatigue (ie, upper airways resistance syndrome).[12,13] This and the other associations and complications of snoring are discussed in more detail below. The assessment and management of snoring is, therefore, important not only to silence the acoustic annoyance, but also to improve health and quality of life.

## Pathogenesis

### Airflow Resistance

The inspiratory noise of snoring is caused by vibration of the soft tissues of the oropharynx, due to collapse of this airway during sleep.[1] Patency of the upper airways is determined by the balance between the pressures surrounding the airway (Figure 1). The negative intraluminal pressure during inspiration tends to collapse the airway, and is counteracted by the outward pressure of the dilatory pharyngeal muscles which contract with each inspiration.[28,29] The compliance of the pharynx will influence the net negative pressure required to obstruct airflow,[30,31] while mucosal stickiness may affect the ease with which the airway reopens.[32] A number of anatomical and functional factors may be responsible for producing airway collapse, but the common underlying abnormality is increased upper airway resistance.

With increased airways resistance, an increased inspiratory effort is required to maintain airflow. This negative pressure generated in the chest has the effect of pulling down the laryngotracheobronchial tree, and lengthening and narrowing the oropharynx.[1] The increased flow further reduces intrapharyngeal pressure. This negative pressure, occuring concurrently with the pharyngeal muscle hypotonia associated with sleep, may cause airway collapse and the vibrations of the pharyngeal soft tissues perceived as snoring. The degree of collapse will depend to some degree on the compliance of the pharyngeal airway. Patients with OSA appear to have increased compliance and airway collapsibility during wakefulness and sleep compared to snorers without OSA, resulting in more marked airway obstruction and cessation of airflow.[30,31]

A variety of factors may contribute to elevated upper airway resistance in the individual patient, and are discussed in more detail in the following sections. Structural abnormalities, including abnormalities of the pharynx where the airway obstruction responsible for snoring and obstructive apnea occur and obstruction at other levels of the airway producing in-

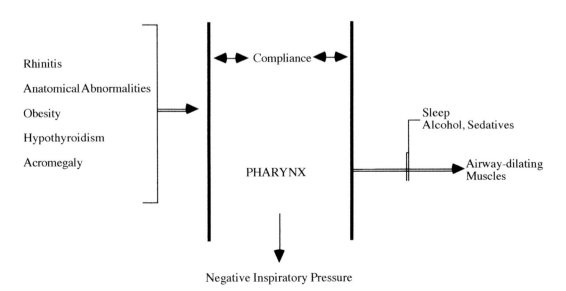

**Figure 1.** Factors influencing upper airway narrowing.

**Table I**

Causes of Increased Upper Airway
Resistance Predisposing to Snoring

**Anatomic Abnormalities**
Rhinitis
Deviated Nasal Septum
Adenoid and Tonsillar Hypertrophy
Glottic Web
Micrognathia
Retrognathia
Lymphoma of Pharyngeal Lymphoid Tissue
**Physiological Effects**
Sleep State
Sleep Deprivation
Body Positioning
Bulbar Incoordination (secondary to poliomye-
     litis, motor neurone disease)
Diaphragmatic Pacing
**Miscellaneous**
Obesity
Hypothyroidism
Acromegaly
Testosterone Administration
Cigarette Smoking
Alcohol
Sedative-Hypnotic Drugs
Familial Trait

creased respiratory efforts, are important. Impaired function of upper airway muscles occurs related to the sleep state. Other factors, such as obesity, hormonal effects, and drugs, may significantly influence upper airway function (Table I).

## Anatomical Factors

The noise of snoring is directly related to the vibratory tissue in the oropharynx.[1] The primary offending tissues are the mucosa and underlying musculature of the soft palate and uvula, the mucosa and underlying musculature of the anterior and posterior tonsillar pillars, the tonsils themselves, and redundant hypopharyngeal mucosa (Figure 2).[33]

Any anatomical factors which affect airflow resistance as described above, can have a secondary effect on snoring. Specifically, narrowed oropharyngeal propor-

tions and a large tongue can significantly contribute to increased airway resistance. Adjacent structures that result in alteration of airflow, such as a deviated nasal septum, nasal polyps, enlarged nasal turbinates, and nasopharyngeal masses, may also secondarily affect the snoring (Figure 3).

Anatomical variations appear to be responsible for the predisposition of some snorers to develop complete airway obstruction and sleep apnea. The relative ratio between upper and lower pharyngeal diameters is important, and those with a narrow velopharynx but large hypopharynx are at increased risk of developing airway collapse.[34] This may be because a narrow hypopharynx damps the inspiratory suction pressure, preventing oropharyngeal collapse.

## Sleep and Breathing

The muscles of the pharynx are responsible for maintaining patency of the upper airway during breathing. Neural control of these muscles is from the same areas of the brain stem that are responsible for controlling motor fibers to the diaphragm and intercostal muscles, known as the respiratory center.[35] The upper airway muscles contract rhythmically with breathing, beginning contraction before and peaking earlier than the diaphragm, stabilizing the airway against the collapsing effect of inspiration.[28,36] During wakefulness, these muscles demonstrate a high level of tonic activity, with some phasic action.

The sleep state is associated with changes in the neural output of the respiratory center, which may affect pharyngeal airway mechanics as well as motor drive to the thoracic pump muscles. Nonrapid eye movement (NREM) sleep is characterized by an increase in thoracic muscle motor drive, although minute volume decreases and $PaCO_2$ rises.[35,37,38] The decreased ventilation may result from increased upper airway resistance due to a loss of tonic activity of the pharyngeal muscles, while a reflex but inadequate

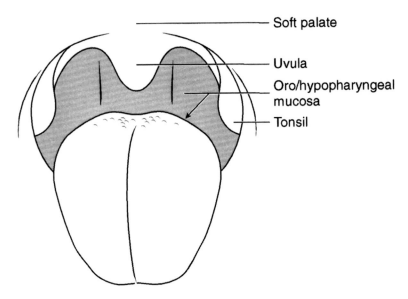

**Figure 2.** Primary snoring tissue.

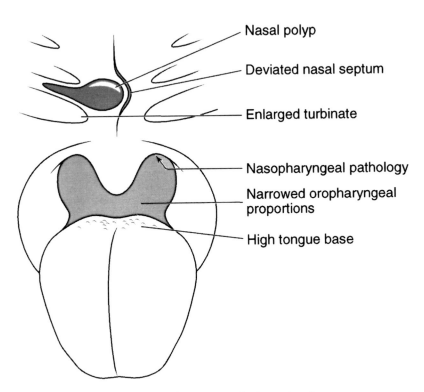

**Figure 3.** Secondary anatomical snoring factors.

compensatory increase in thoracic muscle drive occurs.[38,39] The combination of increased negative inspiratory pressure and pharyngeal obstruction may produce snoring. Snoring may appear as soon as the patient falls asleep, progressing with deepening of NREM sleep.[1] In rapid eye movement (REM) sleep, generalized muscular hypotonia occurs, affecting most muscles except the diaphragm.[35] This hypotonia predisposes to airway collapse, making obstructive apneas common, although snoring tends to diminish.[1,35] This may be because the actual snoring sound depends on the tone of pharyngeal muscles, such as the tensor veli palatini.[1]

The stability of the upper airway depends on the temporal coordination and balanced activity of the dilator muscles of the pharynx and the inspiratory muscles of the chest.[28,29,40] High levels of respiratory drive are associated with a more marked increase in upper airway motor activity compared with chest wall activity. In contrast, low levels of drive, as occur in sleep, result in relatively more marked diaphragmatic motor activity with loss of upper airway tone, predisposing to snoring.[39,41] Other factors have been demonstrated to influence the motor activity of the upper airway muscles. Sleep deprivation causes decreased genioglossus electromyogram activity in older patients and may increase snoring,[42] while similar effects on genioglossus activity have been demonstrated to occur in relation to the ingestion of benzodiazepines[43] and alcohol.[44]

## Other Factors

In addition to the anatomical and functional factors described above, a number of reversible influences may be responsible for aggravating snoring and OSA. Obesity plays an important role in predisposing to snoring.[20,45-47] This may be related to the local deposition of fat adjacent to the pharynx, in the soft palate, in the uvula, and in the submental region.[48-50] The reduction in lung volumes produced by obesity may also play a role in affecting pharyngeal size.[51,52] Increased neck circumference is associated with the presence of OSA, likely due to the dynamic loading of the airway by the weight of fatty tissue in the neck.[53] Hypothyroidism predisposes to snoring and OSA by mechanisms involving obesity and abnormalities in respiratory control.[54] Another hormonal influence is the occurrence of snoring in acromegaly, secondary to macroglossia and anatomical abnormalities.[55]

Nasal obstruction causes an increased negative intrathoracic pressure on inspiration, favoring collapse of the upper airways. Allergic rhinitis, nasal polyps, and other anatomical defects of the nasal passages may predispose to nocturnal breathing disorders.[56,57] Smoking has been associated with snoring in epidemiological studies,[20] and this is due to airways inflammation causing increased airways resistance.[1,20] A variety of drugs may induce or worsen snoring. Alcohol causes mucosal vasodilatation and a selective reduction in the motor neuron activity of the upper airway muscles, resulting in increased nasal and pharyngeal airway resistance.[42,58-60] This, associated with normal diaphragmatic activity, produces snoring and sleep apnea.[58] Benzodiazepines and other hypnotics depress ventilatory drive and may also affect upper airway muscle function.[41,61]

## Diagnostic Approach

The assessment of a patient with snoring involves a detailed history, physical examination, and investigative studies aimed at evaluating the cause and possible complications of this condition (Figure 4). Therapy may be aided by establishing the underlying anatomical and/or functional factors responsible for airway collapse during sleep. The presence of significant complications will determine the extent of the therapeutic interventions.

## History

The snorer without sleep apnea may be asymptomatic, seeking medical atten-

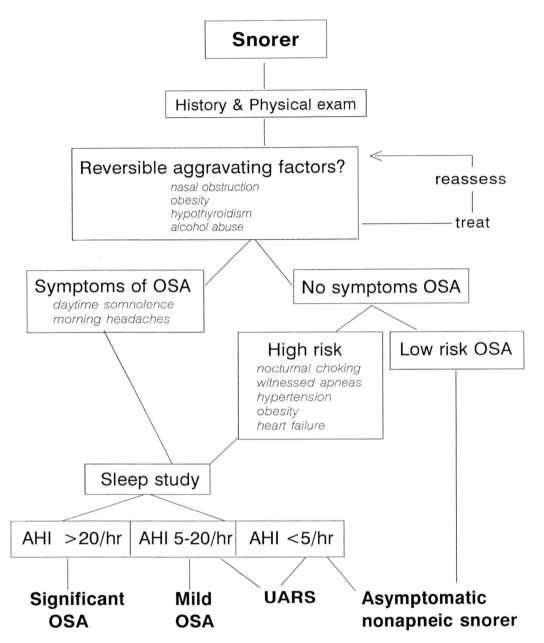

**Figure 4.** Diagnostic algorithm for the management of snoring. AHI = apnea-hypopnea index; OSA = obstructive sleep apnea; UARS = upper airway resistance syndrome.

tion only at the request of the bed partner.[21] A history from those living with the patient is essential in the clinical assessment of snoring. The aims of the history are to assess whether reversible predisposing factors exist, and to evaluate the sever- ity and presence of complications of snoring, including excessive daytime sleepiness, OSA, and cardiovascular disease. Characteristics of the patient's snoring can only be obtained from a partner, while features suggestive of sleep apnea should be elicited from both. Less severe snoring is often continuous occurring on every breath, although postural changes may cause intermittent worsening with increased airflow obstruction occurring in the supine position.[1] Intermittent or cyclic snoring may result from airflow obstruction causing apnea.[1] Features of obstructive sleep apnea which may be reported by a partner include loud, intermittent snoring with periods of apnea terminated by a loud gasp or snort. The patient may awaken due to the noise or with a choking sensation.

While factors, such as age, body mass index, male sex, and daytime somnolence, in association with snoring are predictive of OSA,[62] it is not possible to discriminate between nonapneic snorers and those with sleep apnea based on history.[62–64] A history of daytime sleepiness with nocturnal choking or witnessed apnea is more strongly predictive of OSA.[64] A detailed sleep history, including the degree of sleep disturbance, nocturnal awakenings, restless sleep, diaphoresis, and apneic episodes, should be sought. Social factors disturbing sleep, such as shift work, must be evaluated. Symptoms resulting from sleep fragmentation or sleep disordered breathing should be evaluated. These include excessive daytime somnolence, cognitive dysfunction and memory loss, impotence, and morning headaches.[63,65] Excessive daytime somnolence may occur in association with heavy snoring in the absence of OSA.[12,13,63] The degree of daytime sleepiness varies with the severity of sleep disruption, and may be assessed by the level of activity during which drowsiness occurs.[12] Passive sleepiness occurring while reading or watching TV may be normal while sleepiness occurring during conversation or while driving is very significant.[66] The differential diagnosis of daytime somnolence includes narcolepsy, and inquiry should be made as to a family history or symptoms of this condition. Symptoms include cataplexy (a sudden loss of voluntary muscle tone precipitated by strong emotions), hypnagogic hallucinations (sleep-onset dreams), and sleep paralysis.

A detailed history may elicit factors responsible for precipitating or aggravating snoring. A history of nasal obstruction, nasal surgery, or trauma may be relevant. Smoking, by causing mucosal edema and inflammation, may increase snoring.[20] Snoring may occur only on some nights, due to the use of alcohol or hypnotics.[58,61] Obesity is strongly associated with snoring and OSA, since the lumen of the upper airway is narrowed by excessive adipose tissue[20,16] and recent changes in weight should be determined. The presence of features suggestive of hypothyroidism, such as constipation or cold intolerance, should be evaluated.[54]

Epidemiological studies demonstrate snoring to be associated with hypertension and cardiovascular disease,[14,15] and the presence of such complications may determine whether treatment should be instituted. Complications of OSA, such as polycythemia, cor pulmonale, intellectual deterioration, or impotence, may warrant treatment of only mild OSA. Finally, the social impact of loud snoring should be appreciated and may result in significant family disruption as well as social embarrassment.

## Physical Examination

A complete physical examination is important to assess the upper airway and to exclude reversible conditions predisposing to snoring. Measurement of the patient's height, weight, and blood pressure are necessary. Plethoric skin may indicate polycythemia, suggesting chronic hypoxemia and obstructive sleep apnea. Lethargy and hair-thinning or hair loss may imply hypothyroidism as a causative factor in the patient's snoring.

Careful evaluation of the head, neck, and entire upper airway is essential to assess anatomical variations that may directly or indirectly cause the snoring.[1] Inspection and palpation of the head and neck may reveal a short, thick neck associated with obesity.[53] Masses in the neck may indicate an underlying malignancy of the upper airway as a cause of the snoring.

Airway evaluation begins with assessment of the oral cavity. This includes examination of the mandible and dentition to assess for retrognathia or hypognathia. A large-tongue and high-tongue base are seen more frequently in the snoring than in the nonsnoring patient.[67] The tissues of the oropharynx are the main offenders in snoring. A long, low, thick, soft palate and/or uvula may be seen. The tonsils should be examined for size and position. Vertical pharyngeal folds may be seen indicating redundant mucosa. Asking the patient to snore with the mouth slightly open, often reveals the area of vibrating tissue.

Anterior rhinoscopy will reveal anatomical abnormalities within the nasal cavity which may contribute to airway obstruction, indirectly exacerbating the snoring. The entire nasal cavity should be examined to assess for mucosal pathology, such as hypertrophied turbinates, polyps, or other masses. Nasal decongestants may be required, but should not be used until the nose is examined without medication. The septum is frequently deviated but caution should be exercised before ascribing the septum as the source of the snoring.

Flexible fiberoptic nasolaryngoscopy provides an excellent view of the entire upper airway. The nasopharynx, hypopharynx, and the larynx are quickly and easily visualized with minimal patient discomfort. Once again, the nasal cavity should be evaluated and the nasopharynx may be inspected for narrowing, scarring, or masses. The dorsal aspect of the soft palate and uvula may show thickening. The oropharynx, hypopharynx, and larynx can be evaluated for structural or physiological abnormalities.

Two maneuvers may be used to more accurately determine the site of the snoring. The first involves positioning the tip of the endoscope in the nasopharynx such that the dorsal surface of the soft palate is visualized but not impinged upon. The patient is then asked to snore or snort and the main vibrating tissue may be seen. The second technique involves a Muller's maneuver during nasolaryngoscopy.[67] The flexible fiberoptic nasolaryngoscope is placed through the nose into the oropharynx, the patient is then asked to inhale vigorously with a closed mouth while the examiner occludes the nostrils. This creates a negative pressure within the upper airway. The lateral pharyngeal wall as well as the tongue are observed for collapse and movement. The endoscope is then repositioned in the nasopharynx and the exercise is repeated to assess for collapse in the area of the soft palate.[67] The snoring is thought to be originating from these collapsible parts of the airway.[68]

## Investigations

The investigation of the patient with snoring is aimed at assessing the presence of an underlying treatable condition and excluding complications such as sleep apnea syndrome and cardiovascular disease. In addition to the specific investigations detailed below which may be indicated in certain patients, selected baseline investigations, guided by the clinical findings, may be necessary. In the patient with clinical features of underlying lung disease or obesity-hypoventilation syndrome, investigation with a hematocrit level, arterial blood gas, chest roentgenogram, and pulmonary function tests may be of value. The flow-volume loop has been suggested to be of value in screening patients at risk of obstructive sleep apnea, by demonstrating abnormalities of the inspiratory curve[69] and oscillatory flow termed the "saw tooth" sign.[70] Although this finding has significant specificity for OSA, the sensitivity is poor and it is not a useful screening test.[71,72] Other tests that may be necessary based on the clinical findings include electrocardiography, echocardiography, and tests of thyroid function.

### Sleep Studies

While the majority of snorers do not develop OSA, this complication should be actively identified and treated as it carries significant morbidity and increased mortality.[73,74] A number of studies have assessed the efficacy of screening parameters to identify snorers at risk of OSA. Of significant value are a history of nocturnal choking, the observation by a bed partner of apneic episodes, and the presence of hypertension or obesity.[62,64] Other indications for sleep studies include snorers with co-existing lung disease, those with daytime hypoxemia or pulmonary hypertension, or those with other potential complications of OSA such as excessive daytime sleepiness or unexplained heart failure.[75] Alternative diagnostic approaches, such as clinical observation of the sleeping patient or overnight oximetry, are inadequate for diagnosing OSA, with a sensitivity of only about 65%.[76–78]

A number of variables should be monitored during a sleep study, as noninvasively as possible. A standardized polysomnogram, which is necessary to accurately diagnose and assess the severity of a suspected cardiorespiratory sleep disorder, has been delineated.[75] This involves overnight monitoring of sleep state and respiratory parameters. The assessment of sleep stage is accomplished by monitoring the EEG, rapid eye movements are detected by the electro-oculogram, and submental muscles are usually evaluated with the electromyogram. Respiratory airflow at the mouth and nose and respiratory effort by chest and abdominal inductance plethysmography are used to detect and classify apneas, differentiating obstructive from central. In difficult patients, an esophageal balloon to assess pleural pressure may be necessary to properly classify apneas.[13] Arterial oxygen saturation is measured by pulse oximetry, and cardiac parameters are measured by continuous electrocardiographic monitoring. Electromyogram of the tibialis anterior muscle is used to detect periodic movements during sleep, and body position is monitored.

Data generated by the sleep study include the apnea index (mean apneic events per hour sleep), the apnea-hypopnea index, indices of oxygenation, and sleep architecture.[75,79] While an apnea-hypopnea index of less than 5 events is considered normal[22] and an apnea index

greater than 20 events is associated with increased mortality,[74] the clinical significance of an apnea index between 5 and 20 events is uncertain. The decision to treat a patient with mild OSA in this range would depend on the presence and severity of symptoms, and the degree of associated oxygen desaturation.

## Diagnostic Imaging

Studies involving routine roentgenographic views of the upper airway,[80–82] computer-assisted tomographic scanning,[83] magnetic resonance imaging,[50] and acoustic-reflection techniques to assess pharyngeal area[84] have all been done in an attempt to find a reliable measure to differentiate snorers from nonsnorers with and without sleep apnea. Many cephalometric measurements have been assessed with many conflicting results. The distance from the mandibular plane to the hyoid bone on lateral view of the airway has been shown to differ between apneic and nonapneic snorers but not between nonapneic snorers and nonsnorers.[81] This difference seems to be an effect, rather that a cause for the apnea. Some studies indicate that pharyngeal shape is predictive of snoring,[50] whereas other studies imply the cross-sectional area is the important parameter.[84] At present, there is no simple, reliable diagnostic imaging study which correlates accurately with snoring or OSA.

## Differential Diagnosis

### Asymptomatic Nonapneic Snoring

Although heavy snoring may have significant social implications, the health risk to the asymptomatic, nonapneic snorer is unclear. Acutely, a number of physiological abnormalities occur during episodes of snoring, including transient oxygen desaturation,[1] a small rise in systemic blood pressure,[1,27,85] and transient arousal from sleep.[13] With regard to long-term complications, such as the risk of cardiovascular disease, patients with OSA appear to be at increased risk,[8,25,26,86] while the risk for nonapneic snorers is less clear. Epidemiological surveys of self-reported snorers suggest an increased risk of hypertension, ischemic heart disease, and stroke.[14,15,17-19,22] These data have been criticized in that snoring was self-reported and confounding variables were not considered.[2] Because snoring is strongly associated with other cardiovascular risk factors such as age, obesity, and tobacco smoking,[16] controlling for these confounders is essential. Also, the results of these epidemiological studies are not directly applicable to the nonapneic snorer since polysomnography was not performed in these patients. Prospective studies have demonstrated no association of hypertension or cardiac arrhythmias with nonapneic heavy snorers.[7,8,87] Using an objective measure of snoring, it has been shown that this variable was not a significant determinant of blood pressure, when corrected for OSA and oxygen desaturation. On the other hand, body mass index, age, and OSA were strongly associated with the presence of hypertension.[7] This study did not address asymptomatic patients since all were referred for sleep studies for a variety of reasons. Nevertheless, it is likely that snorers with normal sleep studies are not at increased risk of cardiovascular complications.

## Upper Airways Resistance Syndrome

Excessive daytime somnolence is a common complaint in severe snorers and is often attributed to concomitant obstructive sleep apnea. However, in a significant proportion of heavy snorers, this symptom is not associated with the presence of OSA or nocturnal desaturation.[63] Recently, some cases of daytime sleepiness have been shown to be related to an abnormal breathing pattern during sleep, termed the "upper airways resistance syndrome."[13] A subset of nonobese snorers, who had excessive daytime sleepiness but did not meet criteria diagnostic of OSA on polysomnography was studied.[12,13] Sleep was noted to be fragmented by transient short EEG arousals lasting 3 to 10 seconds not associated with apnea or hypopnea that may be ignored in standard sleep analysis. These arousals were shown to be directly related to an increased inspiratory pressure in the preceding respiratory cycle. It has previously been demonstrated that the mechanism of arousal from sleep due to breathing disorders relates predominantly to increased ventilatory effort.[11] Snoring was often associated with this increased airway resistance, but was neither sufficient nor necessary for identification of the clinical syndrome. The level of sleepiness measured by multiple sleep latency tests (MSLT) correlated with the frequency of the EEG arousals, and treatment with nasal continuous positive airway pressure (CPAP) improved MSLT scores and eliminated respiration-related EEG arousals.[12,13]

In clinical practice, it may be difficult to reliably diagnose this condition. In order to identify short arousals as being respiratory-related, monitoring of intrathoracic pressure with an esophageal balloon is necessary. This is not feasible during routine polysomnography, and the diagnosis of this syndrome would be more inferential. While the routine use of nasal CPAP as long-term therapy of this syndrome is not recommended,[13] it appears reasonable to offer a therapeutic trial of nasal CPAP. If sleep fragmentation and symptoms are improved, continued use may be recommended or consideration given to surgical correction of airway abnormalities.[10]

## Obstructive Sleep Apnea

The upper airway abnormality producing snoring may result in airway occlusion during sleep, leading to ventilatory abnormalities. Complete occlusion will result in the cessation of airflow or apnea, while partial occlusion produces hypopnea with reduced but not absent airflow. Apnea duration averages 20 to 30 seconds, seldom exceeding 60 seconds.[88] Futile respiratory efforts continue until the apnea is terminated by a brief arousal, which activates upper airway muscles, restoring patency of the airway. The stimulus for arousal appears to be the increased ventilatory effort, independent of arterial blood gas abnormalities.[11,89] The patient may snort, gasp, and hyperventilate for a few breaths and then return to sleep. Significant oxygen desaturation may occur during this period of ventilatory disturbance and be worse in patients with underlying lung disease.[89,90] These episodes may recur every few minutes, resulting in significant hypoxemia and sleep fragmentation.

The sleep apnea syndrome is most common between the ages of 30 and 60 years, and the prevalence is conservatively estimated at 4% in men and 2% in women in this age group.[22] Obstructive sleep apnea can be considered part of the spectrum of complications related to snoring. An evolution from asymptomatic snoring through clinically significant OSA to alveolar hypoventilation persisting during wakefulness has been suggested.[1] Factors predisposing to OSA are similar to those described for snoring, namely anatomical factors and functional changes during sleep, aggravated by obesity, hormonal influence, and drugs. While both nonapneic and apneic snorers have diminished pharyngeal cross-sectional areas,[91,92] those with sleep apnea have increased compliance and therefore significant collapsibility of the pharynx.[30,31,84] This collapse may also be related to the fall in lung volume that occurs in the recumbent position and during sleep.[52,87,93]

The diagnosis of OSA depends on the documentation of apneas and hypopneas during sleep by polysomnography. While a distinct cut-off between normal and abnormal has not been demonstrated,[79] an apnea-hypopnea level greater than 5 events per hour[22] to 15 events per hour[77] has been used. An apnea index of more than 5 events per hour (apnea-hypopnea index approximately 10 events per hour) has been shown to be associated with an increased risk of myocardial infarction.[94] Patients with an apnea index greater than 20 events per hour are at significant risk of

complications and increased mortality.[74] Because significant oxygen desaturation as well as arousal may occur during hypopnea, the severity of sleep disturbance is often assessed by the apnea-hypopnea index.[79,88,95] Other factors, such as the degree of nocturnal desaturation, may have an important role in defining disease severity.[1,96] Severe OSA may be associated with an apnea-hypopnea index above 80.[1]

Complications of OSA are many, ranging from daytime sleepiness to significant cardiovascular disease (Table II). Excessive daytime somnolence and cognitive dysfunction occur. These complications are related to both the nocturnal hypoxemia and to the sleep disturbance, which causes fragmentation of sleep and loss of the deeper levels of sleep.[65,97,98] Personality changes, memory loss, and impotence may result. The excessive daytime drowsiness puts these patients at a high risk of causing motor vehicle accidents.[65] Obstructive sleep apnea has been demonstrated to be associated with an increased incidence of hypertension,[8,24–26,86] and may be considered a reversible risk factor

---

### Table II
### Clinical Manifestations of Sleep Apnea

**Nocturnal**
  Restless Sleep
  Witnessed Apneas
  Nocturnal Choking
  Cardiac Arrhythmias
  Seizures
  Enuresis
  Night Sweats
**Daytime**
  Excessive Daytime Somnolence
  Intellectual Deterioration
  Personality Changes
  Morning Headaches
  Impotence
**Long-term Complications**
  Systemic Hypertension
  Pulmonary Hypertension
  Ischemic Heart Disease
  Stroke
  Left Ventricular Dysfunction
  Obesity-hypoventilation Syndrome
  Cor Pulmonale

for cardiovascular disease.[25] An increased incidence of stroke and myocardial infarction has been noted.[18,19,94] Sleep apnea appears to play a role in producing or exacerbating left ventricular dysfunction, and treatment with nasal CPAP can lead to a significant improvement in left ventricular ejection fraction for these patients.[99,100] Cardiac arrhythmias are common in patients with sleep apnea and nocturnal desaturation.[7] Daytime alveolar hypoventilation may occur in obese patients with OSA. The mechanism of this obesity-hypoventilation syndrome is not clear, but is related to abnormal central ventilatory drive and increased mechanical loads on the respiratory system.[96,101,102] The role of OSA in the development of this syndrome is unclear. Pulmonary hypertension and right heart failure generally do not develop in these patients unless daytime hypoxemia, which occurs predominantly in those with co-existing obstructive airways disease, is present.[90] The term "Pickwickian syndrome" usually refers to those patients with severe obesity, OSA, and alveolar hypoventilation complicated by polycythemia, pulmonary hypertension, and right heart failure in the absence of intrinsic lung disease.[102,103]

## Treatment

### Reversal of Aggravating Factors

The initial management of all patients should include the reversal of any identified predisposing factors. Dietary control of weight can have a dramatic effect on snoring and OSA. Moderate weight loss can alleviate sleep apnea, decrease daytime somnolence, and improve sleep architecture.[45–47] Weight reduction programs require a specialized, dedicated service, and the long-term results of the treatment of obesity are not good, with a high incidence of relapse.[104] Relief of nasal obstruction due to allergic rhinitis may lessen the severity of snoring and OSA.[56] This may be accomplished by the use of topical decongestants or inhaled nasal corticosteroids. If the nasal obstruc-

tion is due to an anatomical defect, this should be further evaluated by an ENT surgeon. Surgical correction of upper airway abnormalities, such as deviated nasal septum[57] or tonsillar hypertrophy,[105] may relieve snoring. The discontinuation of smoking, by reducing airway inflammation, can have a beneficial effect.[20] Avoidance of alcohol before bed time may be beneficial,[58] and patients should not receive hypnotic sedatives.[61]

### Drug Therapy

As described in the preceding section, relief of nasal obstruction using topical decongestants or steroids may benefit certain patients. The efficacy of a long-acting lubricating agent, phosphocholinamin, instilled into the nose, has been demonstrated in a small group of patients.[106] Protriptyline hydrochloride, which has been used in the treatment of obstructive sleep apnea and nocturnal desaturation in chronic obstructive airways disease, can lessen the frequency and loudness of snoring.[107] This is likely due to its anticholinergic effects, reducing upper airway edema, as well as increasing upper airway dilating tone.

### Nasal Continuous Positive Airway Pressure (CPAP)

The application of CPAP at the nose is effective treatment for snoring and obstructive sleep apnea.[108–110] This approach was first introduced in 1981 and has become recognized as the treatment of choice for OSA.[108,110] A number of units are now commercially available which produce positive pressure by means of a blower motor, the pressure being delivered to the patient via a tight fitting plastic and silicone nasal mask. This is secured by means of straps extending over the patient's head. The pressure applied to the upper airways acts as a pneumatic splint, passively opening the upper airway preventing airway occlusion.[108,111] An increase in pharyngeal size may also occur through augmentation of lung volumes.[52]

This form of therapy is highly effective and generally well tolerated.[110,112] Long-term compliance is higher in patients with severe daytime somnolence,[113,114] while the long-term effectiveness is poor in patients with snoring alone.[113] Continuous positive airway pressure should be used every night, throughout the night for optimal efficacy.[115] However, excessive daytime somnolence and cognitive function may remain improved with only intermittent use.[112] While intermittent use is associated with persistent sleep apnea during periods off CPAP, the severity of these apneas is somewhat diminished, probably due to a reduction in mucosal edema.[115] In addition to the relief of symptoms, CPAP has been demonstrated to improve survival in patients with moderately severe OSA.[74] A significant benefit has been demonstrated in patients with OSA and congestive heart failure due to left ventricular dysfunction. Nasal CPAP was associated with an improvement in left ventricular ejection fraction after 4 weeks of use.[99]

Since this therapy is very safe and has few contraindications, a therapeutic trial may be undertaken in most patients with diagnosed OSA without the need for other investigations. Continuous positive airway pressure is contraindicated in patients with skull fractures who may be susceptible to barotrauma, and those unable to cooperate.[110] After a diagnostic sleep study, therapy with nasal CPAP is usually initiated with a second sleep study during which the appropriate pressure level is determined. This is usually in the range of 5 to 20 cm $H_2O$.[110] A subtherapeutic pressure may be potentially harmful when a situation occurs where arousal is avoided but hypoventilation persists.[110] Unnecessarily high pressure leads to poor patient compliance. With correct use, improvement in daytime somnolence is rapid, with some benefit being noted after the first night.[116] After 2 weeks of therapy, the MSLT, an indicator of daytime sleepiness, is into the normal range.[117]

Although very effective, nasal CPAP may be difficult to use, and about one third of patients are unable to tolerate it long-term[113,114] while many use it for only a limited number of hours each night.[112] Objectively monitored CPAP use averages only 3.4 hours per night, but this may be sufficient to benefit patients symptomatically.[112] Reasons for discontinuing CPAP include intolerance of the mask due to discomfort, claustrophobia, or the inconvenience of being connected to a machine.[110] Adverse effects include drying of the nasal mucosa, rhinitis, and corneal ulceration related to airleaks around the mask.[118] Intolerance of CPAP can be managed by using a system whereby a low pressure is initially applied, which gradually increases to the preset pressure over a 30-minute period. Alternatively, bilevel positive airway pressure, with a higher inspiratory pressure and lower expiratory pressure, may be better tolerated.[119] Machines providing "intelligent" CPAP, with mask pressures self-adjusted according to the degree of flow-limitation, may soon become available.[110]

## Prosthetic Devices

The main prosthetic devices used in the treatment of snoring attempt to reposition the anatomy to decrease airway resistance. Dental appliances are used to retract the lower teeth, mandible, and tongue anteriorly. These devices are effective in controlling snoring and obstructive sleep apnea in 60% of patients.[120,121] A nasal vestibular dilator has been shown to reduce nasal airway resistance, but no significant effect on the intensity, frequency, or duration of snoring was seen when this apparatus was used during sleep.[122] In some patients, avoidance of the supine position during sleep using a ball sewn into the back of the pajamas, may improve snoring.[123]

## Surgical/Laser Therapy

Prior to proceeding with surgery directly on the offending vibratory tissue, procedures to alleviate nasal or nasopharyngeal airway obstruction should be attempted. Septoplasty, reduction of nasal turbinates, and/or removal of offending nasal or nasopharyngeal polyps or neoplasms should be performed if necessary.[124]

The uvulopalatopharyngoplasty (UPPP) was described by Ikematsu in 1964 as a treatment for snoring, and in 1981, Fujita applied this treatment to sleep apnea. The UPPP is performed with the patient under general anaesthesia. Tonsils, if present, are removed by standard technique and the soft palate is trimmed, including complete resection of the uvula. The tonsillar pillars are also trimmed and the dorsal and ventral aspects of the soft palate are sutured together using an absorbable suture. Reports indicate a 60% to 86% success rate for the procedure, in terms of an acceptable reduction in snoring.[124-127] Complications include hemorrhage, temporary nasopharyngeal regurgitation, and rarely, permanent velopharyngeal insufficiency.

Recently, the laser has been used to provide a variation on the UPPP. The laser-assisted uvula-palatoplasty (LAUP) was described in 1990 by Kamami. The LAUP is usually done as an office procedure with the patient fully awake and sitting upright. After local anesthetic (ie, topical spay, followed by injection) is applied, a carbon dioxide laser with specialized hand pieces is used. Trenches are cut vertically through the soft palate, lateral to the uvula, bilaterally. The edges of the uvula and lateral aspects of the trenches are then treated with the laser to vaporize, thus trimming, this tissue. Care is taken in an attempt to vaporize mainly the underlying muscle, preserving the overlying mucosa as much as possible.

The LAUP usually requires two to three treatments spaced 4 to 6 weeks apart. Up to seven treatments have been described but it is not uncommon to require only one treatment. Since this is a staged procedure, the patient can be evaluated prior to each successive treatment and if there is any indication of impending nasal regurgitation or reflux, further treatments can be suspended. Complications include only minor bleeding, and pain which varies from mild pain lasting only 2 to 3 days to, on occasion, severe pain lasting for as long as 2 weeks. Limited data are available but reports indicate an 84% success in eliminating the snoring with another 7% of patients having reduced snoring to the point where the sleeping partner is satisfied.[68]

Other surgical options for snoring include tracheostomy[124] and mandibular surgery to advance the base of tongue anteriorly. Inferior mandibular osteotomy with hyoid myotomy and suspension has been described as has maxillary, mandibular, and hyoid advancement.[128] These procedures are usually reserved for obstructive sleep apnea sufferers, rather than simple snorers.

## References

1. Lugaresi E, Cirignotta F, Montagna P, et al. Snoring: pathogenic, clinical, and therapeutic aspects. In: Kryger MH, Roth T, Dement WC, eds. *Principles And Practice Of Sleep Medicine.* Philadelphia, Pa: WB Saunders Company 1994:621–629.
2. Waller PC, Bhopal RS. Is snoring a cause of vascular disease? An epidemiological review. Lancet 1989;i:143–146.
3. Hoffstein V, Rubinstein I, Mateika S, et al. Determinants of blood pressure in snorers. Lancet 1988;i:992–994.
4. Hoffstein V, Mateika JH, Mateika S. Snoring and sleep architecture. Am Rev Respir Dis 1991;143:92–96.
5. Wilson K, Mulrooney T, Gawtry RR. Snoring: an acoustic monitoring technique. Laryngoscope 1985;95:1174–1177.
6. Rogelio Perez-Padilla J, Slawinski E, Difrancesco LM, et al. Characteristics of the snoring noise in patients with and without occlusive sleep apnea. Am Rev Respir Dis 1993;147:635–644.
7. Hoffstein V, Mateika S. Cardiac arrhythmias, snoring, and sleep apnea. Chest 1994;106:466–471.
8. Hoffstein V. Blood pressure, snoring, obesity, and nocturnal hypoxaemia. Lancet 1994;344:643–645.
9. Liistro G, Stanescu DC, Veriter C, et al. Pattern of snoring in obstructive sleep

apnea patients and in heavy snorers. Sleep 1991;14:517–525.

10. Strollo PJ, Sanders MH. Significance and treatment of nonapneic snoring. Sleep 1993;16:403–408.

11. Gleeson K, Zwillich CW, White DP. The influence of increasing ventilatory effort on arousal from sleep. Am Rev Respir Dis 1990;142:295–300.

12. Guilleminault C, Stoohs R, Duncan S. Snoring (I). Daytime sleepiness in regular heavy snorers. Chest 1991;99:40–48.

13. Guilleminault C, Stoohs R, Clerk A, et al. A cause of excessive daytime sleepiness. The upper airway resistance syndrome. Chest 1993;104:781–787.

14. Lugaresi E, Cirignotta F, Coccagna G, et al. Some epidemiological data on snoring and cardiocirculatory disturbances. Sleep 1980;3:221–224.

15. Norton PG, Dunn EV. Snoring as a risk factor for diseases: an epidemiological survey. Br Med J 1985;231:630–632.

16. Jennum P, Hein HO, Suadicani P, et al. Cardiovascular risk factors in snorers. A cross-sectional study of 3323 men aged 54 to 74 years: the Copenhagen male study. Chest 1992;102:1372–1376.

17. Gislason T, Benediktsdottir B, Bjornsson JK, et al. Snoring, hypertension, and the sleep apnea syndrome: an epidemiological survey of middle-aged women. Chest 1993;103:1147–1151.

18. Koskenvuo M, Kaprio J, Partinen M, et al. Snoring as a risk factor for hypertension and angina pectoris. Lancet 1985;i:893–896.

19. Koskenvuo M, Kaprio J, Telakivi T, et al. Snoring as a risk factor for ischaemic heart disease and stroke in men. Br Med J 1987;294:16–19.

20. Bloom JW, Kaltenborn WT, Quan SF. Risk factors in a general population for snoring. Importance of cigarette smoking and obesity. Chest 1988;93:678–683.

21. Wiggins CL, Schmidt-Novara WW, Coultas DB, et al. Comparison of self- and spouse-reports of snoring and other symptoms associated with sleep apnea syndrome. Sleep 1990;13:245–252.

22. Young T, Palta M, Dempsey J, et al. The occurrence of sleep-disordered breathing among middle-aged adults. N Engl J Med 1993;328:1230–1235.

23. Partinen M, Palomaki H. Snoring and cerebral infarction. Lancet 1985;2:1325–1327.

24. Fletcher EC, DeBehnke RD, Lovoi MS, et al. Undiagnosed sleep apnea in patients with essential hypertension. Ann Intern Med 1985;103:190–195.

25. Partinen M, Guilleminault C. Daytime sleepiness and vascular morbidity at seven-year follow-up in obstructive sleep apnea patients. Chest 1990;97:27–32.

26. Hoffstein V, Chan CK, Slutsky AS. Sleep apnea and systemic hypertension: a causal association review. Am J Med 1991;91:190–196.

27. Hla KM, Young TB, Bidwell T, et al. Sleep apnea and hypertension. A population-based study. Ann Intern Med 1994;120:382–388.

28. Remmers JE, De Groot WJ, Sauerland EK, et al. Pathogenesis of upper airway occlusion during sleep. J Appl Physiol 1978;44:931–938.

29. Block AJ, Faulkner JA, Hughes RL, et al. Factors influencing upper airways closure. Chest 1984;86:114–121.

30. Brown IG, Bradley TD, Phillipson EA, et al. Pharyngeal compliance in snoring subjects with and without obstructive sleep apnea. Am Rev Respir Dis 1985;132:211–215.

31. Gleadhill IC, Schwartz AR, Schubert N, et al. Upper airway collapsibility in snorers and in patients with obstructive hypopnea and apnea. Am Rev Respir Dis 1991;143:1300–1303.

32. Olson LG, Strohl KP. Airway secretions influence upper airway patency in the rabbit. Am Rev Respir Dis 1988;137:1379–1381.

33. Rodenstein DO, Stanescu DC. The soft palate and breathing. Am Rev Respir Dis 1986;134:311–325.

34. Polo OJ, Tafti M, Fraga J, et al. Why don't all heavy snorers have obstructive sleep apnea? Am Rev Respir Dis 1991;143:1288–1293.

35. Phillipson EA. Control of breathing during sleep. Am Rev Respir Dis 1978;118:909–939

36. Strohl KP, Hensley MJ, Hallett M, et al. Activation of upper airway muscles before onset of inspiration in normal humans. J Appl Physiol 1980;49:638–642.

37. Tabachnik E, Muller NL, Bryan AC, et al. Changes in ventilation and chest wall mechanics during sleep in normal adolescents. J Appl Physiol 1981;51:557–564.

38. Krieger J. Breathing during sleep in normal subjects. In: Kryger MH, Roth T, Dement WC, eds. *Principles And Practice Of*

*Sleep Medicine.* Philadelphia, Pa: WB Saunders Company; 1994: 212–223.

39. Hudgel DW. The role of upper airway anatomy and physiology in obstructive sleep apnea. Clin Chest Med 1992;13: 383–398.

40. Hyland RH, Hutcheon MA, Perl A, et al. Upper airway occlusion induced by diaphragm pacing for primary alveolar hypoventilation: implications for the pathogenesis of obstructive sleep apnea. Am Rev Respir Dis 1981;124:180–185.

41. Brouillette RT, Thach BT. Control of genioglossus muscle inspiratory activity. J Appl Physiol 1980;49:801–808.

42. Leiter JC, Knuth SL, Bartlett D. The effect of sleep deprivation on activity of the genioglossus muscle. Am Rev Respir Dis 1985;132:1242–1245.

43. Leiter JC, Knuth SL, Krol RC, et al. The effect of diazepam on genioglossal muscle activity in normal human subjects. Am Rev Respir Dis 1985;132:216–219.

44. Krol RC, Knuth SL, Bartlett D. Selective reduction of genioglossal muscle activity by alcohol in normal human subjects. Am Rev Respir Dis 1984;129:247–250.

45. Browman CP, Sampson MG, Yolles SF, et al. Obstructive sleep apnea and body weight. Chest 1984;85:435–436.

46. Smith PL, Gold AR, Meyers DA, et al. Weight loss in mildly to moderately obese patients with obstructive sleep apnea. Ann Intern Med 1985;103:850–855.

47. Wittels EH, Thompson S. Obstructive sleep apnea and obesity. Otolaryng Clin North Am 1990;23:751–760.

48. Horner RL, Mohiaddin RH, Lowell DG, et al. Sites and sizes of fat deposits around the pharynx in obese patients with obstructive sleep apnoea and weight matched controls. Eur Respir J 1989;2: 613–622.

49. Stauffer JL, Buick MK, Bixler EO, et al. Morphology of the uvula in obstructive sleep apnea. Am Rev Respir Dis 1989;140: 724–728.

50. Rodenstein DO, Dooms G, Thomas Y, et al. Pharyngeal shape and dimensions in healthy subjects, snorers, and patients with obstructive sleep apnoea. Thorax 1990;45:722–727.

51. Ray CS, Sue DY, Bray G, et al. Effects of obesity on respiratory function. Am Rev Respir Dis 1983;128:501–506.

52. Hoffstein V, Zamel N, Phillipson EA. Lung volume dependence of pharyngeal cross-sectional area in patients with obstructive sleep apnea. Am Rev Respir Dis 1984;130:175–178.

53. Katz I, Stradling J, Slutsky AS, et al. Do patients with obstructive sleep apnea have thick necks?. Am Rev Respir Dis 1990;141:1228–1231.

54. Rajagopal KR, Abbrecht PH, Derderian SS, et al. Obstructive sleep apnea in hypothyroidism. Ann Intern Med 1984;101: 491–494.

55. Mezon BJ, West P, Maclean JP, et al. Sleep apnea in acromegaly. Am J Med 1980;69: 615–618.

56. McNicholas WT, Tarlo S, Cole P, et al. Obstructive apneas during sleep in patients with seasonal allergic rhinitis. Am Rev Respir Dis 1982;126:625–628.

57. Lavie P, Zomer J, Eliaschar I, et al. Excessive daytime sleepiness and insomnia: association with deviated nasal septum and nocturnal breathing disorders. Arch Otolaryngol 1982;108:373–377.

58. Issa FQ, Sullivan CE. Alcohol, snoring and sleep apnea. J Neurol Neurosurg Psychiatry 1982;45:353–359.

59. Robinson RW, White DP, Zwillich CW. Moderate alcohol ingestion increases upper airway resistance in normal subjects. Am Rev Respir Dis 1985;132: 1238–1241.

60. Bonora M, Shields GI, Knuth SL, et al. Selective depression by ethanol of upper airway respiratory motor activity in cats. Am Rev Respir Dis 1984;130:156–161.

61. Guilleminault C. Benzodiazepines, breathing, and sleep. Am J Med 1988(suppl 3A):25S–28S.

62. Viner S, Szalai JP, Hoffstein V. Are history and physical examination a good screening test for sleep apnea? Ann Intern Med 1991;115:356–359.

63. Hillerdal G, Hetta J, Lindholm C-E, et al. Symptoms in heavy snorers with and without obstructive sleep apnea. Acta Otolaryngol 1991;111:574–581.

64. Crocker BD, Olson LG, Saunders NA, et al. Estimation of the probability of disturbed breathing during sleep before a sleep study. Am Rev Respir Dis 1990;142: 14–18.

65. Findley LJ, Barth JT, Powers DC, et al. Cognitive impairment in patients with obstructive sleep apnea and associated hypoxemia. Chest 1986;90:686–690.

66. Findley LJ, Unverzagt ME, Suratt PM. Automobile accidents involving patients with obstructive sleep apnea. Am Rev Respir Dis 1988;138:337–340.

67. Sher AE, Thorpy MJ, Shrpintzen RJ, et al. Predictive value of Muller maneuver in selection of patients for uvulopalatopharyngoplasty. Laryngoscope 1985;95:1483–1487.

68. Krespi Y, Pearlman S, Keidar A. Laser-assisted uvula-palatoplasty for snoring. J Otolaryngol 1994;23:328–334.

69. Haponik EF, Bleecker ER, Allen RP, et al. Abnormal inspiratory flow-volume curves in patients with sleep-disordered breathing. Am Rev Respir Dis 1981;124:571–574.

70. Sanders MH, Martin RJ, Pennock BE, et al. The detection of sleep apnea in the awake patient: the "saw tooth" sign. JAMA 1981;245:2414–2418.

71. Shore ET, Millman RP. Abnormalities in the flow-volume loop in obstructive sleep apnoea sitting and supine. Thorax 1984;39:775–779.

72. Hoffstein V, Wright S, Zamel N. Flow-volume curves in snoring patients with and without obstructive sleep apnea. Am Rev Respir Dis 1989;139:957–960.

73. Phillipson EA. Sleep apnea—a major public health problem. N Engl J Med 1993;328:1271–1273.

74. He J, Kryger MH, Zorick FJ, et al. Mortality and apnea index in obstructive sleep apnea: experience in 385 male patients. Chest 1988;94:9–14.

75. Phillipson EA, Remmers JE. Indications and standards for cardiopulmonary sleep studies. Am Rev Respir Dis 1989;139:559–568.

76. Haponik EF, Smith PL, Meyers DA, et al. Evaluation of sleep disordered breathing: is polysomnography necessary? Am J Med 1984;77:671–677.

77. Douglas NJ, Thomas S, Jan MA. Clinical value of polysomnography. Lancet 1992;339:347–350.

78. Cooper BG, Veale D, Griffiths CJ, et al. Value of nocturnal oxygen saturation as a screening test for sleep apnoea. Thorax 1991;46:586–588.

79. Block AJ, Boysen PG, Wynne JW, et al. Sleep apnea, hypopnea and oxygen desaturation in normal subjects: a strong male predominance. N Engl J Med 1979;300:513–517.

80. Hoffstein V, Weiser W, Hanley R. Roentgenographic dimensions of the upper airway in snoring patients with and without obstructive sleep apnea. Chest 1991;100:81–85.

81. Maltais F, Carrier G, Cormier Y, et al. Cephalometric measurements in snorers, non-snorers, and patients with sleep apnea. Thorax 1991;46:419–423.

82. Zucconi M, Ferlini-Strambi L, Palazzi S, et al. Habitual snoring with and without obstructive sleep apnea: the importance of cephalometric variables. Thorax 1992;47:157–161.

83. Krmpotic-Nemanic J, Vinter I, Marotti I, et al. Possible anatomical base of snoring. Acta Otolaryngol 1991;111:389–391.

84. Bradley TD, Brown IG, Grossman RF, et al. Pharyngeal size in snorers, nonsnorers, and patients with obstructive sleep apnea. N Engl J Med 1986;315:1327–1331.

85. Mateika JH, Mateika S, Slutsky AS, et al. The effect of snoring on mean arterial blood pressure during non-REM sleep. Am Rev Respir Dis 1992;145:141–146.

86. Kales A, Bixler EO, Cadieux RJ, et al. Sleep apnoea in a hypertensive population. Lancet 1984;ii:1005–1008.

87. Rausher H, Popp W, Zwick H. Systemic hypertension in snorers with and without sleep apnea. Chest 1992;102:367–371.

88. Shepard JW. Gas exchange and hemodynamics during sleep. Med Clin North Am 1985;69:1243–1264.

89. Kimoff RJ, Cheong TH, Olha AE, et al. Mechanisms of apnea termination in obstructive sleep apnea: role of chemoreceptor and mechanoreceptor stimuli. Am J Respir Crit Care Med 1994;149:707–714.

90. Bradley TD, Rutherford R, Grossman RF, et al. Role of daytime hypoxemia in the pathogenesis of right heart failure in the obstructive sleep apnea syndrome. Am Rev Respir Dis 1985;131:835–839.

91. Suratt PM, Dee P, Atkinson RL, et al. Fluoroscopic and computed tomographic features of the pharyngeal airway in obstructive sleep apnea. Am Rev Respir Dis 1983;127:487–492.

92. Rivlin J, Hoffstein V, Kalbfleisch J, et al. Upper airway morphology in patients with idiopathic obstructive sleep apnea. Am Rev Respir Dis 1984;129:355–360.

93. Hudgel DW, Devadatta P. Decrease in functional residual capacity during sleep in normal humans. J Appl Physiol 1984;57:1319–1322.

94. Hung J, Whitford EG, Parsons RW, et al. Association of sleep apnoea with myocardial infarction in men. Lancet 1990;336:261–264.

95. Guilleminault C. Clinical features and evaluation of obstructive sleep apnea. In:

Kryger MH, Roth T, Dement WC, eds. *Principles and Practice of Sleep Medicine*. Philadelphia, Pa: WB Saunders Company 1984:667–677.

96. Jones JB, Wilhoit SC, Findley LJ, et al. Oxyhemoglobin saturation during sleep in subjects with and without the obesity-hypoventilation syndrome. Chest 1985; 88:9–15.

97. Guilleminault C, Partinen M, Quera-Salva M, et al. Determinants of daytime sleepiness in obstructive sleep apnea. Chest 1988;94:32–37.

98. Cheshire K, Engelman H, Dreary I, et al. Factors impairing daytime performance in patients with sleep apnea/hypopnea syndrome. Arch Intern Med 1992;152: 538–541.

99. Malone S, Liu PP, Holloway R, et al. Obstructive sleep apnoea in patients with dilated cardiomyopathy: effects of continuous positive airway pressure. Lancet 1991: 338:1480–1484.

100. Bradley TD. Right and left ventricular functional impairment and sleep apnea. Clin Chest Med 1992;13:459–479.

101. Garay SM, Rapoport D, Sorkin B, et al. Regulation of ventilation in the obstructive sleep apnea syndrome. Am Rev Respir Dis 1981;124:451–457.

102. Rapoport DM, Garay SM, Epstein H, et al. Hypercapnia in the obstructive sleep apnea syndrome: a reevaluation of the "Pickwickian syndrome". Chest 1986;89: 627–635.

103. Burwell CS, Robin ED, Whaley RD, et al. Extreme obesity with alveolar hypoventilation: a Pickwickian syndrome. Am J Med 1956;21:811–818.

104. Bray GA. Barriers to the treatment of obesity. Ann Intern Med 1991;115:152–153.

105. Orr WC, Martin RJ. Obstructive sleep apnea associated with tonsillar hypertrophy in adults. Arch Intern Med 1981;141: 990–992.

106. Hoffstein V, Mateiko S, Halko S, et al. Reduction in snoring with phosphocholinamin, a long-acting tissue-lubricating agent. Am J Otolaryng 1987;8:236–240.

107. Series F, Marc T. Effects of protriptyline on snoring characteristics. Chest 1993; 104:14–18.

108. Sullivan CE, Issa FG, Berthon-Jones M, et al. Reversal of obstructive sleep apnoea by continuous positive airway pressure applied through the nares. Lancet 1981;i: 862–865.

109. Berry RB, Block AJ. Positive nasal airway pressure eliminates snoring as well as obstructive sleep apnea. Chest 1984;85: 15–20.

110. Polo O, Berthon-Jones M, Douglas NJ, et al. Management of obstructive sleep apnoea/hypopnoea syndrome. Lancet 1994; 344:6556–6560.

111. Strohl KP, Redline S. Nasal CPAP therapy, upper airway muscle activity, and obstructive sleep apnea. Am Rev Respir Dis 1986;134:555–558.

112. Engleman HM, Martin SE, Deary TJ, et al. Effect of continuous positive airway pressure treatment on daytime function in sleep apnoea/hypopnoea syndrome. Lancet 1994;343:572–575.

113. Waldhorn RE, Herrick TW, Nguyen MC, et al. Long-term compliance with nasal continuous positive airway pressure therapy of obstructive sleep apnea. Chest 1990;97:33–38.

114. Rolfe I, Olson LG, Saunders NA. Long-term acceptance of continuous positive airway pressure in obstructive sleep apnea. Am Rev Respir Dis 1991;144: 1130–1133.

115. Rauscher H, Popp W, Wanke T, et al. Breathing during sleep in patients treated for obstructive sleep apnea: Nasal CPAP for only part of the night. Chest 1991;100: 156–159.

116. Rajagopal KR, Bennett LL, Dillard TA, et al. Overnight nasal CPAP improves hypersomnolence in sleep apnea. Chest 1986; 90:172.

117. Lamphere J, Roehrs T, Wittig R, et al. Recovery of alertness after CPAP in apnea. Chest 1989;96:1364–1367.

118. Weil JV, Cherniack NS, Dempsey JA, et al. Respiratory disorders of sleep: pathophysiology, clinical implications, and therapeutic approaches. Am Rev Respir Dis 1987;136:755–761.

119. Sanders MH, Kern N. Obstructive sleep apnea treated by independently adjusted inspiratory and expiratory positive airway pressures via nasal mask. Chest 1990; 98:317–324.

120. Cartwright RD, Samelson CF. The effects of a nonsurgical treatment for obstructive sleep apnea. JAMA 1982;248:705–709.

121. Miyazaki S. Prosthetic devices in the treatment of obstructive sleep apnea. Oper Tech Otolaryngol Head Neck Surg 1991;2:96–99.

122. Metes A, Cole P, Hoffstein V, et al. Nasal

airway dilation and obstructed breathing in sleep. Laryngoscope 1992;102:1053–1055.

123. Anonymous. Patient's wife cures his snoring. Chest 1984;85:852.

124. Fairbanks DNF. Snoring: surgical vs. non-surgical management. Laryngoscope 1984;94:1188–1192.

125. MacNab T, Blokmanis A, Dickson RI. Long-term results of uvulopalatopharyngoplasty for snoring. J Otolaryngol 1992; 21:350–354.

126. Meyer B, Chabolle F, Chouard C. Re-sultats et complications a long terme de l'uvulopalatopharyngoplastie dans la rhonchopathie sans syndrome d'apnea du sommeil. Ann Otolaryngol Chir Cervico-fac (Paris) 1988;105:291–297.

127. Katsanotis G, Friedman W, Rosenblum B. The surgical treatment of snoring: A patient's perspective. Laryngoscope 1990; 100:138–140.

128. Riley R, Powell N. Maxillofacial surgery and obstructive sleep apnea syndrome. Otolaryngol Clin North Am 1990;23: 809–826.

# 8

# Singultus

J. Mark Madison, M.D.

## Introduction

Singultus, or hiccup, is an abrupt, involuntary contraction of the inspiratory musculature rapidly followed by glottic closure to produce a characteristic sound. The reflex does not serve any known useful or protective function. Brief episodes of hiccup are common and usually do not require medical attention. While recurrent or prolonged episodes of hiccup lasting more than 48 hours are unusual, the symptom may lead to serious medical consequences and may signify the presence of underlying pathology. Therefore, physicians should be knowledgeable about this symptom and how to evaluate it.

## History

Hiccups have been a medical curiosity for centuries. In the time of Hippocrates, the symptom was associated with ailments of stomach and liver.[1, 2] Since then, many potential causes and cures have been suggested but most of the medical literature remains, at best, anecdotal.

It was not until the 1800's that a connection between hiccups and the phrenic nerve was made.[3] This observation contributed to the belief that hiccups must be some type of respiratory reflex. Many studies subsequently reported observations that contributed to understanding the neurologic pathways involved in the reflex.[4,5] Finally, in 1970, observations were made that strongly supported the current consensus that hiccups are not a respiratory reflex.[6]

## Pathogenesis

### Physiology of the Hiccup Reflex

Why the hiccup reflex exists is not known. Mammals other than humans can hiccup and hiccups are known to occur commonly in fetal and neonatal life.[7–11] These observations suggest that hiccups might be a vestige of an obscure primitive reflex or that the reflex has some unknown role in fetal development.[2]

A hiccup starts with an inspiration caused by a sudden involuntary contraction of the diaphragm, external intercostals, and anterior scalene muscles.[6] In some cases, contractions are unilateral with only one leaf of the diaphragm—usually the left—contracting.[4,5] Approximately 35 milliseconds after the onset of diaphragm contraction, there is an abrupt

From Irwin RS, Curley FJ, Grossman RF (eds): Diagnosis and Treatment of Symptoms of the Respiratory Tract. Armonk, New York, Futura Publishing Company, Inc., © 1997.

closure of the glottis and a consequent characteristic sound.[6] Glottic closure is probably due to adductor laryngeal muscle contraction, but may also be due to abrupt negative intrathoracic pressure.

If this sequence of abrupt inspiration followed by abrupt glottic closure occurs for more than approximately seven repetitions,[6, 12, 13] then hiccups tend to become established and a bout of hiccups occurs. That is, some unknown feature of hiccups predisposes toward additional ones. Bouts of hiccup occur more frequently in the evening hours. This suggests that a circadian rhythm may influence the likelihood of bouts.[13, 14] For a given individual, the frequency of successive hiccups is not absolutely fixed but usually is relatively constant, most commonly at a rate between 17 hiccups/min and 24 hiccups/min.[6, 15] Frequency of successive hiccups does not correlate with the strength of the diaphragmatic contraction (amplitude) during each hiccup.[6]

The neural reflex mechanisms that underlie hiccupping are not well established, but several observations suggest that the reflex is not a "respiratory" one.[6] First, hiccups occur at any point in the respiratory cycle, although most commonly during inspiration. Second, unlike respiratory reflexes that are often stimulated by inhalation of carbon dioxide, hiccup frequency is slowed by increased carbon dioxide. Interestingly, although hypercapnia markedly slows the frequency of hiccup, it has little effect on the amplitude of diaphragmatic contraction. Third, also atypical of a respiratory reflex, hypocapnia increases the amplitude of hiccup. Fourth, if the symptom were due to output from the respiratory center in the medulla, one might expect hiccup amplitude to be greatest during inspiration, especially near peak inspiration. However, this is not the case.

Moreover, the ventilatory effects of hiccup are small.[6] The reason for this is that glottal closure occurs 35 milliseconds after the onset of inspiratory muscle effort and persists during the entire inspiratory muscle contraction. Exceptions are patients with tracheostomies in whom hiccup can cause severe hyperventilation.[16]

Possibly, hypocapnia contributes to the persistence of hiccups in these individuals.

The relationships between sleep and hiccup are variable.[17] In some instances hiccup resolves during sleep. In other cases, hiccup persists during both rapid eye movement (REM) and non-REM sleep but at a slower frequency.[18] Interestingly, it has been reported that there may be a high incidence of sleep apnea among male patients with intractable hiccup. Eleven of 16 elderly subjects with chronic hiccups had evidence of obstructive sleep apnea during sleep studies.[17]

## Neuroanatomy Of The Hiccup Reflex

The afferent limb of the hiccup reflex includes the vagus nerve, phrenic nerve, thoracic sympathetic (T-6 through T-12) nerves, and pharyngeal plexus (C-2 through C-4) nerves (Figure 1).[6, 19] The suspected, but poorly established, association between hiccup and some retroperitoneal and pelvic disorders, such as hydronephrosis and prostatitis, suggests that afferents from the pelvic plexus may also contribute to the reflex arc. Irritation of these nerve fibers or the tissues they innervate results in afferent nerve impulses to the central nervous system. Where the "hiccup center" of the central nervous system resides is unestablished. However, it probably resides in the upper medulla in a region distinct from the respiratory center.[6, 19] Some have speculated that hiccup represents an imbalance in the reciprocal inhibition normally present between the "glottis closure complex" (which includes input from the hiccup center) that is normally activated during swallowing and the "inspiratory complex" that is normally activated during inhalation.[20]

Output from the hiccup center in the medulla is probably integrated with other descending tracts in the spinal cord between the third and fifth cervical segments.[4, 5, 17] From these cervical segments, efferent impulses pass via the phrenic nerves to stimulate diaphragm contraction. However, efferent impulses also pass to the glottic musculature via the recurrent

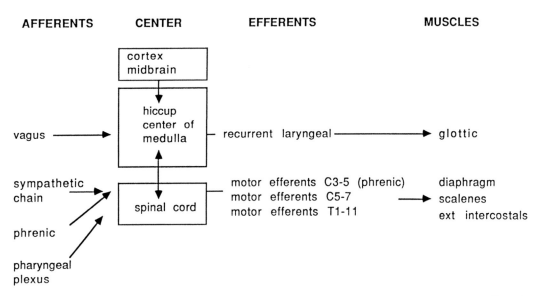

**Figure 1.** The hiccup reflex arc. Afferent input reaches the hiccup center of the medulla. The precise anatomic location of the center is not known but it is probably distinct from the respiratory center. Efferent output from the center is probably integrated with other descending and ascending tracts in the cervical spinal cord. Motor efferent output stimulates the diaphragm via the phrenic nerve and other respiratory muscles via motor nerves of C-5 through T-11.

laryngeal nerve and to the anterior scalene muscles and external intercostal muscles via motor neurons of cervical segments 5, 6, 7 and via motor neurons of thoracic segments 1–11.[19] That inspiratory muscles other than the diaphragm participate in the hiccup reflex is evident from reports of patients with persistent hiccup even after blockade of the phrenic nerves bilaterally.[2]

## Differential Diagnosis

### Disorders Other Than Hiccup

There are other disorders distinct from hiccup that involve the sudden inappropriate contraction of the inspiratory musculature. Leeuwenhoek's disease, or diaphragmatic flutter, is a rhythmic repetitive contraction of the respiratory muscles at a rate of 30 to 300 contractions/min.[21] Besides the frequency of contractions being higher, diaphragmatic flutter is different than hiccups because glottic closure does not occur. Diaphragmatic flutter has been described as a cause of failure to wean from mechanical ventilation following coronary artery bypass grafting.[22]

Less rhythmic contractions of inspiratory muscles have been described as respiratory dyskinesias.[23] These have been observed in patients with neurogenic asthenia and in patients with autonomic dysfunction, as seen in Shy-Drager syndrome and familial dysautonomia. Abnormal oscillations in airflow also occur in Parkinson's disease. Finally, respiratory dyskinesias have been described in patients with choreiform movement disorders and in patients treated with metoclopramide and haloperidol.

### Acute Hiccups

The acute onset of hiccup may occur spontaneously or may seemingly be precipitated by gastric distention, temperature changes, alcohol ingestion, heavy tobacco smoking, or emotional excitement

## Table I
### Causes of Acute Hiccup Bouts

Gastric Distention
Temperature Changes
Alcohol
Tobacco Smoking
Emotional Excitement
Myocardial Ischemia/Infarction
General Anesthesia
   Light Anesthesia
   Neck Hyperextention
   Traction on Viscera or Diaphragm
   Short-acting Barbiturates

(Table I).[2] A bout usually subsides spontaneously after several minutes and has no medical consequences or implications.[2]

However, in some situations, acute bouts may have important medical consequences or implications. For example, hiccups are common in the operating room and postoperative setting.[5,19,24] Hyperextension of the neck for intubation, irritation of the oropharynx during intubation, induction of anesthesia, and irritation of the vagus nerve by manipulation and retraction of abdominal viscera all are causes of hiccups in the operating room.[19,24] Also, the use of short-acting barbiturates has been implicated as a cause of hiccups in the operating room.[19] The consequence of hiccups in this setting may be serious since the bout may interfere with the surgical procedure itself or with ventilation of the patient. In the postoperative setting, gastric distention and ileus are common causes of acute and persistent hiccup.[25, 26] Hiccups commonly complicate intra-abdominal surgery and tend to occur within the first 4 days after surgery.[25] Following intra-abdominal surgery, the symptom may interfere significantly with pain management, wound healing, eating, and sleeping. Hiccups in this setting are often difficult to relieve and may become persistent.[25]

## Persistent Hiccups

There are myriad causes of persistent hiccup (Table II). Many times, the suspected causes are common disorders that uncommonly result in hiccup. Therefore, there is probably a wide variation among individuals with respect to susceptibility to hiccup.

For many of the conditions associated with persistent hiccup, causality remains unestablished. Furthermore, little is known about the relative frequencies of the symptom among the different suspected causes. Overall, intra-abdominal, neurologic, and metabolic causes are the most firmly established and probably are the most frequent organic causes of persistent hiccup. In this regard, it is notable that fully 25% to 30% of persistent hiccups occur in men following surgery.[25] Thoracotomy, laporotomy, and craniotomy all have been linked to persistent hiccups.

### Central Nervous System Causes

Presumably, by altering neural input pathways to the hiccup center in the medulla, a wide range of central nervous system disorders has been associated with chronic hiccup.[2,17] Cerebral trauma,[19] brain neoplasms,[27,28] arteriovenous malformations,[29] brain abscesses, cerebral ischemia,[30] cerebral hemorrhage, meningitis, encephalitis, neurosyphillis, and epilepsy have all been reported causes of hiccup. Following head trauma or in the setting of cerebral neoplasm, there is sometimes a constant periodicity between bouts.[27,31]

Many examples of hiccup secondary to infections of the central nervous system have been described and include meningitis, encephalitis, neurosyphyllis, and brain abscesses.[15,30,32–34] Hiccups have also been linked to parasitic infections of the gut, malaria, herpes zoster, typhoid, rheumatic fever, and influenza.[2,17,35,36]

The link between influenza and hiccups is well documented but most peculiar. Epidemics of recurring bouts of hiccup were reported during the influenza/encephalitis outbreaks between 1919 and 1924.[2,33] For 4 to 5 days, affected patients had 1 hour episodes of hiccup that recurred every 2 to 3 hours. A strain of strep-

---

**Table II**
Suspected Causes of Persistent Hiccup

| | |
|---|---|
| CNS | Thoracic |
|   Trauma |   Empyema |
|   Brain Neoplasms |   Pleuritis |
|   AV Malformations |   Asthma |
|   Brain Abscess |   Bronchitis |
|   Ischemia |   Pneumonia |
|   Hemorrhage |   Tuberculosis |
|   Epilepsy |   Mediastinitis |
|   Neurosyphillis |   Vascular Aneurysm |
|   Meningitis |   Mediastinal Neoplasms |
|   Encephalitis |   Mediastinal Abscess |
|   Hysteria |   Pericarditis |
|   Grief Reaction |   Myocardial Ischemia/Infarction |
|   Personality Disorders |   Neoplasms of Diaphragm |
| Head and Neck |   Neurofibromas of Phrenic Nerve |
|   Pharyngitis |   Diaphragmatic Hernia |
|   Laryngitis | Metabolic |
|   Neoplasms |   Uremia |
|   Irritation of Tympanic Membrane |   Diabetes Mellitus |
| Abdomen |   Alcohol |
|   Esophagitis |   Gout |
|   Esophageal Obstruction |   Hyponatremia |
|   Esophageal Achalasia |   Hypokalemia |
|   Gastric Distention |   Hypocalcemia |
|   Gastroesophageal Reflux |   Hypocarbia |
|   Gastric Neoplasms |   Fever |
|   Gastritis | Drugs |
|   Gastric Ulcer |   Cefotetan |
|   Ileus |   Sulfonamides |
|   Peptic Ulcer |   Short-acting Barbiturates |
|   Bowel Obstruction |   Benzodiazepines |
|   Crohn's Disease |   Dexamethasone |
|   Ulcerative Colitis |   Methylprednisolone |
|   Appendicitis |   Etoposide |
|   Pancreatitis |   Nicotine |
|   Pancreatic Pseudocyst |   Chlordiazepoxide |
|   Hepatitis |   Alpha-methyldopa |
|   Cholelithiasis | Idiopathic |
|   Cholecystitis | |
|   Intraabdominal Abscess | |
|   Peritonitis | |
|   Hydronephrosis | |
|   Prostatitis | |
|   Prostatic Cancer | |
|   Abdominal Aortic Aneurysm | |

AV = arteriovenous; CNS = central nervous system.

---

tococcus (*S singultus*) could be isolated from the throat and urine of afflicted patients, and this strain of streptococcus induced diaphragmatic contractions when injected into animals.[7]

Different psychiatric disorders also have been associated with persistent hiccup. Hysteria, grief reactions, reaction to strong emotional shock, various personality disorders, and malingering have been described as psychogenic causes.[25,37,38] The evidence is usually based on a negative evaluation for organic causes and/or resolution of the symptom after behavioral treatment. However, caution should be exercised when attributing hiccup to psychiatric causes because further investigation often reveals an underlying organic cause and because the symptom itself may precipitate changes in personality and behavior.[17]

### Head and Neck Causes

Hiccup may be precipitated by the stimulation of afferent nerves in the pharyngeal plexus and those afferent fibers that pass through the recurrent laryngeal nerve. Stimulation of these nerves by pharyngitis and laryngitis may both cause persistent hiccup.[35,39] Also, benign or malignant tumors of the neck have been associated causes.[15,40] A hair in the external auditory meatus is well described as a cause of chronic cough, but it also has been linked to cases of hiccup.[41] There is even one reported case of an ant in the external auditory canal causing hiccup.[42]

### Thoracic Causes

Asthma, bronchitis, pneumonia, and tuberculosis have all been described as uncommon causes of intractable hiccup.[25] Hiccups associated with these conditions would presumably be due to stimulation of vagal afferents in the lung. Pleural disease has also been linked to intractable hiccup. Pleuritis[25] and empyema[32] could conceivably precipitate hiccup by irritating the diaphragm or phrenic nerves directly. However, with the possible exception of empyema, these potential causes of persistent hiccup are not well documented. That is, the apparent association is based on few cases, and cause and effect were not established.

Because the mediastinum has many afferent and efferent nerves that participate in the hiccup reflex, it is not surprising that diseases of the mediastinum could precipitate hiccup. Mediastinitis, vascular aneurysms and tumors of the mediastinum, pericarditis, and mediastinal abscess have all been linked to cases of persistent hiccup.[25,32,43]

Myocardial infarction involving the inferior or lateral aspects of the heart is a recognized cause of hiccups.[25,44–47] Presumably, direct irritation of the diaphragmatic surfaces or of the phrenic nerves bordering the lateral aspects of the heart is the underlying mechanism. In some reports, the symptom has interfered with the management of acute myocardial infarction and required phrenic nerve block.[46]

Because of the diaphram's central role in the hiccup reflex, it is not unexpected that a number of diaphragm abnormalities have been causally linked. Tumors of the diaphragm and neurofibromas of the phrenic nerve have been reported as causes of intractable hiccup.[48] In addition, diaphragmatic hernia, a common disorder, has been the suspected cause of hiccup in some cases.[25] Of course, irritation of the diaphragm by adjacent processes in the pleural space or abdominal cavity may also elicit the symptom.

### Abdominal Causes

Gastrointestinal causes of hiccup are probably the most common and particular attention to abdominal and gastrointestinal symptoms is important during the initial evaluation. A history of intra-abdominal surgery is especially significant.[2,17,25]

Esophageal abnormalities have long been suspected to play a role in precipitating many cases of persistent hiccups.[49] Esophagitis, esophageal obstruction, esophageal achalasia, and diaphragmatic hernias have all been implicated.[2,17,50–52] In one report, 9 of 15 patients with achalasia had hiccups and dysphagia in association with meals.[50] Both hiccups and dysphagia improved soon after dilatation of the esophagus in all of the patients.

One common disorder long suspected of being a cause of persistent hiccup is gastroesophageal reflux disease.[51] Presumably reflux of acid into the esophagus could stimulate vagal afferents. However, some patients have had fundoplication with diminution of gastroesophageal reflux events and resolution of heartburn and, yet, had persistent hiccups.[53] Therefore, some have suggested that the association between gastroesophageal reflux and persistent hiccups is a chance association.[53,54] Further complicating the controversy is the fact that hiccups can provoke gastroesophageal reflux.[54] The negative intrathoracic pressure during a diaphragm contraction against a closed glottis creates a pressure gradient between the abdomen and chest, favoring reflux of gastric contents.

Gastric distention, gastric cancer, gastritis, and gastric ulceration have all been linked to persistent hiccups.[15,25,32,55,56] Intestinal causes are peptic ulcer disease, bowel obstruction, Crohn's disease, ulcerative colitis, and appendicitis.[2,15,17] Other causes include disorders of the pancreas, liver, and biliary system including pancreatic cancer, pancreatitis, pancreatic pseudocyst, cholelithiasis, cholecystitis, and hepatitis.[2,17,25]

Intra-abdominal abscess formation and peritonitis are nongastrointestinal abdominal disorders that have been linked to cases of persistent hiccup.[2,17,25] Retroperitoneal and pelvic causes of hiccup also have been suggested although the evidence is not strong. These causes include hydronephrosis, prostatitis, prostatic cancer, and abdominal aortic aneurysm.[2,17,25] Interestingly, some have speculated that the predominance of persistent hiccup in men is due to prostatic disorders.[57] How prostatic and other pelvic disorders could stimulate afferent nerves in the hiccup reflex arc is not known, but possibly, afferents of the pelvic plexus carry input to the medulla or contribute to the integration of the hiccup reflex at the level of the cervical spinal cord.

## Metabolic Causes

Metabolic causes are uremia,[25,58–60] diabetes mellitus,[25] alcohol,[25,51] gout,[17] hyponatremia,[61] hypokalemia,[62] hypocalcemia,[17] hypocarbia,[6] and fever.[17] There may be other metabolic causes yet unidentified. For example, even though no specific cause of hiccups may be identifiable, terminally ill patients not uncommonly have recurring bouts of hiccup lasting hours or days.[17,63] For another example, there also is a report of chronic hiccup occurring with a familial pattern.[64]

## Drugs

Drugs implicated in causing hiccups include the antibiotics cefotetan[65] and the sulfonamides (Table III).[66] The case of cefotetan-induced hiccups occurred within 1 hour of intravenous infusion and lasted 4 to 5 hours and was documented to recur with rechallenge. Other drugs that cause hiccups include the short-acting barbiturates[19,24] commonly used for induction of anesthesia and benzodiazepines.[67,68] Although hiccups are unusual after benzodiazepines, these drugs certainly should be avoided in patients with persistent hiccups. Finally, dexamethasone,[69] methylprednisolone,[70] etoposide,[71] nicotine,[2] chlordiazepoxide,[72] and alpha-methyldopa[2,17] have been implicated as causes of hiccup.

### Table III
#### Drugs That Cause Hiccup

Antibiotics
  cefotetan
  sulfonamides
Steroids
  methylprednisolone
  dexamethasone
Centrally Acting
  benzodiazepines
  short-acting barbiturates
  alpha-methyldopa
Other
  etoposide
  chlordiazepoxide
  nicotine

## Approach To Diagnosis

### Importance of Etiologic Diagnosis

Even though acute hiccups have been reported as an atypical sign of myocardial ischemia,[25,44–47] acute, isolated bouts of hiccup are an experience common to most people and they do not commonly require any evaluation for underlying cause. However, persistent hiccup is an important symptom that should not be discounted. Persistent hiccup is defined as hiccup lasting more than 48 hours or frequent recurring bouts of hiccups.[2,17] For unknown reasons, persistent hiccups occur more commonly in men than women.[25,73]

In general, patients with persistent hiccups should be evaluated for an underlying organic cause of the symptom.[2,17] When bouts have persisted for more than 1 week, spontaneous resolution is rare and simple empiric treatments are usually unsuccessful.[17] Identifying a potential organic cause of hiccup is important since it suggests specific therapy to relieve hiccup and also may have important therapeutic implications in its own right. Specific organic causes for hiccup are identifiable in more than 90% of men with persistent hiccup.[25] Organic causes of persistent hiccup should be sought in women as well, but are reportedly less frequently identifiable.[25]

In assessing the value of a systematic medical evaluation for the cause of persistent hiccup, the potential medical consequences of this symptom should not be underestimated (Table IV). Relief of in-

---

### Table IV
Reported Complications of Persistent Hiccup

Discomfort
Weight Loss
Debilitation
Reflux Esophagitis
Respiratory Alkalosis (posttracheostomy)
Wound Dehiscence
Sleep Deprivation
Psychiatric Disturbances
Death

---

tractable hiccups is important since prolonged attacks are uncomfortable to the patient and may interfere with work, eating, and sleeping. Severe weight loss, reflux esophagitis, debilitation, psychiatric disturbances, sleep deprivation, and even death have been attributed to intractable hiccups.[2,15,17,20,74–76] For patients with a tracheostomy or endotracheal tube for mechanical ventilation, persistent hiccups present a special problem. These patients may develop a severe respiratory alkalosis during hiccups since glottic closure no longer limits the inspiratory effectiveness of diaphragmatic contraction.[16]

### Diagnostic Evaluation

Because the spectrum and frequencies of causes of hiccups remain unestablished and because cases of persistent hiccup are relatively uncommon, there are no widely accepted algorithms for efficient diagnostic evaluation.[17] Nevertheless, a systematic approach based on the anatomy of the hiccup reflex should be effective (Figure 2).

The essence of the diagnostic evaluation is to determine where in the reflex arc there is irritation that could be stimulating hiccup. Because the involved neural pathways are widely distributed anatomically, the differential diagnosis is understandably broad. Irritation or stimulation of any portion of the reflex pathways may precipitate the development of hiccup. Since inputs to the medulla's "hiccup center" can originate in the central nervous system, the head and neck, thorax, diaphragm, and abdomen, the suspected causes of persistent hiccup can be subdivided into these anatomic regions for simplicity.

Evaluation should begin with a careful history detailing the chronology of the hiccups, symptoms associated with hiccups, and any remedies already attempted by the patient. A detailed medication history and drinking history are important because certain medications (eg, alpha-methyldopa, dexamethasone, diazepam) and alcohol can stimulate hiccup. Special attention should be paid to any gastrointesti-

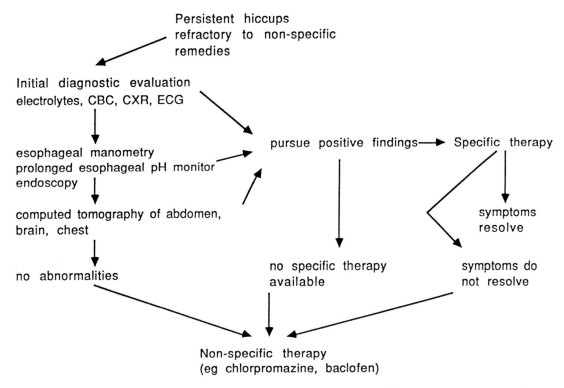

**Figure 2.** Diagnostic approach to persistent hiccup. The differential diagnosis for persistent hiccup is broad. The initial diagnostic evaluation should seek potential metabolic and drug causes of hiccup and seek evidence of organic disease in the central nervous system, head and neck, thorax, abdomen, and pelvis. Positive findings should be pursued to establish a definite diagnosis. A negative initial evaluation should be followed by studies that focus on the gastrointestinal tract since gastrointestinal disorders are common causes of chronic hiccup. Some have recommended computed tomography of the brain, chest, and abdomen if an organic cause of hiccup still is not established. When a cause of hiccup is identified, then specific therapy directed at the underlying diagnosis is begun. If specific therapy does not relieve the symptom, if specific therapy is not available or is contraindicated, or if no diagnosis has been established despite extensive evaluation, then nonspecific therapy with pharmacologic agents is begun. Phrenic nerve disruption is rarely performed for persistent hiccup. CBC = complete blood count; CXR = Chest x-ray; ECG = electrocardiogram.

nal symptomotology. Heartburn, bloating, acid taste in mouth, and sore throat may be indications of gastroesophageal reflux. History of past surgery, especially intra-abdominal surgery, is significant.[17,25] A careful physical exam of the head and neck, thorax, abdomen, and nervous system should be done and any abnormalities pursued. In the oropharynx, evidence of mucosal irritation, such as cobble-stoning of the mucosa, should prompt an assessment of the source of irritation. One cause of irritation in the oropharynx is gastroeso-

phageal reflux and this condition has been associated with chronic hiccup.[51–54] Basic laboratory tests should be done to exclude metabolic causes of persistent hiccups including electrolytes and complete blood count. Because there are mediastinal and other thoracic causes of hiccup, a chest roentenogram is also performed. For patients with recent onset of symptoms, an electrocardiogram should be obtained to rule out atypical presentation of myocardial infarction. Some authors recommend that all patients undergo esophageal studies with prolonged esophageal pH monitoring, manometry, and endoscopy.[17] Any abnormalities discovered in these initial evaluations should be pursued and then specific treatment should be initiated based on the findings. Because most persistent hiccups are due to an underlying organic cause, some recommend, and we concur, that a negative initial evaluation be followed by computed tomography of the abdomen, brain, and thorax .[17]

## Treatment

### Acute Hiccups

More numerous than suspected causes are the recommended cures for acute hiccups (Table V). Since Hippocrates, solemn advice for relief has never been lacking. Most of these common remedies presumably interrupt hiccups by providing counter irritation or blockade of afferent impulses. Many recommended "home remedies" for hiccup are amusing, but of dubious clinical value.

Nasal and pharyngeal stimulation is widely suggested as a cure for hiccups and these methods include inhalation of irritating vapors, swallowing granulated sugar, drinking a large glass of water, pulling on the tongue sharply, and 20 seconds of posterior pharyngeal wall stimulation with a plastic or rubber catheter passed through the nose.[2,5,17,77] The latter has been recommended as a simple nonpharmacologic method of treatment in the operating room or in the early (less than 5 days) postoperative setting.[5]

Respiratory maneuvers such as breath-holding, breathing into a paper bag, or breathing a 5% $CO_2$ mixture have long been advocated as simple means to relieve acute hiccups.[4,15,32,35,78] Also recommended are cough, sneezing, Valsalva maneuver, Müller's maneuver, continuous positive airway pressure (CPAP), and hyperventilation.[2,17,35,78] Hypercapnia decreases the frequency of hiccup and, presumably, relieves bouts of hiccup by

## Table V
### Treatment of Hiccup

Specific Therapy For Organic Cause
Nonspecific Therapy
  Simple Nonpharmacologic
    Irritating Vapors
    Swallowing Sugar
    Drinking Water
    Traction on Tongue
    Breath-holding
    Breathing Into Paper Bag
    Cough
    Sneezing
    Valsalva
    Müller's Maneuver
    Hyperventilation
    Fasting
    Vagal Stimulation
    Bed rest
    Sudden Fright
    Radial Artery Compression
    Acupuncture
    Pinching of Wrists
    Prayer

  Complex Nonpharmacologic
    Posterior pharynx Irritation
    5% $CO_2$ Mixture
    Vomiting by Emetic
    Behavior Modification
    Hypnosis
    Pulmonary Inflation
    Nasal CPAP
    Gastric Lavage
    Ether Into Nose
    Disrupt Phrenic Nerve(s)
  Pharmacologic
    See Table VI

CPAP = continuous positive airway pressure

decreasing the frequency to a low enough level that the hiccups are no longer self-sustaining. Whether and how hyperventilation and other respiratory maneuvers succeed in stopping hiccups is not clear, especially in light of the fact that hiccup is not thought to be primarily a respiratory reflex.

Relief of gastric distention through fasting, aspiration of gastric contents, gastric lavage, and vomiting have relieved hiccup.[32,35] Vagal stimulation by ocular compression and carotid massage also has been recommended.[32,35]

Finally, there are numerous miscellaneous treatment recommendations. These have included bed rest, sudden fright, compression of the patient's radial arteries while gazing in the patient's eyes, digital rectal massage, acupuncture, prayers to St. Jude, pressure on the ears, and pinching of the wrists.[2,17,79]

The onset of hiccups in a patient undergoing surgery may significantly complicate the surgical procedure and the postoperative period.[5,80] In this special setting, many maneuvers have been used to treat hiccups. Often, hiccups abate with deepening of anesthesia[2,17]; however, other measures may be necessary. Stimulation of the nasopharynx with a catheter,[5] instillation of ether,[81] pulmonary inflation,[82] or even nasal CPAP[83] have been employed successfully. Sixteen anesthetized patients had relief of hiccup upon application of 25 to 35 cm $H_2O$ nasal CPAP. Pharmacologic treatment has included atropine, chlorpromazine and metoclopramide, pentobarbital, methylphenidate, edrophonium, ketamine, and pentazocine.[2,17,19,24,35,84,85]

## Persistent Hiccups

### Specific Therapy

In general, when a specific cause of persistent hiccup can be identified, treatment of the underlying problem results in resolution of the symptom.[17] There are no clinical trials that establish the efficacy of specific treatments but, as a general principle, treating the underlying cause of a symptom seems prudent. However, if no cause for hiccup can be found or if specific treatment either fails to resolve the hiccups or is unavailable, then nonspecific therapy is warranted. Nonspecific therapy for persistent hiccup can be either non-pharmacologic or pharmacologic.

### Nonspecific Therapy

**Nonpharmacologic Therapy:** Most patients with persistent hiccups have tried many simple measures (Table V) to relieve hiccup before seeking medical advice. Therefore, more vigorous nonpharmacologic measures can be tried such as 5% $CO_2$ inhalation,[6] pharyngeal stimulation,[5] gastric aspiration and lavage, and vagal maneuvers (eg, carotid sinus massage, supraorbital pressure).[32,35] However, if hiccups have persisted for more than 1 week, these methods are likely to provide transitory relief at best.[2,17] Notably, however, some success has been reported with psychiatric methods including hypnosis.[37,38,86]

Disruption of the phrenic nerves is a drastic, nonpharmacologic approach to hiccup relief that has a long history.[2,17,87] Generally, it is no longer recommended because the method has serious potential complications and is not always successful even when the phrenic nerves are interrupted bilaterally. Also, the loss of phrenic nerve function may cause severe respiratory failure. Methods to disrupt phrenic nerve activity have included nerve blockade with novocaine, cooling of the nerves, electrical stimulation, nerve crush, and transection. In the rare instance that these methods are contemplated, fluoroscopy should be performed first to assess which leaf of the diaphragm is contracting during the hiccups.[2,17,88] In many instances, only one diaphragmatic leaf is contracting and usually it is the left one.[15]

**Pharmacologic Therapy:** A variety of agents have been suggested for the relief of hic-

## Table VI
### Pharmacologic Therapy for Persistent Hiccup

| Dopamine Antagonists | Other |
|---|---|
| chlorpromazine | nifedipine |
| haloperidol | amitriptyline |
| metoclopramide | amantadine |
| Antispasticity | quinidine |
| baclofen | apomorphine |
| Anticonvulsants | amyl nitrite |
| diphenylhydantoin | edrophonium |
| valproic acid | atropine |
| carbemazepine | scopolamine |
| Muscle Relaxants | pentazocine |
| mephenesin | ketamine |
| orphenadrine | |

cups when specific etiologic therapy is either unavailable or fails (Table VI). The pharmacologic treatment of hiccup is based largely on case report studies only. No double-blind, controlled, randomized trials have been conducted.

The strategy for pharmacologic treatment is to try different agents for a brief trial until an effective drug is found. Chlorpromazine has traditionally been a first-line agent but many would now start with baclofen (see below).[17] If unsuccessful, alternative drugs should be tried. No guidelines exist for selecting the order of agents for therapeutic trial, and failure with one agent does not necessarily predict failure with other agents. The trial of any one drug should not be longer than 3 to 4 days since success usually occurs within that interval. Usually symptoms stop abruptly in response to drug therapy, but in some cases the frequency and amplitude of hiccups gradually decrease. Once symptoms have resolved, the medication should be withdrawn after 7 to 10 days of therapy to determine whether maintenance treatment is necessary.[2,12,17] The value of combining agents in treatment is not known.

Chlorpromazine has long been used to relieve persistent hiccups.[2,12,19,89-92] Since several drugs with dopaminergic antagonism have efficacy in treating hiccups, it is felt that the dopaminergic antagonist properties of chlorpromazine probably underlie its efficacy in treating persistent hiccups. Studies suggest that approximately 80% of patients experience relief with chlorpromazine and an additional 10% experience temporary relief.[91,92] Chlorpromazine has been used as a 25 to 50 mg intravenous infusion over 1 to 3 hours or, alternatively, as a 25 to 50 mg intramuscular dose. This is followed by an oral maintenance dose of 25 to 50 mg three or four times daily.[12] Important side effects of chlorpromazine are systemic and postural hypotension, especially when the drug is administered intravenously.

Other dopaminergic antagonists used to treat persistent hiccups include metoclopramide[12,19,39,93] and haloperidol.[63,90,94] Metoclopramide has been used at an initial dose of 10 mg, intravenously or intramuscularly, followed by an oral maintenance dose of 10 to 20 mg, q.i.d.[12,17,47,56] Haloperidol was found highly effective in one study when administered intramuscularly (2 to 5 mg) followed by maintenance therapy with 1 to 4 mg, orally t.i.d.[63,90,94]

For some authors, baclofen, a gama-amino-butyric acid (GABA) agonist, has recently emerged as the agent of choice for the treatment of persistent hiccup.[17] The drug appears to relieve or partially relieve hiccup in more than two thirds of patients and has infrequent severe side effects.[12,64,95-97] Baclofen should be started at a low daily dose (5 mg, orally 2 or 3 times daily) and gradually increased with the maximum daily dose not exceeding 60 mg.[17] The drug has been used successfully to treat hiccups due to uremia, although it should be noted that renal mechanisms are important for baclofen elimination. The drug should not be withdrawn from patients abruptly since rapid withdrawal may induce hallucinations and seizures.[17]

Other agents used successfully have included the calcium channel antagonist, nifedipine.[98,99] In one study, nifedipine (30 to 60 mg daily) relieved hiccup in four out of seven subjects, although hiccup returned upon withdrawal of the medication.[98] Other drugs have included the anticonvulsants carbamazepine,[100] diphenylhydantoin,[101] and valproic acid.[102,103] Valproic acid may act by enhancing GABA activity in the central nervous system and therefore may have a mode of action similar to baclofen. Also employed successfully are the muscle relaxants, mephenesin and orphenadrine citrate.[2,12,17,104] Finally, amitriptyline hydrochloride,[105,106] amantadine hydrochloride,[107] quinidine, apomorphine hydrochloride, amyl nitrite, edrophonium chloride, atropine, scopolamine, pentazocine, and ketamine reportedly have been successful agents, but experience is limited.[2,12,17]

## References

1. Hippocrates. Aphroisms. In: *Hippocrates, IV*: The Loch Classical Library, WHS Jones. Cambridge, MA: Harvard University Press;1962.
2. Lewis JH. Hiccups: causes and cures. J Clin Gastroent 1985;7:539–552.
3. Shortt T. Hiccup, its causes and cure. Edinburgh Med Surg J 1833;39:305.
4. Bailey H. Persistent hiccup. Practitioner 1943;150:173–177.
5. Salem MR, Baraka A, Rattenborg CC, et al. Treatment of hiccups by pharyngeal stimulation in anesthetized and conscious subjects. JAMA 1967;202:126–130.
6. Newsom Davis J. An experimental study of hiccup. Brain 1970;93:851–872.
7. Rosenow EC. Diaphragmatatic spasms in animals produced with a streptococcus from epidemic hiccup: preliminary report. JAMA 1921;76:1745–1747.
8. Dearlove J. Intrauterine hiccup. Br Med J 1978;2:1716.
9. Dunn AM. Fetal hiccups. Lancet 1977;2:505.
10. Brouillette RT, Thach BT, Abu-Osba YK, et al. Hiccups in infants: characteristics and effects on ventilation. J Pediatr 1980;96:219–225.
11. Fuller GN. Hiccups and human purpose. Nature 1990;343:420.
12. Kolodzik PW, Eilers MA. Hiccups (singultus); review and approach to management. Ann Emerg Med 1991;20:565–573.
13. Anthoney JR, Anthoney SL, Anthoney DJ. On temporal structure of human hiccups: ethology and chronobiology. Int J Chronobiol 1978;5:477–492.
14. Halberg, F. Chronobiology. Anim Rev Physiol 1969;31:675–725.
15. Samuels L. Hiccup: a ten year reviw of anatomy, etiology, and treatment. Can Med Assoc J 1952;67: 315–322.
16. Campbell LA, Schwartz SH. An unusual cause of respiratory alkalosis. Chest 1991;100:1159.
17. Launois S, Bizec JL, Whitelaw WA, et al. Hiccup in adults: an overview. Eur Respir J 1993;6:563–575.
18. Askenasy JJM. Sleep hiccup. Sleep 1988;11:187–194.
19. Nathan MD, Leshner RT, Keller AP. Intractable hiccups. Laryngoscope 1980;90:1612–1618.
20. Askenasy JJM. About the mechanism of hiccup. Eur Neurol 1992;32:159–163.
21. Phillips JR, Eldridge FL. Respiratory myoclonus (Leeuwenhoek's Disease). N Engl J Med 1973;289:1390–1395.
22. Hoffman R, Yahr W, Krieger B. Diaphragmatic flutter resulting in failure to wean from mechanical ventilator support after coronary artery bypass surgery. Crit Care Med 1990;18:499–501.
23. Aldrich TK, Rochester DF. The Lungs and Neuromuscular Diseases. In: Murray JF, Nadel JA, eds. *Textbook of Respiratory Medicine*. Philadelphia, Pa: WB Saunders Company; 1994.
24. Butt HR Jr, Hanleberg W, Jacoby J. Hiccup: its possible cause and treatment in anesthesia. Anesth Analgesia 1961;40:182–185.
25. Souadjian JV, Cain JC. Intractable hiccup: etiological factors in 220 cases. Postgrad Med 1968;43:72–77.
26. Popescu C, Minea O, Manescu GH. Incoercible post-operative gastrogenic hiccup. Right splanchnicectomy. Rom Med Rev 1969;13:56–59.
27. Stotka VL, Barcray SJ, Bell HS, et al. Intractable hiccup as the primary manifestation of brain stem tumor. Am J Med 1962;32:313–315.
28. Kozik M, Owsianowska T. Persistent hiccoughs as the predominent symptom with a tumour of the medulla oblongata. J Neurol 1976;212:91–93.
29. Laing TJ, Morarin MA, Malik GM. Intractable hiccups and a posterior fossa arteriovenous malformation: a case report. Henry Ford Hosp Med J 1981;29:145–147.
30. Al Deeb S, Sharif H, Al Moutaery K, et al. Intractable hiccup induced by brainstem lesion. J Neurol Sci 1991;103:144–150.
31. Stalnikowicz R, Fich A, Troudart T. Amitriptyline for intractable hiccups. N Engl J Med 1986;315:64–65.
32. Noble EC. Hiccup. Can Med Assoc J 1934;31:41.

33. Rosenow EC. Further studies on the etiology of epidemic hiccup (singultus) and its relation to encephalitis. Arch Neurol Psychiat 1926;15:712–734.

34. Jansen PH, Joosten EMG, Vingerhoets HM. Persistent periodic hiccups following brain abscess: a case report. J Neurol Neurosurg Psychiat 1990;53:83–84.

35. Gigot AF, Flynn PD. Treatment of hiccups. JAMA 1952;150:760–764.

36. Eisenstadt HB. A case of hiccups. JAMA 1967;202:915.

37. Bobele M. Interactional treatment of intractable hiccup. Fam Process 1989;28:191–206.

38. Theohar C, McKegney FP. Hiccups of psychogenic origin: a case report and review of the literature. Compr Psychiat 1970;11:377–384.

39. Wagner MS, Stapczynski JS. Persistent hiccups. Ann Emerg Med 1982;11:24–26.

40. Stromberg BV. The hiccup. Ear Nose Throat J 1979;58:51–58.

41. Cardi E. Hiccups associated with hair in the external auditory canal—successful treatment by manipulation. N Engl J Med 1961;265:286.

42. Lossos IS, Breuer R. A rare case of hiccups. N Engl J Med 1988;318:711–12.

43. Loewenberg SA, March HC. Persistent hiccoughs as the sole symptom of thoracic aneurysm. Am Heart J 1937;13:624–626.

44. Swan HR, Simoson LH. Hiccups complicating myocardial infarction. N Engl J Med 1952;247:726–728.

45. Weiss MM. Hiccup as complication of acute coronary artery occlusion. Ann Intern Med 1939;13:187–188.

46. Ikram H, Orchard RT, Read SE. Intractable hiccuping in acute myocardial infarction. Br Med J 1971;2:504.

47. Douthwaite AH. Intractable hiccup in myocardial infarction. Br Med J 1971;2:709.

48. Burcharth F, Agger P. Singultus: a case of hiccup with diaphragmatic tumour. Acta Chir Scand 1974;140:340–341.

49. Cabane J, Derenne JP. Le hoquet. Concours Medical 1988;110:2829–2832.

50. Seeman H, Traube M. Hiccups and achalasia. Ann Intern Med 1991;115:711–712.

51. Gluck M. Chronic hiccups and gastroesophageal disease: the acid perfusion test as a provocative maneuver. Ann Intern Med 1986;105:219–220.

52. Kauffman HJ. Hiccup: an occasional sign of esophageal obstruction. Gastroenterology 1982;82:1443–1445.

53. Marshall JB, Landreneau RJ, Beyer KL. Hiccups: esophageal manometric features and relationship to gastroesophageal reflux. Am J Gastroenterology 1990;85:1172–1175.

54. Fisher J, Mittal RK. Hiccups and gastroesophageal reflux: cause and effect? Dig Dis Sci 1989;348:1277–1280.

55. Weeks C. Surgery of the phrenic nerve in the treatment of intractable hiccup. Ann Surg 1931;93:811–815.

56. Madanagopolan N. Metoclopramide in hiccup. Curr Med Res Opin 1975;3:371–374.

57. Mayo CW. Hiccup. Surg Gynecol Obstet 1932;55:700–708.

58. Gibbs AE. Two cases of persistent hiccup treated with orphenadrine citrate. Practitioner 1963;191:646.

59. Korczyn AD. Hiccup. Br J Med 1971;2:590–591.

60. Krahn A, Penner SB. Use of baclofen for intractable hiccups in uremia. Am J Med 1994;96:391.

61. Jones JS, Lloyd T, Cannon L. Persistent hiccups as an unusual manifestation of hyponatremia. J Emerg Med 1987;5:283–287.

62. Pines A, Goldhammer E. Hiccups as a presenting symptom of hypokalemia. Harefuah 1982;102:65–66.

63. Driscoll CE. Symptom control in terminal illness. Prim Care 1987;14:353–363.

64. Lance JW, Bassil GT. Familial intractable hiccup relieved by baclofen. Lancet 1989;2:276–277.

65. Morris JT, McAllister CK. Cefotetan-induced singultus. Ann Intern Med 1992;116:522–523.

66. Efrati P. Obstinate hiccup as a prodromal symptom in thoracic herpes zoster. Neurology 1956;6:601–602.

67. de Medonca MJ. Midazolam-induced hiccoughs. Br Dent J 1984;157:49.

68. Greenblatt DJ, Shader RI. Benzodiazepines in clinical practice. New York, NY: Raven Press, 1974: 203.

69. Lewitt PA, Barton NW, Posner JB. Hiccup with dexamethasone therapy. Ann Neurol 1982;12:405–406.

70. Baethge BA, Lidsky MD. Intractable hiccup associated with high-dose of intravenous methylprednisolone therapy. Ann Intern Med 1986;104:58–59.

71. Umeki S. Intravenous etoposide therapy and intractable hiccups (letter). Chest 1991;100:887.

72. Winstaed DK. Hiccup following ingestion

of oral chlordiazepoxide. Am J Psychiat 1976;136:719.

73. Fisher CM. Protracted hiccup: a male malady. Trans Am Neurol Assoc 1967;92:231–233.

74. Shay SS, Myers RL, Johnson LF. Hiccups associated with reflux esophagitis. Gastroenterology 1984;87:204–207.

75. Triadafilopoulos G. Hiccups and esophageal dysfunction. Am J Gastroenterol 1989;84:164–169.

76. Fleet W, Morgan HJ, Morello PJ. A fatal case of hiccups. J Tenn Med Assoc 1990;83:79–80.

77. Engleman EG, Lankton J, Lankton B. Granulated sugar as treatment for hiccups in conscious patients. N Engl J Med 1971;285:1489.

78. Bellingham-Smith E. The significance and treatment of obstinate hiccoughs. Practitioner 1938;140:166–171.

79. Odeh M, Bassan H, Oliven A. Termination of intractable hiccups with digital rectal massage. J Intern Med 1990;227:145–146.

80. Santos G, Cook WA, Frater RWM. Reclosure of sternotomy disruption by hiccup. Chest 1974;66:189–190.

81. Moses JA, Ramachandran KP, Surendran D. Treatment of hiccups with instillation of ether in nasal cavity. Anesth Analg 1970;49:367–368.

82. Baraka A. Inhibition of hiccup by pulmonary inflation. Anesthesiology 1970;32:271–273.

83. Satto C, Gristina G, Cosmi EV. Treatment of hiccups by continuous positive airway pressure (CPAP) in anesthetized subjects. Anesthesiology 1982;57:345.

84. Shantha T. Ketamine for the treatment of hiccups during and following anesthesia: a preliminary report. Anesthesiology 1973;52:822–824.

85. Macris SG. Methylphenidate for hiccups. Anesthesiology 1971;34:201.

86. Bendersky G, Baren M. Hypnosis in the termination of hiccups unresponsive to conventional treatment. Arch Intern Med 1959;104:417–420.

87. Eisele JH, Noble MIM, Katz J. Bilateral phrenic nerve block in man. Technical problems and respiratory effects. Anesthesiology 1972;37:64–67.

88. Benzon HJ, Prasad YS, Barthwell DA. The value of fluoroscopy before performing a phrenic nerve block. Anesthesiology 1981;55:469–470.

89. Williamson B, Macintyre I. Management of intractable hiccup. Br Med J 1977;2:501–503.

90. Lamphier T. Methods of management of persistent hiccup (singultus). Md Med J 1977;11:80–81.

91. Friedgood CE, Ripstein CB. Chlorpromazine (Thorazine) in the treatment of intractable hiccups. JAMA 1955;157:309–310.

92. Davignon A, Laurieux G, Genest J. Chlorpromazine in the treatment of persistent hiccough. Union Med Can 1955;84:282.

93. West T. Drug control of common symptoms in terminally ill patients. S Afr Med J 1977;51:415–418.

94. Ives TJ, Flemming MF, Weart CW, et al. Treatment of intractable hiccup with intramuscular haloperidol. Am J Psychiat 1985;142:1368–1369.

95. Bhalotra R. Baclofen therapy for intractable hiccoughs. J Clin Gastroenterol 1990;12:122.

96. Yaqoob M, Prabhu P, Ahmad R. Baclofen for intractable hiccups. Lancet 1989;2:562–563.

97. Burke AM, White AB, Brill N. Baclofen for intractable hiccup. N Engl J Med 1988;319:1354.

98. Lipps DC, Jabbari B, Mitchel MH, et al. Nifedipine for intractable hiccups. Neurology 1990;40:531–532.

99. Mukhopadadhyay P, Osman MR, Wajima T, et al. Nifedipine for intractable hiccups. N Engl J Med 1986;314:1256.

100. McFarling DA, Susac JO. Carbamazepine for hiccoughs. JAMA 1974;230:962.

101. Petroski D, Patel AN. Diphenylhydantoin for intractable hiccups. Lancet 1974;1:739.

102. Jacobson PL, Messenheimer JA, Farmer TW. Treatment of intractable hiccups with valproic acid. Neurology 1981;31:1458–1460.

103. Zimmerman HJ, Ishak KG. Valproate-induced hepatic injury; analysis of 23 fatal cases. Hepatology 1982;2:591–597.

104. Finch JW. Rapid control of persistent hiccups by orphenadrine citrate. Med Times 1966;94:485–488.

105. Parvin R, Milo R, Klein C, et al. Amitriptyline for intractable hiccup. Am J Gastroenterol 1988;63:1007–1008.

106. Stalnikowicz R, Fich A, Troudart T. Amitriptyline for intractable hiccups. N Engl J Med 1986;315:64–65.

107. Askenasy JJM, Boiangiu M, Davidovitch S. Persistent hiccup cured by amantadine. N Engl J Med 1988;318:711.

# 9

# Sneeze

Oren P. Schaefer, M.D.
Richard S. Irwin, M.D.

## Introduction

Stimulation of the nasal mucosa has been shown to produce dramatic reflex responses.[1,2] Sneezing, or sternutation, is part of a generalized reflex response to abnormal stimulation of the nasal mucosa, and it is the most common respiratory reflex arising from the nose. Like the apnea and diving reflex, it helps to protect the lower respiratory tract from the entrance of irritants and fluids. Though sneezing is very rarely the sole presenting complaint, it is often part of a complex of symptoms that commonly brings a patient to the physician's office. While sneeze is not usually associated with significant morbidity, it can at times become intractable and interfere with one's occupation, lifestyle, and sense of well being. Though often a minimized complaint today, sneeze holds a prominent place in the history of medicine. This chapter will serve to review the anatomy and physiology of the sneeze reflex and its causes, and offer a diagnostic approach to the evaluation and the treatment of sneeze, often as part of its greater symptom complex.

## Historical Aspects of Sneeze

Nearly all ancient people felt the sneeze to be sacred. Greek philosophers of the fourth century BC considered sneezing to be holy, a divine sign of great importance.[3] Of all other types of air emanating from the body, only the sneeze held such prominence, and it was rationalized that sneeze emanated from the most divine organ.[4] Hippocrates (460 to 377 BC) felt sneezing to be dangerous before or after lung illness, but was beneficial to other diseases.[3] He felt it was a cure for the hiccup. Discorides described a case of epilepsy occurring after "copious sneezing," and others felt it heralded menstruation.[4] In the Jerusalem Talmud, sneezing is described as one of the six bodily functions which help the sick. A tale is related of a Shunamite woman who appeared to have died of sunstroke and sneezed seven times and opened her eyes.[3] Amongst Jewish belief, there is a legend that there was no illness in the world. Whenever it came for a healthy person to die, he sneezed and his soul would leave him through his nose.[5] In Genesis 49:18, when Jacob began to bless his sons, he began to sneeze and, in anticipation of his imminent death, he said, "Give me enough time to bless my sons." Thus, when a person sneezes, he is obligated to thank God that he remains alive.[4]

Sneeze took on a negative aspect in the middle ages when the Bubonic Plague

From Irwin RS, Curley FJ, Grossman RF (eds): Diagnosis and Treatment of Symptoms of the Respiratory Tract. Armonk, New York, Futura Publishing Company, Inc., © 1997.

afflicted Rome in the period 590 to 610 AD. In this epidemic, people suddenly died while sneezing. One victim of the epidemic was Pope Pelagius II who reportedly died while sneezing. At that time, Pope Gregory VII asked his people to say "May God bless you," following the sneeze.[3] Such a blessing remains to this day. Additionally during this time a children's nursery rhyme emerged in reference to the Plague,[5] a rhyme, though perhaps altered, is still uttered by children today: "Ring around the rosy [refers to the ring rash]/ Pocket full of posy/ Achew! Achew!/ All fall down [dropping dead]"

## Anatomy of Sneeze

The nose is the superior portion of the respiratory tract. It is a complex organ capable of multiple functions, including not only olfaction but the specialized respiratory functions of humidification and temperature modification, regulation of the volume and speed of airflow, and trapping of airborne particles. And clearly, the nose has a central role in the sneeze reflex. What follows is a brief overview of the neuroanatomy of the nose involved in this reflex.

### Nasal Mucosa

The nasal respiratory mucosa is supplied by free subepithelial and intraepithelial nerve endings. They respond to mechanical and chemical stimuli and, possibly, to temperature and airflow.[6–8] The sensory nerves of the nose are derived from the ophthalmic and maxillary divisions of the trigeminal nerve. The nasociliary branch of the ophthalmic division divides into the anterior and posterior ethmoidal nerves which supply the upper and anterior areas of the lateral wall and the nasal septum. The maxillary division supplies the posterior and inferior areas. Branches of the maxillary nerve include the posterior lateral and septal branches to the inferior and middle turbinates, the

nasopalatine nerve to the lower anterior portion of the septum and incisive canal, the major palatine nerve which forms the lower nasal branches, and the anterior superior alveolar nerve which supplies branches to the anterior floor of the nose and the inferior meatus.[6] Some afferent nerves may run in the nervi terminalis in association with the olfactory nerves and could mediate the sneezing caused by strong olfactory irritants.[1] Figure 1 is a schematic representation of the nervous innervation of the nose.

## Nasal Blood Vessels and Glands

The postganglionic parasympathetic fibers supplying the nasal blood vessels and glands are derived from the pterygopalatine ganglion. These fibers reach their supply area primarily with the branches of the trigeminal nerve. The sympathetic vasomotor fibers are derived from the superior cervical ganglion and travel with arteries and veins and also with branches of the trigeminal nerve.[6] The nasal vascular bed has both a sympathetic and parasympathetic nerve supply. All the components of the nasal glands receive cholinergic parasympathetic input. The blood vessels that supply these glands have the same dual autonomic innervation as other nasal vasculature, and, in this way, the secretory activity of the glands is partly under sympathetic influence.[6]

## Mediators of Sneeze

Substance P, a neuropeptide, as well as a dense distribution of substance P–containing nerves have been observed immunohistochemically in the nasal mucosa.[9–12] Substance P is a potent stimulator of sensory nerves, and intravenous and intranasal capsaicin will cause the release of substance P.[13,14] Intranasal capsaicin has been shown to effectively induce sneeze.[15–17] Capsaicin, the pungent agent in hot pepper, stimulates a specific neural cation channel that allows for $Na^+$ and

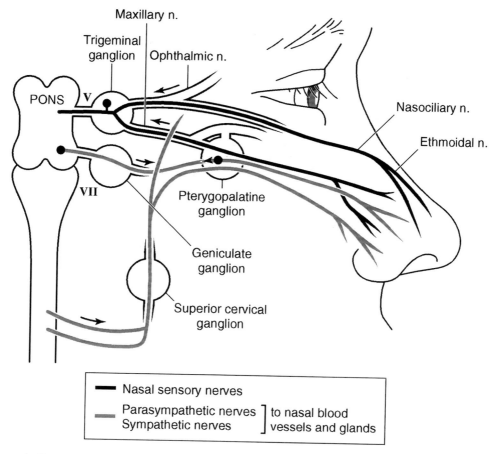

**Figure 1.** Innervation of the human nose. Figure shows major sensory and autonomic pathways of the human nose involved in the sneeze reflex.

$Ca^{2+}$ ions to enter and $K^+$ to leave the cell, thereby leading to neural depolarization.[18] Capsaicin-sensitive nerves are generally assumed to be unmyelinated, chemosensitive afferents. Repeated, high, or systemic doses of capsaicin will result in substance P depletion[9,16] and the inhibition of the sneeze response.[15,16,19,20] This suggests that at least a portion of the afferent limb of the sneeze response is mediated via C fiber afferents and is probably involved in the sneeze associated with allergic rhinitis, as well as that associated with irritants such as cigarette smoke, formalin, and nicotine.[21] Nonetheless, there are clearly afferent pathways that are capsaicin-resistant that do play a role in sneeze formation; sneeze induced by mechanical stimulation is one such stimulus, and nicotine will cause sneeze by a non–capsaicin-sensitive mechanism as well.[21]

Nasal inhalation of histamine is a very effective stimulus of sneeze,[22–24] and is thought to be the primary mediator of the sneeze of allergic rhinitis.[24] A provocative dose of histamine resulted in sneezing within 1 minute of its application when sprayed into the nostril of an atopic individual.[23] The effect is mediated through the $H_1$-histamine receptor.[23,24] Since histamine has been shown to cause release of substance P from sensory nerves,[25,26] it is possible that the sneeze response to histamine may be mediated by substance P. Imamura and Kambara[27] demonstrated that a $3\times10^8$-fold greater concentration of histamine over substance P was needed to induce sneeze in sensitized guinea pigs. Capsaicin treatment of normal or sensitized guinea pigs significantly inhibited the sneezing induced by either antigen challenge or by application of histamine.[20,28] These data suggest that histamine released as part of the allergic response results in sneeze by causing the stimulation of substance P–containing C afferent fibers. In patients with nonallergic rhinitis, obstruction, rhinorrhea, and sneezing were all reduced after local treatment with a capsaicin aerosol,[29] suggesting the importance of a substance P–related mechanism in sneeze in a more generalized group.

Serotonin induces a variety of nasal responses including sneeze[30]; this compound may play a role in rhinitis,[31] though its role in the initiation of sneeze appears small, if any. Terfenadine, which has no antiserotonergic activity[32,33] abolished sneeze in allergen-challenged atopic volunteers.[24] Electrical stimulation of the ethmoidal nerves, Vidian nerve, or greater petrosal nerve can produce sneezing.[34,35] The optic nerve may have a role as well[36] and is discussed in greater detail below.

## Physiology of Sneeze

Like cough, the sneeze is a complex respiratory reflex (Table I). However, unlike cough, the sneeze cannot be produced voluntarily. Despite being more common than the other nasal reflexes (eg, diving or apnea reflex), the sneeze has been much less studied. This may in part be due to the fact that the reflex is easily suppressed with anesthesia,[1,37] making its controlled study more difficult. Sneeze is one of several motor acts in which the sequence of movements appears to be centrally patterned; once set in motion, the act continues to its predetermined end without the need for continuing input or feedback from the periphery.[38] Numerous stimuli can trigger the response and appear to do so through a final common pathway.

Sneeze occurs in two distinct phases, termed the nasal, or sensory phase and the

**Table I**
Sneeze and Cough: Similarities and Differences

*Similarities*
Both are complex respiratory reflexes.
Both protect the lower respiratory tract from potentially harmful agents.
Both involve closure of the glottis to increase intrathoracic pressure prior to expulsion of air.
Both involve high expiratory velocities of air.
*Differences*
Sneeze is involuntary. Cough can be both voluntary and involuntary.
The pharynx is constricted just before expiration only during sneeze.
New inspiratory neurons are only recruited during sneeze.
Only sneeze is associated with a complex behavior pattern (eg, lacrimation, contraction of facial muscles, involuntary closure of the eyes, and head and body movements).

respiratory or efferent, phase. Stimuli in the anterior portion of the nose or elsewhere send impulses to the pons and medulla by way of the trigeminal nerve. The impulses ultimately converge on a "sneezing center" in the medulla. Sneeze-evoking regions in the cat have been located along the ventral portion of the trigeminal nucleus and the pontine-medullary lateral reticular formation.[39,40] In a 1991 study, a patient who was unable to sneeze despite a sensory urge to do so was described with a medullary neoplasm.[41] The tumor was located in an area that could interfere with the proposed sneezing center, which suggests that its location in humans is similar to that in the cat.

From the medulla, preganglionic fibers pass the impulse to the greater petrosal nerve, via the nervus intermedius. From there the signal goes to the sphenopalatine ganglion. Postganglionic fibers then stimulate glands and blood vessels in the nasal mucosa that result in edema of the membranes and production of a clear nasal secretion and edema. Experimentally induced sneezes following nasal vasodilatation and secretion were produced by stimulation of the greater superficial petrosal nerve.[42] Such concludes the nasal phase.[43,44]

The respiratory phase begins with stimulation of the trigeminal nerve by the nasal edema and secretions. Impulses are again passed to the pons and medulla to stimulate the respiratory center at the floor of the fourth ventricle. Once stimulated, inspiratory neurons in the ventrolateral nucleus of the tractus solitarius lead to activation of the phrenic and other nerves which results in inspiration. When transdiaphragmatic pressure (Pdi) was measured in experimental animals during induced sneeze, it reached or exceeded $Pdi_{max}$.[45] This is in distinction to a Pdi of about 12% maximum during quiet tidal breathing.[45] It is likely that during nonventilatory behaviors that abdominal muscles are also activated and possibly contribute to the measured Pdi response by causing a lengthening contraction of the diaphragm. Therefore, the maximal or supermaximal response does not entirely reflect diaphragmatic activity. In distinction to cough though, new inspiratory neurons are recruited in sneeze, in which the inspiratory efforts are faster.[46]

Inspiration is then followed by the expiratory phase. The magnitudes of the two components are linked. How the two phases are matched is uncertain. It probably involves vagal feedback from pulmonary stretch receptors; though, multiple interacting mechanisms cannot be excluded.[34,38] In airway defense reflexes characterized by the alteration of inspiratory and expiratory efforts, both the mean and maximum frequency of firing of inspiratory and expiratory neurons increases significantly as compared with control breathing.[46]

Study of the expiratory neurons located in the caudal medulla has found the following: Acceleration of previously active expiratory neurons, earlier firing of late expiratory units, and recruitment of latent expiratory neurons.[47] It appears that the latent units may be essential for the generation of active expiration, but all contribute to the force of the expiratory thrust.[47] These same expiratory units are involved in cough and sneeze. Recruit-

ment of new expiratory neurons with a different amplitude from spontaneously active expiratory units and with a higher excitability threshold have been observed, and termed "latent" expiratory neurons.[46] They appear regularly during different types of active expiration and are nonspecific. It is assumed that the ventral respiratory group contains large numbers of expiratory neurons that are activated and linked in many respiratory processes associated with active expiration.[46] Data indicate that various afferent systems activate a common pool of expiratory neurons.[47]

Just before expiration, the palate is raised and the superior constrictor muscle of the pharynx is contracted so that respiratory passages are shut off from the nose. In distinction from cough, the pharynx is constricted.[43,44] Activation of the laryngeal adductors[34,48] along with activation and contraction of the abdominal muscles, causes an increase in intrapulmonary pressure. Monitoring of both the triangularis sterni and transversus abdominus muscles in dogs revealed a marked augmentation of both the peak and rate of rise of expiratory muscle electromyograms[49] during the expulsive phase of both sneeze and cough. The pattern of recruitment of the two muscles during both of these reflexes differed from what occurred during rest and $CO_2$-stimulated breathing.[49,50] Such data suggest a difference in the central pattern generator that controls expiratory muscle activity during breathing and that which regulates expulsive respiratory acts.[49]

The strength of the expiratory effort in sneeze is enhanced by the preceding large inspiration by a vagal inflation reflex, similar to that seen with a cough.[1,47] This reflex enhancement is presumably mediated by slowly adapting pulmonary stretch receptors.[1] Enhancement of the active expiration also occurs because of the added elastic recoil of the lung and the stretch of the expiratory muscles. Theoretically, this preceding deep inspiration may have the effect of increasing inhalation of the irritant substance. Presumably, this is compensated for by the added mechanical efficiency of the subsequent expulsive effort.[8]

With the rising pressure developed by active expiration, the nasopharynx is forced open, and air is driven out, primarily through the nose but through the mouth as well. This results in a highly atomized naso-oral discharge. Like in cough, high expiratory air velocity is achieved, reaching 30 to 40 m/sec (66 to 83 mph) or more[43,51,52] with peak airflow approaching 6 L/sec.[53] An involuntary closure of the eyes, as well as lacrimation, contraction of the facial and nasal muscles, and head and body movements appear to be part of a complex behavioral pattern that completes the sneeze.

There appears to be a threshold or trigger mechanism that regulates a sneeze. Stimulation of the nasal mucosa may only create the desire to sneeze, and under these circumstances, it is possible to precipitate a sneeze by superimposing additional stimuli, even of another nature (see below).[54] Such a sneeze threshold may be lower in atopic individuals.[55]

Numerous stimuli will provoke a sneeze. Sneezing may result from any condition that causes an increase in nasal mucous production, perhaps most commonly, the "common cold." Similarly, sneezing is very common in those afflicted with hay fever or sensitized to other aeroallergens, as well as those with rhinitis of a nonallergic nature. Other stimuli that can precipitate sneezing include cooling of the body,[1] irritation of the scalp or ear,[51] bright light,[36] nasal or aural foreign bodies,[44,51] epilepsy,[56] psychogenic factors,[57,58] male orgasm,[44,59,60] and fullness of the stomach.[61,62] This wide variety of stimuli most likely do not have a common afferent pathway. It has been suggested that the afferent limb of the sneeze reflex converges on a "sneeze center," or, alternatively, that these factors all cause nasal mucosal hyperemia, and mucous secretion, which then may secondarily activate the nasal receptors responsible for sneeze.[1,36,43]

## Differential Diagnosis of Sneeze

In considering the differential diagnosis of sneeze, it is important to remember the anatomic/physiologic basis of the reflex. Stimulation of a number of areas can result in sneeze. The differential is broken into the following four general categories: irritative, autonomic, psychologic, and central nervous system (CNS) disease.

### Irritative

The most common causes of sneeze fall into this first group. Sneezing is commonly associated with allergic rhinitis. The cause of the sneeze appears to be due to the release of histamine as a result of local deposition of a specific allergen,[22,23] though a number of other mediators (leukotrienes, prostoglandin $D_2$, kinins, TAME-esterase) are recovered after nasal challenge as well,[18,63] and have been correlated closely with sneeze.[64] Commonly inhaled allergens include tree and grass pollens, weeds, mold spores, dust mites, and animal dander. Sneeze may also be a manifestation of a more severe allergic disorder, such as anaphylaxis.[65-68]

Infectious agents such as rhino- and adenovirus, and those causing pertussis and measles can elicit sneeze. Nonspecific irritants can result in sneeze as well. Such agents include powder, pepper, snuff, chemical agents, foreign bodies, and nasal hairs.[21,44,69] Sneeze can be aggravated by other nonspecific factors such as nasal polyps, nasal septum deviation, and mucosal ulcers. The above fall under the heading of nonallergic rhinitis (Table II). A case of paroxysmal sneeze felt to be secondary to a parathyroid adenoma that impinged upon the recurrent laryngeal nerve has been reported.[70] Inhaled corticosteroids and cromolyn sodium, both effective in the treatment of sneeze, can themselves cause sneeze in 3% to 10% of those using the medication.

### Autonomic

Factors that may trigger the sneeze reflex via autonomic pathways have already been mentioned and are outlined in Table

## Table II
### Nonallergic Rhinitis

Atrophic Rhinitis
Cystic Fibrosis
Dyskinetic Cilia Syndrome
Drugs
    Antihypertensives
    Aspirin/Nonsteroidal Anti-inflammatory drugs
    Cocaine
Granulomatous Rhinitis
    Sarcoidosis
    Wegener's Granulomatosis
    Relapsing Polychondritis
    Midline Granuloma
    Granulomatous Infection
Gustatory Rhinitis
Hormonal
    Pregnancy
    Oral Contraceptives
    Conjugated Estrogens
    Cyclic Hormonal Change/Menopause
Infectious Rhinitis
Nasal Foreign Body
Nasal Malignancy
Nasal Polyposis
Nonallergic Rhinitis with Eosinophilia (NARES)
Perennial Nonallergic Rhinitis (without eosino-
    philia)
Rhinitis Medicamentosa
Systemic Disease
    Hypothyroidism
    Uremia
    Diabetes Mellitus
Vasomotor Rhinitis

## Table III
### Autonomic Sneezes

Photic Sneeze
Menstruation
Pregnancy
Sexual Intercourse
Narcotic Withdrawal
Strong Odor*
Temperature Change*
? Thyroid Disease

* May be due to mechanism similar to irritant stimuli.

III. The photic sneeze reflex, discussed later in the chapter, would fall into this category. Sneeze has also been elicited by strong odors, chilling of the body, menstruation and pregnancy, sexual intercourse, narcotic withdrawal, and following the ingestion of wine.[36,44,71,72] Some can argue that odors and temperature change may act as irritant stimuli. Sneezing has been associated with the rhinitis of thyroid disease (hyper and hypo), and its cause may fall under this grouping.[73]

## Psychologic

Psychologic sneezing most often occurs in the teenage years. It is usually par-oxysmal, and often protracted (see below). It has no seasonal disposition, and no physical stimulant is found after the history and physical examination (Table IV). Emotional stimuli influence sneeze in other ways. Fear will result in shrinkage of the nasal mucosal membranes, presumably from the adrenergic response. A variety of other emotions, such as grief or frustration, may result in hyperemia and nasal congestion. It is interesting that the lack of sneezing, termed "asneezia," has been associated with a variety of psychiatric illnesses, particularly endogenous depression. The incidence of "asneezia" of approximately 1% to 2% has been reported in an uncontrolled study of Indian populations.[69,74] That "asneezia" is an unrecognized psychiatric symptom has been refuted,[75] and there have been no similar reports of a similar symptom in Western culture.

## Table IV
### Characteristics of Psychogenic Sneeze

The majority of intractable sneezers.
More common in adolescents.
More common in females.
Many atypical features which include:
    Little/no inspiratory phase
    Little/no aerosolization of mucous secretions
    Lack of sneeze during sleep
    Artificial rate (up to 2000/day)
    Lack of eye closure.
Lack of physical findings.
Significant psychopathology often found.

## Central Nervous System Disease

Sneezing may be a sign of CNS disease, most notably, temporal lobe epilepsy.[56,76] However, this is often accompanied by other more typical seizure activity. Stimulation of the temporal lobe during surgery can produce a sneeze.[44] Very rarely though, sneezing may be the only manifestation of a seizure disorder.[56,77] It is of historical note that sneezing was associated with seizures as far back as the first century BC.[3] In addition to seizures, sneeze has been reported to occur with other forms of CNS disease, including mild encephalitis, poliomyelitis, and tabes dorsalis.[78]

## Specific Sneezes

### Photic Sneeze

Sneeze in response to the exposure to bright light, usually sunlight, termed the photic sneeze,[36] or photosternutory reflex,[79] was first described more than 100 years ago (Table V).[71] Everett[36] was the first to try to characterize these patients. In a questionnaire study of 75 college students, medical students, and hospitalized patients, he found an average frequency of photic sneeze of almost 11% (23% in the group of medical students), with a clear male predominance. Others report a similar-to-somewhat higher incidence, up to 36%.[80–83] Buckley notes the reflex to be frequent among babies.[84] It is interesting that effected individuals believe light to be a common precipitant of sneeze, while those unaffected individuals have rarely, if ever, heard of the reflex!

A familial tendency to sneeze when exposed to bright light appears to exist. Collie et al.[85] studied four kindreds (their own!) and showed evidence of an autosomal dominant pattern of inheritance. They gave the reflex the acronym ACHOO (Autosomal-dominant Compelling Helio-Ophthalmic Outburst) syndrome. This mode of inheritance has since been suggested by others.[80–82,86] The condition is clearly benign, though one can imagine it might be troublesome in certain occupations, such as airline and fighter pilots, truck drivers, and ballplayers, to name a few.

The mechanism of this reflex is unclear. In the first review of the subject, Everett[36] put forth three explanations. The first he termed optic-trigeminal summation. Association between the optic nerve and fifth cranial nerve, especially in the mesancephalon may enhance irritability of one nerve, when the other is stimulated.[87] He suggested that optic stimulation may produce referred sensation in the nasal branches of the fifth cranial nerve, producing or enhancing nasal stimulation enough to produce a sneeze. Photophobia may be due to such a mechanism via an afferent optic nerve and an efferent trigeminal (ophthalmic branch) limb.[72]

Another possibility suggested by Everett was termed parasympathetic generalization; stimuli that excite one specific branch of the parasympathetic nervous system tend to activate other branches. Such an example would be a bright light that leads to pupillary constriction (cranial nerve III) that also produces lacrimation (cranial nerve VII). Should such parasympathetic activity become sufficiently generalized, nasal secretion and congestion (like lacrimation, mediated through cranial nerve VII and the sphenopalatine ganglion) may result. Nasal congestion

---

**Table V**
Characteristics of Photic Sneeze

Frequency 11% to 36%.
Autosomal dominant inheritance pattern.
Sneeze occurs in response to change in light intensity.
Sneeze is not dependent on specific wavelength.
Long refractory period suggests polysynaptic reflex.
Proposed causes include:
  Optic-trigeminal summation
  Parasympathetic generalization
  Parasympathetic hypersensitivity/hyperreactivity.

may then trigger the respiratory phase of the sneeze.

The last possibility offered by Everett was that of hypersensitivity and/or hyperreactvity of the parasympathetic system in the nasal mucosa. Such a mechanism appears to play a role in vasomotor rhinitis, possibly in allergic rhinitis, and in nasal mucosal responses to various emotional states. However, there does not appear to be a higher incidence of the photic sneeze reflex in patients with allergic rhinitis or asthma.[36,83]

The photic sneeze reflex is frequently noted by ophthalmologists during opthalmoscopy or slit lamp examination. Interestingly, there appears to be a high frequency of the reflex in patients with nephropathic cysteinosis, a disorder which is characterized by crystal deposition in the cornea.[88,89] Deposition of cysteine crystals in the basal epithelium of the eye possibly interferes with regional neuronal connections which may result in trigeminal irritation and supersensitivity to a photic stimulus.[72,88] Lewkonia[90] described a patient with the photic sneeze reflex who he treated for corneal edema and vascularization after an alkali burn. The frequency of sneeze diminished as the condition improved, which again suggests abnormal irritability of the trigeminal branches. Keratitis has been reported to enhance the photic sneeze reflex by others.[71,79]

Sédan, a French ophthalmologist, documented not only sunlight as a stimulus for the photosternutatory reflex, but the light from a photographic flash, slit lamp, and Wood's lamp as well. The response does not appear to be mediated by specific wavelengths of light but rather the change in its intensity.[91] Sédan also found that a sneeze occurred only after the first exposure to light, and never upon repetitive photic stimulation.[79] This observation is consistent with other reports that describe a refractory period, suggesting that the reflex is polysynaptic. A patient being evaluated for a seizure disorder was noted to sneeze after photic stimulation was administered as part of the electroencephalogram protocol.[92]

Electroencephalographic recordings in this patient found a latency on average of 9.9 seconds. Forrester[80] has reported the latency of the response to be 2.5 to 15 seconds. Such a long latency period suggests that the phenomenon is not due to reflex activity mediated by the pregeniculate branches from the optic nerve to the brain stem tectile region. It is more likely that the reflex is secondary to stimulation of the trigeminal nerve by indirect means, such as tearing or squinting.[86] Such a hypothesis is supported by the observation that hair pulling, facial touching, and eyebrow plucking may lead to sneeze in affected patients. Why some are prone to photic sneeze, whereas others are not is not clear.

Finally an interesting hypothesis has been put forth by Pies.[93] He questions whether there is an association between the photic sneeze reflex and Seasonal Affective Disorder, a psychiatric condition that appears to respond to photic therapy. Depression may involve supersensitivity of a central muscarinic mechanism,[94] and bright light appeared to subsensitize central cholinergic receptors in rats.[95] Pies[93] questioned whether similar cholinergic mechanisms are involved in the photic sneeze reflex. There are no data to support (or refute) this possibility.

## Intractable Sneeze

Though yet to be clearly defined, there exists a small body of literature on protracted sneezing. Table VI[51,56–59,77,96–111] summarizes these reports. Approximately 30 cases of intractable, paroxysmal sneeze, are reported in the literature. The entity was first described by Shilkret in 1949.[58] The majority of these cases appeared to occur in adolescents, and in the great majority, no pathophysiologic trigger mechanisms were elucidated. A psychogenic cause was responsible for most of the reported cases. A specific cause was found in only six cases. These have included epilepsy,[56] tuberculous adenitis,[112] triethanolamine sensitivity,[107] atopy,[101] sexual stimulation,[59] and multifactorial causes.[98]

**Table VI**
Intractable Sneeze—Causes and Therapy

| Case | Age | Sex | Duration | Atopy | Cause | Treatment | Ref. |
|------|-----|-----|----------|-------|-------|-----------|------|
| 1 | 11 | F | 10 mo | Neg | Psychogenic | Psychotherapy | 96 |
| 2 | 13 | F | 7 d | Neg | Psychogenic | Psychotherapy | 97 |
| 3 | 11 | F | 22 d | Pos | Psychogenic | Psychotherapy | 98 |
| 4 | 13 | F | 3 mo | Pos | Psychogenic | Psychotherapy | 99 |
| 5 | 9 | F | ? | Neg | Psychogenic | Psychotherapy | 100 |
| 6 | 11 | F | ? | ? | ? | ? | 101 |
| 7 | 10 | F | >7 d | Pos | ? Allergic | Immunotherapy | 101 |
| 8 | 11 | F | 2 mo | Neg | Psychogenic | Psychotherapy | 56 |
| 9 | 39 | M | 20 yrs | Neg | Seizures | Anticonvulants | 56 |
| 10 | 11 | F | 22 d | Pos | Multifactorial | Multiple | 98 |
| 11 | 15 | M | ? | ? | Psychogenic | Psychotherapy | 102 |
| 12 | 13 | F | 5 d | Pos | Psychogenic | Hypnotherapy | 103 |
| 13 | 21 | F | ? | Neg | Tuberculosis | Meds/surgery | 104 |
| 14 | 11 | F | 6 d | ? | Psychogenic | Self-resolution | 105 |
| 15 | 12 | F | 2 d | Neg | Psychogenic | Psychotherapy | 105 |
| 16 | 9 | M | 10 hr | Pos | Psychogenic | Psychotherapy | 105 |
| 17 | 10 | M | 4 d | Neg | Psychogenic | Psychotherapy | 105 |
| 18 | 13 | F | ? | Neg | Psychogenic | Self-resolution | 106 |
| 19 | 13 | M | 10 mo | Pos | Psychogenic | Psychotherapy | 77 |
| 20 | 15 | F | 1 mo | Pos | Psychogenic | Psychotherapy | 77 |
| 21 | 12 | M | 10 d | Pos | Psychogenic | Behavioral Therapy | 77 |
| 22 | 11 | F | 10 mo | Neg | Psychogenic | Psychotherapy | 96 |
| 23 | 8 | F | months | Neg | Immune hypersensitivity | Avoidance | 107 |
| 24 | 14 | M | 33 d | Pos | Psychogenic | Psychotherapy/hypnosis | 57 |
| 25 | 40 | F | ? | Neg | Psychogenic | Suggestive Therapy | 58 |
| 26 | 13 | F | ? | ? | Psychogenic | Isolation | 51 |
| 27 | 17 | F | ? | ? | Psychogenic | Psychotherapy | 96 |
| 28 | 69 | M | ? | ? | ? Orgasm related | ? | 59 |
| 29 | 14 | F | ? | ? | Psychogenic | Psychotherapy | 108 |
| 30 | 14 | F | ? | ? | Psychogenic | Psychotherapy | 108 |
| 31 | 16 | F | ? | Neg | Psychogenic | Psychotherapy | 109 |
| 32 | 6 | M | ? | Neg | Psychogenic | Suggestive Therapy | 109 |
| 33 | 60 | F | 139 d | Neg | Psychogenic | Haloperidol | 110 |
| 34 | 10 | F | 4 d | ? | Psychogenic | Diazepam | 111 |

d = days; F = females; hr = hours; M = males; mo = months; neg = negative; pos = positive; Ref. = reference; yrs = years.

Evaluation clearly requires a careful history and physical examination, as well as selected laboratory tests aimed at identifying one or more of the known causes of sneeze.

Psychogenic sneeze (Table IV) is more common in adolescents and more common in females than males. The sneeze has atypical features, such as a lack of sneeze during sleep and its unnatural, artificial, and atypical rate; sneezing has been reported to occur as frequently as 6 to 60 times per minute and lasts from days to months.[77,98,113] One reported patient had 700 "violent" sneezes in one 30-minute period,[56] another, 2000 sneezes in a single day.[99] There often is a lack of associated facial and other expressions, such as lack of eye closure during the sneeze.[77,106] Sneeze is often "aborted," and is termed a pseudosneeze. There is often little or no inspiratory phase, and little or no aerosolization of the nasal mucous secretions.[105] Commonly, there is a lack of specific physical findings, and it is refractory to a wide variety of medical treatments. Significant psychopathology can often be identified.

## Complications of Sneeze

Sneeze is most often a rarely considered symptom and is felt to be inconsequential at least and annoying at most. However, during a sneeze, as in cough, very high intrathoracic pressures are generated. This is felt to be the cause of significant, albeit rare, consequences of a sneeze (Table VII[5,44,52,113–127]). Less dramatic than those noted in the table, but probably of more clinical significance, is the spread of infection that potentially results from this reflex act.

Droplets, with a diameter of 0.1 to 2 mm moving at a velocity of 45 m/sec, are released during a sneeze and, on average, travel 1.5 to 5.5 ft.[44] Most of these come from the mouth, though certainly larger droplets are released from an unprotected nose. These larger drops contain greater numbers of pathogenic organisms, but because of their size quickly settle out of the air. They can impinge on clothing and hard surfaces and can be infective.[52] Of greater importance in the airborne spread of infection, most clearly evidenced by the spread of tuberculosis, are small respiratory droplets (1 to 3 $\mu$m) termed droplet nuclei. Though naturally infected patients do shed virus from the nose in high titers during sneeze, many viruses lose their infectivity by drying in air.[128–130] This, in combination with the larger droplets expelled from the nose, make the sneeze a less likely mode of transmission of infection than is commonly thought.

## Diagnostic Evaluation of Sneeze

It is unusual for patients to present solely for evaluation of sneeze. More commonly, it is just one complaint among a collection of symptoms. However, there will be patients who find the sneeze more than a mere annoyance. There is no published systematic, anatomic, diagnostic protocol for the evaluation and treatment of sneeze as there is for cough.[131,132] Nevertheless, in evaluating these patients, the physician's knowledge of the differential diagnosis of sneeze gives him or her a framework on which to approach the patient. A careful history and physical examination will often suggest the cause of the sneeze. Clearly, a careful examination of the nose must be performed.

Figure 2 offers an algorithm that can be followed in the diagnostic evaluation of sneeze. This algorithm was constructed with the medical adage, "common diseases do occur commonly" in mind. In this light, the irritative causes of sneeze are clearly the most common. Among these, and the first condition to be considered, is allergic rhinitis. The prevalence in this country of allergy to airborne antigens is about 20%.[133] History may suggest a seasonal preference or a specific trigger such as cat exposure. The allergic patient will often not only complain of sneeze but of rhinorrhea, nasal congestion, and ocular irritation as well. Nasal examination may reveal the classic pale, bluish mucous membranes, though this finding is neither very sensitive, nor specific. The turbinates

## Table VII
### Complications of Sneeze

Acquired Chiari Malformation[113]
Acute Blindness[5]
Acute Glaucoma[114]
Cervico-mediastinal Hemorrhage[115,116]
Conductive Hearing Loss[117,118]
Cerebrospinal Fluid Rhinorrhea[119]
Epistaxis[44]
Fractures*[44,120]
Hemiparesis[5,121,122]
Infection[44,52]
Myocardial Infarction[123]
Retinal Detachment[120]
Spontaneous Abortion[120]
Syncope[124,125]
Vaginal Vault Laceration[126]
Vertebral Artery Dissection[127]
Vertigo[117]

* Nasal, rib, shoulder, thyroid cartilage, sinus, middle ear.

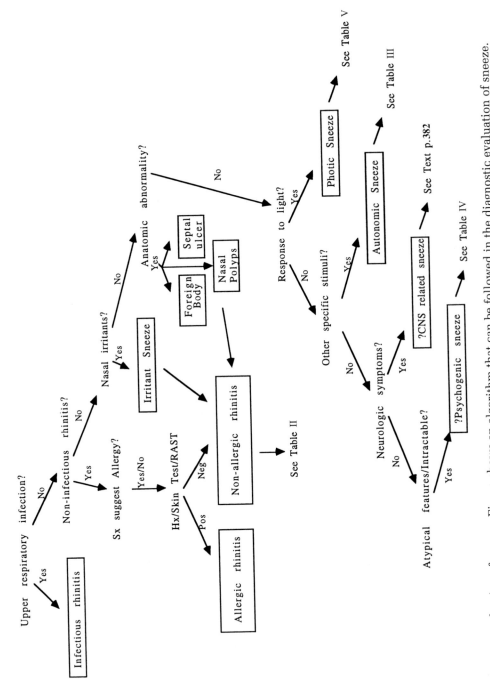

**Figure 2.** Evaluation of sneeze. Figure shows an algorithm that can be followed in the diagnostic evaluation of sneeze. CNS = central nervous system; Hx = history; RAST = radioallergosorbent test; Sx = symptoms.

are often hypertrophied, and other stigmata of atopic disease may be present (eg, allergic shiners and conjunctival inflammation, asthma, and atopic dermatitis).

Laboratory testing is nonspecific and usually not helpful. The use of nasal smears for cytologic evaluation has declined. Its clinical utility may be to differentiate infectious (neutrophilic) from allergic (eosinophilic) rhinitis. Eosinophilia suggests allergy but is nondiagnostic as it is seen in nonallergic rhinitis with eosinophilia (NARES).[134] Prick skin testing to common aeroallergens can be very useful when considering a diagnosis of allergic rhinitis. A radioallergosorbent test (RAST) for immunoglobulin E (IgE), though not as sensitive, can be performed in those with contraindications to skin testing or significant dermatographism.

Should skin testing or RAST be unrevealing, the differential of nonallergic rhinitis should then be considered (Table II). If these conditions are found not to be present, evaluation of the remaining conditions under the "Irritative" heading must then follow. Consideration should be given to performing fiberoptic rhinoscopy. Search should be made for nasal mucosal hypertrophy, nasal polyps, septal abnormalities such as deviation or ulceration, and nasal foreign bodies. In young children, nasal foreign bodies clearly must be excluded.

Other causes of sneeze (Autonomic, Psychologic, and CNS Disease) are much less common (Tables III & IV). Pointed historical evaluation can usually sort through this differential.

## Treatment

Sneeze most often presents as part of a symptom complex, most likely related to infection (eg, common cold) or inhalant allergies. Nonetheless, one must consider the differential diagnosis as described above in an attempt to determine the cause of the sneeze and offer specific treatment. In approaching the therapy of sneeze, it is again useful to consider the four major categories of sneeze as described previously—Irritative, Autonomic, Psychologic and CNS disease. This provides a framework on which to base appropriate therapy.

## Treatment for Sneeze by Irritative Causes

The irritative causes of sneeze are clearly the most common. Sneezing associated with upper respiratory tract infections (infectious rhinitis) is common and is most often self-limited. Though the symptoms of the common cold do not appear to be mediated by histamine, sneeze (and other symptoms) may be ameliorated with the use of antihistamine-decongestant preparations, an effect most likely due to nonhistaminergic properties of the drug.[135,136] Centrally active antitussives of the codeine-type strongly suppress expiratory efforts, not only in cough but also in sneeze,[46] though clinical efficacy in humans has never been demonstrated for sneeze.

After infectious rhinitis, the most common irritative causes of sneeze fall under the aegis of allergic and nonallergic rhinitis. Therapeutic agents aimed at the sneeze associated with allergic rhinitis, and for the most part with nonallergic rhinitis as well, are limited but effective. However, before a discussion of medical therapy, it must be stressed that nonmedical environmental control measures, so-called avoidance therapy, can play a great role in the treatment of sneeze related to allergic rhinitis. Such measures are reviewed elsewhere.[137,138]

If history, skin tests, or RAST IgE do not suggest atopy, one should consider the various entities of nonallergic rhinitis (Table II). Consideration must be given to medications a patient may be taking, particularly antihypertensive drugs (eg, reserpine, clonidine hydrochloride, labetalol hydrochloride) commonly associated with rhinitis,[134] over-the-counter nasal decongestants, as well as occult aspirin ingestion or illicit drug use. Systemic illness involving the nose also must be excluded. A careful nasal examination to look for anatomic abnormalities is important, and if suggestive, an ear, nose, and throat evaluation is recommended. This may be particularly important in the case of young children in whom nasal foreign bodies are common. Identifying such factors will allow for more specific treatment of the sneeze.

The pharmacologic options available to treat sneeze associated with both allergic and nonallergic, noninfectious rhinitis are efficacious. As discussed previously, histamine plays a prominent role in the symptom complex of allergic rhinitis. It, therefore, is not surprising that antihistamines, specifically $H_1$ antagonists, are effective therapy for sneeze associated with this condition. There are six classes of $H_1$ histamine antagonists (Table VIII), and

physicians should become familiar with agents from each class. The first generation antihistamines have other receptor effects, and this may result in unwanted side effects from the medication. These include dry mucous membranes, and cognitive or performance impairment and sedation. Perhaps the most bothersome effects result from the inhibition of cholinergic receptors. The alkylamines may be the least sedating of the traditional antihistamines.[139,140] Adaptation to the sedative effects usually occurs. This bothersome, and often limiting side effect can be minimized by initiating therapy with a small bedtime dose, increasing it slowly until a salutary effect is reached. It is worthy to note that cholinergic stimulation of the nasal mucosa does result in nasal hyperse-

**Table VIII**
Major Groups of Antihistamines

| Drug Name | Trade Name |
| --- | --- |
| Ethanolamine Derivatives | |
| Diphenhydramine hydrochloride | Benadryl |
| Carbinoxamine | Rondec |
| Clemastine | Tavist |
| Ethylenediamine Derivatives | |
| Pyrilamine | Triaminic |
| Tripelennamine hydrochloride | PBZ |
| Piperazine | |
| Hydroxyzine hydrochloride | Atarax |
| Hydroxyzine pamoate | Vistaril |
| Piperidine | |
| Cyproheptadine | Periactin |
| Azatadine | Trinalin |
| Diphenylpyraline | Nolahist |
| Phenindamine | |
| Phenothiazine Derivatives | |
| Promethazine hydrocloride | Phenergan |
| Trieprazine tartrate | |
| Alkylamine Derivatives | |
| Chlorpheniramine maleate | Chlor-Trimeton Allergy |
| Brompheniramine maleate | Bromfed |
| Triprolidine | Actifed |
| Dexchlorpheniramine maleate | |
| Nonsedating Long-acting | |
| Astemizole | Hismanal |
| Loratidine | Claritin |
| Fexofenadine | Allegra |
| Cetirazine | Zyrtec |

**Table IX**
Inhaled Nasal Steroid Preparations

| Drug | Trade Name | Recommended Dose |
|---|---|---|
| Beclomethasone dipropionate | Beconase | 1 to 2 sprays b.i.d. |
| | Vancenase | same |
| Beclomethasone dipropionate, monohydrate | Beconase AQ | same |
| | Vancenase AQ | same |
| Triamcinalone acetonide | Nasacort | 2 sprays q.i.d. |
| Flunisolide | Nasalide | 2 sprays b.i.d. |
| Budesonide | Rhinocort | 4 sprays q.i.d |
| Dexamethasone sodium phosphate | Decadron Tubinaire | 2 sprays b.i.d. |
| Fluticasone propionate | Flonase | 2 sprays q.i.d. |

AQ = aqueous; b.i.d. = twice daily; q.i.d. = four times daily.

cretion[18,54]; potentially the anticholinergic effect of the drug may be useful in combating nasal congestion and secretions, and the sneeze that might result from this.

Newer second generation antihistamines appear to have pure antihistamine effects and therefore are less sedating, though they may be less efficacious as well.[33,140] Agents available in the United States at this time include fexofenadine (Allegra), astemizole (Hismanal®), and loratidine (Claritin®). Others in this class include azelastine and cetirizine. Prior to prescribing, one must consider adverse drug interactions when a patient is also taking a macrolide antibiotic or ketoconazole since a prolongation of the QT interval may occur. The dosage should never exceed that which is recommended.

Inhaled (topical) nasal steroids have proven very effective in the treatment of symptoms such as sneeze associated with both allergic and nonallergic rhinitis.[134,141,142] Steroids have a variety of pharmacologic actions which include decreasing inflammation, decreasing intercellular edema, and suppressing neutrophil chemotaxis the mast cell-mediated late-phase reaction. Use of nasal steroids results in significant inhibition of mediator-release from the nose on provocative challenge with antigen, diminishing both the early- and late-phase responses.[143] However, the exact mechanism(s) of their effectiveness remains uncertain. Inhaled steroid preparations have the benefits of systemic corticosteroids, but lack the systemic toxicity of the oral preparations, when used in appropriate dosage (Table IX). The primary side effects of such preparations include nasal irritation and headache, as well as a variety of other nonspecific nasopharyngeal complaints, including sneeze. Intranasal steroids other than dexamethasone, when used in appropriate doses, can be administered over a prolonged period of time without the fear of systemic absorption and adrenal suppression.[134] Patients must be told to expect a latency period of about 4 days before symptom improvement is noted, with a maximal effect seen only after 2 weeks of therapy.[106] See Table IX for a compilation of commercially available nasal steroid preparations in the United States and their recommended doses.

Oral or intramuscular (systemic) steroids, for example, 20 to 40 mg of prednisone, or its equivalent, given daily over 5 to 7 days, have clear efficacy in the treatment of allergic rhinitis. However, their use in the control of inhaled allergic symptoms, particularly sneeze, is very limited, and should not be routinely considered.

Cromolyn sodium, a mast cell stabilizing agent, can prevent the release of histamine (among other mediators) thereby inhibiting both the immediate- and late-phase mast cell– mediated reactions following nasal allergen challenge. It, therefore, is useful as a prophylactic agent. It tends to be effective against the nasal symptoms associated with allergic rhinitis, particularly so in those with high titers of IgE[144]; however, it is not suggested for the treatment of sneeze associated with nonallergic rhinitis. Surprisingly, nasal cromolyn (Nasalcrom®) has been associated with up to a 10% incidence of sneezing from use of the product! This adverse occurrence is likely due to cromolyn acting as an irritant. Its efficacy is similar to that of the inhaled nasal steroids, though often the product has to be used more frequently (4 to 6 times per day), making it less convenient than topical nasal steroids. Nedocromil sodium, an anti-inflammatory pyranoquinoline chemically distinct from cromolyn, but similar in its inhibition of inflammatory mediator-release, available in the United States only for use in asthma, is available outside the United States as a nasal preparation.

Lastly, in the control of the symptoms associated with inhaled aeroallergens, immunotherapy, or desensitization, has been quite effective.[145,146] Data support its use in the control of rhinitis due to grass and tree pollens, ragweed, and cat allergens.[147–149] There also are data suggesting its efficacy in the control of symptoms in dust mite–sensitive and mold-sensitive individuals.[149–151] It must be emphasized that immunotherapy is not a cure. However, approximately 60% to 90% of properly selected patients will experience a significant beneficial effect.[147] Such benefits will persist once immunotherapy is discontinued in 60% to 80% of treated patients.[145]

## Treatment for Sneeze by Autonomic Causes

While autonomic-associated sneezes are not common, history often points to this diagnosis. Specific therapy, such as the avoidance of noxious odors, should be instituted. There is no proven effective therapy for the photic sneeze. Dark, polarized lenses may be helpful though have never been evaluated. Prophylactic topical nasal decongestants have been recommended for the sneeze associated with sexual intercourse.[59] Consideration should be given to the diagnosis of hyper- and/or hypothyroid disease (as with nonallergic rhinitis), and if present, appropriately treated.

## Treatment for Sneeze by Psychogenic Causes

Should the complaint be that of protracted, frequent sneeze, and should the clinical description and demographic profile fit the diagnosis of psychogenic sneeze, that entity, though rare, should be considered, and early psychiatric intervention sought before extensive, expensive, and possibly morbid therapy is applied. Individual psychotherapy and family therapy, as well as hypnosis and suggestive therapy have all been successfully employed to treat sneeze of psychogenic origin.[96,98,103,105]

In cases of intractable sneeze of both psychiatric or other origin, a variety of nonspecific agents have been used with greater or lesser success. Such agents have included topical sympathomimetics, cocaine and other local anesthetics, subcutaneous epinephrine, benzodiazepines, neuroleptics, and tricyclic antidepressants.[96,97,99,101,112]

## Treatment for Sneeze by CNS Causes

Lastly, the sneeze associated with CNS disease is extremely rare. Therapy is directed at the underlying disorder, most likely seizures. Therapy with anticonvulsants in such cases has been successful.[56]

## Summary

In summary, sneeze is the most common nasal reflex, though its mechanism has not been studied in as much detail as other respiratory reflexes, such as the apnea reflex or cough. Clinically, sneeze is a common complaint of patients seeking medical care, though it is almost always a part of a complex of upper airway symptoms. The cause of sneeze is broad, but can be narrowed effectively by a careful history and physical examination. The medical therapy available to treat sneeze is most often very effective.

## References

1. Widdicombe JG. Reflexes from the upper respiratory tract. In: *Handbook of Physiology, Section 3: The Respiratory System, II.* Bethesda, Md: American Physiological Society; 1986: 363–394.

2. Widdicombe JG. Respiratory reflexes and defenses. In: Mathew OP, Sant' Ambrogio G, eds. *Lung Biology in Health and Disease, Vol. 35. Nasal and pharyngeal reflexes. Protective and respiratory functions.* New York, NY: Marcel Dekker Inc; 1988: 233–258.

3. Askenasy JJM. The history of sneezing. Postgrad Med J 1990;66:549–550.

4. Rosner F. The sneeze (letter). JAMA 1983; 250:3281.

5. Kavka SJ. The sneeze—blissful or baneful. JAMA 1983; 249:2304–2305.

6. Cauna N. Blood and nerve supply of the nasal lining. In: Proctor DF, Andersen IB, eds. *The Nose, Upper Airway Physiology And The Atmospheric Environment.* New York, NY: Elsevier Biomedical Press; 1982: 45–69.

7. Burrow A, Eccles R, Jones AS. The effects of camphor, eucalyptus and menthol vapour on nasal resistance to airflow and nasal sensation of airflow. Acta Otolaryngol 1983;96:157–161.

8. Widdicombe JG. Respiratory reflexes and defenses. In: Braun JD, Proctor DF, Reid LM, eds. *Lung Biology in Health and Disease, Vol . 5: Respiratory Defense Mechanisms.* New York, NY: Marcel Dekker Inc; 1977: 593–630.

9. Holzer P, Bucsics A, Lembeck F. Distribution of capsaicin sensitive nerve fibers containing immunoreactive substance P in cutaneous and visceral tissue of the rat. Neurosci Lett 1982;31:253–257.

10. Lundblad L, Änggård A, Lundberg JM. Capsaicin-sensitive substance-P nerves: Antidromic vasodilation and increased vascular permeability in the nasal mucosa. Br J Pharmacol 1982;77:378P.

11. Lundblad L, Lundberg JM, Brodin E, et al. Origin and distribution of capsaicin-sensitive substance P–immunoreactive nerves in the nasal mucosa. Acta Otolaryngol 1983;96:485–493.

12. Uddman R, Malm M, Sundler F. Substance-P-containing nerve fibers in the nasal mucosa. Arch Otolaryngol 1983; 238:9–16.

13. Buck SH, Burks TF. The neuropharmacology of capsaicin: Review of some recent observations. Pharmacol Rev 1986; 8: 179–226.

14. Jessel TM, Iversen TL, Cuello AC. Capsaicin-induced depletion of substance P from primary sensory neurons. Brain Res 1978;152:183–188.

15. Geppetti P, Fusco BM, Marabini S, et al. Secretion, pain and sneezing induced by the application of capsaicin to the nasal mucosa in man. Br J Pharmacol 1988;93: 509–514.

16. Janscó N, Janscó-Gábor A, Takáts J. Pain and inflammation induced by nicotine, acetylcholine and structurally related compounds and their prevention by desensitizing agents. Acta Physiol Acad Sci Hung 1961;19:113–132.

17. Lundblad L, Saria A, Lundberg JM, et al. Increased vascular permeability in rat nasal mucosa induced by substance P and stimulation of capsaicin-sensitive trigeminal neurons. Acta Otolaryngol 1983;96: 479–484.

18. Baraniuk JN, Kaliner M. Neuropeptides and nasal secretion. Am J Physiol 1991; 261:L223-L235.

19. Kokumai S, Imamura T, Masuyama K, et al. Effect of capsaicin as a neuropeptide-releasing substance on sneezing reflex in a type I allergic animal model. Int Arch Allergy Appl Immunol 1992;98:256–261.

20. Lundblad L, Lundberg JM, Änggård A. Local and systemic capsaicin pretreatment inhibits sneezing and the increase in nasal vascular permeability induced by certain chemical irritants. Naun Schmeid Arch Pharmacol 1984;326:254–261.

21. Lundblad L. Protective reflexes and vascular effects in the nasal mucosa elicited by activation of capsaicin-sensitive P-immunoreactive trigeminal neurons. Acta Physiol Scan 1984;529 (suppl):1–49.

22. Naclerio RM, Meier HL, Adkinson NF, et al. *In vivo* demonstration of inflammatory mediator release following nasal challenge with antigen. Eur J Respir Dis 1983; 64 (Suppl 128):26–32.

23. Shelton D, Eiser N. Histamine receptors in the human nose. Clin Otolaryngol 1994;19:45–49.

24. Wagenmann M, Baroody FM, Kagey-Spbotka A, et al. The effect of terfenadine on unilateral nasal challenge with allergen. J Allergy Clin Immunol 1994;93:594–605.

25. Tani E, Senba E, Kokumai S, et al. Histamine application to the nasal mucosa induces release of calcitonin gene-related peptide and substance P from peripheral terminals of trigeminal ganglion: A morphological study in the guinea pig. Neurosci Lett 1990;112:1–6.

26. Saria A, Martling C-R, Yan Z, et al. Release of multiple tachykinins from capsaicin-sensitive sensory nerves in the lung by bradykinin, histamine, dimethylphenyl piperazinium, and vagal nerve stimulation. Am Rev Respir Dis 1988;137:1330–1335.

27. Imamura T, Kambara T. Substance P as a potent stimulator of sneeze responses in experimental allergic rhinitis of guinea pigs. Agents Action 1992;37:245–249.

28. Kokumai S, Imamura T, Masuyama K, et al. Effects of capcaisin as a neuropeptide-releasing substance on sneezing reflex in type I allergic animal model. Int Arch Allergy Immunol 1992;98:256–261.

29. Lacoix JL, Burelot JM, Polla BS, et al. Improvement of symptoms of nonallergic chronic rhinitis by local treatment with capsaicin. Clin Exp Allergy 1991;21:595–600.

30. Tønnesen P. Mygind N. Nasal challenge with serotonin and histamine in normal persons. Allergy 1985;40:350–353.

31. Tønnesen P. Effect of topically applied atropine, methysergide and chlorpheniramine on nasal challenge with serotonin. Allergy 1985;40:616–619.

32. McTavish D, Goa KL, Ferrill M. Terfenadine. An updated review of its pharmacological properties and therapeutic efficacy. Drugs 1990;39:552–574.

33. Simons FE, Simons KJ. Second-generation H1-receptor antagonists. Ann Allergy 1991;66:5–19.

34. Batsel HL, Lines AJ. Neural mechanisms of sneeze. Am J Physiol 1975;229:770–776.

35. Wallois F, Gros F, Condamin M, et al. Postnatal development of the anterior ethmoidal nerve in cats: unmyelinated and myelinated nerve fiber analysis. Neurosci Lett 1993;160:221–224.

36. Everett HC. Sneezing in response to light. Neurology 1964;14:483–490.

37. Angel James JE, Daly MD. Nasal reflexes. Proc Roy Soc Med 1969;62:1287–1293.

38. Batsel HL, Lines AJ. Discharge of respiratory neurons in sneeze resulting from ethmoidal nerve stimulation. Exp Neurol 1978;58:410–424.

39. Batsel HL. Trigeminal and reticular neurons concerned with sneezing. Physiologist 1969;12:171.

40. Nonaka S, Unno T, Ohta Y, et al. Sneeze-evoking region within the brainstem. Brain Res 1990;511:265–270.

41. Martin RA, Handel SF, Aldama AE. Inability to sneeze as a manifestation of medullary neoplasm. Neurology 1991;41:1675–1676.

42. Malcomson KG. The vasomotor activities of the nasal mucous membrane. J Otolaryngol 1959;73:73–98.

43. Brubaker AP. The physiology of sneezing. JAMA 1919;73:585–587.

44. Stromberg BV. Sneezing: Its physiology and management. Eye Ear Nose Throat Monthly 1975;54:449–453.

45. Sieck GC, Fournier M. Diaphragm motor unit recruitment during ventilatory and nonventilatory behaviors. J Appl Physiol 1989;66:2539–2545.

46. Jakus J, Tomori Z, Stransky A. Activity of the bulbar respiratory neurones during cough and other respiratory tract reflexes in cats. Physiol Bohemoslovaca 1985;34:127–136.

47. Price WM, Batsel HL. Respiratory neurons participating in sneeze and in response to resistance to expiration. Exp Neurol 1970;29:554–570.

48. Rudomin P. The electrical activity of the cricothyroid muscles of the cat. Arch Intern Physiol Biochem 1966; 74:135–153.

49. Van Lunteren E, Haxhiu MA, Cherniak NS, et al. Role of triangularis sterni during coughing and sneezing in dogs. J Appl Physiol 1988;65:2440–2445.

50. Van Lunteren E, Haxhiu MA, Cherniak NS, Arnold JS. Rib cage and abdominal expiratory muscle responses to $CO_2$ and esophageal distention. J Appl Physiol 1988;64:846–853.

51. Birch CA. Sneezing. Practitioner 1959;12:122–124.

52. Anonymous. Editorial: Spread of colds. Br Med J 1973;4(885):123–4.

53. Widdicombe JG, Sterling GM. The autonomic nervous system and breathing. Arch Intern Med 1970;126:311–329.

54. Eccles R. Neurological and pharmacological considerations In: Proctor DF, Andersen IB, eds, *The Nose, Upper Airway Physiology And The Atmospheric Environment.* New York, NY: Elsevier Biomedical Press; 1982: 191–214.

55. Van Lier LAJ. The influence of non-specific factors on the nasal mucous membranes in patients with rhinitis vasomotoria. Acta Allerg 1959;13:507–509.

56. Kofman O. Paroxysmal sneezing. Can Med Assoc J 1964;91:154–157.

57. Murray N, Bierer J. Prolonged sneezing. A case report. Psychosom Med 1951;13: 56–58.

58. Shilkret HH. Psychogenic sneezing and yawning. Psychosom Med 1949;11: 127–128.

59. Questions and Answers. Paroxysmal sneezing following orgasm. JAMA 1972; 219:1350–1351.

60. Hobbs AG. Some amusing instances of nasal reflex. JAMA 1897;28:789–790.

61. Forrai G, Antal J, Balogh A. Sneezy twins. Acta Paed Hung 1985;26:323–326.

62. Teebi AS, Al-Saleh QA. Autosomal dominant sneezing disorder provoked by fullness of the stomach. J Med Genet 1989; 26:539–540.

63. Norman PS, Naclerio RM, Creticos PS, et al. Mediator release after allergic and physical nasal challenges. Int Arch Allergy Appl Immunol 1985;77;57–63.

64. Naclerio RM, Meier HL, Kagey-Sobotka A, et al. Mediator release after nasal airway challenge with allergen. Am J Respir Dis 1983;128:597–602.

65. Hollingsworth HM, Giansiracusa, Upchurch KS. Anaphylaxis. J Intensive Care Med 1991;6:55–70.

66. Halperin LS. Sneezing as an early indicator of allergy to fluorescin dye. Am J Ophthalmol 1991;112:601–602.

67. Segars LW, Threlkeld KR. Clindamycin-induced lip and nasal passage swelling. Ann Pharmacother 1993;27:885–886.

68. Schenk FX, Bellinger, MF. The "innocent" cough or sneeze: a harbinger of serious latex allergy in children during bladder stimulation and urodynamic testing. J Urol 1993;150:687–690.

69. Shukla GD. 'Asneezia"-A hitherto unrecognised psychiatric symptom. Br J Psychiatry 1985;147:564–565.

70. Foster AH, Nichol WW. Parathyroid adenoma: A case report with unusual clinical features. Ann Surg 1957;145:279–281.

71. Watson WC. *Diseases of the Nose and its Accesory Cavities.* London, England: Lewis; 1875: 343–344.

72. Whitman BW, Packer RJ. The photic sneeze reflex: Literature review and discussion. Neurology 1993; 3:868–871.

73. Hubert L. A study of the mechanism and treatment of rhinorrhea and sneezing—a local manifestation of some metabolic disorder, with an analysis of thirty four cases. Ann Otol Rhinolaryngol 1924; 33: 824–841.

74. Shukla GD. 'Asneezia'—some further observations. Br J Psychiatry 1989;154: 689–690.

75. Akhtar S, Verma SH. Asneezia (let). Br J Psychiatry 1990;156:285.

76. Kavka SJ. The sneeze (letter in reply). JAMA 1983;250:3281.

77. Kaplan MJ, Lanoff G. Intractable paroxysmal sneezing. A clinical entity defined with case reports. Ann Allergy 1970;28: 24–27.

78. Shapiro SL. Paroxysmal sneezing. Ears Nose Throat Monthly 1967;46:1532–1538.

79. Sédan J. Photosternutory reflex. Rev Otoneurophthalmol 1954;26:123–126.

80. Forrester JM. Sneezing on exposure to bright light as an inherited response. Hum Hered 1985;35:113–114.

81. Beckman L, Nordenson I. Individual differences with respect to the sneezing reflex: An inherited physiological trait in man? Hum Hered 1983;33:390–391.

82. Peroutka SJ, Peroutka LA. Autosomal dominant transmission of the "photic sneeze reflex." N Engl J Med 1984;310: 599–600.

83. Lang DM. Solar sneeze reflex (letter). JAMA 1987;257:1330–1331.

84. Buckley B. Photic sneezing. Arch Dis Child 1991;66:908.

85. Collie WR, Pagon RA, Hall JG, et al. ACHOO syndrome (autosomal dominant compelling helio-ophthalmic outburst syndrome). Birth Defects 1978;14:(6B) 361–363.

86. Morris HH. ACHOO syndrome. Prevalence and inheritance. Cleveland Clin J Med 1987;54:431–433.

87. Eckhardt LB, McLean JM, Goodell H. The genesis of pain from the eye. Assoc Res Nerv Mental Dis Proc 1943;23:209–207.

88. Katz B, Melles RB, Swenson MR, et al. Photic sneeze reflex in nephropathic cystinosis. Br J Ophthalmol 1990;74: 706–708.

89. Smith R. Photic sneezes. Br J Ophthalmol 1990;74:705.

90. Lewkonia I. An infrequent response to slit-lamp examination. Br J Ophthalmol 1969;53:493–495.

91. Breitenbach RA, Swisher PK, Kim MK, et al. The photic sneeze reflex as a risk factor to combat pilots. Military Med 1993;158: 806–809.

92. Morris HH. ACHOO syndrome: laboratory findings. Cleveland Clin J Med 1989; 56:743–744.

93. Pies R. Seasonal affective disorder and the photic sneeze response (let). Am J Psychiatry 1990;147:1094.

94. Dilsaver SC. Cholinergic mechanisms in depression. Brain Res Rev 1986; 11: 285–316.

95. Dilsaver SC, Marjchrzak MJ. Bright artificial light subsensitizes a central muscarinic mechanism. Life Sci 1987;41: 2607–2614.

96. Keating MU, O'Connell EJ, Sachs MI. Intractable paroxysmal sneezing in an adolescent. Ann Allergy 1989;62:429–431.

97. Shenker IR, Nussbaum M, Abramson AL, et al. Intractable paroxysmal sneezing: A conversion reaction of adolescence. Int J Ped Otorhinolaryngol 1979;1:171–175.

98. Co S. Intractable sneezing. Case report and literature review. Arch Neurol 1979; 36:111–112.

99. Weiner D, McGrath K, Patterson R. Factitious sneezing. J Allergy Clin Immunol 1985;75:741–742.

100. Vogel DH. Otolaryngologic presentation of tic-like disorders. Laryngoscope 1979; 89:1474–1477.

101. Shapiro RS. Paroxysmal sneezing in children: Two new cases. J Otolaryngol 1992; 21:437–438.

102. Zolov B. Intractable paroxysmal sneezing (abstract). Ann Allergy 1972;30:230.

103. Elkins M, Milstein JJ. Hypnotherapy of pseudo-sneezing: A case report. Am J Clin Hypnosis 1962;4:273–275.

104. Kammermeier R. Cited by Shapiro SL. Paroxysmal sneezing. Ears Nose Throat Monthly. 1967;46:1532–1538.

105. Bergman GE, Hiner LB. Psychogenic intractable sneezing in children. J Pediatr 1984;105:496–498.

106. Aggarwal J, Portnoy J. Intractable sneezing with a specific psychogenic origin. Ann Allergy 1986;56:345–346.

107. Herman JJ. Intractable sneezing due to IgE-mediated triethanolamine sensitivity. J Allergy Clin Immunol 1983;71:339–344.

108. Zolov B. Cited in Shenker IR, Nussbaum M, Abramson AL, Ebin E. Intractable paroxysmal sneezing: A conversion reaction of adolescence. Int J Ped Otorhinolaryngol 1979;1:171–175.

109. Galia LJ, Roscoe G. Intractable sneezing. Trans Pa Acad Ophthalmol Otolaryngol 1981; 34:164–168.

110. Davison K. Pharmacologic treatment for intractable sneezing. Br Med J 1982; 284: 1163–1164.

111. Gervis JH. Pharmacologic treatment for intractable sneezing (letter). Br Med J 1982;284:1560.

112. Sturm JT. Status sternuens (continual sneezing). N Engl J Med 1986;315:1488.

113. Sullivan LP, Stears JC, Ringel SP. Resolution of syringomyelia and Chiari I malformation by ventriculoatrial shunting in a patient with pseudotumor cerebri and a lumboperitoneal shunt. Neurosurgery 1988;22:744–747.

114. Sharir M, Huntington AC, Nardin GF, et al. Sneezing as a cause of acute-angle closure glaucoma. Ann Ophthalmol 1992; 24:214–215.

115. Macdonald RG, Kelly J. Cervico-mediastinal haematoma following sneezing. Anaesthesia 1975;30:50–53.

116. Sandor F, Cooke RT. Spontaneous cervico-mediastinal haematoma. Br J Surg 1964;51:682–686.

117. Schuknecht HF, Witt RL. Suppressed sneezing as a cause of hearing loss and vertigo. Am J Otolaryngol 1985;6: 468–470.

118. Azem K, Caldarelli DD. Sudden conductive hearing loss following sneeze. Arch Otolaryngol 1973;97:413–414.

119. Shugar JMA, Som PM, Eisman W, et al. Non-traumatic cerebrospinal fluid rhinorrhea. Laryngoscope 1981;91:114–120.

120. Kavka SJ. The sneeze. In reply (letter). JAMA 1983; 250:3281.

121. Bradley WG Jr, Bank WO, Fischbeck KH. Sneeze induced hemiparesis from unruptured intracranial aneurysm. J Neuroradiol 1982;9:323–327.

122. Fischbeck KH, Bradley WG, Bank WO. Sneeze-induced hemiparesis. Ann Neurol 1982;11:105–106.

123. Therrien ML, Moreno B, Korr KS, et al. Acute myocardial infarction associated with prolonged sneezing. Am J Cardiol 1987;59:364–365.

124. Bardella L, Maleci A, DiLorenzo N. Drop attack as the only symptom of type 1 Chi-

ari malformation Riv Pat Ner Ment 1984; 105:217–222.

125. Corbett JJ, Butler AB, Kaufman B. 'Sneeze syncope,' basilar invagination and Arnold-Chiare type I malformation. J Neurol Neurosurg Psychiatry 1976;39:381–384.

126. Morrison J. Vault laceration due to sneezing. J Obstet Gynaecol Br Commonw 1967;74:773.

127. Gutowski NJ, Murphey RP, Beale DJ. Unilateral upper cervical posterior spinal artery syndrome following sneezing. J Neurol Neurosurg Psychiatry 1992;55: 841–843.

128. Buckland PE, Tyrrell DAJ. Loss of infectivity on drying various viruses. Nature 1962;195:1063–1064.

129. Hendley JO, Wenzell RD, Gwaltrey JM. Transmission of rhinovirus colds by self innoculation. N Engl J Med 1973;288: 1361–1364.

130. Riley RL. Airborne infection. Am J Med 1974;57:466–475.

131. Irwin RS, Curley FJ, French CL. Chronic cough. The spectrum and frequency of causes, key components of the diagnostic evaluation, and outcome of specific therapy. Am Rev Respir Dis 1990;141: 640–647.

132. Irwin RS, Corrao WM, Pratter MR. Chronic persistent cough in the adult: the spectrum and frequency of causes and successful outcome of specific therapy. Am Rev Respir Dis 1981;123:413–417.

133. Settipane GA. Allergic rhinitis—update. Otolaryngol Head Neck Surg 1986; 94: 470–475.

134. Druce HM. Allergic and nonallergic rhinitis. In: Middleton E, Reed CE, Ellis EF, Adkinson NF Jr, Yunginger JW, Busse WW, eds. *Allergy. Principles and practice.* 4th ed. Boston:Mosby; 1993: 1433–1454.

135. Hendeles L. Efficacy and safety of antihistamines and expectorants in nonprescription cough and cold preparations. Pharmacotherapy 1993; 13:154–158

136. Smith MBH, Feldman W. Over-the-counter cold medications. A critical review of clinical trials between 1950 and 1991. JAMA 1993; 269:2258–2263.

137. Klein GL, Ziering RW. Environmental control of the home. Clin Rev Allergy 1988; 6:3–22.

138. Squillace SP. Environmental control. Otolaryngol Head Neck Surg 1992; 107: 831–834.

139. Marshall KG, Attia EL. *Disorders of the Nose and Paranasal Sinuses. Diagnosis and Management.* Littleton, Ma: PSG Publishing Company Inc; 1987: 174–181.

140. Drouin MA. $H_1$ antihistamines: Perspective on the use of the conventional and new agents. Ann Allergy 1985;55: 747–752.

141. Mygind N. Intranasal corticosteroid treatment of rhinitis. Eur J Respir Dis 1982; 63(suppl 122):192–196.

142. Okuda M, Sakguchi K, Ohtsuka H. Intranasal beclomethasone: Mode of action in nasal allergy. Ann Allergy 1983;50: 116–120.

143. Siegal SC, Katz RM, Rachelefsky GS, et al. Multicentric study of beclomethasone diproprionate nasal aerosol inadults with seasonal allergic rhinitis. J Allergy Clin Immunol 1982;69:345–353.

144. Welsh PW, Yunginger JW, Kern EB et al. Preseasonal IgE ragweed antibody level as a predictor of response to therapy of ragweed hay fever with intranasal cromolyn sodium solution. J Allergy Clin Immunol 1977;60:104–109.

145. Bush RK, Ritter MW. Allergen immunotherapy for the patient with allergic rhinitis. Immunol Allergy Clin North Am 1992;12:107–124.

146. Van Metre TE Jr, Adkinson NF. Immunotherapy for aeroallergen disease. In: Middleton E, Reed CE, Ellis EF, Adkinson NF Jr, Yunginger JW, Busse WW, eds. *Allergy. Principles and Practice.* 4th ed. Boston, Ma: Mosby; 1993: 1489–1510.

147. Satterson R. Clinical efficacy of allergy immunotherapy. J Allergy Clin Immunol 1979;64:155–158.

148. Wood RA, Eggleston PA. Management of allergy to animal danders. Immunol Allergy Clin North Am 1992;12:69–84.

149. Cleveland CH, Metzger J. Immunotherapy with pollens and fungi. Immunol Allergy Clin North Am 1992;12:39–52.

150. Scinto JD, Bernstein DI. Immunotherapy with dust mite allergens. Immunol Allergy Clin North Am 1992;12:53–67.

151. Platts-Mills TAE, Chapman MD. Dust mites: Immunology, allergic disease, and environmental control. J Allergy Clin Immunol 1987;80:755–775.

# 10

# Globus Sensation

Martyn Mendelsohn, M.B., B.S.
Arnold Noyek, M.D.

## Introduction

Globus pharyngeus is the commonly used term for the sensation of a lump in the throat in the absence of definable disease. Most patients present with a chief complaint of "a lump in the throat." In our view, the historic broadly used term "globus pharyngeus" might better presently be referred to as "globus sensation." Generally, we understand globus pharyngeus to represent a specific globus sensation due to muscle contraction, tension, anxiety, stress, or psychosomatic conversion.

Globus sensation is a common symptom, comprising between 3% to 20% of the chief complaints of new referrals in otolaryngologic practice.[1,2,3] Although it is often recognized after a few minutes of history taking, ultimately it is a diagnosis of exclusion. The diagnosis of an organic disease precludes the diagnosis of globus pharyngeus and determines the pathophysiologic basis of the globus sensation.

Globus hystericus was first described by Hippocrates over 2000 years ago.[4] Many terms have been used in association with this condition: globus hystericus,[4,5] globus sensation,[6,7] globus symptom,[1] and globus syndrome.[8] Unlike globus pharyngeus, the terms globus sensation or globus symptom indicate a feeling of a lump in the throat which may occur due to an organic disease.

The term globus hystericus was replaced by globus pharyngeus and now should be replaced by globus sensation. The sensation of a lump in the throat is usually perceived anywhere from the suprahyoid neck to the thoracic inlet, with the low neck being the common site (Figure 1). Globus sensation, accurately reflects the nature of the condition, the feeling of a lump in the throat, without suggesting a hysterical cause which remains unproven. Indeed, emphasis is placed upon managing what is perceived by the patient as a very real symptom. Most times, the hypopharynx and upper esophagus are the anatomic sites of pathologic abnormality, usually in conjunction with dysphagia. The investigation of globus sensation from an upper gastrointestinal perspective is detailed below. However, a neck mass, such as a thyroid nodule, can give rise to globus sensation and should be considered in the diagnostic algorithm.

From Irwin RS, Curley FJ, Grossman RF (eds): Diagnosis and Treatment of Symptoms of the Respiratory Tract. Armonk, New York, Futura Publishing Company, Inc., © 1997.

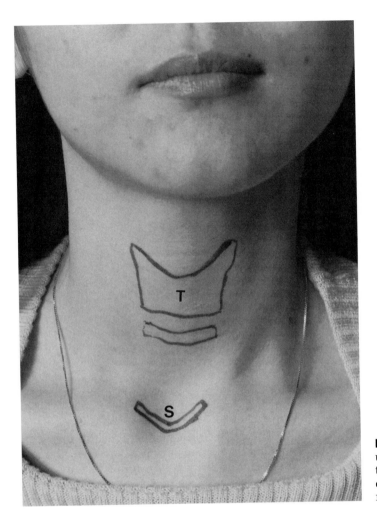

**Figure 1.** Globus symptoms are usually felt in the lower half of the throat, between the thyroid cartilage (T) and the sternal notch (S).

## Etiology and Pathogenesis

A variety of theories have been advanced throughout history as explanation for the feeling of a lump in the throat. The ancient Greeks believed that the womb was a floating organ, and that the lump in globus hystericus represented the uterus rising into the throat. It was believed to be a manifestation of hysteria, occurring exclusively in females. In fact, true hysteria is rarely associated with globus.[5] In 1707, John Purcell stated that globus was due to contraction of the strap muscles against the thyroid cartilage.[9] In the early 20th century, psychiatrists believed it represented a subconscious desire for oral sexual practices.[10] More recent research has focused upon the role of gastroesophageal reflux. Despite a substantial literature, the cause of the globus sensation (globus) has defied a unified theory and is probably multifactorial. The diseases that have been reported to cause the globus sensation have arisen within the head, neck, and thoracic regions.

Although gastroesophageal reflux has been implicated as a cause of globus, the literature is replete with conflicting evidence. Several authors have found a positive link between globus and reflux in up to 90% of patients,[11–18] whereas other studies could not support these findings.[1,19–21] Reflux is a common condition in the general population. Most patients who have abnormal amounts of gastroesophageal reflux do not develop globus sensation.

Reflux may be associated with globus sensation through three possible mechanisms. Globus may be due to referred discomfort from esophagitis, direct local irritation of the pharyngeal mucosa from pharyngeal reflux, or cricopharyngeal hypertension in response to esophageal acid exposure.[17] A patient may have one or more of these abnormalities. Patients with globus have a high incidence of supine reflux.

Despite the feelings of muscle tightness, manometric studies have not reliably defined cricopharyngeal hypertonicity in this condition either at rest or during stress.[6,17,19,20,22,23] Koufman[17] has documented a single case in which globus was associated with a hypertensive upper esophageal sphincter. The symptom resolved once the sphincter pressure returned to normal after treatment of the gastroesophageal reflux.[17] Others have suggested that esophageal or pharyngeal dysmotility, primary or secondary to reflux, may be a factor.[18,22,24,25]

Some studies have suggested that globus pharyngeus may be related to psychopathology,[8,19,26] especially when occurring in men.[5] The globus sensation is a common response to emotional stimuli in the general population.[8,27,28,29] Many patients find that their symptoms are worse during periods of stress. However, the mechanism in which stress causes globus is unclear. Stress does not cause a significant rise in pressures at the upper esophageal sphincter.[6]

Wilson et al.[19] argue that globus pharyngeus has many features which characterize a conversion disorder. Investigators have found globus patients had higher levels of depression,[5,6,30] anxiety,[6,19] obsessiveness,[31] and hypochondriasis.[5] Brown[32] found some success in using antidepressant medication. There has been a link in patients who also have irritable bowel syndrome, suggesting further evidence for a psychosomatic link.[25]

Puhakka[8] demonstrated a significant reduction in globus symptoms by improving dental occlusive abnormalities in a double blind study of 22 patients. Despite demonstrating a major improvement, little further work has been reported, and the link seems unclear.

## Differential Diagnosis

The conditions which commonly give rise to a feeling of a lump in the throat are listed in Table I. The presence of an organic illness precludes the diagnosis of globus pharyngeus.

### Gastroesophageal Disease

Gastroesophageal reflux disease may present with traditional symptoms, such

---

**Table I**
Differential Diagnosis

**Gastroesophageal**
  Gastroesophageal Reflux Disease
  Esophageal Web
  Lower Esophageal Ring
  Esophageal Stricture
  Barrett's Esophagus
  Hypertensive Upper Esophageal Sphincter
  Hiatus Hernia
  Pharyngeal or Esophageal Motility Disorders
  Achalasia
**Inflammatory**
  Pharyngitis
  Pharyngeal or Lingual Tonsillitis
  Epiglottitis
  Esophagitis (Viral, monilial)
  Cervical Lymph Nodes
  Sinusitis with Postnasal Drip
**Structural**
  Mucus Retention Cyst
  Cervical Osteophytes
  Zenker's Diverticulum
  Foreign Body (external, ingested, or inhaled)
  Lingual Thyroid
  Long Uvula
  Neck Trauma
**Benign or Malignant Tumor**
  Thyroid, Pharyngeal, Cervical Soft Tissue, Mediastinal
  Cervical Lymph Nodes, Cyst
**Other**
  Vascular (aberrant cervical vessel, aortic aneurysm)
  Temporomandibular Joint Dysfunction

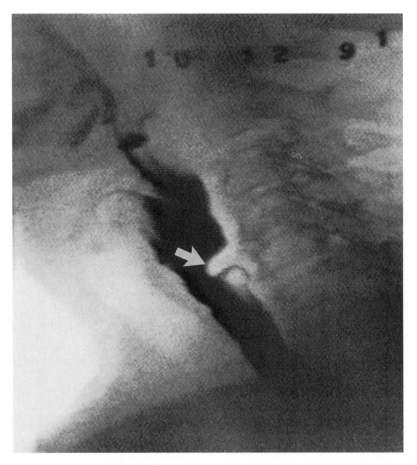

**Figure 2.**  An asymptomatic cricopharyngeal bar outlined on barium swallow (arrow).

as heartburn or regurgitation, or it may be clinically occult. Gastroesophageal reflux disease may also cause associated chronic sore throat, chronic cough, hoarseness, throat-clearing, and halitosis. The management of this condition is discussed below.

Other gastroesophageal conditions are more likely in patients with difficulty in swallowing food, chest pain, odynophagia, regurgitation, or aspiration. These symptoms mandate further investigation.

There has been no correlation between globus pharyngeus and a cricopharyngeal bar (Figure 2). Demonstration of a cricopharyngeal bar is likely to be a chance finding, but myotomy could be carried out as a last resort in patients with significant symptoms.

## Inflammatory

Unlike globus pharyngeus, acute inflammatory conditions of the pharynx usually have a significant pain component, causing odynophagia and dysphagia. Chronic tonsillitis is characterized by tonsillar hypertrophy, halitosis, and development of tonsilloliths. Response to antibiotics and antiseptic gargles is variable, and tonsillectomy may be indicated. Lingual tonsil hypertrophy may be deceptive unless careful evaluation of the tongue base is carried out during indirect laryngoscopy. This condition may be controlled by antibiotics, antiseptic gargles, or removal by diathermy or laser.

Chronic monilial esophagitis is most likely to occur in the immunocompromised patient. It is usually characterized by true dysphagia and odynophagia. Barium swallow may be suggestive and endoscopy with biopsy diagnostic. Oral antifungal treatment is usually effective.

Chronic pharyngitis may occur secondary to chronic postnasal drip. It may be aggravated by chronic mouth-breathing and occupational chemical or dust inhalation. Treatment is aimed at control of the sinonasal disease. For further discussion, see Chapter 1, "Cough" and Chapter 15, "Nasal Obstruction, Rhinorrhea, and Postnasal Drip," section on postnasal drip.

## Structural

Mucous and epidermoid retention cysts are not uncommon in the pharynx and tonsil. The vallecular cyst is readily diagnosed on indirect laryngoscopy. Large cysts may pose an airway hazard during drainage or during intubation. Tongue-base lesions may be lingual thyroid, lymphoma, or other tumor. Examination of this area requires digital palpation, close inspection using indirect or fibreoptic pharyngolaryngoscopy (Figure 3) and may require imaging techniques to delineate

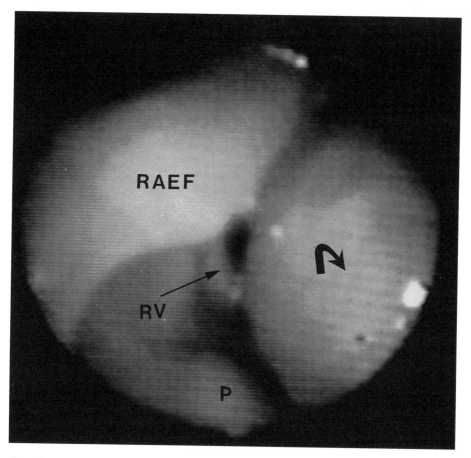

**Figure 3.** A large solid mucocele of the left aryepiglottic fold (large, curved arrow) is well seen by flexible telescope. The patient presented with globus symptoms. This photograph, taken at flexible fiberoptic telescopic examination, is oriented so that the anterior portion of the larynx is located toward the bottom of the photograph. P = petiolus of epiglottus; RAEF = right aryepiglottic fold; RV = right true vocal cord. (Courtesy: Dr. Ian Witterick, Department of Otolaryngology, Mount Sinai Hospital, Toronto, Canada)

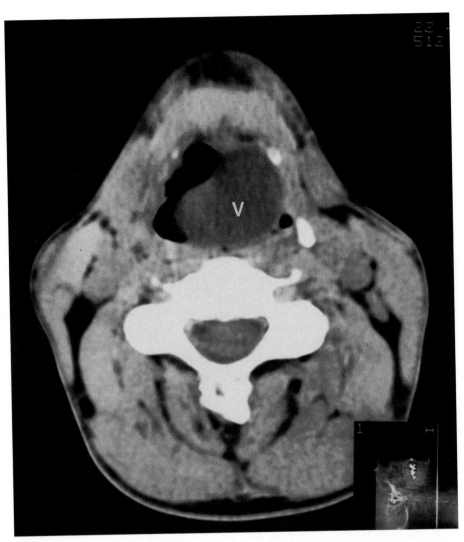

**Figure 4.** A large vallecular cyst (V) seen on computed tomography scan causes globus symptoms.

the size, location, and nature of the lesion prior to any intervention (Figure 4).

Cervical osteophytes are common, but rarely attain a size that interferes with normal functioning of the throat (Figure 5). They present as a broad swelling in the pharynx and may be removed should they be symptomatic, which is rare.

Zenker's diverticulum usually presents with dysphagia, regurgitation, gurgling, and sometimes aspiration. The barium esophagram finding is diagnostic of retained contrast in the hypopharyngeal or Zenker's pulsion diverticulum (Figure 6). The patient is invariably older than 60 years of age. Treatment, when necessary, can be accomplished by endoscopic or external surgical means.

## Malignant

Malignant disease of the aerodigestive tract, thyroid gland, and neck must be actively excluded in every patient. This can usually be achieved based upon the his-

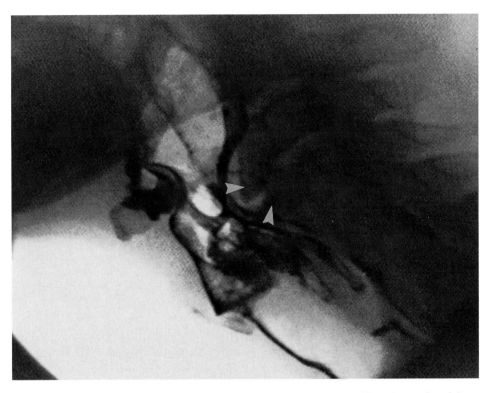

**Figure 5.** Lateral view of anterior cervical osteophytes on barium swallow (arrowheads) interfering with deglutition.

tory and physical examination alone. Patients who are high risk or who have any abnormal physical signs, such as dysphagia for food, pain, a mass, or vocal palsy, must be investigated. Postcricoid cancer must be excluded by endoscopy in patients with Plummer-Vinson syndrome (glossitis, iron deficiency anaemia, achlorhydria, postcricoid web).

Malignancies usually present with progressing symptoms over a period of weeks to months. Aerodigestive tract malignancy is more likely in a patient who smokes cigarettes or has significant alcohol intake. Cervical lymphadenopathy may occur during an upper aerodigestive tract infection. But a clinical suspicion of a metastatic disease involving deep cervical lymph nodes should trigger a search for a mucosal primary carcinoma. The Delphian lymph node lies in the midline anterior to the cricoid cartilage. This node is far

less frequently enlarged than the laterally placed deep cervical lymph nodes.

## Diagnostic Approach

The diagnostic process aims to elicit the presence of any specific organic disease located within the head, neck, and thoracic regions. This is made more challenging by the vague nature of the symptoms and the difficulty in assessment of the hypopharynx.

### History

Patients with globus frequently have difficulty in defining their symptoms. The condition may appear vague and changeable. The clinician needs to show concern

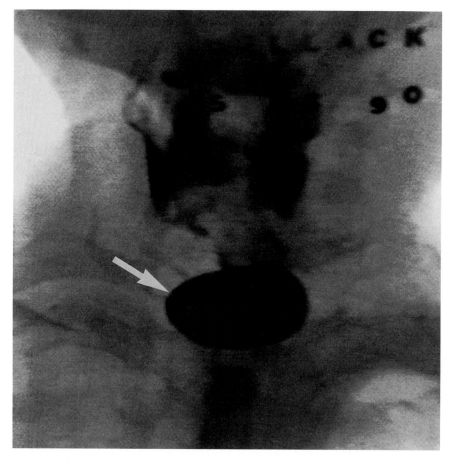

**Figure 6.** Anterior view of Zenker's diverticulum filled with barium (arrow).

and interest in helping the patient to clarify the symptoms.

The condition has been documented in adults between 14 and 75 years of age, with a female preponderance.[1,5,16] Apart from feelings of a lump in the throat, patients may complain of throat tightness or feelings of choking. Throat-clearing is common, in up to 74% of patients.[16] Difficulty in swallowing requires careful discussion. The clinician must define whether the patient has true dysphagia for solid or liquid food. Dysphagia for food is likely to indicate either a structural or neuromuscular disorder and requires appropriate investigation.[33] Patients with globus may describe a feeling of something which is blocking the swallowing of their saliva.

However, they deny any difficulty in swallowing solid or liquid food. Odynophagia, pain on swallowing food, is not a feature of globus pharyngeus. Globus pharyngeus may be aggravated by stress and alcohol.[16]

Most patients cannot identify a precipitating cause triggering the globus. A preceding life event may suggest a psychological basis for the condition.[30]

The site of the lump is usually between the thyroid cartilage and the root of the neck (Figure 1).[16] Symptoms occurring higher in the throat, or in the chest suggest an alternative condition. The symptoms are usually but not always midline. The condition may be episodic or continuous. In some cases, the feeling is eased by swallowing food.[14,15] Progressive deterioration of symptoms suggests an alternative diagnosis.

As globus is a diagnosis of exclusion, alternate diagnoses must be explored. The presence of true dysphagia for food or liquids usually indicates organic illness. The presence of heartburn and regurgitation indicates gastroesophageal reflux disease. Other features of reflux may include chronic cough, chronic sore throat, chronic throat-clearing, and hoarseness. The presence of associated postnasal drip, nasal airway obstruction, and sinusitis suggests sinonasal pathology. The presence of pain suggests an inflammatory condition. Change in the voice requires exclusion of a vocal cord palsy or a mass in the laryngopharynx.

## Physical Examination

An absence of physical signs is essential for the diagnosis. Nevertheless, these patients require a thorough head and neck examination to exclude organic pathology, as listed under differential diagnosis.

The physical examination begins with assessment of vocal quality during the interview. Hoarseness requires exclusion of organic disease. The tongue base should be palpated to exclude an occult tumor. The lingual tonsils, lateral pharyngeal walls, piriform fossae, and postcricoid region must be thoroughly assessed by indirect laryngoscopy. Presently, fiberoptic evaluation of the larynx and hypopharynx is nearly always required. Pooling of saliva, mucosal asymmetries, or vocal cord abnormalities (eg, mass, reduced mobility) requires further investigation.

Reflux frequently occurs in the presence of a normal larynx. Signs of reflux laryngitis include inflammation or thickening of the posterior larynx (ie, pachyderma laryngis), vocal granuloma, vocal ulcer, edema and inflammation of the vocal cords, and thickened laryngeal mucus.[17,34]

Evaluation of the nose and postnasal space may identify features to suggest sinonasal dysfunction, such as deviated nasal septum, swollen turbinates, nasal polyps, nasal pus, postnasal mucus, and pharyngitis of the postnasal space.

Neck examination must be systematic. Enlarged lymph nodes require further investigation with either fine-needle biopsy or imaging. The larynx should be grossly mobile over the prevertebral fascia (ie, Trotter's sign). In health, laryngeal crepitus can be heard as the laryngeal cartilaginous framework is moved from side to side over the prevertebral muscle and fascia. The thyroid gland must be examined in detail.

The presence of dysphagia or pooling can be evaluated further by swallowing nasolaryngoscopy (Figure 7).[33] This procedure involves having the patient swallow colored puree or water or something solid, such as a chocolate-covered wafer, while observing the laryngopharynx through the nasolaryngoscope. This test may define a functional swallowing disorder or possible aspiration.

## Investigations

When globus pharyngeus occurs without any other localizing symptoms, the incidence of positive findings after investigations is extremely low.[35] Many patients require no investigation. However, the list of possible investigations of globus sensation is extensive (Table II). Investiga-

---

**Table II**
Investigations

Modified Barium Swallow
Barium Swallow

Thyroid Scan
Thyroid Ultrasound
Thyroid Function Tests

Lateral Airways X-ray
Chest X-ray
CT Scan
Fine-needle Biopsy
Endoscopy
Angiography
MRI

24-Hour Esophageal pH Monitoring (single- or dual-probe)
Esophageal Manometry
Psychiatric Inventory

---

CT = computer-assisted tomographic scanning; MRI = magnetic resonance imaging.

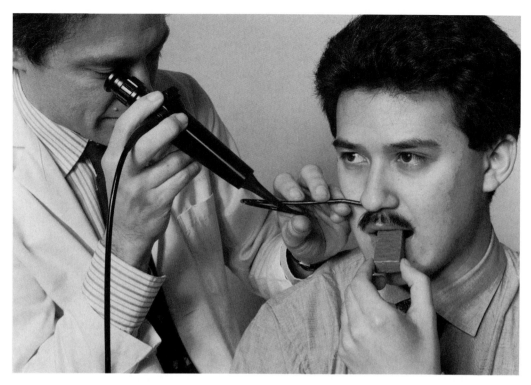

**Figure 7.** Evaluation of deglutition using the fibreoptic nasolaryngoscope.

tions are mandatory under the following circumstances:

(i) Difficulty in swallowing solid food or drinks (This indicates that a structural or neuromuscular disorder is likely and should be investigated with a modified barium swallow, a routine barium swallow, and possibly manometry and endoscopy.);

(ii) A strong history of smoking and drinking alcohol (The patient should be considered for endoscopy and a chest x-ray to exclude an upper aerodigestive tract malignancy.);

(iii) The presence of a palpable neck mass, or abnormality seen on indirect laryngoscopy (A nonpulsatile neck mass requires a fine-needle aspiration biopsy. Other investigations that may be required include chest x-ray, computed tomography, magnetic resonance imaging, angiography, endoscopy, and thyroid function tests.).

Frequently, the patient has no suspicious clinical features. Occult gastroesophageal reflux disease may be a cause of globus sensation in this group. Koufman reported only 43% of a reflux population had gastrointestinal symptoms of heartburn or regurgitation.[17] Single-probe 24-hour esophageal pH monitoring can quantify the amount of reflux, and correlate the reflux with the timing of symptoms while the patient carries out a normal daily routine. In the normal subject, the pH of the lower esophagus may drop to less than 4 for 6.3% upright, 1.2% supine, and 4.2% total time per day.[36] However, any reflux to the level of the pharynx is considered abnormal. Thus, pharyngeal reflux may occur in the presence of a normal amount of esophageal reflux. Detection of the pharyngeal reflux requires a second probe placed in the hypopharynx. Dual-probe 24-hour pH monitoring is the only test that can detect pharyngeal reflux (Figure 8).

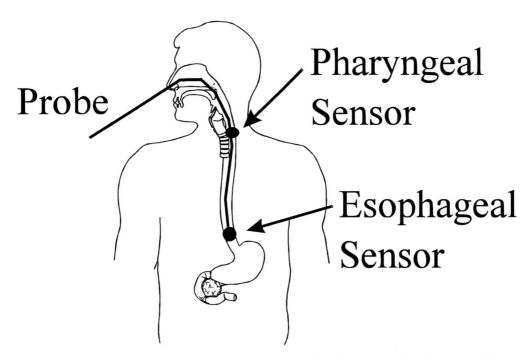

**Figure 8.** The dual-probe pH system has a sensor in the pharynx and the lower esophagus.

Other investigations for gastroesophageal reflux disease and motility disorders include endoscopy, biopsy, manometry, and barium swallow. These investigations are the preferred modalities when evaluating the esophageal complications of reflux or in the patient with true dysphagia.

A diagnostic algorithm using history, physical examination, and laboratory investigations is depicted in Figure 9.

## Treatment

Treatment of globus sensation begins once specific organic disease is excluded. All patients require reassurance that their symptoms are real and not a sign of hysteria. Most patients are relieved to know that they do not have a malignancy. For many patients, a thorough evaluation combined with firm reassurance is enough. Others, greatly disturbed by this persistent symptom and convinced that a lump must be present, demand further investigation and treatment.

All patients with a short history should be reassessed subsequently to exclude the development of a specific organic illness.

A lack of a specific treatment and poor cure rates frustrate the clinician. Complete response rates vary widely from 25% to 88%.[1,14–17] Factors that are likely to produce a better prognosis include male sex, symptom duration of less than 3 months, and no associated throat symptoms.[16]

Many patients are sufficiently disturbed by their symptoms that they request further management. As globus is likely to be multifactorial, treatment may require several approaches before improvement is noted. As discussed under pathogenesis, conditions which may be etiologically associated with globus include gastroesophageal reflux disease, anxiety, and occult postnasal drip.

Results of reflux treatment for globus

DIAGNOSTIC ALGORITHM FOR GLOBUS SENSATION

1. Full ENT exam to exclude local disease →

2. If local disease or neck mass or heavy smoker or heavy alcohol intake →
   CT scan neck, thyroid and/or neck ultrasound, barium swallow, chest x-ray,
   MRI neck, endoscopy and biopsy as required

3. If dysphagia →
   Routine barium swallow or modified barium swallow

4. If postnasal discharge on telescopic examination nasal cavities →
   CT paranasal sinuses (coronal cuts), allergy workup

5. Otherwise →
   Treat for gastroesophageal reflux for one month

6. If no improvement →
   After one month, or if GI symptoms - full ENT exam again

7. If abnormal →
   repeat 2,3,4 or 5

8. If normal →
   Dual probe 24 hour esophageal pH study, possible endoscopy, barium swallow,
   esophageal manometry

**Figure 9.** Diagnostic algorithm for globus sensation. CT = computed tomography; ENT = ear, nose, and throat; GI = gastrointestinal; MRI = magnetic resonance imaging.

have varied significantly.[13–17] At this stage, the weight of evidence supports treatment of occult or overt reflux in the patient with globus where symptomatic control is desirable. Treatment includes weight reduction, smoking cessation, elevation of the head of the bed, and commencement of antacids or $H_2$ blocking agents and/or prokinetic drugs. Dietary control includes reduction in alcohol, chocolate, spicy foods, fatty foods, mint, orange juice, and carbonated drinks. Treatment should be continued for no less than 3 months, and some patients may prefer maintenance treatment.[15] This therapy has produced a strong placebo effect in two uncontrolled trials.[1,21] See Chapter 1, "Cough," for further discussion of treatment of reflux disease.

Although the heartburn may respond quickly to antireflux treatment, globus symptoms may take weeks to settle. Should this regimen fail, dual-lumen 24-hour esophageal pH monitoring, and possibly other reflux investigations, should be carried out to confirm the diagnosis before more aggressive treatment of reflux is instituted.

Although globus pharyngeus has been associated with increased levels of anxiety, depression, obsessiveness, and hypochondriasis, there has been a swing away from psychiatric treatment. This parallels the name change from globus hystericus to globus pharyngeus. Nevertheless, some patients may have psychological disturbances that aggravate the condition. A precipitating life event may suggest a psychological basis for the condition.[30] Success with antidepressants has been reported.[32] Treatment of anxiety may involve stress management counselling, relaxation therapy, speech pathology, and possibly psychiatric referral.

Sinonasal problems may respond to treatment. The patient may be unaware of postnasal drip or nocturnal mouth-breathing. Evaluation and treatment of rhinosinusitis may yield positive results. For further discussion, see Chapter 1, "Cough" and Chapter 15, "Nasal Obstruction, Rhinorrhea, and Postnasal Drip," section on postnasal drip.

Patients often complain of a feeling of thick mucus and the need to clear the throat. Many patients feel that these symptoms are related to milk ingestion, although the mechanism for this is unclear.[37,38] The symptoms may respond to cessation of milk and other dairy products. Thickened mucus may also respond to improving hydration by increasing water intake, steam inhalations, reduction of diuretics such as coffee and alcohol, and changing dehydrating medications. Mucolytics may help. Patients who work in a dusty environment should wear a filtering mask. Improvements in nasal airflow are important to reduce the drying effect of mouth-breathing.

Finally there will be a group of patients who will not respond to any form of treatment. These patients feel globus sensation is a very real physical condition. They become tormented by its failure to resolve. The clinician, unable to cure the problem, may find it tempting to minimize or deny the symptoms. This approach, which is certain to aggravate the patient's distress, must be avoided. These patients require a great deal of patience, reassurance, and due diligence to ensure that an organic lesion is not missed.

## Acknowledgment:

This work was supported by the Saul A. Silverman Family Foundation and Temmy Latner/Dynacare as a Canada-International Scientific Exchange Program in Otolaryngology (CISEPO II) Project.

## References

1. Moloy PJ, Charter R. The globus symptom. Arch Otolaryngol 1982;108:740–744.
2. Vandeleur T. Globus. Aust J Otolaryng 1993;1:257–259.
3. Malcomson KG. Globus Hystericus vel pharyngeus. J Laryngol Otol 1968;82:219–230.
4. Hippocrates. *The genuine works, Vol 1.* London, England; 1849:77.
5. Pratt LW, Tobin WH, Gallagher RA. Office evaluation by psychological testing with the MMPI. Laryngoscope 1976;86:1540–1551.
6. Cook IJ, Dent J, Collins SM. Upper esophageal sphincter tone and reactivity to stress in patients with a history of globus sensation. Digest Dis Sciences 1989;34:672–676.
7. Moser G, Vicariou-Granser GV, Schneider C, et al. High incidence of esophageal motor disorders in consecutive patients with globus sensation. Gastroenterology 1991;101:1512–1521.
8. Puhakka HJ, Kirveskari P. Globus hystericus: globus syndrome? J Laryngol Otol 1988;102:231–234.
9. Purcell J. *A Treatise Of Vapours Or Hysteric Fits.* 2nd ed. London, England; 1707.
10. Ferenczi S; Suttle JI, trans. The phenomenon of hysterical materialisation. In: *Further Contributions to the Theory and Technique of Psychoanalysis* (Int. Psychoanalytical Library No. 11); London, England: L & V Woolf.; 1926:90–104.
11. Delahunty, Ardran GM. Globus hystericus—a manifestation of reflux oesophagitis. J Laryngol Otol 1970;84:1049–1054.
12. Cherry J, Siegel CI, Margulies SI, et al. Pharyngeal localisation of symptoms of gastroesophageal reflux. Ann Otol Rhinol Laryngol 1970;79:912–915.
13. Freeland AP, Ardran GM, Emrys-Roberts E. Globus hystericus and reflux oesophagitis. J Laryngol Otol 1974;88:1025–1031.
14. Batch AJG. Globus pharyngeus (Part I). J Laryngol Otol 1988;102:152–158.
15. Batch AJG. Globus pharyngeus (Part II), Discussion. J Laryngol Otol 1988;102:227–230.
16. Timon C, Cagney D, O'Dwyer T, et al. Globus pharyngeus: Long-term follow-up and prognostic factors. Ann Otol Rhinol Laryngol. 1991;100.351–354.
17. Koufman JA. The Otolaryngologic manifestations of gastroesophageal reflux disease (GERD): A clinical investigation of 225 pa-

tients using ambulatory 24-hour ph monitoring and an experimental investigation of the role of acid and pepsin in the development of laryngeal injury. Laryngoscope 1991;101:1–78.

18. Ossakow SJ, Elta G, Colturi T, et al. Esophageal reflux and dysmotility as the basis for persistent cervical symptoms. Ann Otol Rhinol Laryngol 1987;96:387–392.

19. Wilson JA, Deary IJ, Maran AGD. Is globus hystericus? Brit J Psych 1988;153:335–339.

20. Wilson JA, Pryde A, Piris J, et al. Pharyngoesophageal dysmotility in globus sensation. Arch Otolaryngol Head Neck Surg 1989;115:1086–1090.

21. Mair IWS, Schroder KE, Modalsli B, et al. Aetiological aspects of the globus symptoms. J Laryngol Otol 1974;88:1033–1054.

22. Flores TC, Cross FS, Jones RD. Abnormal oesophageal manometry in globus hystericus. Ann Otol 1981;90:383–386.

23. Caldarelli DD, Andrews AH, Derbyshire AJ. Oesophageal motility studies in globus sensation. Ann Otol Rhinol Laryngol 1970; 79:1098–1100.

24. Linsell JC, Anggiansah A, Owen WJ. Manometric findings in patients with the globus sensation. 1987;28:1378–1380.

25. Watson WC, Sullivan SN. Hypertonicity of the cricopharyngeal sphincter: a cause of globus sensation. Lancet 1974;2: 1417–1419.

26. Mohun M. Globus Management. Laryngoscope. 1955;65:73–79.

27. Heartburn and globus. Pathological, functional or normal? (Editorial) Lancet 1982; 54:832–835.

28. Thompson WG, Heaton KW. Heartburn and globus in apparently healthy people. CMA Journal 1982;126:46–48.

29. Glaser JP, Engel GL. Psychodynamics, psychophysiology and gastrointestinal symptomatology. Clin Gastroenterol 1977;6: 507–531.

30. Deary IJ, Smart A, Wilson JA. Depression and 'hassles' in globus pharyngis. Br J Psychiatry 1992;161:115–117.

31. Lehtinen V, Puhakka H. A psychosomatic approach to the globus hystericus syndrome. Acta Psychiatrica Scandinavica. 1976;53:21–28.

32. Brown SR, Schwartz JM, Summergrad P, et al. Globus hysterics syndrome responsive to antidepressants. Am J Psychiatry 1986; 143:917–918.

33. Mendelsohn MS. New concepts in dysphagia management. J Otolaryngol 1993;22: 5–24.

34. Ward PH. Berci G. Observation on the pathogenesis of chronic non specific pharyngitis and laryngitis. Laryngoscope 1982;92: 1377–1382.

35. Wilson JA, Murray JAM, von Haacke NP. Rigid endoscopy in ENT practice appraisal of the diagnostic yield in a district general hospital. J Laryngol Otol 1987;101: 286–292.

36. Castell DO. Ambulatory monitoring in esophageal disease. Dig Dis. 1989;21:1–4.

37. Arnay WK, Pinnock CB. Appetite. 1993;20: 53–60.

38. Pinnock CB, Graham NM, Mylvaganam A, et al. Relationship between milk intake and mucus production in adult volunteers challenged with rhinovirus-2. Am Rev Respir Dis 1990;141:352–356.

# 11

# Sore Throat

B.C. Papsin, M.D., M.SC.
J.S. Chapnik M.D.

## Introduction

Sore throat results from inflammation of the mucosal and submucosal structures of the pharynx and represents one of the most common reasons for visits to doctors.[1] Ten percent of all office visits to primary care physicians and 50% of all outpatient antibiotics used are for sore throats.[2] Commonly, infection plays a major role in this inflammatory process. The structures involved, by virtue of their generous innervation, are highly symptomatic making the "sore throat" a common presenting complaint. Furthermore, because of the high concentrations of lymphoid tissue in this region, these sites are prone to reactive changes especially in response to viral and bacterial challenge. In addition, lymphoproliferative and epithelial neoplasms may present first with pharyngeal involvement. A common endpoint, the local release of kinins,[3] correlates strongly with the perception of pharyngeal pain resulting in presentation with sore throat.

In this chapter, the anatomy, physiology, and pathology of the pharynx will be reviewed and the approach to "sore throat" will be described.

## Anatomy

The throat comprises the structures of the nasopharynx, oropharynx, and hypopharynx (Figure 1). In total, it is a 12- to 14-cm musculomembranous tube extending from the base of the skull and the back of the mouth and nose to the level of the sixth cervical vertebra. The pharynx is widest at the base of the skull, posterior to the eustachian tube orifices. It narrows to the level of the palate and then widens again in the oropharynx only to narrow as it nears the beginning of the esophagus.[4-6]

The oropharynx (Figure 2) extends from the vallate papillae, tonsillar fossae, and inferior soft palate to join the hypopharynx at the level of the arytenoid cartilages. The hypopharynx continues inferiorly to the postcricoid region where the esophagus begins. The oropharynx communicates anteriorly with the mouth and superiorly with the nasopharynx. Inferiorly, it communicates with the hypopharynx which is contiguous further distally with the cervical esophagus.

The lining of the pharynx is stratified squamous epithelium[7] and the mucous membrane contains a considerable amount of elastic tissue and many glands,

From Irwin RS, Curley FJ, Grossman RF (eds): Diagnosis and Treatment of Symptoms of the Respiratory Tract. Armonk, New York, Futura Publishing Company, Inc., © 1997.

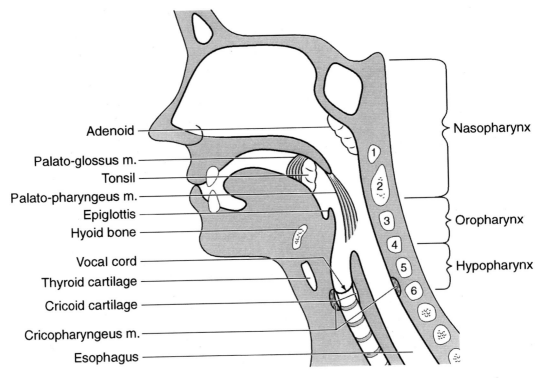

Adenoid

Palato-glossus m.

Tonsil

Palato-pharyngeus m.

Epiglottis

Hyoid bone

Vocal cord

Thyroid cartilage

Cricoid cartilage

Cricopharyngeus m.

Esophagus

Nasopharynx

Oropharynx

Hypopharynx

**Figure1.** Cross-section of the head showing the three divisions of the pharynx—nasopharynx, oropharynx, and hypopharynx.

mainly mucous in type. There are many subepithelial collections of lymph tissue into which the epithelium descends to form narrow crypts or pits. This lymph tissue is similar to that of a lymph node but differs from it because it has only efferent vessels. Collections of this lymphoid tissue form the palatine and lingual tonsils in the oropharynx. Together, the lymph tissue of the nasopharynx and oropharynx forms an almost complete ring, called Waldeyer's ring, which provides an ideal physiologic collection system allowing the organism to sample, analyze, and process incoming antigens.[8]

The musculature of the pharynx is predominantly made up of the three constrictor muscles which are curved sheets forming the posterior and lateral walls of the pharynx.[4, 5] They overlap each other from below upwards. These muscles all insert in the midline posteriorly at the medial fibrous pharyngeal, raphe which descends from the pharyngeal tubercle on the base of the skull. The pharyngeal plexus of the glossopharyngeal and vagus nerves with an additional supply to the inferior constrictor from the external branch of the superior and recurrent laryngeal nerves supply the pharyngeal musculature.

Three additional longitudinal muscles pass obliquely from their origins into the pharyngeal wall. The palatopharyngeus, which forms the posterior tonsillar pillar, runs from the palate to the posterolateral oropharyngeal wall. The salpingopharyngeus muscle runs from the nasopharyngeal orifice of the eustachian tube to blend anteriorly with the palatopharyngeus muscle. The stylopharyngeus muscle runs from the medial base of the styloid process to the posterolateral pharyngeal wall between the superior and middle constrictors.

The pharynx is bounded laterally by

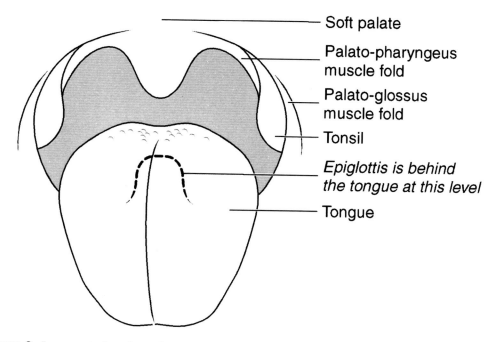

Soft palate

Palato-pharyngeus
muscle fold

Palato-glossus
muscle fold

Tonsil

*Epiglottis is behind
the tongue at this level*

Tongue

**Figure 2.** In an anterior view, the oropharynx is bounded by the soft palate, the palatoglossus muscles, and the tongue base. Note that the tonsils, which are posterior to the palato-glossus muscles, are anatomically a part of the pharynx.

the buccopharyngeal fascia, but beyond this partition certain important spaces and planes lie through which infection or tumors may spread. Posteriorly, the pharynx is separated from the prevertebral fascia by loose connective tissue, allowing easy movement of the pharynx in swallowing and forming the retropharyngeal space.[9] This space is bounded laterally by the carotid sheaths. Laterally, loose connective tissue is also found but here is bounded by the pterygoid muscles and the thick deep parotid fascia. This lateral connective tissue forms the parapharyngeal space which descends from the base of the skull to an apex at the level of the hyoid bone and is limited by the submandibular gland's fascial attachments to the stylohyoid and posterior digastric muscles.

The pharynx receives its arterial blood supply predominantly from the external carotid artery via the ascending pharyngeal artery, dorsal branches from the lingual artery, tonsillar branches of the facial artery, and palatine branches from the maxillary artery.[4–5] The pharyngeal veins communicate superiorly with the pterygoid and vertebral plexus of veins and drain inferiorly into the jugular vein.

Lymphatic drainage from the oropharynx empties into the retropharyngeal, the superior deep cervical, and the jugular lymph nodes. The hypopharynx drains into the retropharyngeal, lateral pharyngeal, and deep cervical and jugular nodes. The specialized lymphatic structures in the pharynx, the faucial or palatine tonsils, contribute significantly to pharyngeal immunocompetence and are often the site of symptomatic inflammation. The palatine tonsils are paired generally ovoid masses on the lateral walls of the oropharynx innervated by the glossopharyngeal nerve and some branches of the lesser palatine nerves via the sphenopalatine ganglion. The deep surface of the tonsil is attached to the fascia overlying the superior constrictor muscle, and it is bounded anteriorly by the palatoglossus muscle and posteriorly by the palatopharyngeus muscle.

The internal carotid artery lies about 2 cm posterolateral to the deep aspect of the tonsil. The palatine tonsils drain primarily into the superior deep cervical and jugular lymph nodes.

## Physiology

The pharynx is intimately involved with activity critical to human survival: deglutition, respiration, communication, and immune surveillance. These varied activities are often undertaken simultaneously and require considerable coordination to avoid catastrophic consequences. The pharynx performs these functions in tight coordination with the airway musculature under strict neurological control.

### Deglutition

The swallowing mechanism is divided into oral, pharyngeal, and esophageal phases.[10] Briefly, the oral phase involves chewing and preparation of food including a mixture of the bolus with saliva. During this phase, the soft palate is actively pulled anteriorly and downwards by the palatoglossus muscle to contact the tongue and prevent premature loss of food into the pharynx. Next, the tongue propels the bolus towards the pharynx by establishing tongue-palate contact which progresses posteriorly.[11] The oral phase of swallowing is primarily under voluntary cortical control.

Once the bolus passes the back of the tongue the pharyngeal swallow is triggered and the base of the tongue moves backwards to make contact with the posterior pharyngeal wall.[12] The tongue base movement propels the bolus through the pharynx involuntarily mediated via medullary centers. During this phase, the palate is elevated (ie, levator palati muscle) and drawn posteriorly (ie, palatopharyngeus) and the posterior pharyngeal wall moves anteriorly (ie, Passavant's ridge) to close the connection between the nasopharynx and the oropharynx. The ad-

enoid pad may contribute to this closure. Failure to close this opening would result in nasal regurgitation of food. Once propelled into and through the pharynx, the food bolus is directed into the esophagus by a series of coordinated movements of both the larynx (ie, elevation and epiglottic closure) and the upper esophageal sphincter (ie, cricopharyngeal muscle relaxation) which result in bolus transfer into the esophagus.[13]

### Respiration

The laryngeal inlet has as its primary function, the prevention of the ingress of anything other than air into the lungs.[14] The pharynx contributes little to respiratory protection other than taking part in coordinated swallowing as noted above, and merely acts as a conduit for the passage of air into the lungs via the laryngeal airway.[15] During inspiration when the negative pressure within the pharynx would tend to close the lumen, muscular contraction of the genioglossus, geniohyoid, and anterior belly of the digastric muscles pulls the base of the tongue and the hyoid bone anteriorly.[9] It is precisely at this point in the airway that collapse can occur in a somnolent person resulting in snoring and possibly apnea during sleep.[16]

### Communication

Although the larynx is the principal component of speech production, human voice results from coordinated interaction of the larynx, lungs, diaphragm, abdominal muscles, neck muscles, lips, tongue, buccinators, soft palate, and the pharynx.[17] Phonation results from vocal cord vibration-induced by expiratory airflow in the larynx.[18] Resonance of the laryngeal sound output results from induced vibration in the chest and pharynx and selective amplification of certain frequencies depending on pharyngeal shape and size.[17] It is resonance, a primarily pharyngeal function, which gives voice its characteristic timbre and provides amplification. Resonance is controlled by altering the pharyngeal shape and volume and by varying the amount of sound transmitted through the nasopharynx. Articulation also depends on the shape of the pharynx, jaw, mouth, and nasopharynx. The importance of the pharynx in voice production is clearly seen in postlaryngectomy patients who develop intelligible speech emanating from an intact pharynx and mouth resonating the vibration generated either by the pharynx itself as with the Blom et al.[19] artificial tracheoesophageal fistula prosthesis or an extrinsic vibrator such as an electrolarynx.

## Immune Surveillance

The mucosa of the aerodigestive tract represents the first line of defense for an organism exposed constantly to new antigens in food and in the environment. A mucous layer which acts as a weak mechanical barrier lines the entire pharynx. Surface protection also depends on the presence of secretory IgA which is quite acid stable and resistant to digestion.

The tonsils are unique in that they are involved in both local immunity and immune surveillance for the development of the body's immunologic defense system.[8] Each tonsil contains up to $10^9$ lymphoid cells.[20] As stated above, in contrast to lymph glands elsewhere in the body, the tonsils of the pharynx have no afferent lymphatics but rather have only mucosal exposure to provide afferent input. Chronic infection in the tonsils and adenoids can result in increased local antibody levels, shifts in B- and T-cell ratios and changes in serum immunoglobulin levels, which return to normal after tonsillectomy.

The key to the immunologic defense apparatus of the pharynx is the close approximation of antigen and lymphoid tissue which is made possible by the arrangement of epithelial-lined crypts in the tonsillar tissue. Secretory IgA is produced as a result of the proliferation of B cells in response to exposure to an antigen.[21] The

tonsils act as antigen processors. Antigen is transported through the crypt epithelium and eventually to the center of the lymphoid follicle where a B response is generated. High-antigen doses can induce a polyclonal B-cell proliferation.[22] Regulation of the immune response is the function of the extranodular T lymphocytes. T cells also play a role locally in the tonsil. Sensitized T cells are important in defense against viruses and fungi. In addition, lymphokine production (ie, interferon gamma) within the tonsils results from T-cell activation.

The most heated debate concerning pharyngeal tonsillar defense surrounds the issue of whether the removal of tonsillar tissue affects the immunocompetence of the patient. No specific adverse effects have been seen after tonsillectomy or adenoidectomy, although the removal of pharyngeal lymphoid tissue should only be performed for clearly defined clinical disease.[23]

## Pathogenesis

Pharyngeal inflammation can result from a number of different etiologic agents. These agents have in common the release of mediators into the richly innervated mucous membrane of the throat. The pain associated with the sore throat correlates closely with physical findings, including oropharyngeal erythema, exanthems, and the presence of cervical adenopathy.[24] The degree of throat pain is independent of its cause (ie, viral versus bacterial).[25] Importantly, concomitant cough intensifies sore throat possibly by mechanically irritating the mucosa already inflamed by the causing agent.[24]

Kinins specifically have been shown to induce sore throat in direct relation to their pharyngeal concentration.[3] Kinins are vasoactive peptides which increase vascular permeability resulting in nasal obstruction and rhinorrhea in addition to causing sore throat in subjects unilaterally challenged by topical application. Furthermore, the specificity of kinin-release in sore throat is demonstrated by its ab-

sence in allergic rhinitis wherein mediators released from mast cells predominate.
Kinins have been isolated from secretions
in patients with rhinovirus infections in
whom other inflammatory mediators were
absent[26] and in experimentally induced
rhinovirus colds.[27]

## Differential Diagnosis, Causes, and Treatment of Sore Throat

The differential diagnosis of sore
throat is broad; it is outlined in Table I.
Sore throat may result from a number of
different types of diseases both local or
systemic. The generous pharyngeal sensory innervation results in early and often
severe local symptoms. In addition to the
structures within the pharynx, "sore
throat" can represent disease in areas with
common innervation such as the teeth,
gums, and cervical spine resulting in referred throat discomfort.

Commonly, sore throat results from
infection. Bacterial, fungal, and viral
agents all cause pharyngitis and represent
a common presentation to physicians concerned with the aerodigestive tract. In addition, neoplasia, systemic disease,
trauma, foreign body ingestion, motility
disorders, and structural abnormalities
can cause pharyngitis. In this next section
we will examine the common groups of
diseases that cause pharyngitis and discuss some of the more important entities
in detail.

---

### Table I
Differential Diagnosis of Sore Throat

Infection
Granulomatous Disease
Connective Tissue Disease
Malignancy
Gastroesophageal Reflux Disease
AIDS-related Conditions
Chronic Irritation
Conditions Causing Referred Pain

---

AIDS = acquired immunodeficiency syndrome.

## Infections

Sore throat most commonly follows
infection, but the exact incidence of infectious pharyngitis is impossible to calculate
since the majority of patients do not present for treatment of this self-limited malady. It has become clear with the use of
rapid antigen detection techniques that
sore throat can result from a number of
bacterial or viral pathogens occurring
alone or in combination.[25] Although common pathogenic bacterial agents were isolated frequently, in approximately one
third of cases, no microbe was found and
in close to another third of cases, viruses
were isolated. The viral "common cold"
still represents the most frequent causative
agent in sore throat.

### Viral

Viral infections of the pharynx commonly present with sore throat and often
appear similar to bacterial infections. Differentiation can be made by examination
which reveals the absence of exudative
tonsillitis, diffusely enlarged but minimally tender cervical lymph nodes and
systemic symptoms (eg, fatigue, arthral-
gia). Most viral sore throats are self-limited
in immunocompetent hosts.[28]

The common cold is a self-limited
viral infection characterized by nasal obstruction, rhinorrhea, and sore throat and
is often associated with cough, lacrimation, and fever. It usually resolves within
7 days but may last up to 14 days even in
an uncomplicated infection.[29] Transmitted by aerosolized particles, the common
cold spreads effectively in crowded environments, but is even more efficiently
transmitted by hand contact and self-inno-
culation. Although the rhinovirus infection is most commonly isolated, in up to
50% of infections no microbe is identified.
Other infective agents isolated include in-
fluenzas A, B, and C, parainfluenza, respiratory syncytial virus, coronavirus, adenovirus, coxsackievirus A and B, and various
enteric cytopathogenic human orphan viruses (ECHO).

The common cold is best treated preventively by careful hand-washing and hygiene.[29] Symptomatic treatment with nasal decongestants and medications with atropinelike effects can diminish nasal obstruction and rhinorrhea, respectively. Salt-water gargles, increasing environmental humidity, and the use of topical and systemic analgesics,[2] lessen the discomfort associated with this infection.

In measles (ie, rubeola), pharyngotonsillitis occurs along with coryza and conjunctivitis followed by exanthematous buccal mucosal lesions (ie, Koplick's spots) and the pathognomonic generalized cutaneous rash. Treatment is symptomatic only. In children, this infection is benign, though in adults and in immunocompromised patients, the morbidity is higher.

Herpes simplex virus (HSV) infects the aerodigestive tract in both its primary and recurrent forms.[30] In primary infection, HSV commonly causes gingivostomatitis but may present as a "sore throat."

Frequently, primary infection occurs in children between 10 months and 3 years of age though adult cases are common and generally more severe. After a short incubation period following inoculation by saliva or mucous, fever, malaise, and sore throat develop. Examination reveals clusters of vesicular lesions which ulcerate and are quite painful (Figure 3). Treatment is usually symptomatic. Antiviral therapy (ie, topical and/or systemic) may diminish the severity of the infection if initiated early in its course and also may be useful in patients with inadequate immune function.[31] In immunocompromised patients with recurrent HSV infections, the prophylactic administration of acyclovir, an acyclic guanosine derivative highly selective for viral DNA polymerase, is more effective than treatment of established lesions.[32]

Epstein-Barr virus, another herpesvirus, also causes sore throat. Its primary target is the B lymphocyte. This virus has the

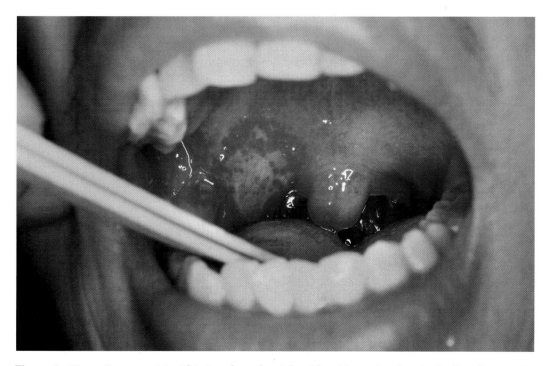

**Figure 3.** Herpetic stomatitis. This involves the right side of the soft palate including the anterior tonsillar pillar and although similar to aphthos stomatitis tends to be more diffuse. (Courtesy of Dr. M. Hawke, Toronto)

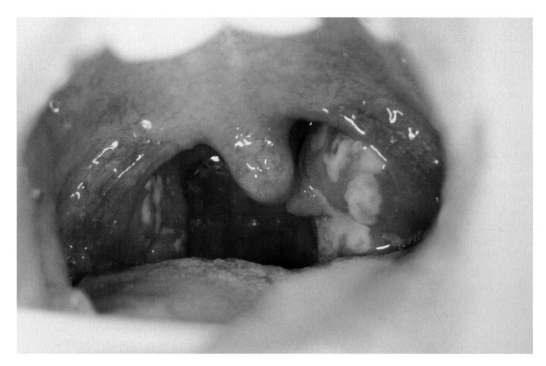

**Figure 4.** Infections mononucleosis. Tonsil and pharyngeal involvement. Unlike that in acute follicular tonsillitis, the white discoloration presents as a superficial membrane that may cover the entire tonsillar surfaces. (Courtesy of Dr. M. Hawke, Toronto)

ability to transform human B lymphocytes into cells capable of indefinite growth in culture. Epstein-Barr virus DNA has also been found in specimens from patients with nasopharyngeal carcinoma and Burkitt's lymphoma, but the virus's exact role in malignancy is not known. Pharyngitis secondary to Epstein-Barr virus infection is, in contrast, very common.

The common clinical entity associated with Epstein-Barr virus infection is infectious mononucleosis, which is a systemic illness primarily affecting adolescents who present with sore throat, fever, malaise, and posterior and anterior cervical adenopathy.[33] The posterior cervical adenopathy is a most useful clinical finding since it occurs rather infrequently in pharyngitis caused by other common pathogens. Hepatomegaly and splenomegaly are also commonly present as well as adenopathy at other, non–head and neck sites. The pharyngitis is typically exudative (Figure 4). Diagnosis is based on clinical findings, lymphocytosis, and the presence of atypical lymphocytes in the peripheral blood smear. The heterophile agglutination test (patients' antibodies to horse red blood cells) is confirmatory but may remain falsely negative early in the disease course for up to 1 month.

Cytomegalovirus (CMV) is a herpesvirus with several antigenically distinct strains.[34] It can cause congenital and acquired infection and usually is manifest as an asymptomatic or mild infection in an immunocompetent host. It is transmitted in secretions, blood infusion, and human milk. Cytomegalovirus mononucleosis refers to infection in which there is violent exudative tonsillitis and negative heterophile antibody tests in the presence of rising CMV titers.[35] The most sensitive diagnostic method is identification of virus in the urine after inoculation of human diploid tissue culture.[34] Virus in urine retains its infectivity for 7 days at 4°C. Serodiagnosis and complement fixation testing can also be used.

Treatment of mononucleosis is supportive including rest and fluids. Antibiotics are often indicated for treatment of bacterial superinfection but the use of ampicillin is contraindicated due to the invariable development of a morbilliform rash after administering this agent in either Epstein-Barr virus or CMV mononucleosis patients.

### Bacterial

Bacterial pharyngitis is usually an acute infection often secondary to or associated with a viral infection in the paranasal sinuses or the nose. The commensal flora of the upper respiratory tract can cause clinical disease. These bacteria are the gram-positive aerobes, including alpha and gamma-hemolytic streptococci, in ad-

dition to several anaerobic organisms, including *Peptostreptococcus, Fusobacterium,* and *Bacteroides* species.[36] Mixed infections with gram-positive, gram-negative, and anaerobic organisms are common. Pathogens, such as *Staphylococcus aureus, Hemophilus influenzae, Diplococcus pneumoniae, Streptococcus pyogenes, Corynebacterium diptheriae,* and *Bordetella pertussis* commonly play a role in mixed infections.

The most common bacterial pharyngeal pathogen is Group A beta-hemolytic Streptococcus (GABHS) which causes acute tonsillitis, especially in children.[37] After a short incubation period ranging from 12 hours to 4 days, the infection manifests with sore throat, dysphagia, fever, pharyngeal inflammation, and a diffuse or follicular exudate (Figure 5). Cervical lymphadenopathy is present in as many as 60% of patients. These nodes are often quite tender on palpation. Diagnosis can be established by culture, and antibiotic

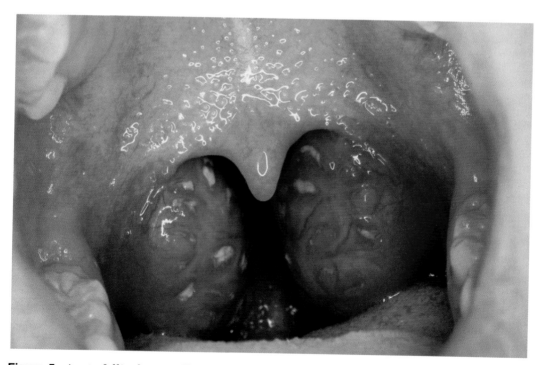

**Figure 5.** Acute follicular tonsillitis. Note the bilateral enlargement and redness of the tonsils and the punctate white areas of purulent inflammation in the tonsillar crypts. (Courtesy of Dr. M. Hawke, Toronto)

therapy is curative.[38] This results in rapid improvement even, interestingly, in patients in whom cultures turn out to be negative. With the exception of cervical adenitis with abscess and peritonsillar abscess, significant complication is rare. There is no role for tonsillectomy in acute tonsillitis, except in the rare case of peritonsillar abscess that does not resolve with incision and drainage along with antibiotic therapy or for airway obstruction.

Interestingly in adults, *Mycoplasma pneumoniae* and chlamydia TWAR are isolated almost as frequently as beta-hemolytic streptococci.[25] This calls into question the usefulness of performing only a streptococcal culture or procedure to detect group A streptococcal antigen in patients in whom there is a suspicion of bacterial sore throat. Huovinen et al.[25] demonstrated a significant number of cases in which there were both viral and bacterial microbes present. Clearly, detection of beta-hemolytic streptococci alone is insufficient for making a thorough and complete assessment of the patient with presumed bacterial sore throat.

Penicillin continues to be the first-line antibiotic in acute tonsillitis due to GABHS[39] despite the fact that some streptococci resistant to this antibiotic have been isolated.[40] Recent studies indicate that cephalosporins are superior in treating acute tonsillitis resulting from GABHS,[41] but question whether the benefits cephalosporins offer are clinically relevant in the majority of cases.[42] Therefore, although cephalosporins and macrolides[43] offer some therapeutic advantage, first-line treatment with penicillin remains the standard in acute tonsillitis.

Recurrent tonsillitis (with multiple episodes per year) and chronic tonsillitis (prolonged tonsillar inflammation/infection unrelieved by antibiotic therapy), however are associated with the presence of a higher percentage of resistant organisms, including beta-lactamase–producing strains of both aerobic and anaerobic bacteria.[44] The pathogenicity of these organisms is related to their ability to both survive penicillin therapy and protect penicillin-susceptible pathogens from that drug. Therefore, chronic or recurrent tonsillitis treatment should commence with an antibiotic having a broader spectrum of activity and the ability to eradicate beta-lactamase–producing bacteria. The use of cephalosporins,[45] amoxicillin-clavulanate,[46] and clindamycin hydrochloride[47] have been shown to be superior to penicillin in this group of patients.

The lingual tonsils may be involved in disease processes that are similar to those affecting the palatine or pharyngeal tonsils.[48] The lingual tonsil may increase in size following repeated infections or may grow after palatine tonsillectomy. Patients may present with no symptoms or may complain of odynophagia, sore throat, and a lump in the throat. In acute lingual tonsillitis, ptyalism and "hot potato voice" may be present and progression of airway compromise can occur. Lateral soft tissue radiographs are useful to objectively document the soft tissue changes.[49] Treatment is the same as for palatine tonsillitis and may include antibiotics in addition to topical analgesia (Tantum oral rinse). Lingual tonsillectomy is occasionally indicated in cases of respiratory embarrassment and consists of a posterior-limited glossectomy.[50] This operation can be performed with electrocautery or $CO_2$-laser excision. Bleeding can be significant and must be meticulously controlled to protect the airway postoperatively,

Patients with chronic or recurrent tonsillitis unrelieved by antibiotic therapy are candidates for surgery.[51] Tonsillectomy versus prolonged or prophylactic antibiotic therapy is best recommended after careful consideration of each patient. Absolute indications for tonsillectomy are limited to the relief of airway obstruction and for excisional biopsy and treatment of tonsillar malignancy. There are no absolute indications for surgery in tonsillitis causing only sore throat.

Relative indications for tonsillectomy are extensive and include recurrent and chronic tonsillitis, halitosis, multiple antibiotic allergies, snoring, and recurrent peritonsillar abscess(es).[52] Clearly, the decision to undertake surgical treatment occurs after considering the impact of the symptoms on the patient and family and the morbidity and mortality associated with surgery. In general, tonsillectomy is safe and effective and postoperative morbidity is often no worse than an episode of acute tonsillitis.

An important variant of an acute streptococcal infection is scarlet fever. Here, the pharyngitis is accompanied by a rash which results from the production of an erythrogenic toxin.[37] This red punctate rash usually appears on the second day of the illness and spreads over the entire body within hours typically sparing the palms and the soles of the feet. It fades within 1 week. Another characteristic finding is that of strawberry tongue, which describes the swollen red and mottled appearance of an affected tongue. Treatment of this disease is with intravenous penicillin or a suitable substitute in patients allergic to penicillin. A scarlatiniform rash can also occur with *Corynebacterium hemolyticum*, a disease which closely resemble streptococcal pharyngitis but occurs in a slightly older patient population.[53] These bacteria are best diagnosed by identifying pleomorphic gram-positive bacilli on gram stain or by culturing the microbes on rabbit or human blood agar. The treatment is intramuscular benzathine penicillin G (one dose) or a course of oral erythromycin. The important feature of this disease is that it frequently remains undetected due to its fastidious growth requirements and therefore requires increased suspicion when diagnosing scarlatiniform rashes in teenagers and young adults.

Although uncommon since the availability of antibiotics, complications of streptococcal infections, including arthritis, heart disease, and glomerulonephritis, still exit. There has, in fact, been a recent re-emergence of acute rheumatic fever in parts of the United States[54] and, interestingly, these recent cases have affected patients who in the past would have been unlikely to acquire this disease. They include children of high- to middle-income parents with ready access to medical care and adults with no clinical history of streptococcal pharyngitis.[55] Fortunately, penicillin is still very effective in treating streptococcal pharyngitis, and aggressive treatment and prophylaxis of pharyngitis is recommended.[56]

Another common throat pathogen is *Hemophilus influenzae* type B, especially in children 2 to 5 years of age.[37] This encapsulated coccobacillary gram-negative organism can also cause illness in adults and is the most common cause of acute epiglottitis in all ages. Pharyngitis caused by this agent is similar to that caused by the Group A beta hemolytic streptococcus. Acute epiglottitis caused by *H influenzae* type B however is dramatically different and is characterized by the rapid onset of severe pharyngitis, high fever, marked dysphagia, and rapidly progressive airway obstruction. Clinically, a fiery red epiglottis is seen, and treatment centers around airway maintenance (eg, observation, intubation, or tracheotomy) and infusion of antibiotics.[57] Ampicillin and chloramphenicol have been widely used in the past to treat acute epiglottitis, but the incidence of beta-lactamase enzyme production by *H influenzae* in North America is now approximately 20% and traditional antibiotic therapy has become obsolete. In the place of the aminopenicillins, cefuroxime (a second generation cephalosporin) and ceftriaxone (a third generation cephalosporin) are now widely used as they are effective against beta-lactamase– producing bacteria and have good penetration into the cerebrospinal fluid.[58,59]

With the common use of Haemophilus influenzae b (Hb) vaccine, the incidence of acute epiglottitis in children has fallen dramatically although the adult incidence has remained the same.[60] Though similar to children in the rapidity of onset and severity of the pharyngeal symptoms, adults infrequently require airway intervention and often can be managed without intubation in hospital where they can be closely observed. The use of racemic epinephrine inhalation, heliox, and corticosteroids in addition to appropriate intravenous antibiotics is recommended in cases of adult epiglottitis managed with observation and no airway intervention.[61]

*S aureus* infection may also cause pharyngitis and is associated specifically with mucopurulence, mucosal edema, and severe erythema. Pustules in the tonsils are characteristic of this infection, but are common to all of the common pharyngeal pathogens. Another uncommon pharyngeal pathogen is *Neisseria gonorrhoeae* (gram-negative diplococcus) and if suspected it can be cultured on chocolate agar for definitive identification.[62] Effective treatment is penicillin or tetracycline. Some penicillinase-producing strains are sensitive to trimethoprim-sulfamethoxazole.[63]

In the past, *Corynebacterium* species had been a common cause of pharyngitis but in North America are exceedingly rare now. Unfortunately, the human disease caused primarily by *C diphtheriae* is still common in countries without vaccination programs. These gram-positive, nonfilamentous rods infect the pharyngeal surfaces and after a short incubation period (ie, 2 to 4 days) produce a severe infection with tissue necrosis secondary to exotoxin production.[64] This necrosis of the tonsillar mucosa results in the characteristic grayish membrane which covers the mucous membrane. Extension of the infection can cause progressive airway obstruction and inability to clear secretions. Antitoxin is the specific treatment while antibiotics (eg, penicillin, erythromycin) are used as adjuvant therapy in both infected patients and asymptomatic carriers.

Less commonly infection with *Treponema pallidum* in its primary, secondary, or tertiary phases can cause sore throat.[65] The primary chancre appearing 3 to 90 days after inoculation may present as a papule that later ulcerates causing pain. The tonsils are a commonly involved site.[66] In the secondary stage, cervical lymphadenopathy may accompany pharyngotonsillitis and painless gray mucosal patches may be seen in the oral cavity.[67] The treatment of syphilis is still penicillin. For those allergic to penicillin, tetracycline or erythromycin are effective alternatives.

## Fungal Infection

The immunocompetent host fungal infections causing sore throat are uncommon. In debilitated, diabetic, or immunocompromised patients, *Candida albicans* frequently produces symptomatic infection. Fungal infections can occur after prolonged treatment with inhalant steroid sprays in healthy patients with normal immunocompetence. This organism can invade pharyngeal mucosa and cause severe dysphagia and sore throat.[68] Typically, a creamy mucosal lesion is seen (Figure 6) and gram stain of the exudate shows budding yeast and pseudohyphae. Treatment with oral nystatin or ketoconazole along with acidification of the pharynx (eg, with dilute vinegar gargle) is appropriate for local disease. Amphotericin B is reserved for systemic infection. Other mycotic infections are exceptionally rare causes of sore throat.

## Granulomatous Diseases of the Head and Neck

For patients in whom sore throat fails to respond to appropriate antibiotic therapy, consideration must be given to granulomatous disease. Granulomas in the head and neck occur as chronic inflammatory responses defined histologically by the presence of macrophages surrounded by other inflammatory cells.[69] Coalescence results in giant cells. These granulomata form in response to foreign material and to specific micro-organisms, including mycobacterium, cat scratch bacillus, some fungi, *Treponema pallidum,* and *Actinomyces bovis.* Alternatively, they can occur in systemic diseases, such as sarcoidosis or Wegener's granulomatosis,[70] neoplasia, and Crohn's disease. In the pharynx, granulomatous sore throat will usually occur with accompanying adenopathy and possibly systemic manifestations. The diagnosis is based on the clinical findings and biopsy results. Causes of sore throat due to granulomatous tissue disease are shown in Table II.

## Connective Tissue Disease

Another uncommon cause of sore throat is connective tissue disease. This

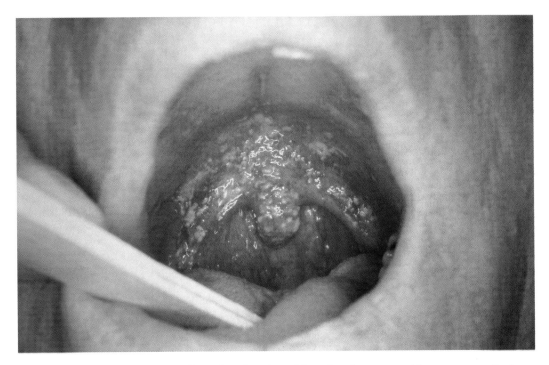

**Figure 6.** Monilial stomatitis. The soft palate is reddened and is covered by a creamy discharge containing *Candida albicans.* (Courtesy of Dr. M. Hawke, Toronto)

group of disorders has in common the inflammation of normal host tissue (often with altered immunologic characteristics) as a result of a systemic immunologic reaction. The most common connective tissue diseases resulting in sore throat are bullous diseases and even these diseases occur infrequently.

Pemphigus vulgaris and pemphigus

vegetans originate in the oral mucosa and produce vesicles and bullae which are characteristically friable and are easily abraded, revealing the underlying dermal tissue (ie, Nikolsky's sign).[71] This denuded layer is exceptionally painful and gives rise to the sore throat or mouth. The lesions typically show disruption at the dermal-epidermal junction. Autoantibodies (IgG directed towards the desmosomes) are demonstrable at this location[72] using immunohistochemical stains and immunofluorescence.[73] The treatment of these diseases includes systemic steroids and cyclophosphamide and the course varies greatly, from indolence to lethality.

In contrast, cicatricial pemphigoid is a benign vesiculobulous lesion predominantly affecting middle-aged women.[74] The lesions in this disease are typically less friable, though they also cause considerable pain until healed. Oral and conjunctival lesions are common, and treatment is symptomatic. Bullous pemphigoid, a disease of older patients, also occasionally

**Table II**
Granulomatous Disease Causing
Sore Throat

Tuberculosis
Leprosy
Parasitic Infection (*Leishmania brasiliensis, Toxoplasma gondii*)
Sarcoidosis
Wegener's Granulomatosis
Crohn's Disease
Malignancy (Hodgkin's, non-Hodgkin's lymphoma, metastases)

## Table III
### Connective Tissue Diseases Causing Sore Throat

Stevens-Johnson Syndrome
Keratosis Follicularis
Kawasaki Disease
Dyskeratosis Congenita
Pemphigus
Cicatricial Pemphigoid
Bullous Pemphigoid
Epidermolysis Bullosa
Dermatitis Herpetiformis
Acrodermatitis Enteropathica
Systemic Lupus Erythematosis
Scleroderma
Tangier's Disease
Sjögren's Syndrome

can present with oral lesions although this is far less common. Treatment is once again symptomatic only. Other causes of sore throat due to connective tissue disease are shown in Table III.

Autoimmune disease may also rarely cause sore throat. An exception is aphthous ulceration of the mouth and pharynx. These nontraumatic ulcers are more common in upper socioeconomic groups.[75] Their cause is unknown but several agents have been implicated, including viruses (eg, HSV), bacteria (eg, *Streptococcus sanguis*), hormonal or nutritional alterations, and stress. Evidence points to an autoimmune mechanism and autoantibodies to oral mucosal membranes have been identified that react to the prickle cell layer rather than the basal cell membrane. Alternatively, there may be a defect in the cell-mediated immune response, evidenced by an increased number of helper T cells and a decreased number of suppressor T cells.[76]

Three types of aphthous ulcers commonly occur: minor aphthous ulcers, major aphthous ulcers and herpetiform ulcers. Minor ulcers measure less than 1.0 cm in diameter and have well-demarcated erythematous halos. They are heralded by

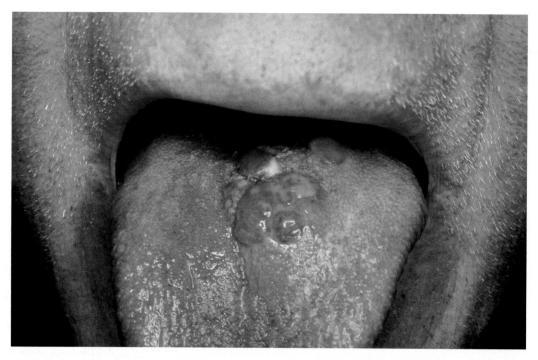

**Figure 7.** Carcinoma of the base of the tongue. These are metastatic lesions from a renal carcinoma. (Courtesy of Dr. J. L. Freeman, Toronto)

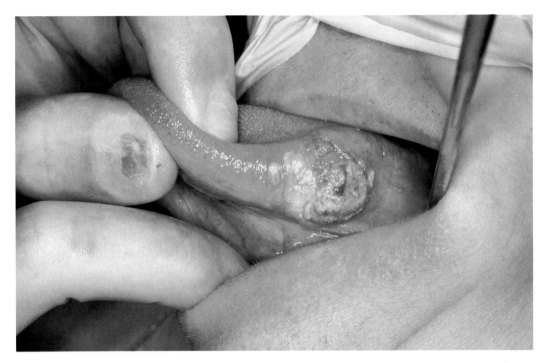

**Figure 8.** Carcinoma of the left posterior, lateral tongue margin. This area and the retromolar trigone are common sites for persistent sore throat. (Courtesy of Dr. J. L. Freeman, Toronto)

a burning sensation prior to eruption and last 7 to 10 days. Recurrence is highly variable. Major ulcers (eg, Sutton's disease) are much less common than minor ulcers but are more severe. They can be up to 3 cm in diameter and last from 6 weeks to several months. Herpetiform ulcers present as an exquisitely painful crop of 20 to 200 small ulcers of 1 to 3 mm in diameter. They differ from true herpetic lesions in that they have no vesicular stage and no HSV has been cultured from them. Treatment of aphthous ulcers consists of analgesia, topical steroids, and topical suspensions of tetracycline (200 mg/5 mL po q6h days). In severe major aphthous ulceration, systemic steroids are occasionally required.[77]

## Malignancy

Malignancy of the oral cavity and pharynx is unfortunately not an uncommon finding in patients presenting with sore throat. This is most exasperating in our North American society, where the risks of tobacco and alcohol consumption are well known and the relationship to aerodigestive tract malignancy is clearly documented. Epithelial cancer of the mouth and throat is predominantly squamous cell (Figure 7), although lymphoreticular lesions, mesenchymal tumors, and salivary gland malignancies also occur. Neoplasia causes symptoms by the disruption of normal oral and pharyngeal function (eg, dysphagia, speech abnormality) but usually only causes throat pain when there is mucosal ulceration. This occurs rarely with benign tumors which rarely present as "a sore throat." Common sites of malignancies causing pain are the floor of the mouth, lateral tongue (Figure 8), retromolar trigone, and tonsillar fossa (Figures 9A and 9B). Due to a shared sensory innervation, lesions of the base of the tongue, vallecula, larynx, and hypopharynx often present with throat pain radiating to the ear.

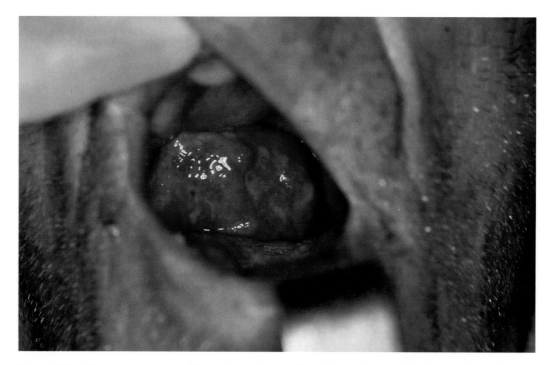

**Figure 9A.** A large squamous cell carcinoma has replaced the right tonsil and extends well across the midline to abut on the normal left tonsil. (Courtesy of Dr. I. J. Witterick, Toronto)

Although the outcome of malignancy of the upper aerodigestive tract is less than ideal, great gains in detection and reconstructive surgery have allowed aggressive surgical treatment to be carried out with the preservation of form and function.

### Gastroesophageal Reflux Disease

An increasingly diagnosed cause of sore throat is gastroesophageal reflux disease (GERD). Previously, patients with GERD with "globus" and chronic vague sore throat symptoms went undiagnosed or were treated symptomatically without success. This clinical disease has evolved, with our increasing understanding, into an extremely common disorder which now recognizably affects the throat causing pain.[10] The disorder results from incompetence at the lower esophageal sphincter secondary to increased intra-abdominal pressure due to excessive weight, de-

creased lower esophageal sphincter tone due to the chemical content of the stomach (eg, alcohol, coffee, chocolate) or diminished neuromuscular tone, and finally, increased gastric volume (possibly due to decreased gastric emptying). Though usually retrosternal, the pain may be present in the throat and may be the sole presenting complaint. Gastroesophageal reflux disease must be considered in those cases where sore throat is accompanied by the symptom of a foreign body sensation in the throat along with excessive throat clearing. The history is most helpful and includes throat pain in the morning often aggravated by alcohol ingestion or other dietary indiscretion in the previous 24 hours.

Relatively noninvasive investigatory options include dual-probe ambulatory 24-hour esophageal pH monitoring, barium swallow to document reflux, and esophageal manometry.[78] Ambulatory 24-hour pH monitoring is the diagnostic test with the highest sensitivity and specific-

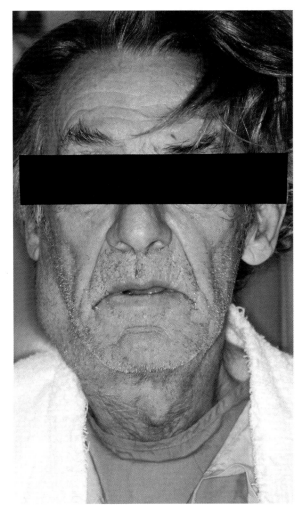

**Figure 9B.** The patient shown in figure 9A demonstrates an obviously enlarged cervical lymph node containing metastatic tumor. (Courtesy of Dr. I. J. Witterick, Toronto)

ity.[79] Direct laryngoscopy with a nasopharyngoscope is easily carried out in the office and if a reddened posterior larynx is visualized,[80] a trial of $H_2$ antagonist therapy, or proton pump inhibitor can obviate the need for further investigation.

Conservative therapy includes education, weight loss, elevation of the head of the bed, and the avoidance of the precipitating dietary components and habits (eg, late eating). This regimen usually relieves symptoms rapidly. $H_2$ antagonists or proton pump inhibitors also relieve symptoms although they have no effect on reflux itself but rather decrease the toxicity of the refluxed material. Prokinetic agents accelerate gastric emptying and increase tension in the lower esophageal sphincter.

## Sore Throat in Acquired Immunodeficiency Syndrome

The oral mucosa can be involved in acquired immunodeficiency syndrome (AIDS) with ulceration, pain, and secondary infection. The most common cause of

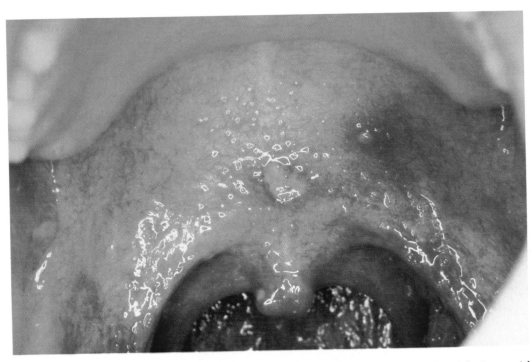

**Figure 10.** Aphthous stomatitis. Note the three white "punched out" superficial lesions with surrounding redness involving the tip of the uvula and the soft palate in the midline and right sides.

sore throat in these patients is mucosal candidiasis or thrush. The presentation and appearance is much the same as in the immunocompetent host.[81] The less common variants of mucosal thrush, the atrophic or chronic hypertrophic forms are also seen in this patient population. Although the diagnosis and initial therapy are the same as in the non–AIDS patient. Often in patients with AIDS, the initial therapy is ineffective and systemic antifungals may be required. Similarly, herpes infections can occur in immunosuppressed patients and tend to produce a more severe infection. Large ulcers form from coalescence of the smaller vesicles and result in huge denuded patches of oral or pharyngeal mucosa. Treatment with acyclovir may speed ulcer healing.[31] Aphthous ulcers (Figure 10), are also common in patients with AIDS and can be managed with intralesional steroid injections.[82]

The violaceous lesions of Kaposi's sarcoma are commonly present in the throat with a predilection for the hard palate (Figures 11A and 11B). Up to 40% of patients with the dermatologic manifestations of Kaposi's sarcoma have oral lesions as well.[83] The oral mucosal lesions are more resistant to radiotherapy than the skin lesions. The management is primarily palliative. Laser ablation and photodynamic therapy are treatment options.

Waldeyer's ring can be the source of sore throat resulting from the lymphadenopathy which often occurs in the course of AIDS infection. Tonsillar hypertrophy can develop with histopathologic follicular hyperplasia.[84] Lymphatic tissue may also ulcerate causing pain with non–Hodgkin's lymphoma, the second most common neoplasm associated with AIDS.[85] The tonsils are primarily affected, but the tongue or other oropharyngeal mucosa can be involved as well. The course of non–Hodgkin's lymphoma in patients with AIDS is more aggressive and is usually of a higher grade when compared with

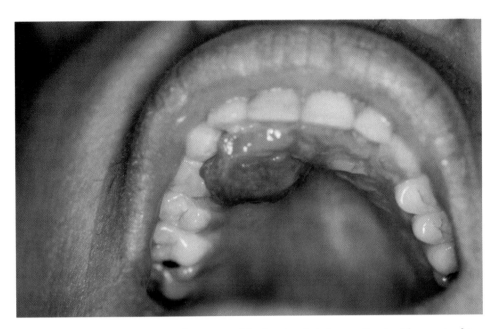

**Figure 11A.** Kaposi's sarcoma. Involvement of the hard palate in a patient with acquired immune deficiency syndrome (AIDS). Note the purple blue discoloration of this obvious lesion. (Courtesy of Dr. I. J. Witterick, Toronto)

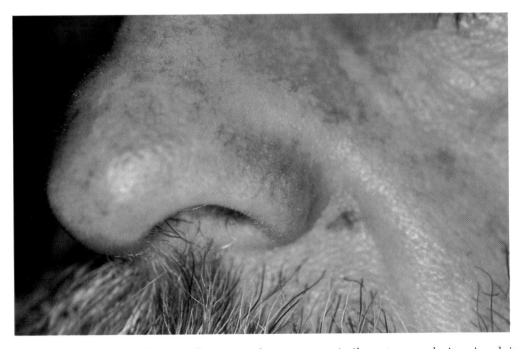

**Figure 11B.** The patient shown in figure 11A demonstrates similar cutaneous lesions involving the left upper lip and tip of the nose. The nasal lesion extends inward to involve the nasal vestibule.

that in patients without HIV infection. Although treatment with chemotherapy and occasionally radiotherapy is initially successful in controlling this disease, recurrence is common.

Hairy leukoplakia commonly develops in patients with HIV most likely related to infection with the Epstein-Barr virus. The probability of developing clinical AIDS is 50% at 16 months and up to 80% at 30 months after the first appearance of hairy leukoplakia.[86] Aggressive periodontal disease also commonly occurs in the course of HIV infection. The gingivitis that results is painful and leads to marked gingival recession. Despite the administration of oral antibiotics and diligent oral hygiene, the course of this periodontal disease remains progressive.[87]

## Irritative Sore Throat

Sore throat can occasionally present when no clear cause can be determined.

The irritative sore throat encompasses the vast majority of these cases. Often these patients present in the winter months when heating systems are used without appropriate humidification. Presentation in summer also occurs in patients who work in a controlled or air-conditioned environment. Symptoms are often worse in the morning when, after a night of mouth-breathing, the pharyngeal mucosa is dried (Figure 12). There are usually no signs on examination and importantly, there is absence of cervical adenopathy. Cultures show commensal flora only. Treatment is directed at modification of the environmental irritants including humidification, increasing the intake of water, and gargling with salt water. Recently, $H_2$-receptor antagonists have been used to give relief to patients with chronic irritative pharyngitis with an excellent response rate, possibly by treating underlying reflux.[88]

Tobacco smoke in the environment is a commonly cited irritant causing sore throat in addition to rhinitis, nasal ob-

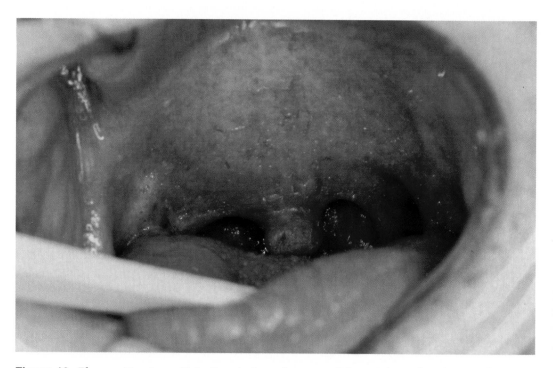

**Figure 12.** Pharyngitis sicca. Note the obvious dryness of the uvula, soft palate, and tongue. (Courtesy of Dr. M. Hawke, Toronto)

struction, and conjunctival irritation.[89] This response is not allergic as evidenced by the lack of increased histamine levels after smoke exposures nor is it mediated by kinins since there is no increase in the nasal concentration of these peptides after smoke exposure. Animal studies have demonstrated that the upper respiratory inflammatory response to tobacco smoke occurs through stimulation of chemosensitive C fiber neurons by the organic vapor-phase component of the smoke.[90] It is possible that tobacco smoke sensitivity represents an increased response to C fiber stimulation in some people.

Irritative sore throat can also occur following exposure to spiced foods, commercial mouth washes, throat astringents, and disinfectants.[91] Industrial solvents and particulate matter can also lead to irritative sore throat.[92, 93] Again the presentation is indistinguishable from inflammatory or infectious pharyngitis, but importantly, there is no adenopathy and cultures are negative for pathogens. Airway protection and work-space ventilation are usually helpful once the source of the problem has been identified. Contact pharyngitis can occur during caustic ingestion, thermal injury,[94] and as a result of mucosal trauma from a foreign body. Sore throat often follows endotracheal intubation,[95] pharyngeal suctioning,[96] and transesophageal echocardiography.[97] Mucosal ulceration from a dissolving lodged pill, such as acetylsalicylic acid, will produce exquisite pain.

## Conditions Causing Referred Sore Throat

Any structure that shares a common innervation with the pharynx can cause referred pain to the throat without oral findings. Although usually occurring with other findings, angina pectoris or pericarditis are serious conditions that can present with radiated pain to the throat. More commonly diseased structures in the central compartment of the neck, such as the trachea, thymus, mediastinum, or thyroid gland can present with throat pain. The throat pain that accompanies acute suppurative thyroiditis is usually associated with redness and swelling in the area of the gland.[98] The pain of laryngeal disease, can be referred to the throat, the ear, or both.

Eagle's syndrome is defined as the elongation of the styloid process or ossification of the stylohyoid ligament, causing recurrent nonspecific throat discomfort.[99] It is usually worsened when the head is turned towards the involved side. Positional dysphagia may be present. The only effective treatment is surgical shortening of the styloid process.

Infections of the deep fascial spaces of the neck can also present with throat pain. The retropharyngeal space is most commonly involved. This potential space lies behind the mucosa and the buccopharyngeal fascia and in front of the alar layer of the prevertebral fascia.[100] In children this space contains lymph nodes that can enlarge and suppurate secondary to infection in the nasal cavity, oropharynx, or vertebral bodies. The abscess can present after the primary infection has resolved, making the diagnosis more difficult. Although airway compromise is the usual presenting symptom, throat pain can occur in the absence of airway compromise. In patients with airway compromise or in those in whom treatment with intravenous antibiotics (eg, clindamycin or penicillin plus metronidazole) has failed, a computed tomography scan is used to identify and delineate an abscess.[101, 102] Surgical drainage is recommended for true abscesses,[103] while antibiotics and analgesia are successful for retropharyngeal cellulitis alone. Of interest, although retropharyngeal abscesses usually occur in the pediatric population, the incidence in the adult population is increasing[104] due to the increase of vertebral tuberculosis and other infections in immunocompromised patients (eg, AIDS, transplant recipients).

Infection of the parapharyngeal space more commonly causes trismus but can present with pain referable to the tonsil or posterior pharyngeal wall. As well, malignant parotid neoplasms (eg, adenoid cystic carcinoma) and other benign lesions in this space (eg, schwannoma) can produce throat discomfort secondary to nerve involvement.

## Diagnostic Approach to the Sore Throat

Based on the frequency with which it occurs, the treatment of pharyngitis should presumably be straightforward. This is not the case since there is still considerable disagreement regarding methods of diagnosis and treatment for the sore throat.[105] Treatment ranges from empiric antibiotics for all patients to obtaining cultures in all patients and reserving treatment for those in whom there is a specific bacterial agent identified. On the one hand, treating all patients with antibiotics is costly, often needless, and requires patient compliance for therapeutic effect. On the other hand, routine culture, administering rapid latex agglutination antigen tests (which range in sensitivity from 55% to 75%), or enzyme-linked immunosorbent assay (ELISA) diminishes the morbidity of antibiotic administration but adds considerable cost to the diagnostic process.[106] Even with tests, such as the optical immunoassay,[107] offering higher sensitivity (97%) and specificity (95%) for the detection of group A streptococcal carbohydrate antigen, routine testing is of questionable value as a first-line measure because of the considerable variation in the spectrum of the causative infectious agents.[25, 108] Since there is no single diagnostic maneuver available, even in the presumably "simple" acute sore throat, some degree of judgement must be exercised in deciding what tests to order and when to order them (Table IV).

Importantly, the temporal course of the sore throat must be determined. Sore throat of less than 2 weeks duration is an acute problem and those lasting longer than 6 weeks represent a chronic condition. The temporal characteristics of the sore throat in addition to the context in which the patient presents (eg, recent immunosuppression, radiation, exposure to

**Table IV**
**Investigations Available in Sore Throat**

General
  Cultures and sensitivity (with specific media where appropriate—eg, chocolate agar)
  Gram's stain, methylene blue stains (gonorrhea)
  Viral cultures
Routine Blood Tests
  CBC, ESR
  Blood smear (mononucleosis)
Urine
  CMV (urine culture and serology)
Serologic Tests
  VDRL, RPR, FTA-ABS for syphillis
  Immunoelectrophoresis (Epstein-Barr virus)
  Antigen titre (Epstein-Barr virus, other viral)
Immunohistochemistry
  ELISA (HSV, HIV)
Molecular Biologic Methods
  Polymerase chain reaction (HPV subtypes, HSV)
Radiologic
  Lateral neck film (epiglottitis)
  Barium swallow (GERD), ± a modified barium swallow
Biopsy
  Incisional, fine-needle aspiration
  Excisional
Special Tests
  Dick test (scarlet fever)
  24-hour dual-probe pH monitoring (GERD)

CBC = complete blood cell; CMV = cytomegolovirus; ELISA = enzyme-linked immunosorbent assay; ESR = erythrocyte sedimentation rate; FTA-ABS = fluorescent treponemal antibody absorption; GERD = gastroesophageal reflux disease; HIV = human immunodeficiency virus; HPV = human papillomavirus; HSV = herpes simplex virus; RPR = rapid plasma reagin test.

sick family members) are helpful diagnostic aids.

The sore throat of short duration with a clear history of infection and confirmatory physical findings is initially treated with symptomatic and supportive therapy. This consists of analgesics and antiinflammatory agents such as aspirin or acetaminophen. Salt-water rinses, anaesthetic gargles (4% xylocaine or Tantum oral rinse), and lozenges (containing benzocaine) can be used to relieve discomfort.[2] Antibiotics are added if bacterial infection is present. The clinical features suggestive of bacterial pharyngitis include fever, intense sore throat, exudate, tender adenopathy, an elevated white blood cell count, and possibly a scarlatiniform rash. In doubtful cases, a throat swab, latex agglutination antigen testing, ELISA for GABHS, viral serology can be carried out while antibiotics are withheld pending test results or until the patient shows evidence of bacterial infection. After an appropriate history is taken and a physical examination is carried out, further management will depend upon the oropharyngeal findings.

The possible physical findings include mucosal ulceration, violaceous lesions, exudate, vesicles, erythema, or no findings. For each of these categories, a suggested management approach can be undertaken (Figure 13).

In patients with a persistent or acute sore throat without physical findings (Figure 14), the presence of dysphagia is important. If dysphagia is present, flexible nasopharyngoscopy is carried out in the office with topical analgesia. This allows visualization of all parts of the upper aerodigestive tract including the hypopharynx[80] and larynx. Redness of the posterior larynx suggests reflux, which can be confirmed by dual-probe 24-hour pH monitoring.[79] Modification of diet and treatment with antacids, $H_2$ antagonists or proton pump inhibitor can be initiated. The barium swallow with or without a cine study and esophageal manometry are still useful in evaluating motility disorders which can occasionally present as "a sore throat." Those patients who do not respond rapidly and completely with conservative antireflux, antispasmodic, and antacid therapy require esophagoscopy.

At endoscopy, if white lesions are present, *Candida* species infection is suspected and scrapings are obtained for culture. If these are confirmatory, topical antifungal suspensions or lozenges are initiated. Systemic treatment may be required for severe esophageal candidiasis when pain prevents oral nutritional and fluid intake. If the white lesion is not felt to be candidial, a biopsy is taken.

If no abnormalities are identified on examination or with invasive testing, psychogenic causes of "globus hystericus" are considered. Empiric antacid treatment may still be used while the patient is being followed.

In cases where there is no symptom of dysphagia or abnormal physical findings on examination, environmental irritants and allergy should be considered, investigated, and treated. A therapeutic trial of antihistamines, or avoidance of the aggravating environmental factor, be it dust or dairy product, is prescribed along with improved humidification. If improvement is not forthcoming, then referred pain, be it from the cervical spine, teeth, thyroid gland, esophagus, heart, mediastinum, or stylohyoid ligament, is investigated further.

Mucosal ulceration or ulcerations will alter the management (Figure 15). Upon initial evaluation, the lesion or lesions are cultured, and serology is requested if indicated. At the same time, an assessment of the dentures and dentition is carried out to exclude mechanical ulceration. Dentition and dental hygiene must be evaluated, especially when partial dentures or prosthetics are used. Commonly, patients present without their dental prosthetics owing to ill fit or pain. Similarly, alcohol and tobacco abuse in addition to dietary habits (eg, beetlenut, snuff, spicy foods) must be considered.

Superinfection should be treated prior to confirming a diagnosis, although for obvious malignancy, a biopsy can be done initially. A 10-day course of antibiotics can be initiated along with symptomatic and supportive therapy. Follow-up is critical since the antibiotic is used only to facilitate further evaluation. The small number who improve should be followed. In patients with continued mucosal ulceration, a biopsy of the ulcer with a margin of normal tissue is taken and assessed histologically and microbiologically. The next phase of treatment depends on the pathology, but ongoing supportive therapy should continue.

If granulomata are identified, a systemic evaluation is undertaken in consul-

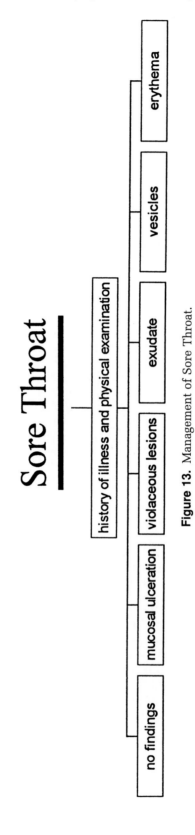

**Figure 13.** Management of Sore Throat.

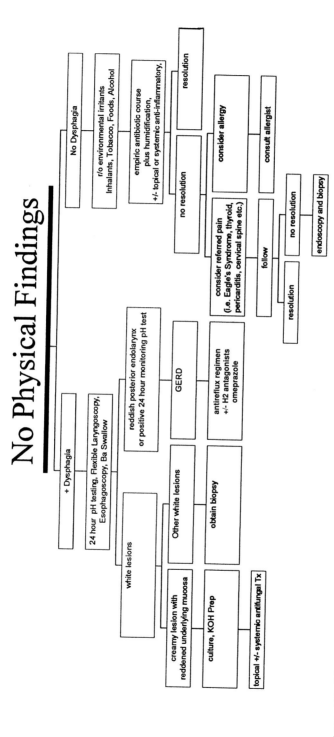

**Figure 14.** Management of Sore Throat: No Physical Findings. Ba = Barium; GERD = gastroesophageal reflux disease; KOH = potassium hydroxide; Tx = treatment.

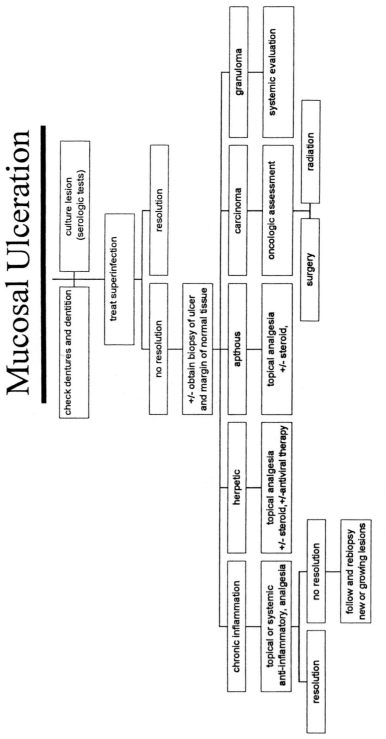

**Figure 15.** Management of Sore Throat: Mucosal Ulceration.

# Violaceous Lesions

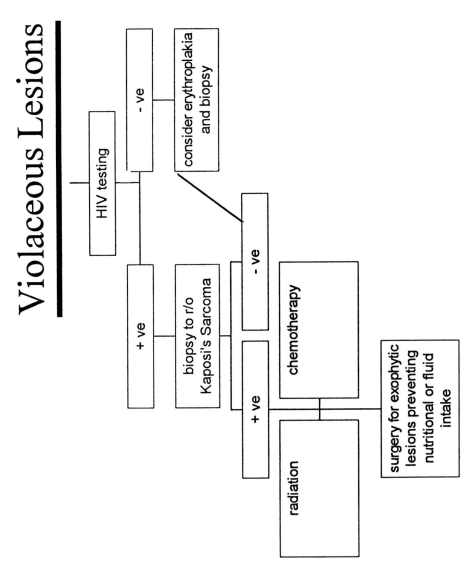

**Figure 16.** Management of Sore Throat: Violaceous Lesions. +ve = positive; −ve = negative; HIV = human immunodeficiency virus.

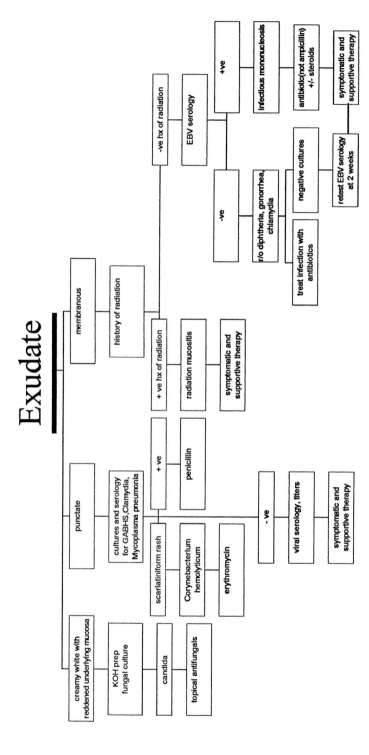

**Figure 17.** Management of Sore Throat: Exudate. +ve = positive; −ve = negative; EBV = Epstein-Barr virus; GABHS = Group A beta-hemolytic *Streptococcus*; hx = history; KOH = potassium hydroxide.

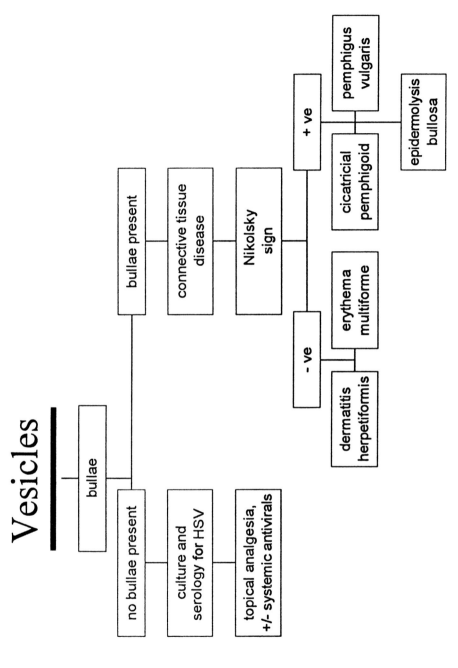

**Figure 18.** Management of Sore Throat: Vesicles. +ve = positive; −ve = negative; HSV = herpes simplex virus.

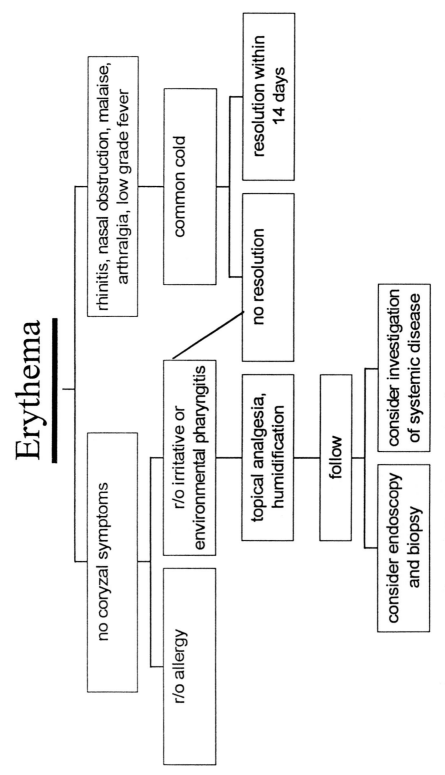

**Figure 19.** Management of Sore Throat: Erythema.

tation with an infectious disease specialist, rheumatologist, or respirologist. Further biopsies of the nose in Wegener's granuloma, of the mouth in Sjogren's syndrome, or of the lymph nodes in patients with sarcoidosis may be required.

Carcinoma of the upper aerodigestive tract is treated with surgery, radiation, or a combination of the two. The treatment of malignant lymphoma will depend upon the staging of the disease.

Aphthous ulcers are often diagnosed without a biopsy and are treated symptomatically with topical analgesics and topical and occasional intralesional steroids. Herpetic ulcers are also managed symptomatically with the addition of topical or systemic antiviral therapy for severe cases or for immunocompromised patients.

A histologic diagnosis of chronic nonspecific inflammation presents a not uncommon dilemma. Such patients are managed with symptomatic treatment, close observation, and repeat biopsy. Despite a negative biopsy a malignancy is suspected while symptoms persist.

The violaceous lesion (Figure 16) is evaluated initially by establishing the HIV status of the patient. Biopsy to confirm Kaposi's sarcoma may be helpful in treatment planning. Surgical excision or debulking is rarely necessary unless the lesion is interfering with oral intake. Cases in which there is a negative HIV status still require biopsy to exclude erythroplakia, which usually progresses to frank carcinoma. Vascular malformations can appear violaceous, but are rarely painful.

Pharyngeal exudates can be membranous, punctate, or creamy (Figure 17). Membranous exudates often occur after radiation and are treated symptomatically. If severe, hospitalization may be required for hydration and nutrition. Infectious mononucleosis is the most common cause of sore throat with membranous exudate. Serologic tests should be carried out in addition to treatment of the bacterial superinfection, which is commonly present. Oral or parenteral steroids may be required if tonsillar hypertrophy is massive. Negative serology for Epstein-Barr virus requires testing for other common pharyngeal pathogens, but in most cases retest at a later date yields positive serology for mononucleosis. Treatment of other confirmed pathogens, such as diphtheria, streptococcal pharyngitis, Vincent's angina, and gonorrhea, necessitates antibiotic therapy tailored to eradicate the specific infection.

Punctate exudate is most commonly bacterial and is caused by *M pneumonia*, *C hemolyticum* or chlamydia. Although viral agents may be implicated, a creamy white exudate is strongly suggestive of candidal infection. Fungal culture and a potassium hydroxide preparation can be performed and treatment consists of topical, and/or oral antifungal agents and acidification.

Vesicular lesions in patients's with sore throat (Figure 18) are subdivided initially by the presence or absence of bullae. If bullae are present, connective tissue disease is suspected and the presence or absence of Nikolsky's sign further subdivides the causes. Pemphigus is treated with steroids. If there are no bullae, the possibility of early HSV infection should be considered. These crops of lesions typically burst soon in the course of the infection, leaving ulcers that are quite painful. Management has been discussed above with the other ulcerative causes of sore throat.

Pharyngeal erythema (Figure 19) associated with coryzal symptoms is a common manifestation of the common cold and is treated symptomatically. If, however, the erythema persists, follow-up and consideration of irritative or allergic pharyngitis must be considered, investigated, and treated. Pharyngeal erythema, if marked and not associated with coryza, may also be of viral or bacterial origin. Finally persistent erythema may be a manifestation of an underlying systemic disease and should be managed as such.

## References

1. Mandel JH. Pharyngeal infections: causes findings and management. Postgrad Med 1985; 77:187–193, 196–199.

2. Jackler RK, Kaplan MJ. Sore throat. In: Tierney LM, McPhee SJ, Papadakis MA, eds. *Current Medical Therapy*. Norwalk, Conn: Appleton and Lange; 1995.

3. Proud D, Reynolds CJ, Lacapra S, et al. Nasal provocation with bradykinin induces symptoms of rhinitis and a sore throat. Am Rev Respir Dis 1988; 137: 613–616.

4. Hollingshead WH. *Anatomy for Surgeons, Vol. 1*. 3rd ed. New York, NY: Harper and Row Publishers; 1982.

5. Cunningham DJ. Romanes GJ, ed. *Manual of Practical Anatomy, Vol. 3*. 15th ed. New York: Oxford University Press; 1986.

6. Hermanek P, Sobin LH, eds). *TNM Classification of Malignant Tumours*. New York, NY: Springer-Verlag; 1987.

7. Bloom W, Fawcett DW. *A Textbook of Histology*. 10th ed. Philadelphia, Pa: W B Saunders Company; 1975.

8. Brodsky L, Moore L, Stanievich JF, et al. The immunology of tonsils in children: The effects of bacterial load on the presence of B and T cell subsets. Laryngoscope 1988;98:93–98.

9. Paonessa DF, Goldstein JC. Anatomy and physiology of head and neck infections (with emphasis on the fascia of the face and neck). Otolaryngol Clin North Am 1976;9:561–580.

10. Mendelsohn M. New concepts in dysphagia management. J Otolaryngol Suppl. 1993;22:5–24.

11. Dantas RO, Dodds WJ, Massey BT, et al. Manometric characteristics of the glossopalatal sphincter. Dig Dis Sci 1990;35: 161.

12. Shawker TH, Sonies B, Stone M, et al. Real time ultrasound visualization of tongue movement during swallowing. J Clin Ultras 1983;11:485–490.

13. Jacob P, Kahrilas P, Logemann J, et al. Upper esophageal sphincter opening and modulation during swallowing. Gastroenterology 1989;97:1469–1478.

14. Fink R, Demarest R. *Laryngeal Biomechanics*. Cambridge Ma: Harvard University Press

15. Brancatisano A, Engel LA. Role of the upper airway in the control of respiratory flow and lung volume in humans. In: Mathew OP, Sant'Ambrogio G, eds. *Respiratory Function of the Upper Airway*. New York, NY: Marcel Dekker; 1988.

16. Krespi YP, Pearlman SJ, Keidar A. Laser-assisted uvula-palatoplasty for snoring. J Otolaryngol 1994; 23:328–334.

17. Aronson AE. Anatomy and physiology of phonation. In: *Clinical Voice Disorders*. New York, NY: George Thieme; 1990

18. Hirano M. Morphological structure of the vocal cord as a vibrator and its variations. Folia Phoniatrica. 1974;26:89–94.

19. Blom ED, Singer MI, Hamaker RC. Tracheastoma valve for post-laryngectomy voice rehabilitation. Ann Otol Rhinol Laryngol 1982;91:576–578.

20. Piffko P, Koteles GJ, Antoni F. Biochemical properties of tonsillar lymphocytes. Pract Oto-Rhino-Laryngol 1970;32: 350–355.

21. Richtsmeier WJ, Shikhani AH. The physiology and immunology of pharyngeal lymphoid tissue, Otolaryngol Clin North Am 1987;20:219–228.

22. Siegel G. Theorectical and clinical aspects of the tonsillar function. Int J Pediatr Otorhinolaryngol 1983;6:61–75.

23. Brodsky L. Tonsillitis, tonsillectomy, and adenoidectomy. In: Bailey BJ, ed. *Head and Neck Surgery—Otolaryngology*. Philadelphia, Pa: J.B. Lippincott Co; 1993.

24. Schachtel BP, Fillingim JM, Beiter DJ, et al. Subjective and objective features of sore throat. Arch Intern Med 1984; 144: 497–500.

25. Huovinen P, Lahtonen R, Ziegler T, et al. Pharyngitis in adults: The presence and coexistence of viruses and bacterial organisms. Ann Intern Med 1989;110: 612–616.

26. Proud D, Naclerio RM, Gwaltney JM, et al. Kinins are generated in nasal secretions during natural rhinovirus colds. J Infect Dis 1990;161:120–123.

27. Naclerio RM, Proud D, Lichtenstein LM, et al. Kinins are generated during experimental rhinovirus colds. J Infect Dis 1988; 157:133–142.

28. Tyrell DA. Some advances in the diagnosis of respiratory virus infections. J Roy Coll Phys (London) 1987;21:210–213.

29. Irwin RS, Hollingsworth HM. The upper respiratory tract. In: Bone RC, Dantzker DR, George RB, Matthay RA, Reynolds HY, eds. *Pulmonary and Critical Care Medicine. Vol. 1*. Chicago, Ill: Mosby Year Book Inc; 1992:1–28.

30. Evans AS. *Viral Infections in Humans, Epidemiology and Control*. 3rd edition. New York, NY: Plenum Medical Book Company: 1989.

31. Wade JC. Day LM. Crowley JJ. et al. Recurrent infection with herpes simplex virus after marrow transplantation: role of spe-

cific immune response and acyclovir treatment. J Infect Dis 1984;149:750–756.

32. Epstein JB, Sherlock C, Page JL, et al. Clinical study of herpes simplex virus infection in leukemia. Oral Surg Oral Med Oral Pathol 1991; 70:38–43.

33. Brown NA. The Epstein-Barr virus (infectious mononucleosis, B-lymphoproliferative disorders). In: Feigin RD, Cherry JD, eds. *Textbook of Pediatric Infectious Diseases.* Philadelphia, Pa: W B Saunders Company; 1987: 1566–1577.

34. Hanshaw JB. Cytomegalovirus infections. In: Feigin RD, Cherry JD, Eds. *Textbook of Pediatric Infectious Diseases.* Philadelphia, Pa: W B Saunders Company; 1987.

35. Isenhower D, Schleuning AJ III. Otolaryngologic manifestations of systemic disease. In: Paparella MM, Shumrick DA, Gluckman JL, Meyerhoff WL, eds. *Otolaryngology.* 3rd ed. Philadelphia, Pa: W B Saunders Company: 1991.

36. Brook I. The clinical microbiology of Waldeyer's ring. Otolaryngol Clin North Am 1982; 20:259–272 .

37. Cherry JD. Pharyngitis. In: Feigin RD, Cherry JD, Eds. *Textbook of Pediatric Infectious Diseases.* Philadelphia, Pa: W B Saunders Company; 1987.

38. Klein JO. Management of streptococcal pharyngitis. Ped Inf Dis 1994;13:572–575.

39. Markowitz M, Gerber MA, Kaplan EL. Treatment of streptococcal pharyngotonsillitis: reports of penicillin's demise are premature. J Pediatr 1993;123:679–685.

40. Stjernquist-Desatnik A, Orrling A, Schalen C, et al. Pencillin tolerance in group A streptococci and treatment failure in streptococcal tonsillitis. Acta Otolaryngol Suppl (Stockh) 1992;492:68–71.

41. Disney FA, Dillon H, Blumer JL, et al. Cephalexin and penicillin in the treatment of group A beta-hemolytic streptococcal throat infections. Am J Dis Child 1992;146:1324–1327.

42. Pichichero ME. Cephalosporins are superior to penicillin for treatment of streptococcal tonsillopharyngitis: is the difference worth it? Pediatr Infec Dis J 1993; 12(4):268–274.

43. Hamill J. Multicentre evaluation of azithromycin and penicillin V in the treatment of acute streptococcal pharyngitis and tonsillitis in children. J Antimicrob Chemother 1993; 31(Suppl E):89–94.

44. Brook I. Penicillin failure and copathogenicity in streptococcal pharyngotonsillitis. J Fam Pract 1994;38:175–179.

45. Pichichero ME. The rising incidence of penicillin treatment failures in group A streptococcal tonsillopharyngitis: an emerging role for the cephosporins?. Pediatr Infect Dis J 1991;10 (10 Suppl): S50–55.

46. Argen K, Lundberg C, Nord CE. Effect of amoxicillin/clavulanic acid on the aerobic and anaerobic tonsillar microflora in the treatment of recurrent tonsillitis. Scand J Infect Dis 1990;22(6):691–697.

47. Jensen JH. Larsen SB. Treatment of recurrent acute tonsillitis with clindamycin. An alternative to tonsillectomy? Clin Otolaryngol 1991;16:498–500.

48. Ballenger JJ. *Diseases of the Nose, Throat, Ear, Head and Neck.* 14th ed. 1991.

49. Willatt D, Youngs R. The value of soft-tissue radiography in the assessment and treatment of lingular tonsillar hypertrophy. J Laryngol 1984;98:1217–1219.

50. Kornblut AD. Non-neoplastic diseases of the tonsils and adenoids. In: Paparella MM, Shumrick DA, Gluckman JL, Meyerhoff WL, eds. *Otolaryngology.* 3rd ed. Philadelphia, Pa: W B Saunders; 1991.

51. Paradise LJ, Bluestone CD, Bachman RZ, et al. Efficacy of tonsillectomy for recurrent throat infections in severely affected children: results of a parallel randomized and non-randomized clinical trials. N Engl J Med 1984;310:674.

52. Paradise JL. Tonsillectomy and adenoidectomy. In Bluestone CD, Stool SE, eds. Pediatric Otolaryngology. Philadelphia, Pa: W B Saunders Company; 1990: 915.

53. Miller RA, Brancato F, Holmes KK. *Corynebacterium hemolyticum* as a cause of pharyngitis and scarlatiniform rash in young adults. Ann Intern Med 1986;105: 867–872.

54. Congeni BL. The resurgence of acute rheumatic fever in the United States. Pediadr Ann 1992;21:816–820.

55. Ayoub EM. Resurgence of rheumatic fever in the United States. The changing picture of a preventable illness. Postgrad Med 1992;92:133–136, 139–42.

56. Sergent JS. Acute rheumatic fever. Transactions of the American Clinical & Climatological Association 1992;104:15–23, (discussion) 23–25.

57. Andreassen UK, Baer S, Nielsen TG, et al. Acute epiglottitis—25 years experience with nasotracheal intubation, current management policy and future trends. J Laryngol Otol 1992;106(12):1072–1075.

58. Justo RN, Masters IB. Towards short

course single daily dose ceftriaxone in epiglottis. Pediatr Infect Dis J 1992;10: 477.

59. Crysdale WS, Sendi K. Evolution in the management of acute epiglottis: A 10-year experience with 242 children. International Anesthesiology Clinics 1988;26: 32–38.

60. Frantz TD, Rasgon BM. Acute epiglottitis: changing epidemiologic patterns. Otolaryngol Head Neck Surg 1993;109: 457–460.

61. Shih L, Hawkins DB, Stanley RB. Acute epiglottitis in adults: A review of 48 cases. Annals Otol Rhinol Laryngol 1988;97: 527–529.

62. Tice AW, Rodriguez VL. Pharyngeal gonorrhea. JAMA 1981;246:2717–2719.

63. Washington AE. Update on treatment recomendations for gonococcal infections. Rev Infect Dis 1982;4:S758.

64. Feigin RD, Stechenberg BW. Diptheria. In: Feigin RD, Cherry JD, eds. Textbook of Pediatric Infectious Diseases. Philadelphia, Pa: W B Saunders Company; 1987.

65. Martinez SA, Mouney DF. Treponemal infections of the head and neck. Otolaryngol Clin North Am 1982;15:613–620.

66. Fiumara NJ, Walker EA. Primary syphillis of the tonsil. Arch Otolaryngol 1982;108: 43–44.

67. Harstock RJ, Halling LW, King FM. Luetic lymphadenitis. A clinical and histologic study of 20 cases. Am J Clin Pathol 1970; 53:304–314.

68. Zegarelli DJ. Fungal infections of the oral cavity. Otolaryngol Clin North Am 1993; 26:1069–1090.

69. Batsakis JG. Pathology of tumors of the oral cavity. In: Thawley SE, et al., eds. Comprehensive Management of Head and Neck Tumors. Philadelphia, Pa: W B Saunders Company; 1987: 480.

70. Kornblut AD, Wolff SM, deFries HO, et al. Wegener's granulomatosis. Otolaryngol Clin North Am 1982;15:673–683.

71. Bernier LJ, Tiecke RW. Pemphigus. J Oral Surg 1951;9:253.

72. Shklar G, Cataldo E. Histopathology and cytology of oral lesions of pemphigus. Arch Dermatol 1970;101:635.

73. Daniels TE, Quadra-White C. Direct immunoflorescence in oral mucosal disease. A diagnostic anaysis of 130 cases. Oral Surg Oral Med Oral Path 1981;51:38–47.

74. Person JR, Rogers RS III. Bullous and cicatricial pemphigoid. Clinical, histological, and immunological correlations. Mayo Clin Proc 1977;52:54.

75. Regezi JA, Sciubba JJ. Oral Pathology: Clinical Pathologic Correlations. Philadelphia, Pa: W B Saunders Company; 1989.

76. Landesberg R, Fallon M, Insel R. Alterations of T helper/inducer and T suppressor/inducer cells in patients with recurrent apthous ulcers. Oral Surg Oral Med Oral Pathol 1990;69:205–208.

77. Birt BD, From L, Main J. Diagnosis and management of long-standing benign oral ulceration. Laryngoscope 1980;90: 758–768.

78. Bremner RM, Bremner CG, DeMeester TR. Gastroesophageal reflux: The use of pH monitoring. Curr Prob Surg 1995;32: 429–568.

79. Koufman JA, Wiener GJ, Wu WC, et al. Reflux laryngitis and its sequelae: The diagnostic role of ambulatory 24-hour pH monitoring. J Voice 1988;2:78–89.

80. Lorenz R, Jorysz G, Clasen M. The globus syndrome: value of flexible endoscopy of the upper gastrointestinal tract. J Laryngol Otol 1993;107:535–537.

81. Marcusen DC, Sooy CD. Otolaryngologic manifestations of acquired immunodeficiency syndrome. Laryngoscope 1985;95: 401–405.

82. Liang GS, Daikos GL, Serfling U, et al. An evaluation of oral ulcers in patients with AIDS and AIDS-related complex. J Am Acad Dermatol 1993;29:563–568.

83. Patow CA, Steis R, Longo DL, et al. Kaposi's sarcoma of the head and neck in the acquired immune deficiency syndrome. Otolaryngol Head Neck Surg 1984;92:255–260.

84. Kraus DH, Rehm SJ, Orlowski JP, et al. Upper airway obstruction due to tonsillar lymphadenopathy in human immunodeficiency virus infection. Arch Otolaryngol Head Neck Surg 1990;116:738–740.

85. Rosenberg RA, Schneider KL, Cohen NL. Head and neck presentations of acquired immunodeficiency syndrome. Laryngoscope 1984;94:642–646.

86. Tami TA, Lee KC. Manifestations of the acquired immunodeficiency syndrome. In: Bailey BJ, ed. Head and Neck Surgery—Otolaryngology. Philadelphia, Pa: J B Lippincott Co; 1993.

87. Rutherford GW, Lifson AR, Hessol NA, et al. Course of HIV-1 infection in a cohort of homosexual and bisexual men: and 11

year follow-up study. Br Med J 1990;301: 1183–1188.

88. Zaidi SH. A study of H2 receptor antagonists in the treatment of chronic intractable pharyngitis. Pakistan Med Assoc 1990;40:217–219.

89. Bascom R, Kulle T, Kagey-Sobotka A, et al. Upper respiratory tract environmental tobacco smoke sensitivity. Am Rev Respir Dis 1991;143:1304–1311.

90. Lundblad L, Lundberg JM. Capsaicin sensitive sensory neurons mediate the response to nasal irritation induced by the vapour phase of cigarette smoke. Toxicology 1984;33:1–7.

91. Wenig B, Kornblut AD. Pharyngitis In: Bailey BJ, ed. *Head and Neck Surgery—Otolaryngology*. Philadelphia, Pa: J B Lippincott Co; 1993.

92. Kowalska S, Sulkowski W, Bazydlo-Golinska G. Diseases of the upper respiratory tract in furniture industry workers. Medycyna Pracy 1990;41:137–141.

93. Sesline D, Ames RG, Howd RA. Irritative and systemic symptoms following exposure to Microban disinfectant through a school ventilation system. Arch Environ Health 1994;46:439–444.

94. Riccio JC, Abbott J. A simple sore throat? Retropharyngeal emphysema secondary to free-basing cocaine. J Emerg Med 1990; 8:709–712.

95. Christensen AM, Willemoes-Larsen H, Lundby L, et al. Postoperative throat complaints after tracheal intubation. Br J Anaes 1994;73:786–787.

96. Fuller J, Lu G, Dain S. The contribution of pharyngeal suction devices to sore throat after endotracheal anaesthesia. Can J Anesth 1990;37:S157.

97. Owall A, Stahl L, Settergren G. Incidence of sore throat and patient complaints after intraoperative transesophageal echocardiography during cardiac surgery. J Cardiothorac Vasc Anesth 1992;6:15–16.

98. Strakosch CR. Thyroiditis. Aust N Z J Med 1986;16:91–100.

99. Baugh RF, Stocks RM. Eagle's syndrome: a reappraisal. Ear Nose Throat 1993;72: 341–344.

100. Grodinski, Holyoke. Am J Anat 1938;63: 367–408.

101. Lazor JB, Cunningham MJ, Eavey RD, et al. Comparison of computed tomography and surgical findings in deep neck infections. Otolaryngol Head Neck Surg 1994; 111:746–750.

102. Ravindranath T, Janakiraman N, Harris V. Computed tomography in diagnosing retropharyngeal abscess in children. Clin Pediatr 1993;32:242–244.

103. Levitt GW. Cervical fascia and deep neck space infections, Otolaryngol Clin North Am 1976;9:703–716.

104. Har-El G, Aroesty JH, Shaha A, et al. Changing trends in deep neck abscess. A retrospective study of 110 patients. Oral Surg Oral Med Oral Path 1994;77: 446–450.

105. Del Mar C. Managing sore throat: a literature review. I. Making the diagnosis. Med J Australia 1992;156:572–575.

106. Tunik MG, Fierman AH, Dreyer BP, et al. Latex agglutination for the rapid detection of streptoccocal pharyngitis: Use by housestaff in a pediatric emergency service. Pediatr Emerg Care 1990;6:93–95.

107. Harbeck RJ. Novel, rapid optical immunoassay technique for detection of group A streptococci from pharyngeal specimens: Comparison with standard culture methods. J Clin Microbiol 1993;31:839–844.

108. Timon CI, McAllister VA, Walsh M, et al. Changes in bacteriology of recurrent acute tonsillitis: 1980 vs. 1989. Resp Med 1990; 84:395–400.

# 12

# Halitosis

Lipa Bodner, D.M.D.
Dan M. Fliss, M.D.
David R. Goldfarb, B.SC., M.D.
Arnold M. Noyek, M.D.

## Introduction

Halitosis (ie, bad breath, oral malodor, fetor ex ore, fetor oris) is a general term for unpleasant breath arising from oral and systemic sources, associated with pathologic or nonpathologic causes. The principal underlying reason for the occurrence of halitosis in different individuals is usually related to one specific source. However, as the halitus (ie, expired breath) is emitted through the oral cavity, it is blended with malodor emerging from the oral cavity. Thus, the oral malodor is a contributing or frequently dominant component of halitosis.

Halitosis is a common complaint that may periodically affect most of the adult population.[1,2] In most cases, halitosis originates in the oral cavity[1-13] as the result of microbial metabolism.[3,4] Halitosis of oral causes may result from microbial metabolism on the dorsum of the tongue, gums, and retained detritus in cryptic tonsils. It is modulated by salivary flow rate, food impaction, and diet.[5-7] Nonoral etiologies[14-26] may include upper and lower respiratory tract conditions, gastrointestinal disorders, various systemic diseases, and the use of certain drugs.[8-9]

It is the purpose of this chapter to review oral and regional factors, systemic factors, differential diagnosis, and the diagnosis, treatment, and prevention of halitosis.

## Etiology And Pathogenesis

### Oral and Regional Factors

Halitosis arising in the upper aerodigestive tract is a result of the production of volatile compounds through the putrefactive action of micro-organisms on exogenous and endogenous substrates, such as exfoliated oral epithelium, food debris, saliva, and blood.[1,3,10] Proteins undergo proteolysis to peptides and constituent amino acids, which are further degraded to highly volatile compounds causing an offensive odor to the breath.[11] This process occurs in the mouth of all individuals.

When underlying pathology such as tissue necrosis is present, this malodorous process is accentuated. Therefore condi-

From Irwin RS, Curley FJ, Grossman RF (eds): Diagnosis and Treatment of Symptoms of the Respiratory Tract. Armonk, New York, Futura Publishing Company, Inc., © 1997.

tions like gingivitis, periodontitis, ulcerations, sinusitis, rhinitis, pharyngitis and tonsillitis are frequently associated with halitosis.[12] Other conditions which may produce halitosis include oroantral fistulae, necrotic tumors of the oral cavity, pharynx, trachea and bronchi. Nasal foreign bodies and rhinoliths are a common cause of halitosis in childhood, as is tonsillar and adenoid hypertrophy with resultant airway obstruction with stasis of secretions. Structural changes following pharyngeal flap surgery can also produce halitosis.[8,9,13]

In the oral cavity, halitosis is usually the result of microbial action on the tongue dorsum and periodontium. The putrefactive action of the microorganisms on available substrates, such as exfoliated oral epithelium, salivary proteins, food debris, and blood, occurs in the mouths of all individuals. However, the process is modulated by the rate of salivary secretion, food impaction, diet, and oral hygiene.[1,3,9,10,27]

The most objectionable odor, regardless of the health status of the oral cavity, is usually seen when there is reduced salivary flow and lack of food and fluid intake (eg, early morning air sample[1] after overnight sleep). During sleep, the rate of salivary flow is very low[28] and there is more than adequate time for putrefaction to occur.[29] Conversely, during meals and the chewing process, there is movement of the tongue, cheek, lips, and teeth and a high rate of salivary flow; this helps to remove food debris and, consequently, helps to decrease the intensity of halitosis. Food impaction usually occurs in areas of dental decay or crowded teeth and can lead to halitosis. This can be easily prevented by routine dental care. Vegetable food impaction causes halitosis of a lesser degree than meat impaction since there are fewer and less objectionable degraded waste protein byproducts in vegetables. The periods of objectionable breath attributed to normal physiological causes are transient in duration and can be readily reduced to socially acceptable levels by appropriate oral hygiene measures.[6]

The coated tongue is a particularly common source of bad breath. The desquamated epithelium of the tongue provides an ideal environment for trapping minute food particles and bacteria capable of emitting offensive odors. Therefore, oral hygiene should include brushing the dorsum of the tongue.[7]

Dentures usually encourage accumulation of food debris and can cause a type of halitosis known as "denture breath."[30] Certain age groups present a characteristic mouth odor. Young children, 2 to 5 years old, have a sweet fetid mouth odor, whereas middle-aged men and women tend to suffer more severe morning breath odor.[30] Xerostomia due to aging[31] or radiation therapy to the head and neck[24,26] can reduce salivary secretion and oral self-cleansing with consequent halitosis. Disease within the lungs or lower respiratory tract, such as infections or cancer, are reported to produce malodor.[18-21] Zenker's (hypopharyngeal) diverticulum is often associated with halitosis because of retained undigested food content. Halitosis can originate from gastric content, during regurgitation, belching, or vomiting.[30]

## Systemic Factors (Table I)

A variety of systemic conditions may give rise to "bad breath."[6,8,14] These include, among many others, diabetes mellitus,[15] chronic renal failure,[16] and cirrhosis of the liver.[17] These diseases are examples of how oral odors may serve as diagnostic indicators of aberrations of systemic metabolism. Each systemic condition usually has a characteristic malodor. For example, the "ketonic breath" of the patient with diabetic ketoacidosis is produced by acetone and other ketones.[15] The "fishy odor" of ammonia in uremia and kidney failure is produced by dimethylamine or trimethylamine.[16] The "fetor hepaticus" characteristic of liver failure in cirrhosis of the liver is generated by aliphatic acid, methylmercaptan, ethamethiol, and dimethylsulfide.[17]

Halitosis can also occur in toxemia, gastrointestinal disorders, or hemorrhage at any level of the gastrointestinal tract. Neuropsychiatric disorders may also fea-

**Table 1**
Systemic Etiologies of Halitosis

| Etiology | Characteristics |
| --- | --- |
| Diabetes Mellitus | Acetone, Ketonic Breath |
| Cirrhosis of the Liver and Liver Failure | "Fetor Hepaticus," Decomposed Blood |
| Kidney Failure | "Fishy Odor," Ammonia, Urine |
| Blood Dyscrasias, Anticoagulant Therapy, Internal hemorrhage | Decomposed Blood |
| Fever, dehydration, Sjögren's Syndrome, Xerostomia | Malodor Due to Dry Mouth and Poor Hygiene |
| Eosinophilic Granuloma, Letterer-Siwe Disease, Hand-Schüller-Christian Disease | Fetid Breath, Unpleasant Taste |

ture the complaint of halitosis (real or imagined).[8] In the nonlipid reticuloendothelioses—such as eosinophilic granuloma, Letterer-Siwe disease, and Hand-Schüller-Christian disease—halitosis, unpleasant taste, and sore mouth are among the chief complaints.[22] Acute or chronic scurvy due to vitamin C deficiency may produce bad breath, probably due to gingival bleeding.[22] In hematologic disorders, such as macroglobulinemia, hemophilia, von Willebrand's disease, leukemia, and thrombocytopenia, and in patients taking anticoagulants, halitosis results from the decomposition of blood from spontaneous bleeding in the upper aerodigestive tract.[23]

Drugs containing iodine or chloral hydrate can reach the breath.[12,23] Antineoplastic agents, antihistamines, tranquilizers, diuretics, phenothizides, and atropinelike drugs diminish salivary production and thus decrease self-cleansing of the oral cavity.[24,25] In addition, several antineoplastic drugs, such as methotrexate, actinomycin D, adriamycin, and bleomycin, can cause candidiasis, gingival bleeding. and oral ulceration with consequent malodor. Dimethyl sulfoxide (DMSO) is a colorless and odorless prescribed drug for muscle pain or interstitial cystitis[25] which is metabolized and reduced to dimethyl sulfide, the chemical essence of garlic. Consequently a garliclike odor is given-off through the breath.

Xerostomia (ie, dry mouth) results from systemic drug administration, and several systemic conditions, such as Sjögren's syndrome and Mikulicz's disease.

Systemic breath odors may result from pulmonary excretion of metabolites originating from ingested foods. A vegetarian has less tendency to produce halitosis than an excessive meat-eater because there are fewer degraded waste byproducts of proteinaceous substances in vegetables. Meat also contains fat and stimulates volatile fatty acids to be produced in the gastrointestinal system which are absorbed into the bloodstream and finally excreted in the breath.[12,30] Garlic, onion, leek, and certain spices are known to produce malodorous breath. They are absorbed from the intestine, metabolized in the liver, and gradually released into the bloodstream and excreted via the lungs, as well as by other routes.[30,32] Increased oral malodor can occur in some women during menstruation and especially with dysmenorrhea. The reason is elevation of production of volatile sulphur compounds around menstruation which reach a peak 3 to 5 days after onset of menses.[6] From time to time, one may experience "hunger odor" with hunger sensation. It has been suggested that the odor might be due to putrefaction of pancreatic juice in the stomach during hunger periods.

**Differential Diagnosis (Table II)**

Halitosis is socially embarrassing and always easy to recognize. However, the

**Table II**
Differential Diagnosis

| | |
|---|---|
| Oral | — Dental Carries |
| | — Dental Abscess |
| | — Chronic Gingivitis |
| | — Vincent's Angina |
| | — Candidiasis |
| | — Carcinoma (tongue, floor of mouth) |
| | — Osteoradionecrosis |
| | — Oroantral Fistula |
| | — Xerostomia |
| | — Acute Suppurative Parotiitis |
| Pharynx | — Acute Follicular and Membranous Tonsillitis |
| | — Acute Pharyngitis |
| | — Infectious Mononucleosis |
| | — Retained Detritus in Cryptic Tonsils |
| | — Carcinoma (tongue base, larynx, hypopharynx, tonsil) |
| | — Zenker's Diverticulum |
| | — Diphtheria |
| Nasal and Sinus | — Foreign Body |
| | — Rhinolith |
| | — Leprosy |
| | — Atrophic Rhinitis (ozena) |
| | — Acute and Chronic Purulent Sinusitis |
| | — Malignant Tumors |
| Lower Respiratory Tract | — Pulmonary Abscess |
| | — Bronchiectasis |
| | — Foreign Body |
| | — Bronchogenic Carcinoma |
| Esophagus/Stomach | — Malignant Tumors |
| | — Upper Gastrointestinal Bleeding |
| | — Gastroesophageal Reflux Disease |
| Systemic | — Ketoacidosis |
| | — Uremia |
| | — Hepatic Failure |
| | — Drugs |
| | — Nonlipid Reticuloendothelioses |
| | — Foods |

exact cause may be difficult to identify. The most common causes are found in the mouth. If none is found, then an extra-oral source should be sought. It is possible to differentiate between intra-oral and extra-oral factors, by asking the patient to exhale through the nose with mouth closed or alternatively exhale through the mouth with the nose blocked.

Though halitosis may be multifactorial a useful differential diagnosis is listed in Table II.

## Diagnosis

Halitosis is a diagnostic challenge to the clinician. The oral and systemic component can make the diagnosis quite complicated. After evaluation for potential, life-threatening causes have failed to reveal the diagnosis, a systematic search for upper aerodigestive, lower respiratory, and systemic causes should ensue (Figure 1). A good dental and otolaryngology assessment, appropriate laboratory tests,

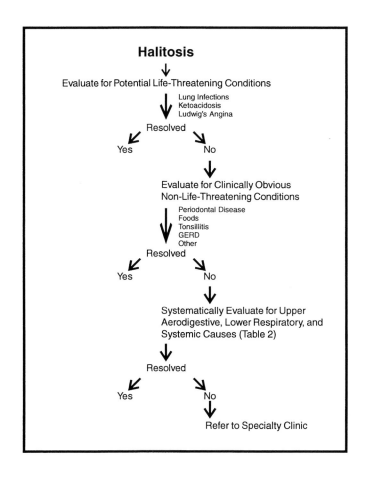

**Figure 1.** Diagnostic approach to determine the cause of halitosis. GERD = gastro-esophageal reflux disease.

and diagnostic imaging (eg, dental x-rays, paranasal sinus x-rays [conventional, computed tomographic scanning], barium esophagram) should be helpful. While the breath normally consists of odors originating from both the oral cavity and the lungs, it may be possible to differentiate the odor from the lungs from that of the oral cavity. The clinician should ask the patient to seal his lips tightly and then forcibly blow through the nostrils. Odor detected in this way is likely to be from the lower respiratory or systemic factors.[9] In order to detect odor from the mouth, the patient should be asked to pinch the nose with the fingers, stop breathing for a moment with lips sealed, and then exhale gently by opening the mouth. The odor detected this way is likely to be from the oropharyngeal cavity.

A record of the patient's food intake over a period of several days may disclose a diet that could possibly be contributory to the oral malodor. Abdominal cramps or diarrhea may suggest a malabsorption problem which might possibly be contributory. A careful head and neck examination, emphasizing the oral cavity, pharynx, nasopharynx, and sinuses, should identify states causing or contributing to malodor.

It is possible to measure and analyze halitosis, largely through industrial methodologies, although this is rarely used clinically. The most simple and commonly used approach to sample and measure halitosis is direct nasal sniffing of expelled mouth air. This is referred to as "organoleptic assessment." This approach closely simulates the everyday situations in which bad breath is detected. However, such organoleptic measurements are strictly subjective raising several problems such as variations between judges on ranking of malodor; reliability and reproducibility of the measurements; sex of the odor judge (odor perception is more developed in women than in men); age of the judge (there is a increase in the ability to perceive odors with increasing age); and adaptation to the odor (the dentist or otolaryngologist may have adapted to oral malodor).[1,6,33]

Over the past three decades, research has developed instrumental analysis of oral malodor using gas chromatography coupled with flame photometric detection.[1,6,7] These methods led to the conclusion that oral malodor is associated primarily with volatile sulphur compounds. Gas chromatography measurement is able to demonstrate malodor reduction after use of mouth rinses or oral hygiene techniques.[6,7]

Gas chromatographic measurement of malodor has several advantages as compared with organoleptic measurement which include the ability to separate and quantitatively measure individual gases and the ability to measure extremely low concentrations of gases. The main disadvantages of such instruments are the relatively high cost, the need for skilled personnel, the lack of portability, and the time required for measurement.

Recently, the application of an industrial sulfide monitor for measuring gases associated with oral malodor has been reported.[27,33] Measurements using the sulfide monitor have been shown to be more reproducible than organoleptic measurements and very sensitive to reduction in malodor following mouth-rinsing. This monitor is inexpensive, can be operated by unskilled personnel, and is portable. The main disadvantage of the instrument is its inability to distinguish between individual sulfides.

The variability of oral malodor measurements and the difficulties in assessing oral malodor[33,34] directly from the oral cavity have led investigators to employ indirect methods. The approach that has been most widely used is the measurement of malodor and volatile sulfides in putrefying saliva samples.[1,2,6,7] In most cases,

saliva obtained directly from the mouth possesses little or no foul odor, but after several hours of in vitro incubation, malodor is easily detected, due to breakdown of particulate matter by micro-organisms.[7] However, the odor of putrefied saliva may differ appreciably from directly sampled oral malodor.[33]

## Treatment and Prevention

Since most halitosis is caused by local factors, elimination of these factors should be the first step in the treatment approach, especially in those cases with a noncontributory medical history. Comprehensive dental care, thorough oral hygiene, and prophylaxis should solve most cases of halitosis. Periodontists have reported that a day-long reduction of oral malodor can be achieved following a two-phase oil-water mouth rinse.[27] The tongue, one of the main foci of micro-organisms in the mouth, should be included in the routine oral hygiene procedures.

Many patients with halitosis chew gum, suck sour candy, or take chlorophyll preparations as a solution to the problem. Sucking sour candy can increase saliva flow, thereby facilitating the removal of food debris, as well as reducing stagnation and putrefaction of saliva. Gum-chewing involves activity of the muscles of the mastication, the cheek, and tongue and increases salivary flow, thus helping in the self-cleansing of the oral cavity. However, it does not solve the underlying problems of halitosis. Chlorophyll masks the underlying odor but, again, does not solve the underlying problem.

Patients with halitosis due to xerostomia could use a sialagogue to stimulate salivary flow; however salivary reserve may be lacking. A salivary substitute may be used to moisten the oral cavity. If halitosis results from drug administration, an alternative medication may be sought. Even if the cause of halitosis is drug-related, meticulous oral hygiene can keep the halitosis minimal.

Halitosis due to systemic disease is usually more intense and persistent and remains until the systemic disease is controlled. Halitosis from dietary habits (eg, frequent garlic or onion intake) or impaired digestion of fats could be treated by educating the patient and adjusting the patient's diet.

## Summary

Although the causes of halitosis are multifactorial, oral causes predominate. Measures that reduce oral bacteria will favorably alter most instances of halitosis. The three most common sites of pathology that cause halitosis are all upper aerodigestive—dental/gingival, tonsillar, and nasal/sinuses. In the diagnostic algorithm, the clinician should consider all the possible causative factors, including the systemic ones, when managing the patient with halitosis.

## Acknowledgements:

Supported by the Saul A. Silverman Family Foundation and Temmy Latner/Dynacare as a Canada-Israel Scientific Exchange Program in Otolaryngology (CISEPO) project.

## *References*

1. Tonzetich J. Production and origin of oral malodor: a review of mechanisms and methods of analysis. J Periodontal 1977;48:13–20.
2. Kleinberg I, Westboy G. Oral malodor. Crit Rev Oral Biol Med 1990;1:247–259.
3. McNamara TF, Alexander JF, Lee M. The role of micro-organisms in the production of oral malodor. Oral Surg Oral Med Oral Pathol 1972;34:41–48.
4. Claesson R, Edlund MB, Persson S, et al. Production of volatile sulfur compounds by various fusobacterium species. Oral Microbiol Immunol 1990;5:137–142.
5. Kostelc JG, Preti G, Zelson PR, et al. Oral odors in early experimental gingivitis. J Periodontal Res 1984;19:303–312.
6. Tonzetich J. Oral malodor: An indicator of health status and oral cleanliness. Int Dent J 1977;28:309–319.
7. Yaegaki K, Sanada K. Biochemical and clinical factors influencing oral malodor in periodontal patients. J Periodontal 1992;63:786–792.
8. Attia EL, Marshall KG. Halitosis. Can Med Assoc J 1982;126:1281–1285.
9. Bogdasarian RS. Halitosis. Otolaryngol Clin North Am 1986;19:111–117.
10. Kleinberg I, Westbay G. Salivary and metabolic factors involved in oral malodor formation. J Periodontal 1992;63:768–775.
11. Tonzetich J, Carpenter PAW. Production of volatile sulphur compounds from cystein, cystine and methionine by human dental plaque. Arch Oral Biol 1971;16:599–607.
12. Sponge ID. Halitosis. A review of its causes and treatment. Dent Pract 1964;14:307–317.
13. Finkelstein Y, Talmi YP, Zohar Y, et al. Endoscopic diagnosis and treatment of persistent halitosis after pharyngeal flap surgery. Plast Reconst Surg 1993; 92: 1176–1178.
14. Preti G, Clark L, Cowart BJ, et al. Non-oral etiologies of oral malodor and altered chemosensation. J Periodontol 1992;63:790–796.
15. Booth G, Ostenson S. Acetone to alveolar air and control of diabetes. Lancet 1966;II:1102–1105.
16. Simenhoff ML, Burke JF, Saukkonen JJ, et al. Biochemical profile of uremic breath. N Eng J Med 1977;247:132–135.
17. Chen S, Mahadevan V, Zieve L. Volatile fatty acids in the breath of patients with cirrhosis of the liver. J Lab Clin Med 1970; 75:622–627.
18. Lorber B. Bad Breath. Presenting manifestation of anaerobic pulmonary infection. Am Rev Respir Dis 1975;112:875–877.
19. McGregor IA, Watson JD, Sweeney G, et al. Tiniazole in smelly oropharyngeal tumours. Lancet 1982;I:110.
20. Gordon SM, Szidon JP, Krotoszynski BK, et al. Volatile organic compounds in exhaled air from patients with lung cancer. Clin Chem 1985;31:1278–1282.
21. Preti G, Labows JN, Kostelc JG, et al. Analysis of lung air from patients with bronchogenic carcinoma and controls using chromatography mass spectrometry. J Chromatogr 1988;432:1–11.
22. Oral Aspects of Metabolic Disease. In: Shaffer WG, Hine MK, Levy BM, eds. *Textbook of Oral Pathology*. 3rd edition. Philadelphia, Pa: WB Saunders Company; 1974: 508–557.

23. Burket LW. *Oral Medicine, Diagnosis and Treatment.* 7th edition. Philadelphia, Pa: JB Lippincott Co; 1977: Chapters 7 and 19.

24. Baum BJ, Bodner L, Fox PC, et al. Therapy-induced dysfunction of salivary glands: implication for oral health. Special Care in Dentistry 1985;5:274–277.

25. Goodman, Gilman A, Rall TW, et al. *Goodman and Gilman's: The Pharmacological Basis of Therapeutics.* 8th edition. New York, NY: Pergamon Press; 1990.

26. Bodner L. Transport of alpha-aminoisobutyric acid into rat parotid after x-irradiation. Int J Rad Biol 1989;55:653–660.

27. Rosenberg M, Gelernter I, Barki M, et al. Day-long reduction of oral malodor by a two-phase oil: water mouth rinse as compared to chlorhexidine and placebo rinses. J Periodontol 1992;63:39–43.

28. Schneyer LH, Pigman W, Hanahan L, et al. Rate of flow of human parotid, sublingual and submaxillary secretions during sleep. J Dent Res 1956;35:109–112.

29. Berg M, Burrill DY, Fosdick LS. Chemical studies in periodontol disease. J Dent Res 1947;26:47.

30. Massler M. Fetor ex ore and Halitosis. Compend Contin Educ Dent 1981;2: 113–115.

31. Bodner L, Baum BJ. Characteristics of stimulated parotid gland secretion in the aging rat. Mech Aging Dev 1985;31:337–342.

32. Blakenhorn MA, Richards CE. Garlic breath odour. JAMA 1936;107:409–410.

33. Rosenberg M, McCulloch CAG. Measurement of oral malodor; current methods and future prospects. J Periodontol 1992;63: 776–782.

34. Kozlovsky A, Gordon D, Gelev I, et al. Correlation between the BANA test and oral malodor parameters. J Dent Res 1994;73: 1036–1042.

# 13

# Hoarseness

Dan M. Fliss, M.D.
Jeremy L. Freeman, M.D.

## Introduction

### Definition and Prevalence

Hoarseness is a voice change wherein vocal quality is rendered uncharacteristically "rough," "gruff," "rasping,"or "croaking" by a pathological or psychological process. In the general practice of medicine or in specialties focusing on disorders of phonation, hoarseness is seen with great prevalence. The management of patients presenting with hoarseness, whether a child with vocal exuberance or an adult with laryngeal cancer, frequently occurs in a general otolaryngology practice or a head and neck oncology practice. In this chapter, we will attempt to give a comprehensive overview of the larynx and management of hoarseness.

### Embryology

The larynx together with the trachea, bronchi, and lungs originate from a midline ventral diverticulum of the foregut, called the laryngotracheal groove, during the fourth week of embryonic life. The groove is located posterior to the hypobranchial eminence and in close proximity to the third, fourth, and sixth branchial arches/pharyngeal pouches (Figure 1). The presence of the fifth branchial system is still controversial, but if there is such an apparatus this is also involved. The tracheoesophageal septum which separates the laryngotracheal groove from the esophagus is established by fusion of the laryngotracheal groove in a caudal to cephalad manner. As maturation takes place, two separate tubular structures are formed: the esophagus and the laryngotracheal apparatus. By the fifth to sixth week, the sagittal primitive laryngeal orifice becomes "T" shaped by the growth of three tissue formations. The hypobranchial eminence is of mesodermal origin and is situated in an anteromedian position just posterior to the copula. This structure will give rise to the forcula which later develops into the epiglottis. Laterally arytenoid masses appear at the fifth week. The cuneiform and corniculate cartilages will later mature from two additional swellings located on each primordial arytenoid.

Supported by the Saul A. Silverman Family Foundation and Temmy Latner/Dynacare as a Canada-Israel Scientific Exchange Program in Otolaryngology (CISEPO)
The authors acknowledge Eiji Yanigasawa, MD for kindly providing laryngeal endoscopic photographs.

From Irwin RS, Curley FJ, Grossman RF (eds): Diagnosis and Treatment of Symptoms of the Respiratory Tract. Armonk, New York, Futura Publishing Company, Inc., © 1997.

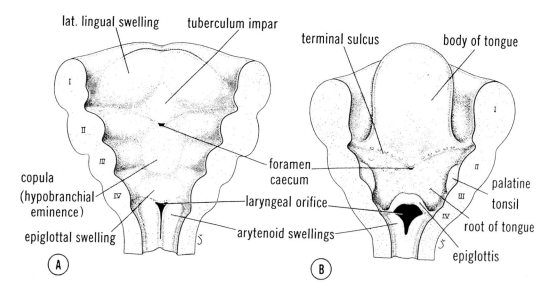

**Figure 1.** Ventral aspect of the pharyngeal arches (I→IV)of the foregut at (A) 5 weeks and (B) 5 months to show the development of the larynx. Note the formation of the "T"-shaped laryngeal orifice with the surrounding epiglottis and arytenoid swellings. Reproduced by permission from Williams and Wilkins Publishers in Medical Embryology by Jan Langman, MD.

As these three masses develop, approximately between the fifth and seventh week, the laryngeal aditus is temporarily obliterated. The recanalization of the larynx occurs from caudal to cephalad and from anterior to posterior. Failure to recanalize results in atresia, stenosis, or webs. By the eighth week, the thyroid cartilage derived from the fourth branchial arch, and the cricoid, arytenoid, and cuneiform cartilages derived from the fifth and sixth branchial arches are easily distinguished. At 10 weeks, the vocal folds are evident. Cephalad to the vocal folds, a vestibular sinus forms. This will later become the laryngeal ventricle. A condensation of mesenchymal tissue within the substance of the primordial vocal folds will give rise to the vocal ligament. The laryngeal muscles are derivatives from mesoderm of the epicardial ridge and are innervated by the branchial nerves of the fourth and sixth arches, namely the superior laryngeal and the recurrent laryngeal nerves. Because of the persistence of ductus arteriosus, a sixth arch artery on the left side and the recurrent laryngeal nerve pass posteriorly.

## Functions of the Larynx

The larynx is situated at the crossroads of the food and air passages. This unique organ performs three important functions: **protection** of the lungs by acting as a valve and preventing the passage of secretions, food, and other foreign materials into the upper respiratory tract; **respiration** hence serving as a conduit for air and waste gases from the lungs; and **phonation**. Negus[1] in 1948 described the phylogenetic modifications of the primitive larynx in order to serve the human needs. The primitive larynx found in the Bichir (polypterus) lungfish functions basically as a simple sphincter that protects the lower airway from the intrusion of foreign material. In the African lungfish (protopterus), in addition to the sphincteric musculature, the first active laryngeal dilator consisting of discrete muscular fibers which draw the valvular margins apart is noted. Lateral cartilages form bars on the sides of the glottis and provide anchorage for the dilator muscles, also developing a ring structure analogous to the cricoid cartilage in mammals. These modifications are noted in certain amphibians, such as the Mexican axolotl (amlyostoma) which incorporate these additional functional necessities of phonation and respiratory regulations as seen in the human larynx. Concluding his phylogenetical observations, Negus considers the primary function of the larynx to be that of a sphincter that protects the lower airway from the intrusion of solids or liquids. The secondary function according to this theory is respiratory governed by active muscular dilatation of the laryngeal aperture. Phonation seems to be a late phylogenetic acquisition and, according to this theory, is of tertiary importance. It is also probably the least understood of the larynx's three basic functions. But phonation is so much more than that part of speech that generates raw sounds. It is not only a means of communication in which the essential link is the transmission of information by means of sound waves, but also an indication of the human intellect, emotional state, and cultural background.[2] In other words, this complex mechanism contributes enormously to what makes us *Homo sapiens*.

## Physiology of Speech Production

Speech is produced by many coordinated factors interacting in a fine network of physiologic actions. These include the expiratory blast of high-pressure air, the vibrating mechanism of the larynx, the resonating spaces in the thoracic cavity, pharynx, mouth, and nasal chambers, and the articulators which provide movements of the tongue, teeth, and lips necessary to create different sounds. The underlying basis of speech is voice which is basically a respiratory function. The almost universally agreed upon myoelastic aerodynamic theory of phonation was first proposed by Muler in 1848 and presented again by Vandenberg in 1958.[3] This theory states that the alternating mode of opening and closing of the vocal cords is produced by two forces: the mass tension of the cords and the aerodynamic forces acting on or around the vocal cords by the exhaled air

column. Therefore, vocal sound formation is the result of the interaction between the air flow-air pressure and elasticity of the vocal cords, which is dependent on their length, mass, and tension. The sequence of events is as follows.

The contraction of the expiratory muscles in the thorax and abdominal wall is essential in providing the subglottic high-pressure column of air. At this stage, the vocal cords are tensed and in adduction by the action of the lateral cricoarytenoid and the interarytenoid muscles. The air is forced through the narrowed vocal tract in an accelerated way. This triggers the Bernoulli-phenomenon in which air current flowing through a narrow channel exerts negative pressure upon the channel's walls, thus the vocal folds are sucked together in adduction. As a result, the air pressure beneath the folds rises until the subglottal pressure is greater than the myoelastic forces of the reapproximated cords and the glottic chink is forced open. This allows the expired air to escape through the glottis and into the supraglottic cavities in little puffs producing laryngeal sounds. When the vocal cords start opening from complete closure, they open in a posterior-to-anterior fashion. At this point, the subglottic pressure falls, and the myoelastic forces of the vocal cords exceeds the aerodynamic forces enabling approximation of the vocal folds again. The vocal folds being in contact prevent the escape of air. The subglottic pressure rises again until the vocal cords are forced apart and this cycle repeats itself.

Changes in the vocal parameters of pitch, loudness, and quality are directly influenced by the property of the subglottic column of air (ie, pressure and quantity) and on the elasticity of the vocal cords which lengthen or shorten or become thin and thick (ie, length, mass, and tension). Changes in the pitch of voice are produced by the vocal cords continually altering in response to changes in tension brought about by laryngeal muscle contraction. The loudness of sound is dependent not on the laryngeal muscle changes, but primarily on the pressure of the expiratory air current. The quality of voice is dependent on the sophisticated interaction of all properties as they affect the vocal fold vibratory system. Therefore, in light of the above discussion, hoarsenss may be defined as the vocal quality perceived as a result of the disruption of the normal phonatory process. The various causing factors will be elucidated further in the chapter. An understanding of the basic principles of voice production will permit the clinician to correlate between perceptual and physiologic patterns of abnormal voice.

The cooperation between the otolaryngologist and the speech pathologist is warranted in any comprehensive diagnostic process involving laryngeal disorders.

## The Diagnostic Approach

The purpose of voice evaluation is to determine the basis of the patient's voice disorder and the factors maintaining it. This evaluation should include a comprehensive history of the way in which the patient is using his or her voice-producing mechanism and a thorough testing of potential voice capabilities.

The treatment of laryngeal disorders is dependent on a reasonable working diagnosis and a thorough understanding of the anatomy, pathophysiology, and pathology of the larynx and the adjacent structures. The functional and anatomical integrity of the larynx is of fundamental importance. The most common causes for the laryngeal complaint are changes in the mucosal surfaces followed by vocal cord paralysis. Other causes are inflammatory, infectious, and neoplastic. In addition, familiarity with basic principles of phonation will allow this correlation between perceptual and physiologic features of the abnormal voice. This is especially important in cases in which the larynx is apparently normal on physical examination and other causes, such as psychogenic or neurologic disorders, should be determined.

### History

A carefully taken patient history should always be obtained. The patient should be encouraged to discuss in detail his or her complaint, and the physician should consider the possible role of not only local and systemic conditions, but also emotional and lifestyle-related factors. Although the patient with a rough quality of voice may fear cancer in his larynx, most lesions causing hoarseness are caused by benign changes of the mucosal surfaces. Cardinal points that should be documented in the patient's history include questions about the onset of the first related symptoms and signs, the progression of events leading to the date of evaluation, and details of prior medical evaluations or therapeutic procedures pertaining to the current complaint.

Apart from the vocal complaint, systematic questioning should include information about heavy cigarette and alcohol abuse. The exposure to other irritants, such as chronic use of drugs (eg, angiotensin-converting enzymes inhibitors) including nonprescription drugs or exposure to a dry, dusty, or chemically contaminated environment, should also be investigated.

A thorough investigation of the patient's voice use or abuse should be performed. The purpose (ie, social or professional), intensity, style, and duration of the voice use should be carefully recorded. An upper respiratory tract infection, sinusitis with postnasal drip, or chronic obstructive pulmonary disease may induce pooling of purulent secretions in the larynx which results in chronic inflammation and hoarseness. Gastroesophageal reflux disease is a digestive disorder with many extradigestive complications, such as microlaryngeal inhalations of gastric content into the larynx and trachea. A history of trauma or surgery to the larynx or the thyroid gland should be elicited. The former may induce hoarseness through the mechanism of edema, hematoma, or arytenoid dislocation and the latter by iatrogenic paralysis of the recurrent larynx nerve or hypoparathyroidism and myxedema.

A group of regional and systemic conditions may induce serious alterations of the vocal functions. Musculoskeletal tension syndromes, such as tension headache, diffuse head and neck tension, and temporomandibular joint syndrome should be considered. The possibility of neurologic disorders should also be explored. This group of neuromuscular conditions include focal dystonias, demyelinating diseases, parkinsonism, and cerebrovascular accidents.

## Physical Examination

After obtaining a clinical history, the physician should perform a complete otolaryngologic examination. This should also include a clinical voice assessment in order to evaluate laryngeal and phonatory function. Pitch, breath support, and muscle tension are evaluated by careful observation, palpation, and listening. A complete head and neck examination is in order for the patient with a laryngeal complaint, regardless of the area of complaint.

The nose and nasopharynx should be inspected for signs of allergy, chronic inflammation, obstruction, and mass lesions. Inspection and palpation of the oral cavity and oropharynx is performed in order to rule out mucosal dryness, inflammation tenderness, or neoplastic lesions. Inspection and palpation of the neck should include major lymph node groups, laryngeal cartilages, hyoid bone, trachea, and the thyroid gland.

Indirect examination of the larynx and adjacent structures is performed using three different techniques: the laryngeal mirror (Figures 2 and 3), the rigid fiberoptic telescope, and the flexible nasopharyngoscope (Figure 4). The first attempt to examine the larynx should be made with the use of the **laryngeal mirror**. The patient should be instructed on every aspect of the procedure, since close cooperation is essential in permitting a successful examination. Good visualization is achieved with the patient assuming the "sniffing po-

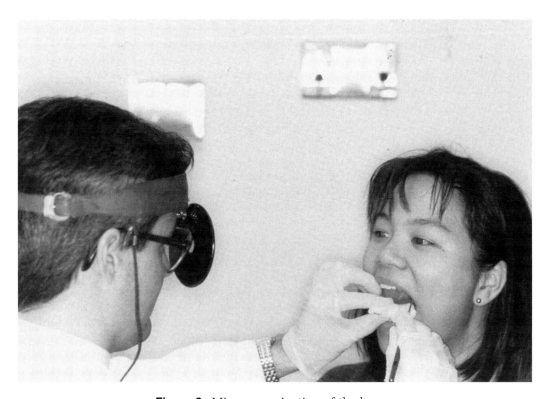

**Figure 2.** Mirror examination of the larynx.

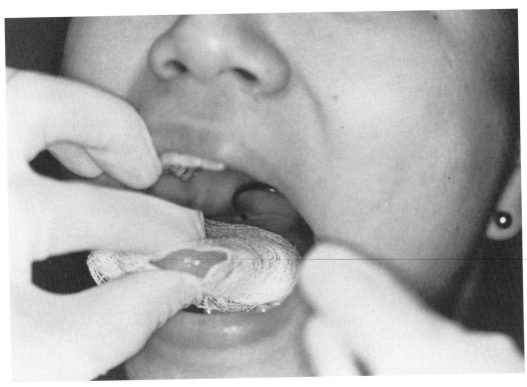

**Figure 3.** The position of the mirror is against the soft palate for visualization of the larynx during mirror examination of the larynx.

sition" in which the neck is flexed on the chest and the head is extended on the neck. The patient is then asked to protrude the tongue which is wrapped with a gauze square sponge. A laryngeal mirror warmed to prevent fogging is then advanced into the oral cavity in order to reach the soft palate and uvula. Often these structures must be displaced posteriorly and superiorly with the back of the mirror in order to bring the larynx and hypopharynx in view. Care should be taken not to touch the tonsils or base of tongue since this will elicit an involuntary gag response.

The base of the tongue, supraglottic larynx, postcricoid area, and pyriform sinuses should be visualized first. Then attention is directed to the false and true vocal cords, first in quiet respiration, then in deep inspiration, and finally during phonation. The subglottis and upper trachea are partially visualized during pauses between vocalization when the glottis is open. Topical anesthetic sprays may be required in patients with a hyperactive gag or overhanging epiglottis. Some patients will not cooperate for the indirect examination under any circumstances. In these cases, the best solution for counteracting the hyperactive gag is the use of fiber-optic devices. A variety of **laryngeal fiber-optic telescopes** have become available in recent years. These are rigid periscopes with self-contained illumination that offer brilliant illumination and fine optics with wide angle magnification of the hypopharynx and larynx. In addition, these instruments permit the performance of photography, videotaping, and stroboscopy and can also be coupled with an observer's post for teaching purposes. Although rigid telescopes facilitate an accurate and detailed examination and documentation of the larynx, their disadvantages include a still relatively large expense and patient intolerance due to gagging. **The flexible naso-**

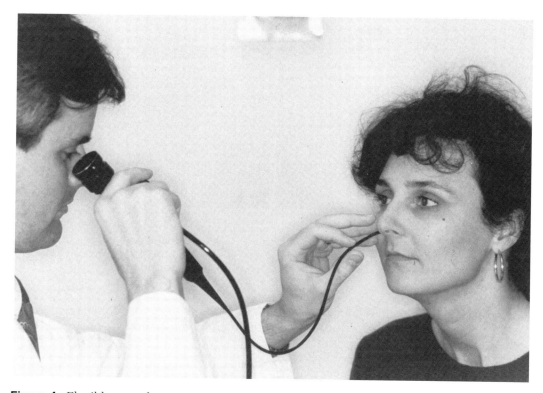

**Figure 4.** Flexible nasopharyngoscope examination of the larynx. The endoscope is introduced through the nose and advanced into the pharynx until the larynx is visualized.

**pharyngoscope** is the most useful instrument in the examination of the larynx. It has the same advantages as the rigid telescope, but in addition, it permits an accurate physiologic examination of the voice since the patient is able to speak and sing during the examination (Figure 5). This is also an excellent technique for the visualization of the nose, nasopharynx, and hypopharynx and is the best-tolerated technique for laryngeal examination especially in children. Diagnostic video stroboscopy and still photodocumentation are available. The nasopharyngoscope is useful in patient education and biofeedback.

## Ancillary Tests

**Videostroboscopy** has become an essential examination for the assessment of vocal function. Stroboscopy is not a new technique,[4] but its acceptance as a routine part of the voice evaluation has not been as forthcoming. The comprehensive behavior of the vibrating mucosal waves of the vocal folds is not visible through indirect laryngoscopy. Stroboscopy creates an illusion of slow motion by generating light flashes at a rate out of synchrony (approximately 2 Hz) coupled with fundamental frequency of phonation. Thus, a typical laryngeal cycle which usually lasts 5 milliseconds is being transformed into a cycle which lasts between 0.25 and 1 second. This "new cycle" represents a montage of many laryngeal cycles rather than the documentation of a single cycle. In order to accurately analyze stroboscopy, knowledge of the vocal fold vibrating physiology is essential.[5-9]

The vocal fold is composed of a loose mucosal cover which vibrates primarily in a vertical dimension and forms a travelling wave. The other component of the vocal

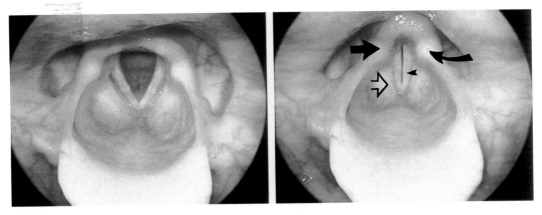

**Figure 5.** View obtained through the flexible nasopharyngoscope of the normal larynx during inspiration (left) and on phonation (right) with the vocal cords in abduction. Straight arrow = right arytenoid; Curved arrow = left arytenoid; Arrowhead (without tail) = left true vocal cord; Hollow arrow = right false vocal cord. Photograph by Eiji Yanagisawa, MD.

fold is the vocalis muscle which provides a stiff underlying body. This muscular body is associated with the transverse movements of the vocal folds. Functionally, the vocal fold has an upper and a lower margin. During phonation, the lower margin separates first. Before the upper margin separates, a subglottic vault confined superiorly by the upper margin and laterally by the lower margins is being filled with a small volume of air. This elliptical volume of air is then released as a puff into the supraglottis as the upper margins move laterally. The delay between the opening of the lower margins and the opening of the upper margins is called "phase delay." The lower margins then return to the midline followed by the gradual closing of the upper margins. The stroboscopic examination provides useful information about this fluidlike movement of the vibrating vocal folds (ie, travelling mucosal wave) and may help differentiate normal from pathologic conditions. Stroboscopy is an excellent technique in assessing alteration of the mucosal waves following trauma or surgery, in differentiating nodules from submucosal cysts, and in assessing superior laryngeal nerve paralysis. It is also useful in diagnosing early spasmodic dysphonia and papillomas and in differentiating adductor spasmodic dysphonia, muscle tension dysphonia, and myoclonus. However, its indications are limited when aperiodicity, hoarseness, and breathiness prevents accurate synchronization of the flashes.[10]

Laryngeal electromyography (EMG) is concerned with prognostic information in the evaluation of patients with vocal cord dysfunction.[11-16] This technique provides an analysis of the electrical activity generated by a motor unit which consists of one alpha motoneuron, the neuromuscular junction, and the muscle fibers innervated by the neuron. When the muscle is activated by a neural impulse, the electrical activity of the motor unit potential can be recorded as an EMG signal. This signal generated by the depolarization of the motor units is referred to as the motor unit action potential.[17] Clinical applications of laryngeal EMG include evaluation of the innervation of the superior and recurrent laryngeal nerves following trauma, iatrogenic injury, idiopathic paralysis cases, and generalized sampling of muscles for evidence of central nervous system and muscular disorders.

The functional integrity of the recurrent laryngeal nerve can be assessed by observing recordings of the thyroarytenoid muscle. This is performed with the use of monopolar or multipolar needles or bipolar-hooked wire electrodes. The placement of the electrodes can be performed by either the peroral or the percutaneous route. Confirmation of the exact placement of the electrode is made by asking the patient to vocalize (activation of the thyroarytenoid) followed by inspiration (decreased muscular activity); a maximal activity is seen with Valsalva's maneuver.

The cricothyroid muscle is the only laryngeal muscle innervated by the superior laryngeal nerve, thus testing of this muscle is an excellent means to assess superior laryngeal nerve function. Cricothyroid muscle EMG is performed transcutaneously. The position of the electrode is confirmed by asking the patient to vocalize at high pitch.

Several laryngeal EMG patterns are observed. Normal motor unit action potentials indicate the entire motor unit is intact. Fibrillation potentials indicate a loss of neural innervation and a poor prognosis. A normal frequency of firing rates with a decrease in the amplitude of the muscle action potential are consistent with loss of muscle function. Furthermore, a loss of nerve function produces a decrease in the frequency of firing rates, but a normal amplitude of some fibers remain. By measuring the timing interval between the onset of audible vocalization and the beginning of contraction of the thyroarytenoid muscle, further information can be obtained about the function of the recurrent laryngeal nerve. If this interval is greater than normal, neuropraxia or weakness of the recurrent laryngeal nerve should be suspected. High amplitude coupled with excessive firing rates during vocalization that would not be normal for that muscle are observed in conditions in which there is an impairment in the central nervous system control of the larynx (eg, spasmodic dysphonia, Parkinson's disease). The differentiation between fixation (posterior commissure stenosis, posterior glottic web) and paralysis of the clinically immobile cord is of utmost importance. In cases of fixation, the performance of laryngeal EMG may reveal a normal tracing and the patient should be a candidate for surgical treatment.

Gastroesophageal reflux disease (GERD) has been implicated in the pathogenesis of certain causes of chronic and acute inflammatory disorders of the upper airway. These include chronic throat-clearing, contact ulcers and granulomata over the arytenoids, globus pharyngeus, cervical dysphagia, cricoarytenoid arthritis, subglottic stenosis, and laryngeal carcinoma. Otolaryngology patients with GERD have a pattern of disease that is different from that of gastroenterology patients with esophagitis. Because of this, the majority of the traditional diagnostic tests, such as barium esophagograms and esophagoscopy with biopsy, are often negative.

**Ambulatory 24-hour pH monitoring** has become the gold standard for the demonstration and measurement of actual reflux.[18–20] Two pH probes are placed. One in the distal esophagus approximately 3 to 6 cm above the lower esophageal sphincter and the other in the hypopharynx just behind the laryngeal inlet approximately at the level of the free margin of the epiglottis. The correct positioning of the electrodes is being confirmed by lateral neck and chest roentgenograms. After calibration of the system, the pH is recorded every 5 seconds on each channel during 24-hour periods. The pH records are analyzed by a PC computer program. A variety of measurements can be chosen the number of episodes of acid reflux, the number of episodes lasting more than 3 minutes, longest period of reflux, lowest pH value, duration of pH under 6, 5, and 4, and finally the fraction of total time with a pH value under 4 and 5. Therefore, 24-hour pH monitoring provides an accurate physiologic measurement that incorporates information obtained over an extended period. It can also test the patient while sleeping, following meals, and in various body positions.

## Diagnosis, Pathogenesis, And Treatment

The Figure 6 algorithm illustrates the diagnostic approach for patients with hoarseness. Additionally, Table I reviews the differential diagnosis of hoarseness.

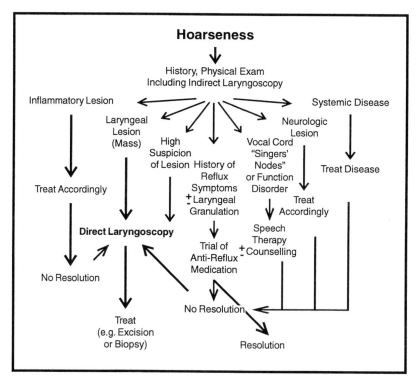

**Figure 6.** Algorithm for the clinical approach to patients presenting with hoarseness.

## Inflammatory Causes In Adults

Inflammatory conditions of the larynx may be produced by a variety of pathogenic organisms, trauma, chemical irritation, ionizing radiation, and allergic reactions. Edema, heat, redness, loss of function, and exudation are the main responses to acute injury leading to hypertrophy and metaplasia of the mucous membranes and in a later phase fibrosis of the underlying tissues. This cascade of limited pathophysiological events will usually take place regardless of the initial offending mechanism and will lead to four major symptoms—hoarseness, dyspnea, dysphagia, and local pain—differing only in the rapidity of onset and the degree and presence of specific systemic causes. Diagnosis is based on history; imaging; and indirect, fiber-optic, and direct examination of the larynx.

### Infectious Inflammatory Causes

***Acute Laryngitis:*** Acute laryngitis is a common condition and may be caused by viral or bacterial infections, allergy, and inhalation of environmental or local irritants.

**Viral laryngitis** is, in most cases, associated with an upper respiratory tract infection. Predisposing factors include voice abuse and the lack of adequate humidification. A number of viruses, especially the rhinoviruses, have been found to be causative. Secondary bacterial infection accompanied by fever may occur. On examination, the laryngeal mucosa is erythematous and edematous especially over the true vocal cords. Since this condition is self-limited, the recommended treatment is symptomatic with humidification, hydration, and voice rest. Antibiotics are recommended only for bacteriologically proven infections.

One of the most common forms of **bac-**

## Table I
### Differential Diagnosis

Inflammatory Causes in Adults
  Infectious Inflammatory Causes
    Acute Laryngitis
      Viral Laryngitis
      Bacterial Laryngitis
    Granulomatous Laryngitis
      Tuberculous Laryngitis
      Syphilis
      Leprosy or Hansen's Disease
      Histoplasmosis
      Blastomycosis
      Actinomycosis
  Noninfectious Inflammatory Causes
    Sarcoidosis
    Wegener's Granulomatosis
    Gastroesophageal Reflux Disease
    Contact Ulcer and Granuloma
Voice Abuse/Misuse/Overuse
Psychogenic Voice Disorders
  Conversion Aphonia/Dysphonia
  Laryngeal and Neck Muscle Tension Dysphonia
Laryngeal Movement Disorders
  Spasmodic Dysphonias
Neoplasms/Masses
  Benign Neoplasms
  Malignant Neoplasms
  Nonneoplastic Laryngeal Masses
  Laryngocele
Neurological Lesions of the Larynx
Trauma
  Blunt and Penetrating Injuries
  Ionizing Radiation
  Foreign Body
  Gaseous or Caustic Injuries
  Intubation Trauma
Laryngeal Maanifestations of Systemic Disease

terial laryngitis is acute epiglottitis.[21–23] This entity usually develops secondary to purulent rhinosinusitis or tracheobronchitis. The pathogen isolated in most cases is *Hemophilis influenzae* B as it is in children, but *Streptococcus pneumoniae* infection and beta-hemolytic streptococcus may be also involved. Characteristically the epiglottis and the supralaryngeal structures appear swollen and bright red (Figures 7 and 8). Fever is usually present and, on lateral neck roentgenogram, the epiglottis appears swollen and the hypopharynx dilated. The disease is clinically manifested by inspiratory stridor, sore throat, muffled voice, and dysphagia. The patient should be closely monitored since airway obstruction can develop rapidly. An intubation or tracheostomy set should be at hand since the primary concern is the airway as soon as the diagnosis is suspected. Until the emergent conditions for airway management are instituted, the administration of Heliox can be performed to facilitate delivery of oxygen in a compromised airway. The diagnosis should be a clinical one, based on visualization of the airway; therefore no imaging is required. Treatment should include conservative measures (as for viral laryngitis) and appropriate parenteral antibiotics; today the antibiotic of choice should be one of the third generation cephalosporins to cover beta-lactamase producing *Hemophilus influenzae*. Although adults can be observed in an intensive care environment, in many instances children require aggressive airway management with intubation and ICU admission. Once the airway is secured, appropriate cultures of the epiglottis and blood can be done. The most serious complication of bacterial epiglottitis is the development of a laryngeal abscess. This is more commonly seen in adults than in children. The clinical course of this complication—severe airway compromise—is fulminant and surgical drainage following tracheostomy should be promptly performed.[24]

***Granulomatous Laryngitis:*** Granulomatous laryngitis is a chronic infectious-inflammatory process involving the larynx and is caused by a variety of micro-organisms. These groups of pathological conditions are almost always controlled by antibiotics or antifungal suspensions and rarely produce the classical protracted disseminated disease patterns of the past.

**Tuberculous laryngitis**[25] is still the most common granulomatous infection of the larynx. Predisposing conditions include pulmonary anthracosilicosis and

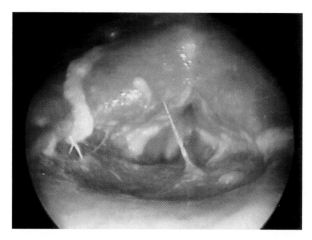

**Figure 7.** Endoscopic appearance of bacterial laryngitis. Note the inflamed larynx with a diffuse exudate. Photogragh by Eiji Yanagisawa, MD.

malnutrition. Tuberculous laryngitis is now almost exclusively associated with pre-existing pulmonary active tuberculous involvement and, therefore, has the same infectivity as the latter. Clinical presentation includes hoarseness, referred otalgia, odynophagia, and airway obstruction in the late phase of the disease. On examination, the involved areas appear edematous and hyperemic, mimicking carcinoma. The most commonly affected areas are the posterior third of the true cord, the arytenoids, and the interarytenoid area. Although the diagnosis may be established by acid-fast–staining organisms in smear or culture of sputum, a biopsy should always be performed since tuberculosus laryngitis may coexist with laryngeal carcinoma or syphilis. Treatment is essentially medical with triple or quadruple antituberculous chemotherapy. Arytenoidectomy or even tracheostomy may become necessary in advanced cases with a fibrotic component.

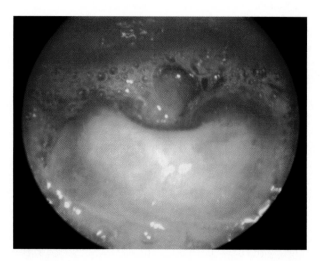

**Figure 8.** Endoscopic appearance of acute epiglottitis. Note the diffuse laryngeal edema and erythema more pronounced in the epiglottis. Photograph by Eiji Yanagisawa, MD.

**Syphilis**[26] may affect the larynx during the secondary and tertiary stages of the disease. During the secondary stage, the laryngeal involvement is characterized by superficial grey areas with fine red margins that heal without scarring. Secondary lymphadenitis often persisting for months is an invariable finding. If the disease is left untreated, gumma formation will lead to the development of granulomas, ulcerations, and ultimately secondary bacterial invasion and perichondritis. The end-stage of the disease consists of scar formation and subsequent stenosis leading to airway obstruction or aspiration. Histopathological examination shows various degrees of vasculitis and obliterative endarteritis. The diagnosis is made serologically. Treatment consists of high doses of intramuscular penicillin.

**Hansen's disease,**[27] or leprosy, may occasionally spread to the larynx. The nose is the first and often the only organ affected. The infection spreads to the larynx probably through the lymphatics. The causative micro-organism is *Mycobacterium leprae*. The supraglottic larynx is usually involved. On examination, the epiglottis and aryepiglottic folds will be seen to be nodular and deformed. In the early stages, the nodules will appear red and edematous, but later may become pallid and ulcerative. Hoarseness is the predominant symptom. The diagnosis is based upon histological findings that show edema, infiltration of chronic inflammatory cells, and the formation of numerous large foam cells. Acid-fast−staining can demonstrate the presence of *M. leprae* in the foam cells. Nasal smears may sometimes be beneficial. Treatment consists of dapsone for 1 to 2 years after the organism can no longer be demonstrated on biopsy.

**Histoplasmosis**[28] is a mycotic infection caused by *Histoplasma capsulatum*. The disease is endemic in certain parts of North America. The primary infection occurs in the lungs since histoplasmosis is caused by inhaling dust containing the spores. The larynx is secondarily involved via the blood stream. Concomitant oral ulcerations are common.

On examination, ulcerated nodular granulomas are seen involving the epiglottis and the false vocal cords. These lesions may become quite painful. Diagnosis is usually made by culturing the fungus or by the complement fixation test. An intravenous antimycotic agent, such as amphotericin B, is the treatment of choice.

**Blastomycosis**[29] is another fungal infection that can involve the larynx. The disease is rare and occurs in two forms. The North American form is due to infection with *Blastomyces dermatitidis* and the South American form is caused by *Blastomyces brasiliensis* infection. Infection occurs by inhalation of the spores, which are usually found in the soil. The lungs are the first affected organ, but the disease may become disseminated by the blood stream. When the larynx becomes involved, there is severe hoarseness and chronic cough. On examination, the lesion is erythematous or nodular and sometimes progresses to microabscesses and ulceration. Pseudoepitheliomatous hyperplasia is often seen in the epithelial layer. The diagnosis is confirmed by biopsy, revealing a tuberculoid granuloma in which fungal cells may be seen. Treatment consists of administration of amphotericin B or ketoconazole.

**Actinomycosis**[30] is a rare multiorgan suppurative condition caused by anaerobic bacteria (*Actinomyces bovis* or *Actinomyces israelii*). The infection is not primarily laryngeal but the initial involvement is in the cervical or mandibular region leading to paralaryngeal and then to laryngeal disease. Local and referred pain, cough, and hoarseness are the main symptoms. On examination, the larynx appears erythematous and edematous with draining sinuses containing sulfur granules. These are aggregations of bacterial colonies. Diagnosis is made by biopsy and identification of the organisms from discharge of the wounds. Actinomycosis requires prolonged penicillin therapy. If deep ulceration or chondritis occurs, repeated debridement should be performed.

*Noninfectious Inflammatory Causes (also see section on "Trauma")*

**Sarcoidosis:** Sarcoidosis[31] involves the larynx in only 5% of the patients with the disease. It is a granulomatous disease without caseation, the typical lesion being a noncaseating granuloma. The disease affects areas rich in lymphatics, thus spares the true vocal cords which are relatively poor in lymphatics and affects the supraglottis which is rich in lymphatics. The clinical presentation is nonspecific hoarseness with various degrees of airway obstruction. Associated constitutional manifestations are rare, but may include fever, hilar lymphadenopathy, erythema nodosum, and arthropathy. Diagnosis is made by excluding tuberculosis and fungal disease. The microscopic appearance is that of a granuloma with epithelioid marcophages and giant cells. The presence of Schaumann's bodies may be a striking feature of the giant cells. Steroids may produce a marked regression of symptoms and signs, and laser surgery is beneficial in cases of obstruction.

**Wegener's Granulomatosis:** Wegener's granulomatosis[32] is a destructive granulomatous disorder which may occasionally involve the larynx. Its laryngeal manifestation is identical to that of midline lethal granuloma. The disease is characterized by systemic involvement. Although the initial lesion is usually found in the nose with nasal crusting and bleeding, necrotizing granulomas and vasculitis usually affect the lungs, kidneys, and other organs. Examination of the larynx shows necrotic ulcerations and pseudoepitheliomatous hyperplasia. Diagnosis is based on the histopathologic features of necrotizing granulomas and fibrinoid necrosis of the small arteries and arterioles. The serum anticytoplasmic autoantibody test is specific for Wegener's granulomatosis. Steroid therapy coupled with immunosuppressive agents have shown some good results in the management of this condition.

**Gastroesophageal Reflux Disease:** Among the causes of laryngeal inflammation, GERD merits special consideration. In recent years, a variety of disorders of special interest to otolaryngologists are being related to this condition. These include posterior laryngitis, cricoarytenoid joint arthritis, subglottic stenosis, hoarseness, hyperkeratosis of the posterior larynx, Plummer-Vinson syndrome, and globus sensation. The pathogenesis of GERD is not well understood. The incompetence of the lower esophageal segment has been attributed to changes in pressure relationships between the stomach and the lower esophageal segment. Transient lower esophageal relaxation, an increase in abdominal pressure, and spontaneous free reflux[33] are the main pathophysiological factors. Other factors include delayed gastric emptying with accumulation of acid/pepsin mixtures in the stomach for longer periods than normal, failure of esophageal clearing with prolonged acid exposure, and motor disorders associated with abnormal esophageal emptying. The tone of the upper esophageal sphincter (cricopharyngeus muscle) prevents ascending reflux and may influence the severity of the extraesophageal disease. Hiatal hernia and local mucosal resistance to refluxed gastric contents may also play important roles in GERD.

The diagnosis of GERD prior to the availability of continuous ambulatory pH monitoring was inferred on the basis of typical otolaryngologic physical findings, indirect diagnostic techniques like barium swallow or endoscopy, and the response to a therapeutic trial. The barium esophagogram and direct esophagoscopy are excellent diagnostic procedures, but in order to establish the diagnosis of GERD significant mucosal lesions must be present. On endoscopy, mucosal erythema alone might not be sufficient, but serious changes as erosions, ulcers, exudate, and stricture may favor the definitive diagnosis. Nevertheless endoscopic results correlate poorly with symptoms; up to one third of patients with chronic GERD symptoms will have normal endoscopic findings.[34] When endoscopy is combined with esophageal biopsy, the diagnosis may be more accurate but the histologic criteria for GERD is still disputed. The barium esophagogram is also not helpful unless the degree of GERD is great and the refluxed material is poorly cleared. In fact, the specificity and sensitivity of these tests as low as 10% to 40%.[35-37] Prolonged intraesophageal pH monitoring has become the most accurate and reliable test for the documentation of GERD. It enables the measurement of the frequency, duration, and cumulative effects of acid exposure as well as the acid clearance in the lower esophagus. This test has a sensitivity and specificity about 90%[19,35]; while this investigatory modality is highly sensitive and specific for GERD, there is less corrrelation of this test pointing to reflux as a causative factor in laryngeal disease. The recent addition of portable computerized data telemetry has permitted a more physiologic and less costly ambulatory test.[38,39]

The treatment of GERD should consist of several recommendations. Posture modifications include the elevation of the head of bed of approximately 6 inches since overnight pH monitoring studies showed reduced acid exposure with this maneuver.[40] For overweight patients, weight reduction is important and always suggested. Dietary considerations include the avoidance of foods that promote reflux or that in themselves are irritants or acids (eg, fat, alcohol, chocolate, carminatives, caffeine, soda, fruit). Patients with GERD should also avoid eating anything 2 hours before bedtime. Antacids are the mainstay of reflux therapy. They buffer the stomach contents, raise the lower esophageal sphincter pressure, and decrease esophageal reflux.[41] Alginic acid is also effective in reducing the effects of reflux. Other medications include cimetidine, ranitidine (both $H_2$ blockers), metoclopramide and cisapride (prokinetic agents), and omeprazole (a proton pump inhibitor).[42]

***Contact Ulcer and Granuloma:*** The perichondrium and cartilage of the vocal process of the arytenoids become inflamed as a result of a forceful opposition of the arytenoids during voicing, chronic coughing, and throat-clearing and as result of reflux esophagitis. The response of the traumatized areas is to either ulcerate or produce a heaped up granuloma. Since the original experiment by Cherry and Margulies,[43] other data have supported the idea that acid reflux of the esophagus is causative in a significant percentage of patients.[44,45] Clinically, patients experience laryngeal discomfort and a foreign body sensation in the throat. They usually have a low-pitched voice in the morning and complain of heartburn. Some blood may occasionally be coughed up if part of the granuloma becomes detached. On examination, contact ulcers and granulomas are unilateral; fresh lesions are partially covered by fibrin and are epithelized at the edges only—mature lesions show thickened epithelial swellings that sometimes may keratinize. Histologically, contact granulomas are identical to pyogenic granulomas.

Diagnosis is usually made by laryngoscopy and 24-hour pH monitoring. If reflux is implicated, a medical regimen should be instituted. This consists of instructing the patient to elevate the head of the bed and prescribing antireflux therapy. In addition to medical treatment, voice rest is also important in order to reduce the constant stress on the vocal processes. Although the medical approach to contact granulomas usually results in healing, the lesions tend to recur at intervals. In these situations, the medical therapeutic regimen should be reinstituted. The role of surgery in the treatment of contact granulomas has been recently minimized because of the observed failure to address the underlying cause. Ablative therapy with $CO_2$ laser has been unsuccessful.

## Voice Abuse, Misuse, and Overuse

The physician is sometimes faced with the responsibility of treating professional voice users. Special consideration, understanding, and compassion are needed in the management of singers, young teachers, trial lawyers and others complaining of imperceptible voice change that is quite intolerable. Often, these patients are seen on a semiurgent basis. The complaint and the physical findings in these patients may differ greatly, but the diagnosis and treatment are usually similar. The trauma inflicted on the larynx is usually due to exuberant or incorrect usage. Because of inappropriate "slapping together" of the vocal cords, a traumatic insult ensues and the sequelae of inflammation results; these findings will be discussed below.

A comprehensive history is essential to establish a proper diagnosis. It is important to determine if the current complaint is acute, recurrent, or chronic. A distinction should be made between hoarseness (coarse or scratchy sound), fatigue (no change in vocal quality), volume disorders (inability to sing loudly or softly), breathiness (excessive loss of air during vocalization), or pain. Other important historical information includes the nature of vocal training, the environment and type of voice performance, exposure to irritants, smoke, alcohol abuse, and drug intake. Information about nutrition, endocrine function, and previous surgery provide essential details for the assessment and treatment of the professional voice user. In addition, physical conditions that might interfere with the normal function of the abdominal musculature should be suspected as a cause of dysphonia. A multisystem review should be conducted in order to determine whether gastrointestinal, pulmonary, or orthopedic problems are present. The presence of reflux esophagitis, diminished pulmonary reserve, and cervical arthritis might have significant effects on the patient's voice use.

The physical examination should include a comprehensive head and neck evaluation. The examination of the larynx begins with the performance of indirect laryngoscopy. Rigid telescopes are very useful and allow for photography and excellent visualization. The findings most often include vocal fold edema, inflammation, or vocal nodules (Figure 9). Vocal fold hemorrhage, mass lesions, contact ulcers, arytenoid erythema, or granulation are other less common findings.

Stroboscopic examination of the larynx adds important information of the laryngeal status in voice users. This, as well as flexible nasopharyngoscopy, is the first line of diagnostic technology. This combination allows magnification, photography, and a detailed assessment of the vocal fold motion. Other diagnostic techniques

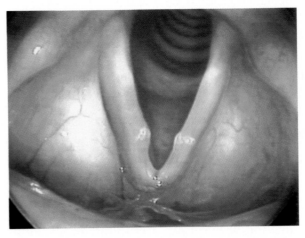

**Figure 9.** Endoscopic appearance of early singer's nodules at the anterior 1/3 of both vocal cords. Note the localized areas of edema which are consistent with vocal overuse or abuse. Photograph by Eiji Yanigisawa, MD.

include electroglottography, phonatory function assessment, and occasionally EMG. The cooperation between the otolaryngologist, a specially trained singing teacher, and the speech therapist is essential in the diagnostic and therapeutic decision-making process concerning voice abuse or technical errors. Before the initiation of any treatment, a complete objective voice analysis and assessment by the combined team should be carried out.

The treatment of voice disorders in professional users should always be conservative. Surgical intervention should be reserved as a last resort and should be undertaken with a great deal of care.

Vocal fold edema or hemorrhage resulting from voice misuse or abuse are managed by voice rest and supportive measures. Restriction of singing and the use of voice only for essential conversation is recommended. Telephone use and whispering is considered harmful. In some cases, this means the modification or cancellation of the performance schedule. The use of humidification and fluid intake is recommended. Mild sedatives may be beneficial in anxious individuals. In some cases, the use of steroids is prescribed but only in short-term courses and in cases in which an inflammatory process is suspected. Antacids are helpful in treating GERD. Voice therapy may be helpful for evaluating vocal abuse and misuse. Therapeutic strategies are applied individually for cases of vocal deviation (ie, vocal overuse). Once acquired by the patient, these techniques may be carried out quite easily.

Surgical therapy for large nodules, polyps, and chronic edema must be undertaken only in extreme situations, when combined conservative measures have been exhausted. The restoration of a singing voice after surgery may sometimes take up to 6 months.

## Psychogenic Voice Disorders

The diagnosis and treatment of psychogenic voice disorders remains one of the most difficult problems in the practice of otolaryngology. These patients are usu-ally referred after being treated for long periods with antibiotics, steroids, antihistamines, or voice therapy. Psychogenic voice disorders may often be misdiagnosed as acute laryngitis, asthma/allergy, or upper respiratory tract infection. This problem is defined as a disproportion between the severity of the patient's dysphonia and objective laryngeal findings. In these cases, the relative influence of vocal misuse, emotional aspects, and environmental features need to be evaluated. The majority of the patients fall within the age range of 18 to 34 years of age, and this condition is reported to be more common in women, with the proportion of 7:1.[46] A comprehensive laryngeal examination is, as usual, the first step toward correct diagnosis and treatment. Some authors[47] differentiate between psychogenic voice disorders associated with benign laryngeal disease (eg, vocal nodules, especially in children, polyps, contact ulcers) and psychogenic dysphonia without laryngeal disease.

Stressful voice use and tense, aggressive, or compulsive personality characteristics may play an important role in the development of the pathological conditions seen in the first group of patients. Although a pathologic process is clearly identifiable in these patients, the severity of dysphonia is disproportionate to the laryngeal findings.

Patients suffering from dysphonia without laryngeal disease present with dysphonia/aphonia, but the laryngeal examination is usually normal. A full case history examination may lead to the understanding of the situation which, although often associated with an event of acute stress, can be the result of relatively minor psychological problems, the relevance of which may not be fully appreciated by the patient.

### Conversion Aphonia/Dysphonia

This disorder is characterized by the loss of the voluntary control over sensory or motor function following an interpersonal conflict.[48,49] This will lead to the inability to express emotions such as fear, to communicate, or to verbalize feelings. The onset is sudden and often associated with a precipitating event. There is no history of prior laryngeal pathology. The voice disorder is stable, not intermittent nor fluctuant. It can manifest either as aphonia, whisper, or severe dysphonia. If any voice is present at all, it will be pitch-locked. Laryngoscopy reveals normal laryngeal anatomy and function. Conversion voice disorder patients are usually responsive to voice therapy. Counselling for the emotional issues involved is often appropriate but should be decided on an individual basis.

### Laryngeal and Neck Muscle Tension Dysphonia

Abnormal and excessive muscle tension in the larynx or the neck as a reaction to emotional stress is often seen in patients with voice disorders. Some patients demonstrate stiff posture with neck and jaw muscle stiffness. In other patients, there is no external evidence of abnormal laryngeal muscle hyperactivity, but a careful palpation of the cervical area may reveal tightening of the suprahyoid musculature.[46, 48, 50, 51] The underlying emotional pathology may emanate from a suppressed conflict to cancerphobia. The symptomatology is intermittent or long-standing fluctuant. There is associated vocal fatigue, reduction in vocal range, and other associated musculoskeletal tension syndromes such as temporomandibular joint syndrome and tension headache. The quality of voice is characterized by a strained, harsh, sometimes pitch-locked, rapid speech. Laryngeal examination is normal. The physical examination reveals abnormal posture, jaw thrust, and neck stiffness. Treatment requires voice therapy—to restore vocal function—and psychological counselling.

## Laryngeal Movement Disorders

**Spasmodic dysphonias** have been defined by Aronson et al.[52] as disorders of phona-

tion characterized by a strained, creaking, and choked vocal attack and a tense squeezed voice sound accompanied by extreme tension of the entire phonatory system.

This chronic and extremely disabling phonatory disorder of unknown origin often creates serious occupational, social, and emotional effects. It was first described in 1871 by Taube as a "spastic form of nervous hoarseness" and, like many dystonias in the past, has been considered primarily psychoneurotic in origin. Aronson et al.[52] proposed that spasmodic dysphonia is a heterogenous disorder with neurologic, psychogenic, and idiopathic subtypes that vary in clinical presentation and in response to therapy. Patients with the condition present with abnormalities in brainstem audiograms, blink reflexes,[53] and the cardiac response to the Valsalva's maneuver.[54, 55] In addition, patients with spasmodic dysphonia also have other forms of dystonias, such as blepharospasm and orofacial dystonias. In cases in which neither a psychologic nor neurogenic cause can be identified, the disease is reported as idiopathic. This differentiation is important since the treatment may differ widely according to the case. Most patients with laryngeal movement disorders have the **abductor** type of spasmodic dysphonia in which the vocal folds approximate too tightly during phonation. A minority of patients present with intermittent breathy dysphonia, or **adductor** spasmodic dysphonia, which is characterized by intermittent breaks in phonation causing brief periods of absence in voicing.

The onset of **adductor spasmodic dysphonia** is in the fourth and fifth decade. There is a slight preponderance of the disease among women in most reported series.[56] The diagnosis is made by presentation of the typical voice pattern. Laryngoscopy reveals a straining of the vocal cords but with normal excursions. Treatment involves[57–72] speech therapy; other maneuvers to correct this problem have been sectioning of the recurrent laryngeal nerve, which has had limited success; a more promising technique has been the injection of botulinum toxin into the nerve.

## Neoplasms/Masses

Neoplasms of the larynx can be classified as either benign or malignant.[73] Any mass lesion of the larynx can cause hoarseness by interfering with vocal cord function.

### Benign Neoplasms

Benign neoplasms of the larynx that interfere with phonation can arise from epithelial or mesenchymal tissue. Although benign neoplasms are rare, the most common epithelially derived lesion is the squamous papilloma.[74] These may occur at any age, but are most frequently encountered in the pediatric population. In addition to causing hoarseness, they may reach sufficient size to obstruct the airway. The human papilloma virus has been implicated in the cause of this problem. The diagnosis is made by examination of the larynx and subsequent biopsy. A variety of treatments have been used over the years, including endoscopic removal with forceps, cryotherapy, radiation as well as systemic therapy such as vaccines and interferon. In recent years the most common modality of treatment is endoscopic removal with the $CO_2$ laser—this has resulted in an excellent chance in resolution if performed by an experienced surgeon.

Benign mesenchymal neoplasms are exceedingly rare and when they occur are classified according to their tissue of origin (eg, hemangioma, fibroma, chondroma). Again, hoarseness is caused by interference with vocal cord function. Diagnosis and treatment is the same as epithelial benign neoplasms except for chondromata which, because of their composition, may require an open laryngeal procedure for removal.

### Malignant Neoplasms

Malignancies of the larynx can be classified[75] into those derived from epithelial and mesenchymal tissues and other special cancers. The vast majority of laryngeal cancer is squamous cell carcinoma. Cancer of the larynx comprises approximately 1.3% of all newly diagnosed malignancies and makes up 20% of all head and neck cancers.[75] The peak incidence is in the seventh decade and the ratio of men to women affected is 5:1. Factors implicated in the cause are tobacco use, alcohol ingestion, ionizing radiation, and possibly GERD.

The first symptom of glottic cancer is voice change or hoarseness. With further growth of the tumor, other symptoms may manifest themselves, such as dysphagia, pain, hemoptysis, otalgia, airway obstruction, and metastatic neck disease.

Examination of the larynx by indirect methods usually raises a high index of suspicion, with the appearance of the characteristic exophytic or ulcerative mass lesion (Figure 10). Any patient with prolonged hoarseness (especially from a "risk group") or with indirect examination evidence of possible malignancy should have a direct examination and biopsy.

Laryngeal cancer should be staged in order to place the patient into correct treatment protocols, for prognostic reporting to the patient and family, and for outcome analysis. The most widely used staging systems are those of the American Joint Committee on Cancer (AJCC) and the Union Internationale Contre le Cancer; they use the TNM (Tumor/Node/Metastasis) system. In addition to clinical and endoscopic appearance, these tumors are staged by imaging (via computed tomographic scanning and/or magnetic resonance imaging).

The treatment of squamous cell carcinoma of the larynx varies with the stage of lesion and with geography. Generally, early carcinomas are managed with external beam radiation, laser surgery, or voice preservation surgery. Advanced disease is usually treated with radiation, radical surgery, or a combination of these. The result of treatment of early lesions is excellent with 5-year survivals of about 80%. Advanced malignancies carry a poorer prognosis with any modality.

Mesenchymally derived malignancies

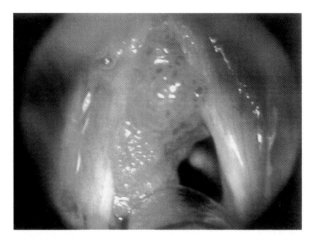

**Figure 10.** Endoscopic appearance of a squamous cell carcinoma of the glottis arising from the right vocal cord. Photograph by Eiji Yanagisawa, MD.

usually present in a similar way to squamous carcinoma and the diagnostic approach is the same. Generally, these tumors are managed surgically with radiation playing an adjunctive role. Other tumors are quite rare and may include oat cell carcinoma, salivary gland malignancies, lymphomas, fibrous histiocytomas, melanomas, carcinoids, and metastases.

### Nonneoplastic Laryngeal Masses

A variety of laryngeal mass lesions may interfere with vocal cord function and present as hoarseness as the first symptom. Vocal nodules due to overuse or improper use have already been discussed earlier in this chapter.

Vocal cord polyps are a common cause of hoarseness.[76] They are usually due to an inflammatory process of the larynx such as an upper respiratory infection, chronic exposure to smoke, or chronic voice abuse. If the process has gone on for a prolonged period of time, both cords may have undergone polypoid degeneration over their whole length. The causative factors are quite apparent on history-taking. Indirect laryngoscopy will reveal a unilateral or multiple areas of discreet edema-

tous masses (Figure 11). Treatment of these includes patient education of the offending agents (eg, voice use-modification, cessation of smoking) and surgical removal of the mass via the endoscopic route. If the polyps involve both cords, staged removal is often necessary to prevent web formation.

Intracordal cysts are sometimes seen as a result of either congenital rests undergoing cystic degeneration or blockage of a secretory gland. Patients present with hoarseness and no provocative factors. The indirect appearance is of a discreet cystic structure on the vocal cord. Treatment is endoscopic removal. The condition of contact granuloma has been covered in a previous section.

### Laryngocele

Laryngocoeles are masses that arise as a result of cystic dilatation of the saccule of the ventricle of the larynx.[77] They are classified as internal if they stay within the confines of the thyrohyoid membrane or external if they extend beyond the membrane. They are usually unilateral and occur most commonly in males. Clinically, they may present as hoarseness, a mass in the neck, or, if they become quite

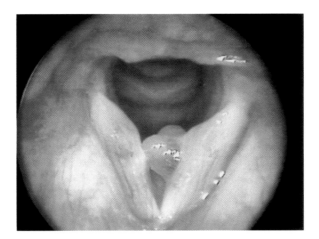

**Figure 11.** Endoscopic appearance of a laryngeal polyp on the left vocal cord. Photograph by Eiji Yanagisawa, MD.

large or infected (laryngopyocele), airway obstruction. Indirect examination of the larynx demonstrates a red mucosal mass consistent with the size on the sidewall of the larynx. Computed tomographic scanning is very helpful in delineating the extent of the lesion.

Treatment is surgical removal of symptomatic laryngoceles (some are incidental findings that merit observation only). Endoscopic removal or marsupialization is performed for small internal laryngoceles while an external approach is done for large external ones.

## Neurological Lesions of the Larynx [78]

Any factor that compromises the motor nervous innervation of the larynx can affect vocal cord movement and result in a dysphonia. With vocal cord movement impaired, vocal quality tends to become "breathy"; however patients perceive this as hoarseness. The disorder is readily recognized on laryngoscopy.

The central origin of the nerve supply to the larynx (ie, the vagus nerve or cranial nerve X) originates in the medulla oblongata. From the nucleus, the vagus nerve descends to the jugular foramen. From here, the vagus nerve descends in the neck within the carotid sheath to the thoracic

inlet. In the neck, the vagus gives off a small motor branch, the external laryngeal nerve, to the cricothyroid muscle. In the chest, the branches to the larynx, the recurrent laryngeal nerves of the vagi, due to embryological development, "recur" to the neck. The right recurrent nerve recurs around the right subclavian artery and the left recurs around the ductus arteriosus.

Intracranial lesions that compromise the central origins of laryngeal innervation must be large and diffuse. They may include infections, vascular compromise, neoplasms, and multiple sclerosis. Patients with intracranial problems present with a spectrum of other clinical findings in addition to their vocal impairment consistent with the extent of neurological involvement. Space occupying lesions of the brain stem at the level of the jugular foramen, such as glomus tumor or neurofibromata, may cause neuropathy of the laryngeal nerve supply.

Lesions in the neck that affect the nerve supply to the larynx are lesions caused by trauma to the nerve (as in thyroid surgery), metastatic carcinoma to the lymph nodes of the neck, or primary tumors of the larynx or thyroid.

Intrathoracic problems may cause paralysis of the recurrent laryngeal nerves. These include primary or secondary mediastinal tumors, penetrating trauma, or iatrogenic sectioning of the nerve.

Large or bilateral lesions in the chest may cause bilateral vocal paralysis.

Systemic diseases such as diabetes mellitus, amyotrophic lateral sclerosis, or myasthenia gravis may also cause unilateral or bilateral vocal cord paralysis.

The patient with dysphonia due to neurological involvement of the larynx presents with the complaint of "hoarseness" and any other manifestation of neurological disorder. The dysphonia is due to the inability of the two cords to appose during phonation. These patients may well have laryngeal incompetence and are subject to aspiration; because of this danger, these patients should be treated expeditiously. The most common presentation of these patients varies as to the specific referral patterns of the receiving laryngologist. For example, a center that is active in chest surgery may expect a large number of patients with recurrent laryngeal nerve impairment due to chest lesions or surgery. In the general laryngeal centers, the most common cause of laryngeal paralysis is idiopathic and is probably attributable to a viral neuropathy.

The diagnosis is made on laryngoscopy (Figure 12). The other ancillary diagnostic tools are helpful in management. Laryngeal EMG is especially beneficial for diagnosis and to predict reinnervation.

If the patient is not aspirating, the treatment of a paralyzed cord may be expectant. Many times, the involved cord will re-innervate if there is a viral neuropathy and this may take up to 18 months. In addition, the uninvolved cord can "compensate" and actually move across the midline to appose the paralyzed cord; this also may take many months.

If significant improvement of voice does not occur or the patient is so compromised vocally that he or she requests intervention, techniques are available to improve vocal quality—these procedures are geared toward allowing the uninvolved cord to approximate the paralyzed one. The two most popular surgical approaches are vocal cord augmentation with Teflon[79] or laryngoplasty.[80]

Teflon is injected into the paralyzed cord to increase its bulk so that apposition is effected by the mobile cord. This is done under a local anesthetic to gauge the amount of Teflon to inject by direct visualization of the glottis and listening to the patient's vocal quality.

With laryngoplasty, either a Silastic bar or a piece of the patient's own cartilage is inserted into a pocket lateral to the true cord via a window in the thyroid cartilage. As with Teflon injection, this procedure is meant to augment the paralyzed cord so the mobile one can appose it.

In bilateral cord paralysis, the primary

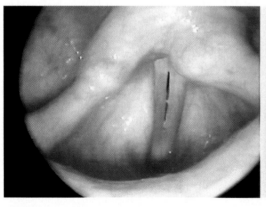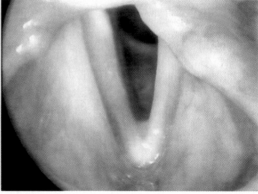

**Figure 12.** Endoscopic appearance of left vocal cord paralysis, (left) on phonation, (right) on respiration. The left cord is immobile with good apposition on phonation by the right. Photograph by Eiji Yanagisawa, MD.

object is to establish an adequate airway. Many times a tracheotomy is necessary. Usually voice is not a concern in this condition.

## Trauma

Trauma to the larynx[81] can cause hoarseness by impairment of proper vocal cord function or actual disruption of the cords. Traumatic injuries can be classified according to the mechanism of the insult. These factors include blunt and penetrating injuries, ionizing radiation, foreign bodies, gaseous or caustic injuries, and iatrogenic intubation trauma.

### Blunt and Penetrating Injuries

Blunt or closed trauma to the larynx is commonly caused by motor vehicle accidents with impact on the dashboard or steering wheel. Other causes of blunt collision with the larynx are fists and sport paraphernalia (eg, balls, sticks). Strangulation and hanging are also sources of blunt trauma. Penetrating injuries are caused by missiles such as bullets, knives, and shrapnel.

The diagnosis is made by the history and characteristic physical findings. Hoarseness is a component of the clinical spectrum. Other symptoms are hemoptysis, airway obstruction, and pain. Examination reveals any or all of hematoma, crepitus, subcutaneous emphysema, and evidence of penetration of a missile. Many times, there are accompanying neck injuries, such as neural injury, vascular, or foodway damage, or impairment at another site, such as chest and abdomen. Examination of the larynx shows edema, laceration, or hematoma.

Computed tomographic scanning is an important diagnostic modality to evaluate the laryngeal injury per se. Many times, other modalities must be utilized in order to elucidate concomitant injuries; these modalities include angiography, barium swallow, and abdominal ultrasound.

Of primary importance in the management of these injuries is adherence to the principle of the "ABCs" (ie, Airway, Breathing, Circulation) of the acutely injured patient. Minimal injuries and nondisplaced fractures with little in the way of symptomatology often require no treatment. However, major disruptions of anatomy, such as cord avulsions or severe fractures of the laryngeal superstructure, mandate open procedures and reconstructions. Failure to do the latter may result in an incompetent larynx with compromise of the airway and/or speech.

### Ionizing Radiation

The larynx may be the recipient of ionizing radiation[82] in the course of therapy to a malignancy in the larynx or to a site in the vicinity. The immediate effects on the vocal cords of radiation are the result of the inflammatory response of the tissues. Hoarseness occurs as a consequence of the edema and hyperemia engendered by the therapy. This is usually a short-lived phenomenon with resolution in a matter of weeks. Sometimes the effects are extremely long-lasting and symptoms may persist for years. In the extreme situation, the radiation can cause chondritis of the larynx with peristent edema, pain, and incompetence of the larynx. For the latter, long-term tracheotomy and/or gastrostomy may be necessary.

The diagnosis of the hoarseness is made in light of the clinical setting. Examination usually reveals an edematous and hyperemic larynx. The major diagnostic dilemma is differentiating the inflammatory response from the primary malignant disease for which the patient was treated.

Management of the hoarseness in this situation is expectant. If there is concomitant airway or foodway compromise due to the swelling, support may require tracheotomy and/or gastrostomy. Direct examination of the larynx is necessary if there is a high index of suspicion of persistent cancer.

## Foreign Body

Foreign bodies[83] are seen in the pediatric as well as the elderly population. Many foreign bodies inhaled come to rest in the tracheobronchial tree, but may have rested on the vocal cords before passing. At times the foreign body may impact on the larynx. The problems related to airway foreign bodies are primarily related to the airway. Impaction on the glottis is an emergent situation and usually requires immediate intervention—such a situation is the so-called "steak house syndrome" or "cafe coronary" where a piece of food may lodge on the larynx giving rise to hoarseness, stridor, and cyanosis. The "Heimlich maneuver" may be a life-saving action for this. Cricothyrotomy may have to be resorted to in extreme situations. If time is not a factor, indirect laryngeal examination may reveal a laryngeal foreign body. Plain radiographs of the upper or lower airway may demonstrate it. If there is a high index of suspicion in the absence of clinical evidence (eg, a persistent wheeze when there is no indication of respiratory disease), direct visualization of the airway with the patient under general anesthesia may be necessary.

## Gaseous or Caustic Injuries

The inhalation of hot air (fire) or irritative burning gases or the swallowing of caustic substances may cause inflammatory damage to the larynx.[83] While the main concern is to the airway, hoarseness may be a component of the whole clinical picture. The diagnosis is made on assessment in light of the clinical presentation, indirect laryngoscopy, and direct visualization of the airway. Treatment is directed towards support of the airway—many times such patients require ventilatory support. With the late effects of scarring on the larynx, secondary procedures to remove scars, webs, and stenoses, either endoscopically or via open approaches, may be required.

Certain patients with chronic lung disease on oral inhalant medication (eg, Ventolin, steroids) may be sensitive to the aerosol and develop an inflammatory response in the laryngeal mucosa with concomitant hoarseness. After the diagnosis is made by history and laryngoscopy, alteration should be made in the medication.

## Intubation Trauma

Intubation for airway support in respiratory failure or in the course of general anesthesia can injure the glottic larynx and result in vocal impairment.[83] The injuries are related to the act of introduction of the tube or the actual presence of the tube.

The placement of the endotracheal tube can damage the larynx by lacerating structures or avulsing major areas of anatomy such as the vocal cord or the arytenoid. Fortunately, the latter is quite rare but tears in the mucosa are common and can result in hoarseness with some frequency. The patient's complaint will be verified on indirect examination, and with minor lacerations, healing is usually spontaneous with no untoward effect. Major avulsions, however, should be treated with open approaches to restore normal anatomy and function. The best manner to deal with this problem is prevention by carefully placing the endotracheal tube and ensuring that the tube is secure in order to avoid mucosal avulsion.

The presence of the endotracheal tube may cause erosion of the abutting mucosa. The common sites are the posterior surface of the vocal cords and the subglottic larynx where the balloon meets the airway. Three consequences may happen: the eroded area may heal without event; granulation tissue may occur as a result of the natural course of wound-healing; or fibrosis of the denuded area may occur in the same vein. The common site of granuloma formation is in the interarytenoid area causing the classic "intubation granuloma" which occurs several weeks after the intubation and result in hoarseness (Figure 13). These granulomata are readily seen on indirect examination and usually disappear spon-

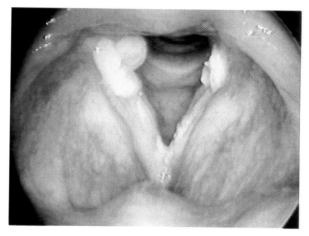

**Figure 13.** Endoscopic appearance of postintubation laryngeal granulomata in the interarytenoid area. Photograph by Eiji Yanagisawa, MD.

taneously within several months; if not, they can be removed endoscopically.

Fortunately, major denudations of mucosa with subsequent fibrosis and resultant stenosis and scarring are rare due to "soft-cuffed tubes" and the policy of early intervention with tracheotomy. In the unusual occasion where they do happen, laser ablation for minor stenoses or open reconstructive procedures for major obstructions are necessary to restore normal voice and airway.

## Laryngeal Manifestations of Systemic Disease

Systemic diseases may have a local effect on the larynx.[84] There are a number of congenital syndromes, such as Cri-du-chat and Down syndrome, in which anatomical anomalies such as vocal paralysis result in vocal impairment. These are apparent shortly after birth with dysfunction of crying or respiratory embarrassment.

General infections, such as tuberculosis, diphtheria, and syphilis, may localize in the larynx. Infiltrative disorders, such as sarcoidosis and amyloidosis, can cause hoarseness by the presence of deposits on the vocal cords.

Immunological diseases, such as rhematoid arthritis and lupus, may cause hoarseness by acute inflammation of the larynx and the late effects of the disease

on the laryngeal mucosa (nodules) and the joints (ankylosis and fixation).

Systemic toxins, such as chemotherapeutic agents (eg, methotrexate, vincristine), may cause hoarseness by mucositis and resultant edema.

Endocrinopathies such as hypothyroidism, acromegaly, and hypoparathyroidism have similar effects on the vocal cords as on the tissues of the body in general.

The diagnosis of these systemic problems is readily made in light of the clinical situation and with laryngoscopy.

## References

1. Negus VE. The Comparative Anatomy and Physiology of the Larynx. London, England: Heinemann; 1949.
2. Perkins WH. Vocal function: A behavioral analysis. In: Travis LE, ed. *Handbook of Speech Pathology and Audiology.* New York, NY: Appleton-Century-Crofts; 1971.
3. Vandenberg JW. Myoelsatic-aerodynamic theory of voice production. J Speech Hear Res 1958; 1: 227–244.
4. Bless DM, Hirano M, Feder RJ. Videostroboscopic evaluation of the learynx. Ear Nose Throat J 1987;66:48–58.
5. Kitzing P. Stroboscopy—a pertinent laryngeal examination. J Otolaryngol 1985;14: 151–157.
6. Hirano M, Kukita Y. Cover-body theory of

vocal fold vibration: In: Daniloff RG, ed. *Speech Science*. San Diego, Calif: College-Hill Press; 1985:1–49.

7. Moore DM, Berke GS, Hanson DG, et al. Videostroboscopy of the canine larynx: the effects of asymmetric laryngeal tension. Laryngoscopy 1987;97:543–553.

8. Zhao R, Hirano M, Tanaka S, et al. Vocal fold epithelial hyperplasia. Arch Otolaryngol Head Neck Surg 1991;117:1015–1018.

9. Serkaz JA, Berke GS, Ming Y, et al. Videostroboscopy of human vocal fold paralysis. Ann Otol Rhinol Laryngol 1992;101:567–577.

10. Kaufman JA. Approach to the patient with a voice disorder. Otolaryngol Clin North Am 1991;24(5):989–998.

11. Blair RL, Berry H, Briant TDR. Laryngeal electromyography—techniques. Applications and a Review of Personal Experience. J Otolaryngol 1977;6:496–504.

12. Gundi GM, Payne JK, Higgenbottam TW. Clinical electromyography in ear, nose, and throat practice. J Laryngol Otol 1981; 95:407–413.

13. Miller RH, Rosenfield DD. The role of electromyography in clinical laryngology. Otolaryngol Head Neck Surg 1984;92:287–291.

14. Parnes SM, Satya-Murti S. Predictive value of laryngeal electromyography in patients with vocal cord paralysis of neurogenic origin. Laryngoscope 1985;95:1323–1326.

15. Blair RL. Laryngeal electromyography. Arch Otorhinolaryngol 1989;246 (5): 395–396.

16. Ludlow CL, Jeh J, Cohen LG, et al. Limitations of electromyography and magnetic stimulation for assessing laryngeal muscle control. Ann Otol Rhinol Laryngol 1994; 103:16–27.

17. Schaefer SD. Laryngeal electromyography. Otolaryngol Clin North Am 1991;24 (5): 1053–1057.

18. Buler AR, Byrne WJ. Twenty-four hour esophageal intraluminal pH probe testing: a comparative analysis. Gastroenterology 1981;80:957–961.

19. Olson NR. Laryngopharyngeal manifestations of gastroesophageal reflux disease. Otolaryngol Clin North Am 1991;24: 1201–1211.

20. O'Sullivan GC, de Meester TR, Smith RB, et al. 24-hour pH monitoring of oesophageal function. Its use in evaluation of symptomatic patients after truncal vagotomy and gastric resection and drainage. Arch Surg 1981;116:581–590.

21. Cavanagh RM, Newsum JK. Supraglottis in children: Evaluation and management. South Med J 1980; 73:1353–1357.

22. Baxter JD. Acute epiglottitis. In: English GE, ed. *Otolaryngology, Vol 3*. Philadelphia, Pa: Harper Rowl; 1984.

23. Mustoe T, Strome M. Adult epiglottitis. Am J Otolaryngol 1983; 4: 393–397.

24. Canalis RF, Jenkins HA, Ostgathrope JD. Acute laryngeal abscess. Ann Otol Rhinol Laryngol 1979;88:275–279.

25. Lell WA. Laryngeal tuberculosis. Diagnosis incidence and present day treatment. Arch Otolaryngol 1954;60:350–356.

26. Caldarelli DD, Friedberg SA, Harris AA. Medical and surgical aspects of the granulomatous disease of the larynx. Arch Otolaryngol 1979;12:767–769.

27. Sandberg P, Shum TK. Lepromatous leprosy of the larynx. Otolaryngol Head Neck Surg 1983;91:216–219.

28. Withers BT. Histoplasmosis primary in the larynx—report of a case. Arch Otolaryngol 1977;25:1963–1967.

29. Snen JY. Blastomycosis of the larynx. Ann Otol Rhinol Laryngol 1980;89:565–568.

30. Koegel L, Tucker HM. Postoperative actinomycosis infection of the larynx. Otolaryngol Head Neck Surg 1983;91:213–217.

31. Tucker HM. Infectious and inflammatory disorders. In: *The Larynx*. Tucker HM, ed. New York, NY: Thieme Medical Publishers; 1993: 231–244.

32. Pashley RT, Levit MN. Some aspects of therapy in the nonhealing granulomas of Wegener. J Otolaryngol 1979;8:53–57.

33. Dodds WJ, Dent J, Hogan WJ, et al. Mechanisms of gastroesophageal reflux in patients with reflux esophagitis. N Engl J Med 1982;307:1547–1552.

34. Behar J, Biancani P, Shehan MB. Evaluation of esophageal tests in the diagnosis of reflux esophagitis. Gastroenterology 1976; 71:9–15.

35. Richter JE, Castell DO. Gastroesophageal reflux: pathogenesis, diagnosis and therapy. Ann Intern Med 1982;97:93–103.

36. Silverstein BD, Pope CE. Role of diagnostic tests in esophageal evaluation. Am J Surg 1980;139:744–751.

37. Ott DJ, Dodds WJ, Wu WC, et al. Current status of radiology in evaluating for gastroesophageal reflux disease. J Clin Gastroenterol 1982;4:365–375.

38. Vitale GC, Cheadler WG, Sadek S, et al. Computerized 24-hour ambulatory esophageal pH monitoring and esophagoduode-

noscopy in the reflux patients. Ann Surg 1984;200:724–728.

39. Contenein P, Narcy P. Gastroesophageal reflux in infants and children. Arch Otolaryngol Head Neck Surg 1992;118: 1028–1030.

40. Ellis FH, Crozier RE. Cervical esophageal dysphagia. Indications for and results of cricopharyngeal myotomy. Ann Surg 1981; 194:279–289.

41. Morrisey JF, Barreras RF. Antacid therapy. N Engl J Med 1974;290:550–554.

42. Kamel PL, Hanson D, Kahrilas PJ. Omeprazole for the treatment of posterior laryngitis. Am J Med 1994;96:321–326.

43. Cherry J, Margulies S. Contact ulcer of the larynx. Laryngoscope 1968;78:1937–1941.

44. Feder RJ, Mitchell MJ. Hyperfunctional, hyperacitic and intubation granulomas. Arch Otolaryngol 1984;110:582–584.

45. Ohman L, Tibbing L, Olofsson J, et al. Esophageal dysfunction in patients with contact ulcer of the larynx. Ann Otol Rhinol Laryngol 1983;92:228–230.

46. Greene M. The voice and its disorders. Philadelphia, PA: J P Lippincott: 1972:130.

47. Harrison-Kay M, Hicks DM. Voice pathology in the larynx. In: *The Larynx.* Tucker HM, ed. New York, NY: Thieme Medical Publishers; 1993: 135–167.

48. Aronson AE. *Clinical Voice Disorders.* 3rd ed. New York, NY: Thieme Medical Publishers; 1990.

49. Kaufman JA, Blalock PD. Functional voice disorders. Otolaryngol Clin North Am 1991;24: 1059–1073.

50. Morrison MD, Rammage LE, Nichol H. Diagnosis and management of psychogenic and other functional dysphonias. In: Johnson J.T., Blitzer A., Ossoff R. et al., eds. *Instructional courses of the American Academy of Otolaryngology-Head and Neck Surgery. Vol. 2.* St. Louis, Mo: C.V. Mosby; 1989: 13.

51. Kaufman JA, Blalock PD. Classification and approach to patients with functional voice disorders. Ann Otol Rhinol Laryngol 1982;91:372–377.

52. Aronson A, McCaffrey V, Litchy WJ. Botulinum toxin injection for adductor spasmodic dysphonia: Patient's self-rating of voice and phonatory effort after three successive injections. Laryngoscope 1993;103: 683–692.

53. Cohen L, Ludlow C, Warden M, et al Blink reflex excitability recovery curves in patients with spasmodic dysphonia. Neurology 1989;39:572–577.

54. Schaefer S, Freeman F, Finitzo-Hieber T. Brainstem conduction abnormalities in spasmodic dysphonia. Ann Otol Rhinol Laryngol 1983;92:59–63.

55. Miller RH, Woodson GE. Treatment options in spasmodic dysphonia. Otolaryngol Clin North Am 1991;24:1227–1235.

56. Cooper M. Recovery from spastic dysphonia by direct voice rehabilitation. Proceedings of the 18th Congress of the International Association of Logopedics and Phoniatrics 1980;1:579–584.

57. Dedo HH. Recurrent laryngeal nerve section for spastic dysphonia. Ann Otol Rhinol Laryngol 1976;85:451–459.

58. Levine H, Wood BG, Batza E, et al. Recurrent laryngeal nerve section for spasmodic dysphonia. Ann Otol Rhinol Laryngol 1979;88:527–530.

59. Aronson AE, De Santo LW. Adductor spastic dysphonia: three years after recurrent laryngeal nerve resection. Laryngoscope 1983;93:1–8.

60. Dedo HH, Izdebski K. Intermediate results of 306 recurrent laryngeal nerve sections for spasmodic dysphonia. Laryngoscope 1983;93:9–16.

61. Crumley R. Regeneration of the recurrent laryngeal nerve. Otolaryngol Head Neck Surg 1990;90:442–447.

62. Isshiki H. *Functional Surgery of the Larynx with Special Reference to Percutaneous Approach.* Tokyo: Maeda Press; 1977.

63. Tucher HM. Laryngeal framework surgery in the management of spasmodic dysphonia. Ann Otol Rhinol Laryngol 1989:98: 52–54.

64. Jankovic J, Ford J. Blepharospasm and cranial cervical dysphonias: Clinical and pharmacological findings in 100 patients. Ann Neurol 1983;13:402–411.

65. Mauriello JA. Blepharospasm, Meige syndrome, hemifacial spasm; treatment with Botulinum toxin. Neurology 1985;35: 1499–1500.

66. Ludlow C, Naunton R, Fugita M, et al. Spasmodic dysphonia: Botulinum toxin injection after recurrent nerve surgery. Otolaryngol Head Neck Surg 1990;102: 122–132.

67. Aronson A, Hartman D. Adductor spastic dysphonia as a sign of essential (voiced) tremor. J Speech Hear Disord 1981;46: 52–58.

68. Hartman DE, Overhold SL, Viswanant B. A case of vocal nodules, masking essential (voice) tremor. Arch Otolaryngol 1982;108: 52–54.

69. Hanson DG, Gerratt BR, Ward PH. Glottographic measurement of vocal dysfunction. Ann Otol Rhinol Laryngol 1983;92:413–420.

70. Darley FL, Aronson AE, Brown JR. *Motor Speech Disorders.* Philadelphia, Pa: W B Saunders Company; 1975: 182–187.

71. Hanson DG, Gerratt BR, Ward PH. Cinegraphic observations of laryngeal function in Parkinson's disease. Laryngoscope 1984;94:348–353.

72. Aronson AE, Olsdon-Ramig L, Winholtz WS. et al. Rapid voice tremor or "Flutter" in amyotrophic lateral sclerosis. Ann Otol Rhinol Laryngol 1992;101: 511–518.

73. Bastian RW. Benign mucosal disorders, saccular disorders and neoplasms. In: Cummings CW, Fredrickson JM, Harker LA, Krause CJ, and Schuller DE, eds. *1965 in Otolaryngology-Head and Neck Surgery.* St. Louis, Mo: CW Mosby; 1986.

74. Alberti PW, Dykun R. Adult Laryngeal Papillomata. J Otol 1981;10:463–470.

75. Sasaki CT, Carlson RD. Malignant neoplasms of the larynx. In: *1987 in Otolaryngology-Head and Neck Surgery.* St. Louis, Mo: CW Mosby; 1986.

76. Kleinsasser O. Pathogenesis of Vocal Cord Polyps. Ann Otol Rhinol Laryngol 1982;91:378–383.

77. DeSanto LW. Laryngocoele, laryngeal mucocoele, large saccules, and laryngeal saccular cysts: a developmental spectrum. Laryngoscope 1974;84:1291–1296.

78. Rontal M, Rontal E. Lesions of the vagus nerve-diagnosis, treatment, and rehabilitation. Laryngoscope 1977;87:72–86.

79. Lewy RB. Experience with vocal cord injection. Ann Otol Rhinol Laryngol 1976;85:440–450.

80. Koufman JA. Laryngoplasty for vocal cord medialization: An alternative to Teflon. Laryngoscope 1986;96:726–731.

81. Cassisi NJ, Isaacs JH, Jr. Trauma. In: *Otolaryngology-Head and Neck Surgery.* St. Louis, Mo: CW Mosby: 1986

82. Salmon LFW. Chronic Laryngitis. In: Ballantyne J, Groves J., eds. *Scott Brown's Diseases of the Ear Nose and Throat. Vol.4.* London, United Kingdom: Butterworths; 1979.

83. Bryce DP. Laryngeal Trauma and Stenosis. In: Ballantyne J, Groves J., eds. *Scott Brown's Diseases of the Ear Nose and Throat. Vol.4.* London, United Kingdom: Butterworths; 1979.

84. Jafek BW, Esses BA. Manifestations of Systemic Disease. In: *1933 in Otolaryngology-Head and Neck Surgery.* St. Louis, Mo: CW Mosby: 1986.

# 14

# Epistaxis

Ian J. Witterick, M.D.
Kris Conrad, M.D.

---

## Introduction

Epistaxis is a common disorder with 60% of people reporting at least one episode in their lifetime.[1,2] The incidence has been estimated to be 30 per 100,000 people per year[3] and the prevalence reported to be 10% to 13% of the general population.[4] It affects all age groups, but is more common in young children and older adults.

Epistaxis is usually of a minor and self-limiting nature with only 5% to 10% of those affected seeking medical attention.[5] The majority of patients suffer from bleeding in the anterior nose from the secondary effects of trauma or drying of the nasal mucosa. This "anterior epistaxis" accounts for approximately 90% of patients and can usually be managed effectively with relatively simple measures.[6] "Posterior epistaxis" is normally diagnosed when anterior rhinoscopy fails to visualize an anterior located bleeding point or a well-placed anterior nasal pack fails to stop the epistaxis.[7] Bleeding in the posterior nasal cavities can be much more difficult to control and can become life-threatening due to uncontrolled hemorrhage with cardiac and respiratory consequences.[8]

## Pathogenesis

### Applied Anatomy

The nasal cavities are designed to perform a number of complex physiological functions, many of which are accomplished by special anatomical and physiological design of the nasal mucosa. In order for the mucosa to fulfill these functions, it has a very rich vascular supply. The nasal septum, the nasal floor, and lateral walls are covered mainly by respiratory epithelium and the nasal vestibule is covered by keratinizing stratified squamous epithelium. The upper most segments of the septum and superior nasal turbinates which are part of the olfactory system are covered by olfactory epithelium.

Blood supply is derived from both the external and internal carotid artery systems. The main arteries of the external carotid system are the maxillary artery and the facial artery, which is the less significant of the two. The maxillary artery is still frequently referred to as the "internal maxillary artery" but current anatomical nomenclature has designated it as the "maxillary artery."[9] Similarly, the "external maxillary artery" is now known as the "fa-

---

From Irwin RS, Curley FJ, Grossman RF (eds): Diagnosis and Treatment of Symptoms of the Respiratory Tract. Armonk, New York, Futura Publishing Company, Inc., © 1997.

cial artery." In addition to the external carotid supply, there are important contributions from the internal carotid artery which may be responsible for refractory epistaxis.[10] The blood supply from the internal carotid artery system is derived via the ophthalmic artery which is the first one to branch out of the internal carotid artery as it arises at the cavernous sinus.

The detailed knowledge of arterial blood supplied to various areas of the nasal cavity and paranasal sinuses is expected of a specialist in head and neck surgery. A general vascular pattern should be known, however, to every physician. It is important to remember that the nasal cavity is the site of multiple anastomoses between the contralateral arterial systems of the head and neck and between the ipsilateral internal and external carotid artery. This special anatomical situation has important clinical significance for managing patients with refractory epistaxis.

## External Carotid Arterial Supply

The major blood supply to the nose is derived from the maxillary artery, which with the superficial temporal artery, is a terminal branch of the external carotid artery. The course of the maxillary artery is usually divided into the mandibular, pterygoid, and pterygopalatine portions (Figure 1). The mandibular portion passes horizontally between the neck of the mandible and the sphenomandibular ligament. It gives off deep auricular, anterior tympanic, middle meningeal, and inferior alveolar branches. In its second portion anterior to the ramus of the mandible (pterygoid portion), the artery passes superficially or very frequently deep to the lower head of the lateral pterygoid muscle. At this stage, the artery gives off muscular branches to the masseter, temporal, buccal, and pterygoid muscles. The third part (pterygopalatine) of the artery enters the pterygopalatine fossa giving off the posterior superior alveolar, infraorbital, pterygoid canal, pharyngeal, descending palatine, and sphenopalatine arteries.[11] The sphenopalatine artery being the final

branch of the internal maxillary artery divides into the lateral branch supplying the lateral wall of the posterior nasal cavity and into the septal branch supplying the posterior aspect of the nasal septum.

The facial artery, which takes origin from the front of the external carotid artery in the carotid triangle just above the lingual artery and above the greater cornu of the hyoid bone, arches upward and finds itself in a groove on the posterior border of the submandibular gland. It then turns downward and forward to cross the lower border of the mandible at the anterior edge of the masseter muscle. On the face, it passes towards the side of the nose where it gives rise to the superior labial artery which courses into the nasal vestibule giving off a septal branch supplying the anterior septum. The septal branch anastomoses with other branches of the external carotid system (sphenopalatine and greater palatine arteries) and with the internal carotid system (anterior ethmoidal artery).

## Internal Carotid Arterial Supply

The internal carotid artery does not have any branches in the neck before it enters the petrous temporal bone (petrous portion) at the skull base. It courses through the cavernous sinus (cavernous portion) and pierces the dura near the anterior clinoid process. The first major branch of the intracranial portion of the internal carotid artery is the ophthalmic artery which arises near the medial side of the anterior clinoid process as the internal carotid artery emerges from the cavernous sinus. It enters the orbit through the optic canal below and lateral to the optic nerve; then crosses obliquely above the optic nerve to reach the medial wall of the orbit. This is where it gives off the posterior ethmoidal artery and anterior ethmoidal artery entering their respective canals (Figure 2). The anterior ethmoidal artery is the more constant and larger nasal branch. The posterior ethmoidal artery supplies the posterior ethmoidal air sinuses and enters the cranium giving off a meningeal

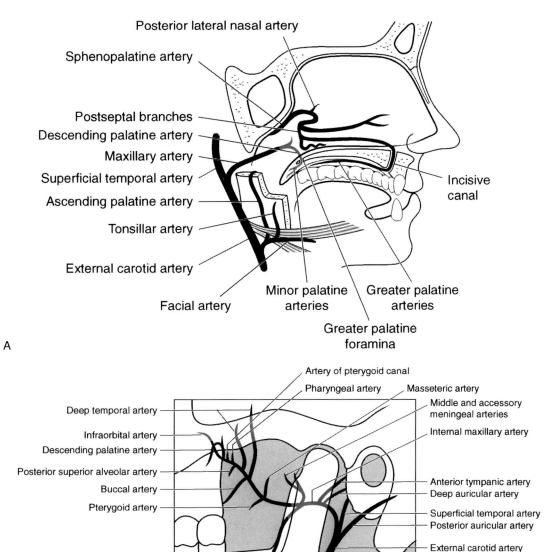

Posterior lateral nasal artery

Sphenopalatine artery

Postseptal branches
Descending palatine artery
Maxillary artery
Superficial temporal artery
Ascending palatine artery
Tonsillar artery

External carotid artery

Incisive canal

Facial artery

Minor palatine arteries

Greater palatine arteries

Greater palatine foramina

A

Artery of pterygoid canal
Pharyngeal artery
Masseteric artery

Deep temporal artery

Middle and accessory meningeal arteries

Infraorbital artery
Descending palatine artery
Posterior superior alveolar artery
Buccal artery
Pterygoid artery

Internal maxillary artery

Anterior tympanic artery
Deep auricular artery

Superficial temporal artery
Posterior auricular artery

External carotid artery

Branch to lingual artery
Inferior alveolar artery

B

**Figure 1.** Course of the maxillary artery. **(A)** Reveals overall relationship of maxillary artery to head; **(B)** shows finer detail of maxillary artery and its branches and relationship to mandible.

branch and nasal branches which find their way into the nasal cavity through the cribriform plate of the ethmoid bone. The ethmoidal arteries anastomose with branches of the sphenopalatine artery. The anterior ethmoidal artery supplies the an-

terior and middle ethmoid sinuses, the frontal sinus, and in the cranium gives off a meningeal branch and nasal branches. The latter enter the nasal cavity descending on the inner surface of the nasal bone and supply branches to the lateral wall and

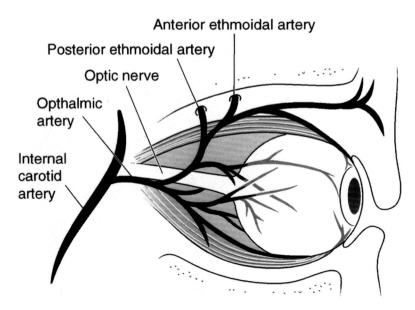

**Figure 2.** Course of the anterior and posterior ethmoidal arteries through the orbit.

the nasal septum superiorly. The terminal dorsal nasal branch appears on the nasal dorsum between the nasal bone and the upper lateral cartilage.

## Nasal Blood Supply

The lateral wall of the nose is thus supplied by the anterior ethmoidal artery in its anterosuperior portion and by the posterior ethmoidal artery in its postero-superior portion (Figure 3). The poster-oinferior part of the lateral nasal wall, including the inferior and middle turbinates, is supplied by the lateral branch of the sphenopalatine artery. The nasal septum in its anterosuperior portion is supplied by the septal branch of the anterior ethmoidal artery and its posterior and middle portion is supplied by the septal branch of the sphenopalatine artery (Figure 4). The anterior portion of the nasal septum derives its blood supply from the septal branch of the superior labial artery. The posterior portion of the nasal septum in the area of the vomer (Figure 4) is supplied by the posterior septal branches of the sphenopalatine artery where they anastomose with the

ethmoidal arteries. One of the branches then descends in a groove on the vomer to the incisive canal and anastomoses with the terminal ascending branch of the greater palatine artery and with the septal branch of the superior labial artery. This is the site known as Little's area or Kiesselbach's plexus, the site of the most common anterior nosebleeds constituting 80% to 90% of all nosebleeds, especially in children and young adults.[1] The facial and maxillary artery anastomose with branches of the opposite side. The maxillary and internal carotid artery anastomose through the ethmoidal arteries. The anastomosis within the external carotid artery systems take place between the ascending pharyngeal artery and palatine branches of the facial artery. The sphenopalatine artery anastomoses with the greater palatine artery (both are branches of the maxillary artery). The greater palatine artery in turn anastomoses with the ascending palatine artery (branch of the facial artery). The superior labial and septal branches of the facial artery also anastomose with the dorsal nasal branch of the ophthalmic artery. Another potentially important anastomosis responsible for

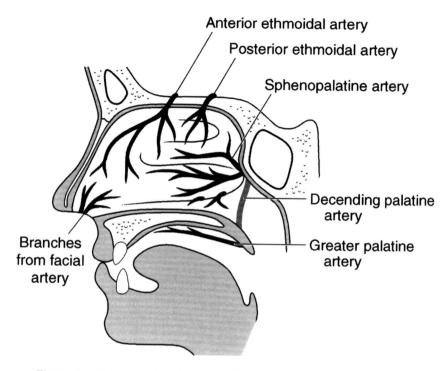

**Figure 3.** Major arterial blood supply to the lateral wall of the nose.

persistent bleeding exists between the ophthalmic artery and the middle meningeal and maxillary arteries.[12] This anastomosis allows persistent bleeding from branches of the maxillary artery to the ethmoid artery or vice versa following single-vessel ligation.

*Venous Drainage*

The veins of the nasal cavity accompany the arteries and drain predominantly to the pterygoid and pharyngeal venous plexuses posteriorly. In addition, some venous drainage passes externally to the anterior facial vein. The important clinical detail about the venous drainage is that the nasal cavity communicates with the facial vein that has no valves. That vein, in turn, communicates freely with the intracranial circulation as well as the deep facial vein that communicates with the pterygoid plexus; the pterygoid plexus communicates with the cavernous sinus as well.

Thrombosis or infectious process in this anatomical location may spread inside the cranium with fatal consequences.

**Pathophysiology**

The main function of the nasal cavity, apart from olfaction, is the preparation of the inspired air before it reaches the delicate complex of the lower respiratory tract. The nasal mucosa allows for recycling of heat and moisture during normal respiratory function. Its special mechanisms allow for cleansing of the air of polluting particles, micro-organisms, and some gases. The nasal mucosa performs this function by being exposed to the environment more than any part of the body. The normal flow of air through the nasal cavity is turbulent and that has certain physiological importance in performing the functions outlined above. Various structural abnormalities may increase the turbulence of the inspired and expired air to the ex-

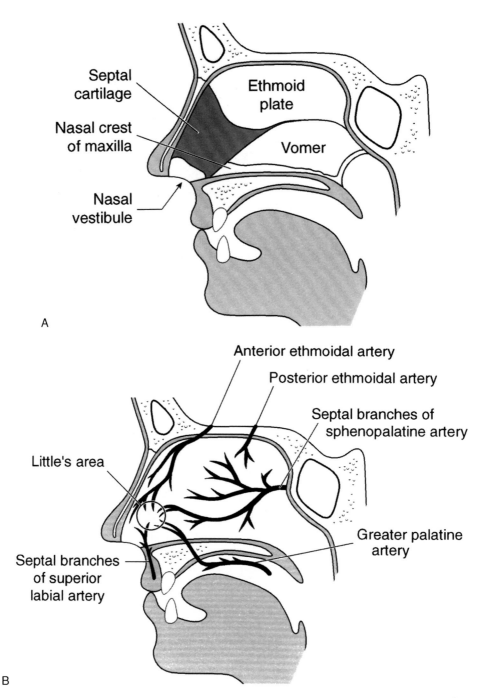

**Figure 4.** Anatomy and major arterial blood supply to the nasal septum. **(A)** shows bony landmarks of the nose; **(B)** and **(C)** show relationship of anatomic variations of arterial blood supply to the nose. **(B)** and **(C)** both show Little's area that contains Kiesselbach's plexus.

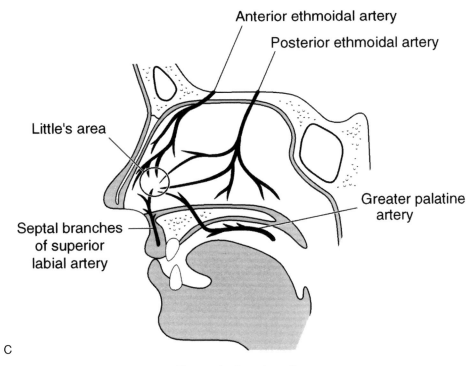

Anterior ethmoidal artery

Posterior ethmoidal artery

Little's area

Greater palatine artery

Septal branches of superior labial artery

C

**Figure 4.** *(continued)*

tent of producing drying of the nasal mucosa and crusting and damage to the surface epithelium. This, in turn, leads to chronic inflammatory changes and, at times, recurrent chronic bleeding. Histologically, the nasal mucosa consists of pseudostratified ciliated columnar epithelium attached to a basement membrane that is adherent to the underlying perichondrium or periosteum. The nasal mucous membrane is characterized by glandular structures, particularly serous glands needed to provide a protective blanket for proper functioning of the cilia and to prevent crusting that may lead to inflammatory conditions and episodic bleeding. In addition, as individuals age, their nasal mucosa becomes atrophic and loses much of its normal physiologic protective properties. This results in crusting and exposure of the underlying blood vessels which are often arteriosclerotic and do not have the same contractile properties to stop bleeding once it has commenced.

## Etiology

Epistaxis has been classified in many ways in an attempt to provide the clinician with a systematic approach to the search for a cause. A simple scheme broadly divides the factors into local and systemic causes (Table I). In most instances, nosebleeds originate in the anterior nasal cavity and are easily manageable by applying pressure; but multiple local and/or systemic causes may coincide to produce life-threatening nasal hemorrhage. In some cases, epistaxis may masquerade as hemoptysis or gastrointestinal bleeding.[13–15]

The major contributing factors associated with refractory epistaxis include hypertension, use of platelet-inhibiting drugs, and liver dysfunction from alcohol abuse.[16] In approximately 10% to 15% of patients, the cause remains unknown.[5]

Environmental factors combined with local or systemic problems can lead to injury of the nasal vasculature. The common

**Table I**
Etiology of Epistaxis

| Local Causes | Systemic Causes |
|---|---|
| Trauma | Deficiency of Clotting Factors |
|   Early |   Congenital |
|   Delayed |     Hemophilia |
|   Self-inflicted |     von Willebrand's Disease |
| Chemical Irritants |     Other (eg, deficiency of factor IX, XI, or XII, fibrinogen, or pro- |
| Septal Deformity |       thrombin) |
| Inflammation/Infection |   Acquired |
| Foreign Bodies |     Vitamin K Deficiency (eg, intestinal malabsorption) |
|   Animate |     Liver Disease |
|   Inanimate |     Anticoagulants (eg, heparin, coumarin derivatives) |
| Granulomatous Disease | Platelet Disorders |
| Neoplasms |   Inadequate Number of Platelets |
| |     Production Defect (eg, chemotherapy, infection) |
| |     Sequestration (eg, splenomegaly) |
| |     Accelerated Destruction (eg, drugs, autoantibodies, infection) |
| |   Poorly Functioning Platelets |
| |     Nonsteroidal Anti-Inflammatory Drugs |
| |     Uremia |
| | Hypertension |
| | Hemorrhagic Hereditary Telangiectasia |

cold and tiredness are frequently experienced before the occurrence of epistaxis.[17] Colder weather,[18] atmospheric pressure, and humidity changes[19] have been implicated in patients with recurrent epistaxis. Epistaxis is more common in the colder winter months because of the more frequent mucosal alterations/inflammation from upper respiratory infections and the nasal lining dries out from the decrease in humidity associated with central heating. Hot, dry climates are also associated with increased rates of epistaxis from the lowered humidity.

## Local Causes of Epistaxis

*Trauma*

Trauma to the nose, maxillary sinus,[20] orbit,[21] base of skull,[22] and middle ear[23] may all manifest as nasal hemorrhage (Figure 5). The nasal mucosa may be traumatized directly from blunt or sharp objects or indirectly from the fractured ends of nasal bone or cartilage. Common sites for mucosal tears include the septum, lateral recesses of the pyriform aperture, and the junction of the upper lateral cartilage with the nasal bones. Nasal or sinus surgery may result in serious primary or secondary hemorrhage.[24] Inferior turbinate operations can result in serious hemorrhage in up to 4% of patients.[25,26] A frequent source of epistaxis, especially in children, is caused by digital trauma of the anterior nasal septum. Participating in activities such as airflight or scuba diving during an upper respiratory tract infection can cause sinus barotrauma with hemorrhage into the affected sinus and, subsequently, into the nose.

Nasal fractures and fractures of the facial bones in general, although frequently associated with nosebleeds, are usually not a serious cause of nosebleeds. It is usually short-lasting and very seldom requires special therapeutic efforts unless there are other predisposing causes. Iatrogenic trauma, on the other hand, associated with nasal surgery or surgery of the paranasal sinuses, may produce severe primary or

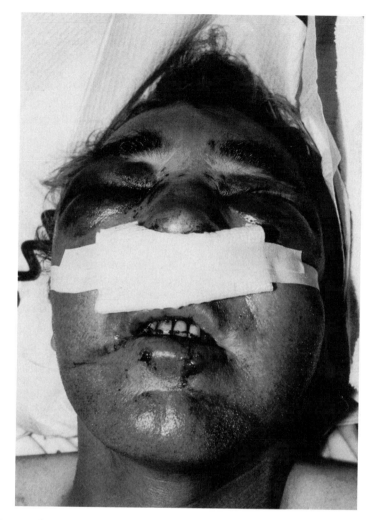

**Figure 5.** Patient with severe epistaxis requiring bilateral nasal packing following maxillofacial trauma.

secondary nosebleeds requiring prolonged nasal packing and supportive therapy.

Craniofacial trauma may injure the external carotid artery[27] or internal carotid artery[28–31] producing severe and life-threatening epistaxis. Injury of the internal carotid artery can cause two types of post-traumatic high-flow communications.[32] The first is a connection between the internal carotid artery and the cavernous sinus resulting in a carotico-cavernous fistula. The second type of injury is a false aneurysm which usually develops in the cavernous portion of the internal carotid ar-

tery but may also develop in the petrous portion.[23,33,34]

Life-threatening massive epistaxis is the most serious complication resulting from these high-flow communications, particularly in false intracavernous aneurysms.[35–40] The resultant epistaxis may be recurrent[30] or delayed for years after the initial trauma.[36,41] Cavernous aneurysms are usually posttraumatic from either blunt or penetrating trauma,[42] sphenoid sinus surgery, or pituitary gland surgery.[35,43] Rare reports of nontraumatic aneurysms of the cavernous portion of the internal carotid artery have been described.[44–46] In addition to epistaxis, there may be signs of one of a variety of cavernous sinus syndromes.[41]

## Chemical Irritants

Toxic and chemical irritants, such as glutaraldehyde, ammonia, gasoline, chromates, sulfuric acid, phosphorous, and printer's ink, can cause epistaxis.[47,48] A major cause of irritation and damage to the nasal lining is the recreational use of cocaine.[49] Topical intranasal steroids may cause mucosal irritation and induce epistaxis that is generally mild.

## Septal Deformity

Chronic inflammatory conditions of the nasal septum leading to septal perforation may be caused by a number of factors, including posttraumatic (eg, nasal fracture, habitual "nose-picker," septoplasty), granulomatous disease, neoplasia (eg, polymorphic reticulosis), and substance abuse (eg, cocaine). Such conditions usually do not lead to severe epistaxis.

Nasal septal abnormality in the form of very superficial and markedly developed capillaries, on the other hand, may be the cause of severe epistaxis especially if associated with drying up of the nasal mucosa caused by abnormal nasal air flow. The latter may be related to septal spurs or deviations which not only contribute to the onset of the crisis but may make the treatment extremely difficult by limiting access to the site where bleeding originates. Emergency septoplasty is warranted in such situations (see "Septoplasty/Submucous Resection" section). Massive epistaxis from the drying effects of nasal continuous positive airway pressure (CPAP) has been described.[50]

## Inflammation/Infection

Viral or bacterial rhinitis and nasopharyngitis predispose to epistaxis from the associated inflammation of the nasal lining.[51,52] Minor irritation from digital manipulation, blowing the nose, or even sneezing may initiate epistaxis. Atrophic rhinitis (ozena) is caused by chronic bacterial infection (*Klebsiella ozaenae*) leading to nasal crusting, mucosal atrophy, and inflammation.[53] During pregnancy, granulation tissue may form as a "pregnancy tumor," usually on the nasal septum, and present with severe or recurrent epistaxis.[54,55]

## Foreign Bodies

Intranasal foreign bodies are usually placed by small children or mentally handicapped individuals and are responsible for unilateral bleeding associated at times with nasal obstruction and purulent or serosanguinous discharge. The foreign body may be inanimate or animate. Some of the organic or inorganic foreign bodies may attract calcium and magnesium salts that will crystallize producing stonelike objects (rhinolith), which after several years may attain large size and create significant difficulties while trying to remove them. The list of inanimate objects that have been found in the nasal cavity could exceed one's imagination. The objects range from beans, nuts, peas, marbles, jewelry, and plastic to screws, bolts, and various parts of toys. A separate category among these foreign bodies are foreign bodies of iatrogenic origin such as broken pieces of instruments, gauze, and cotton sponges as well as forgotten nasal packing. Among the animate category, such conditions as infestation with fly larvae or intestinal worms is mentioned. Fungal infections may produce polypoid masses (*Rhinosporidium*) or granulomatous lesions (*Aspergillus*). Parasitic disease from infestation with *Ascaris lumbricoides* can result in regurgitation of larvae that may enter the nose and paranasal sinuses. Intranasal infestation by leeches has also been reported as a cause for epistaxis.[56–58] The above-described conditions usually occur in immunosuppressed individuals, in tropical climates, and in unsanitary environments.

## Granulomatous Disease

Granulomatous disease of the nose or sinus cavities is uncommon. The disease may be localized to the nose but is usually part of a more generalized process. Wegener's granulomatosis may produce local changes before it becomes a systemic disease and granulomatous conditions related to tuberculosis, syphilis, or sarcoid are mentioned for the sake of completeness but are extremely rare among causes of nosebleeds in North America. The granulomatous inflammation causes mucosal edema, crusting, and friability, leading to symptoms of nasal obstruction, pain, and epistaxis. Destruction of the septal cartilage is common, resulting in a septal perforation that can weaken the supporting framework of the dorsum of the nose leading to a "saddle-nose" deformity (Figure 6).

## Neoplasms

Various benign[59] and malignant neoplasms[60,61] of the nasal cavities, sinuses, nasopharynx, and anterior cranial fossa[62] may present with epistaxis. The classic vascular neoplasm presenting with recurrent or severe epistaxis in adolescent males is the nasopharyngeal angiofibroma.[63] Other vascular neoplasms arising in this region include hemangiomas and hemangiopericytomas.[64,65] It is therefore essential that every attempt be made to rule out a neoplasm as a local cause of epistaxis, especially where the index of suspicion is high because of age, gender, or race of the patient points to the possibility of certain neoplasms. Plain sinus roentgenograms may show bony erosion or expansion but more sophisticated imaging is usually required with computerized tomography (CT), magnetic resonance imaging (MRI), and angiography to fully appreciate the extent of the neoplasm (Figures 7, 8A, and 8B). Caution is advised before biopsying any mass that may have a vascular basis since the ensuing epistaxis can be severe and life-threatening.

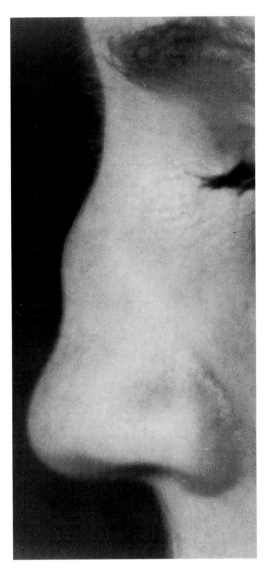

**Figure 6.** Saddle nose deformity from Wegener's granulomatosis involvement of the nasal septum with resultant septal perforation and weakening of the nasal dorsum.

## Systemic Causes of Epistaxis

### Blood Dyscrasia

Blood dyscrasias vary in their ability to cause a hemorrhagic episode. Bleeding may result from a deficiency of clotting factors, inadequate numbers of platelets,

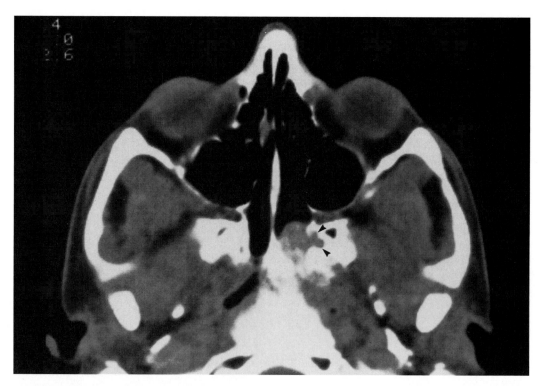

**Figure 7.** Contrast-enhanced CT of an 18-year-old man presenting with recurrent epistaxis demonstrating an enhancing soft tissue mass (nasopharyngeal angiofibroma) in the left nasopharynx causing some destruction of the adjacent medial pterygoid plate (arrowheads). CT = computed tomographic scanning. Photograph courtesy of Dr. E. Kassel, Radiologist-in-Chief, Mt. Sinai Hospital, Toronto, Ontario, Canada.

or poorly functioning platelets. Hereditary forms of easy bleeding, such as hemophilia and von Willebrand's disease, usually present in early life with easy bruising and unexplained prolonged bleeding after minor injury. Parkin et al. found abnormal *in vitro* tests in 53% of patients presenting with symptoms suggesting a mild bleeding disorder including epistaxis.[66] Some patients may have mild, but clinically significant, hemostatic disorders if screened.[67] In many cases, more sophisticated hematologic investigation is required.[68] The common causes of both a blood dyscrasia and epistaxis result from liver disease (usually from alcohol abuse), anticoagulants,[69] nonsteroidal anti-inflammatory medications,[70–72] leukemia, and chemotherapy for malignant disease.[73]

Disorders of coagulation factors may

be congenital or acquired. The most common congenital abnormalities are with factor VIII, where a deficiency in the procoagulant activity results in hemophilia and abnormalities of the von Willebrand protein results in von Willebrand's disease. Other less common congenital deficiencies of coagulation factors include factors IX, XI, and XII; fibrinogen; and prothrombin.

Acquired coagulation disorders may arise from vitamin K deficiency, anticoagulant drugs, and liver disease. Vitamin K is a fat-soluble vitamin essential for the synthesis of normal prothrombin and factors VII, IX, and X. Deficiency of vitamin K usually results from impaired absorption (eg, lack of bile salts in obstructive jaundice, intestinal malabsorption). The common anticoagulant drugs include coumarin derivatives and heparin. The coumarins act by antagonizing the action of vitamin K, whereas heparin inactivates thrombin. Liver disease is one of the most common causes of impaired coagulation. The net result of impaired liver function is a reduction in all levels of coagulation factors except factor VIII.[74] Other less common coagulation problems result from deficiencies of folic acid[75] or vitamin C, heavy metal poisoning, acquired immune deficiency,[76] and the lupus anticoagulant.[77]

Clotting requires an adequate number of functioning platelets. A platelet count below 100,000/mm$^3$ is generally considered to constitute thrombocytopenia. With platelet counts above 40,000/mm$^3$, spontaneous bleeding is uncommon but may occur after injury or surgery. Spontaneous bleeding is common with platelet counts less than 20,000/mm$^3$ and can be severe with counts below 10,000/mm$^3$.[78] Thrombocytopenia can result from a production defect (eg, chemotherapy, radiation, infection, marrow invasion by malignant cells), from sequestration of platelets (eg, splenomegaly), or accelerated destruction of

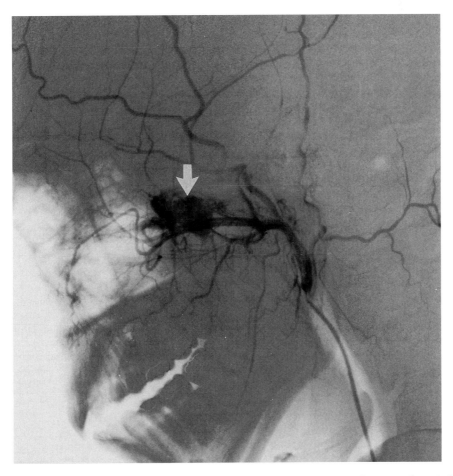

**Figure 8A.** Left external carotid arteriogram of the patient with a nasopharyngeal angiofibroma shown in Figure 7. This lateral view demonstrates abnormal vascularity from the maxillary artery (arrow). Photograph courtesy of Dr. E. Kassel, Radiologist-in-Chief, Mt. Sinai Hospital, Toronto, Ontario, Canada.

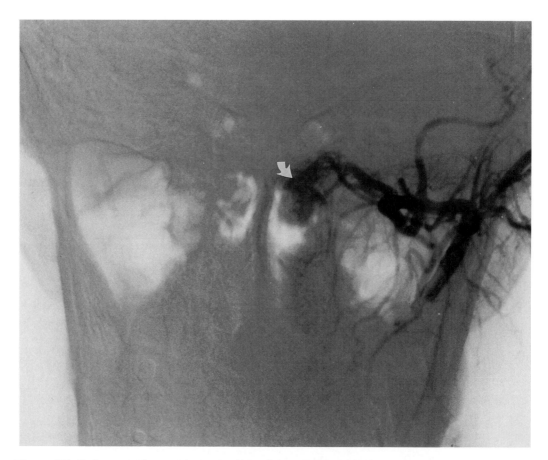

**Figure 8B.** Left external carotid arteriogram of the patient with a nasopharyngeal angiofibroma shown in Figure 7. This frontal projection shows abnormal vascularity high in the left nasopharynx (arrow). The intense blush from contrast enhancement, also visible in Figure 8A, demonstrates the highly vascular nature of nasopharyngeal angiofibromas and the danger of biopsy without appropriate precautions. Photograph courtesy of Dr. E. Kassel, Radiologist-in-Chief, Mt. Sinai Hospital, Toronto, Ontario, Canada.

platelets (eg, autoantibodies, drugs, infection).

Abnormalities of platelet function, even with normal platelet numbers, can initiate or prolong hemorrhage. The most frequent cause responsible for altered platelet function is the ingestion of acetylsalicylic acid or other nonsteroidal anti-inflammatory drugs.[79] These platelet-inhibiting drugs do not produce a bleeding diathesis by themselves but may aggravate an underlying disorder of hemostasis. Uremia also causes a defect in platelet func-

tion with generalized mucosal bleeding which can be reversed by dialysis.[80]

## Hypertension

Hypertension is commonly believed to be a causing factor in epistaxis, particularly refractory posterior epistaxis in the elderly.[81,82] This commonly held belief has been disputed by some authors. Weiss surveyed 6672 subjects to evaluate the relationship of epistaxis to other illnesses and found no relationship between the frequency or severity of epistaxis in patients with hypertension.[83] Shaheen found no relationship between hypertension and the onset of epistaxis but did note that the severity may be related to elevated blood pressure.[84]

### Hereditary Hemorrhagic Telangiectasia (Osler-Rendu-Weber Disease)

Hereditary hemorrhagic telangiectasia (HHT) is an autosomal dominant disorder transferred from either parent to children of both sexes.[85] It is characterized histologically by a lack of contractile elements in blood vessel walls affecting both elastic and muscular tissue elements. This results in arteriovenous fistulae which open spontaneously or with slight trauma or inflammation. Tests of coagulation are normal.

Telangiectasias are common on the face and mucous membranes of the tongue, lips, and nose but can be found almost anywhere on the body. Plauchu studied 324 patients with HHT and noted involvement of the hands and wrists in 41%, the face in 33%, and visceral involvement in 25%.[85] The lungs and central nervous system were more commonly affected in younger patients compared with involvement of the gastrointestinal tract and liver in older patients. Pulmonary arteriovenous malformations were reported in 15% to 20% of patients with HHT by Porteus and collegues.[86]

Epistaxis is the presenting symptom of disease in more than 90% of patients, whereas cutaneous telangiectasias appear 5 to 20 years later.[86] Most episodes of epistaxis start before age 20.[86,87] In Assar's study of 73 patients, the mean onset of epistaxis was 12 years of age, the mean frequency of epistaxis was 18 episodes per month, and the mean duration of bleeding was 7.5 minutes.[87] In two large series, the disease was chronic and stable in 50%, spontaneously resolved in 25%, and became more severe with age in 25% of patients.[88,89] The heaviest and most frequent bleeding seems to occur in middle-aged patients.[85]

## Diagnostic Approach

To determine the cause of epistaxis, perform a history, physical examination, appropriate laboratory investigations, and, on occasions, diagnostic imaging in a systematic manner to assess for the presence of local and systemic factors/diseases (Table I).

### History

The history is important in evaluating any patient with epistaxis but it may have to be taken during or after treatment if the patient is actively bleeding[90] (Table II). Ep-

**Table II**
Essential Features of the Diagnostic Approach to Epistaxis

History
  Anterior or posterior bleeding
  Hypertension
  Trauma/Rhinitis/Foreign body/Cocaine
  Anticoagulants/Nonsteroidal anti-inflammatory medication
  Adolescent male (rule out nasopharyngeal angiofibroma)
Physical Examination
  Good light source
  Remove blood clots
  Vasoconstrict and anesthetize mucosa
  Anterior rhinoscopy $\pm$ fibreoptic telescopes
  Look for bleeding site, septal deviation, or perforation
  Neoplasm
Laboratory Investigation
  Hemoglobin
  Platelets $\pm$ bleeding time
  PT/PTT
Diagnostic Imaging
  CT/MRI if trauma or suspected neoplasm
  Angiography if refractory epistaxis or vascular neoplasm

CT = computed tomography; MRI = magnetic resonance imaging; PT = prothrombin time; PTT = partial thromboplastin time.

istaxis from local causes is often unilateral whereas systemic causes may precipitate more generalized hemorrhage. Postnasal bleeding in an ambulatory patient usually signifies bleeding from the posterior nasal cavity (ie, "posterior epistaxis"), whereas bleeding from the anterior nares may result from either "anterior" or "posterior" epistaxis. Significant unrecognized blood loss may occur from swallowed blood in patients with posterior epistaxis, especially children or patients with an altered level of consciousness.

Local predisposing factors should be sought, such as a history of trauma, rhinitis, foreign body, or chemical abuse (eg, cocaine, intranasal corticosteroids). A benign or malignant neoplasm may present with trivial or severe bleeding and should always be suspected in patients with recurrent or severe epistaxis. Any adolescent male with a history of recurrent or severe epistaxis should be examined for a nasopharyngeal angiofibroma.[63] Bleeding from other areas in the body, a history of easy bruising or bleeding, and a family history of bleeding suggest a systemic disorder of the clotting mechanism. Beran et al. reported a hereditary predisposition in 42% of patients with recurrent epistaxis without any recognizable defect of the clotting mechanism.[17] A history of hypertension or vascular disease may be important. Prescription and nonprescription drugs should be sought since many patients fail to mention the nonprescription drugs which may contain substances such as acetylsalicylic acid or other substances known to prolong hemorrhage.

## Physical Examination

The mucosal surfaces of the nose and nasopharynx should be examined to look for the site of bleeding. In patients who are actively bleeding, anterior rhinoscopy with a nasal speculum and topical vasoconstrictor (eg, 5% cocaine) will localize most cases of "anterior" epistaxis. Flexible and/or rigid fibreoptic telescopes may localize more posteriorly located bleeding sites. In patients not actively bleeding, the

mucosal surfaces are examined for evidence of recent hemorrhage, trauma, inflammation, and neoplasia. Particular attention should be paid to the anterior nasal septum, which is the most frequent site of anterior epistaxis, and the posterolateral nasal wall, which is the most frequent site of posterior epistaxis. Septal deformities or perforations that predispose to epistaxis should be noted. Removing nasal crusts may provoke bleeding, but then the site is identified and can be treated. In addition to the nasal lining, the mucosal surfaces of the oral cavity and pharynx should be examined for any secondary bleeding sources.

## Laboratory Investigation

Screening tests of the hematologic system are warranted in patients with recurrent or severe epistaxis. A hemoglobin or hematocrit level will help in determining blood loss although these tests may be inaccurate immediately following acute bleeding. A normal platelet count helps to rule out thrombocytopenia as a cause of epistaxis. The bleeding time is a useful screening test if there is any question about the qualitative function of platelets. Partial thromboplastin time (PTT) and prothrombin time (PT) are useful screening tests of the intrinsic and extrinsic clotting mechanisms. Consultation with a hematologist is required if any screening investigation is abnormal or the investigations are normal but there is still a question of a systemic clotting problem.

## Diagnostic Imaging

Diagnostic imaging is not required in the vast majority of patients with epistaxis. Plain films of the nose are not usually required to make a diagnosis of a nasal fracture but facial views and CT scans are helpful in determining the full extent of injury in more severe facial fractures. Computed tomography and MRI imaging are helpful in determining the location and full extent of any suspected neoplasm. Digital subtraction angiography of both the external and internal carotid arteries can localize the site of active bleeding in patients with refractory epistaxis.

## Treatment

### General

The management of epistaxis should be individualized based on the severity, site, age, and general health of the patient, history of bleeding or easy bruising, family history of bleeding, and use of medications that alter coagulation (Figure 9). The vast majority of epistaxis can be controlled by compressing the ala nasi, thus applying direct pressure over Little's area (Table III). Surprisingly, this maneuver is performed poorly, even by trained medical personnel.[91] The pressure should be maintained without release for at least 10 minutes. There is no general agreement in the literature on the benefit of an ice pack as adjuvant treatment; although an ice pack on the nape of the neck has been shown to induce reflex constriction of the mucosal vessels of the nose.[92] Ice cubes sucked in the mouth are more effective than forehead ice

packs in lowering the submucosal temperature in the inferior turbinates.[93]

When simple measures do not stop the bleeding, the patient will present to the physician's office or the emergency department. It is essential to ensure that the patient's airway and breathing are stable and to assess for the presence of coagulation abnormalities. If present, they should be corrected. The recognition and rapid treatment of hypovolemia is imperative at the same time as steps are being taken to control the nasal hemorrhage. In the multiple trauma patient, other life-threatening injuries may take precedence but severe epistaxis can be temporarily slowed or stopped by placing one or two Foley catheters transnasally, inflating the balloons in the nasopharynx and pulling the balloons against the posterior choanae to compress potential bleeding sites and protect the airway from blood.[94]

In the hemodynamically stable patient, extra time can be taken to establish rapport and a comfortable upright position as well as to ensure that the essential equipment and assistance are available. Appropriate body fluid precautions should be observed. Good illumination with a head light or mirror is a basic requirement. Clots are removed with a suc-

---

### Table III
#### Treatment Options for Epistaxis

| | |
|---|---|
| General | Ligation |
|   Pressure/Ice pack |   Maxillary Artery |
|   Rest/Humidity/Analgesics |     Transantral |
| Cauterization |     Transoral |
|   Chemical (silver nitrate) |   Ethmoid Arteries |
|   Electrocautery |   External Carotid Artery |
|     Unipolar | Septal Surgery |
|     Bipolar |   Septoplasty |
| Packing |   Septodermoplasty |
|   Anterior Nasal Pack | Endoscopic Cauterization |
|     Absorbable | Angiography and Embolization |
|     Nonabsorbable | Ancillary Techniques |
|     Balloon catheter |   Greater Palatine Block |
|   Posterior Nasal Pack |   Drugs |
|     Gauze Pack |   Cryotherapy |
|     Foley Catheter | |
|     Balloon Catheter | |

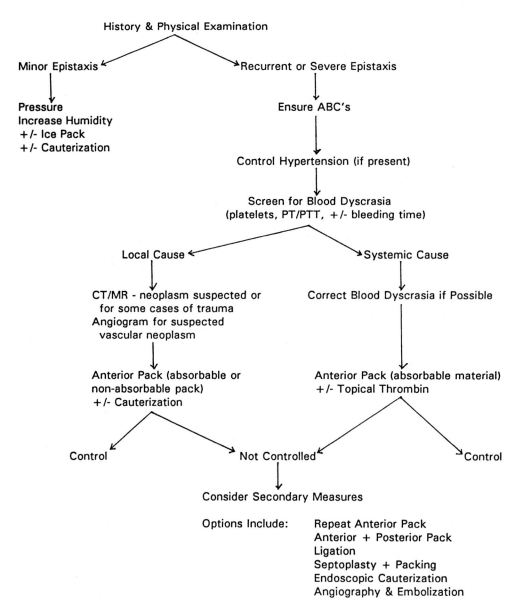

**Figure 9.** Diagnostic algorithm for the management of epistaxis. ABCs = airway, breathing, coagulation; CT = computed tomographic scanning; PT = prothrombin time; PTT = partial prothrombin time; MR = magnetic resonance.

tion catheter or by having the patient blow their nose. A topical vasoconstrictor, such as 4% to 5% cocaine, placed on cotton pledgets will often slow or stop bleeding. Following topical vasoconstriction of the nasal mucosa, the nose is examined to try to isolate the bleeding site which is usually controlled by cauterization or tamponade. One advantage of using cocaine is its topical anesthetic effect in addition to vasoconstriction. The maximum dose of cocaine is 2 to 3 mg/kg of body weight which means the maximum dose for a 70 kg person is approximately 5 mL of a 4% solution or 4 mL of a 5% solution. Overdosage of cocaine can cause pyrexia, tachyarrythmias, and seizures.

Patients are hospitalized if they are hemodynamically unstable, have a posterior pack, require surgical intervention, or have coexisting medical problems that require treatment. Adjunctive treatment measures include increased humidity, rest, analgesics, and, in some patients, mild sedation.[95] Intranasally administered medications and chemicals should be discontinued.

## Cauterization

The two commonly used methods of cauterization are silver nitrate cauterization and electrocautery. A topical vasoconstrictor and anesthetic is applied to slow or stop the bleeding to make cauterization more effective and give some pain relief. Although a topical anesthetic works well, another alternative is the submucosal infiltration of local anesthetic near the bleeding point to provide anesthesia and temporarily tamponade the vessel.

Silver nitrate becomes nitric acid when it comes in contact with a wet surface. The nitric acid causes superficial coagulation and seals the ends of small blood vessels. Silver nitrate is commonly applied from the end of commercially available wooden applicator sticks. It is helpful to cauterize circumferentially around the bleeding point first and then directly on the bleeding point to avoid starting the vessel pumping when it is directly cauterized. The applicator sticks are easy to use in the anterior nose but much more difficult to negotiate through the nose in posterior located bleeding sites or around septal deformities.

Electrocautery uses electrical current to coagulate open vessels with either monopolar or bipolar current. It is commonly applied to the bleeding site through insulated forceps, suction cautery or "hotwires."[96] It is generally believed that silver nitrate works well for mild bleeding in superficial vessels but more active bleeding requires electrocautery because of its deeper level of coagulation.[95] Silver nitrate cauterization and electrocautery have recently been compared in a randomized trial.[97] No significant difference was found in either the control of epistaxis or in the incidence of complications, but the statistical power to detect a difference was low.

With both methods of cauterization, it is important not to cauterize too deeply or in the same location on both sides of the septum at the same time leading to exposure and destruction of the septal cartilage with resultant septal perforation. Application of a topical antibiotic ointment is helpful following cauterization to reduce crusting and inflammation, thereby allowing healing to occur.[98]

## Packing

Nasal packing is commonly used to control epistaxis refractory to simpler measures[99] and for hemostasis following nasal or sinus surgery.[100] The principal reason for using a nasal pack in patients with epistaxis is to apply pressure over the bleeding area to tamponade the vessels. In addition, the pack creates mucosal inflammation and edema which may also help to seal bleeding vessels.[95] Properly placed nasal packing is highly effective in controlling epistaxis in most patients. A frequent reason for packing failing to control epistaxis is poor technique. Other difficulties include poor visualization of the nasal cavities secondary to equipment and lighting, lack of patient co-operation due to apprehension and pain or anatomical barriers (eg, septal deformity) blocking access to the nasal cavities.

### Anterior Nasal Pack

Bleeding in the anterior nose that cannot be controlled by simpler measures such as pressure or cauterization requires packing. Blood clots are cleared from the nose by suctioning or having the patient blow them out and the nose is topically anesthetized and vasoconstricted (eg, 5% cocaine). There are various methods and types of anterior packing. A common form of pack is vaseline gauze (¼- or ½-inch) tightly packed in a layered fashion as far back as possible towards the posterior choanae (Figure 10). The packing is started along the nasal floor and pushed under the inferior turbinate and layered superiorly ensuring only closed loops of gauze are placed posteriorly to prevent strands of packing falling into the nasopharynx. Outfracturing of the inferior turbinate (ie, displacing the inferior turbinates laterally) may be required to properly place the pack. The key to successful anterior packing is adequate visualization and placing the pack in a layered fashion. If the pack is placed "blindly" or only in the vestibule of the nose, it usually fails to control the bleeding.

It is common to place 72 in of packing

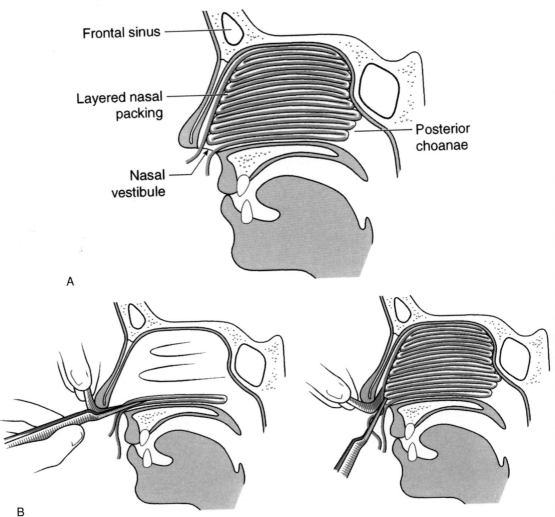

**Figure 10.** Schematic diagram demonstrating the correct placement of anterior vaseline gauze packing **(A)** in a layered fashion starting from inferiorly **(B)** and working superiorly.

in each nasal cavity. Whether one or both nasal cavities are packed will depend on whether the bleeding can be localized to one side and whether a unilateral pack controls the bleeding. The packing is left in place for a minimum of 2 days and sometimes for up to 5 days before it is removed and the nasal cavities reassessed. There are many complications associated with nasal packing, including secondary infections of the middle ear or paranasal sinuses, toxic shock syndrome, hypoxemia and hypercarbia (see "Nasopulmonary Reflex" section below), and necrosis of soft tissues leading to erosion of the nasal septum, columella, or vestibule.[101, 102] Broad spectrum antibiotics are usually given to prevent the secondary infections.

There are many types of packing materials used but nonabsorbable substances such as vaseline gauze are inexpensive and effective. Alternative materials include telfa, gauze strips, absorbable substances, or commercially available balloon catheters. In addition, packing materials are available which can be placed into the nasal cavity and expand greatly in size when liquid (eg, saline) is placed on the pack.[1] It is difficult to compare the effectiveness of one packing material over another as there are few randomized studies. McGashan et al.[103] compared two types of packing, calcium sodium alginate fibre (Kaltostat) and petrolatum gauze impregnated with bismuth tribromophenate (Xeroform gauze), in 40 patients with severe epistaxis and found no difference between the two.

The choice of packing material is important in patients with clotting defects. Traditional packing material may effectively tamponade the bleeding areas while in place but cause excoriation and inflammation of the mucosa. If the clotting abnormality has not been corrected prior to removal of the packing, the bleeding may be aggravated after removal because of the trauma to the mucosa. In these situations, it is advisable to use an absorbable packing material that promotes coagulation and does not need to be removed. There are several excellent choices available including oxidized cellulose preparations (Oxy-cel, Surgicel), absorbable gelatin sponge (Gelfoam), microfibrillar collagen (Avitene),[100,104,105] and tapered strips of porcine packing (salt-cured subdermal fatty tissue or "fat back").[106–108] In addition, application of topical thrombin spray just before the packing is placed can be helpful to arrest the bleeding.

Commercially manufactured balloon nasal packs are available and are popular in some emergency departments.[109] Most of these devices have a larger balloon designed to fill up the anterior nasal cavity and a smaller posterior balloon to fill up the posterior nasal cavity and choanae (Figure 11). The balloons are intended to pneumatically tamponade the bleeding site but cadaver studies have shown the balloons do not conform to the contours of the nasal cavity and they expand along pathways of least resistance prolapsing into the nasopharynx.[110] Accurate nasal tamponade is unlikely to be their true mode of action, and they probably work by a combination of factors. There are arguments for and against the use of these catheters. Their advantages include ease of placement and removal, and they are said to be associated with less risk of hypoxemia and carbon dioxide retention.[109] They are, therefore, useful for clinicians with little experience in the traditional methods of epistaxis control as a definitive measure or temporarily while experienced help is sought. Unfortunately, the balloons are frequently filled with an inflatant considered inappropriate by the manufacturer, and it is not uncommon for balloons designed for water or saline to deflate within 24 hours if filled with air.[111] Traumatic optic neuropathy has been reported with the use of balloon catheters.[112]

## Posterior Nasal Pack

Well-placed anterior packing can generally stop most cases of epistaxis arising from the anterior and posterior nasal cavities. When anterior packing fails to stop the epistaxis, the bleeding site usually involves the sphenopalatine artery or one of its branches and will require posterior

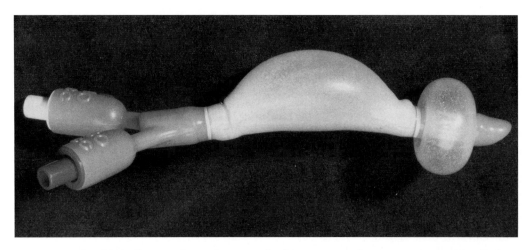

**Figure 11.** Inflatable balloon catheter for use in both anterior and posterior epistaxis. The larger balloon is for inflation in the nasal cavity to control anterior epistaxis and the smaller balloon is for positioning in the posterior nasal cavity/nasopharynx for control of posterior epistaxis (in conjunction with the anterior balloon).

nasal packing. There are several methods of placing a posterior pack but the two commonly used techniques involve placing a wad of rolled gauze or a balloon catheter (eg, Foley catheter) in the nasopharynx and pulling the device anteriorly against the posterior choanae. The functions of a posterior pack are twofold and involve the application of pressure against the posterior choanae to tamponade vessels and the posterior pack also allows anterior packing to be more firmly and tightly packed in the posterior nasal cavity. This last point is the most important and is the reason that posterior packing is almost always accompanied by anterior packing.

The placement of posterior packing can be quite uncomfortable for the patient and usually requires both topical anesthesia and light intravenous sedation. In some instances, general anesthesia may be necessary to properly place the packing. The standard posterior pack involves placing a wad of gauze and cotton in the nasopharynx. There are prefabricated packs available but many clinicians prefer to make their own. This is usually accomplished by taking a piece of gauze and wrapping it around some cotton and forming an oblong gauze roll. Two sutures are placed to come

through the nasal cavities and one is left to retrieve the pack through the mouth. Two red rubber catheters are placed in each nasal cavity and visualized in the oropharynx and the ends brought out through the mouth. The two sutures on the gauze roll are tied to the catheters which are pulled out the nose, thereby placing the sutures through the nose. The pack is guided around the uvula and pushed into the nasopharynx with a finger while the sutures are pulled through the nose. One suture remains attached to the pack through the mouth and is taped to the side of the patient's cheek so the pack can be removed at a later time. An anterior pack is placed against the posterior pack. The two sutures coming out each nostril are tied over a gauze roll in front of the columella to pull the posterior pack against the posterior choanae and anterior pack and provide tension (Figure 12). A posterior pack can be placed through one nasal cavity only if the bleeding is unilateral.

Posterior packing requires admission to an appropriate hospital setting for observation based on the patient's general health, estimated blood loss and impending complications. Oxygen monitoring is recommended because patients are given analgesics for discomfort and sedation,

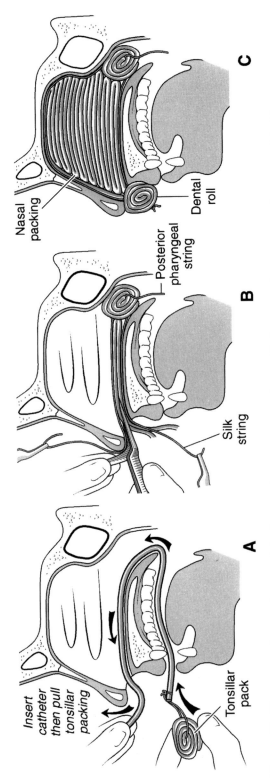

**Figure 12.** Placement of posterior Nasal Packing—The posterior pack is pulled against the posterior choanae and held in position over a gauze roll outside the nostril. An anterior pack is placed buttressed against the posterior pack.

and posterior packing has been associated with abnormalities in respiratory function (see "Nasopulmonary Reflex" section below). Intravenous maintenance of body fluids is important because patients will experience dysphagia while the pack is in place. Calf compression devices can prevent deep venous thrombosis in patients placed on bed rest. Prophylactic systemic antibiotics are given to prevent infection of the middle ear and sinuses.[113] The packing is left in position for 3 to 5 days.

An alternative to the gauze pack is the placement of a number 16 or 18 Foley catheter through one or both nasal cavities, inflating the balloon(s) with 10 to 15 mL of saline or air, and pulling the balloon(s) against the posterior choanae.[114] They can also be used as a temporizing measure to control bleeding while a more traditional pack is being made or when speed is required to control hemorrhage in cases of life-threatening craniofacial injury. The catheter is held in position by a clamp placed across the catheter near the nostril (Figure 13). It is important to place some padding material between the clamp and nostril soft tissues to prevent pressure necrosis.[115,116] Foley catheters have gained acceptance because they are much easier and faster to place and better tolerated by the patient than the traditional posterior gauze roll pack.[109,117] It is useful to periodically check the inflation of the balloon be-

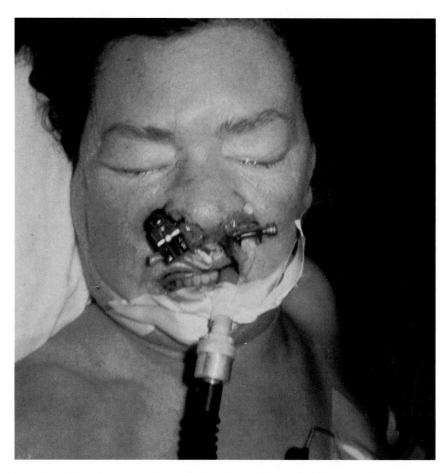

**Figure 13.** Bilateral posterior "packing" with Foley catheters held anteriorly with metal clamps. Bilateral anterior packing with vaseline gauze was also placed.

cause it is not uncommon for the balloon to deflate losing some of its pressure and effectiveness. If the catheter can be pulled anteriorly with little resistance (ie, the balloon is not being resisted by the choanae), then the balloon needs to be inflated more. It is also important not to overinflate the balloon because the resultant pressure can cause necrosis of the adjacent nasopharyngeal tissues and soft palate. Excessive pain is the hallmark of overinflation. Care must be taken in placement with craniofacial injury because of the potential for positioning the catheter in the intracranial cavity.[118]

## Ligation

Posterior epistaxis can be treated by posterior pack, balloon tamponade, arterial ligation, or embolization; each technique has its own technical difficulties, unique complications, and reasons for failure. The existence of multiple techniques for the treatment of posterior epistaxis implies that no one technique is ideal. There is some controversy concerning the order in which these various procedures are best used and when to proceed to the next form of therapy (see "Initial Intervention" discussion in the "Controversies" section at the end the chapter). The method used will depend on the experience of the clinician managing the problem and the available equipment. Since as many as 25% of patients with posterior epistaxis fail conventional packing techniques,[119] selective arterial ligation has been proposed as an alternative form of therapy either initially or after failure of posterior packing. The evidence in favor of early ligation include a shorter hospitalization and reduced cost,[3,120] reduced patient discomfort, fewer complications[3,120,121] and lowered risk of cardiopulmonary problems since nasal packing is removed postligation (see "Nasopulmonary Reflex" section below). The arguments against surgery are the requirements for a general anesthetic and in the majority of cases, conventional packing is effective.

The purpose of arterial ligation is to decrease the pressure gradient to the bleeding vessel to allow a clot to form by normal clotting mechanisms. The closer the ligation is to the bleeding vessel, the more effective the ligation will be since there is less likelihood of collateral vessels revascularizing the bleeding vessel and perpetuating the epistaxis. This point is illustrated in one study where external carotid artery ligation was associated with a rebleeding rate of 45% (9 of 20 patients) compared to 10% (3 of 29 patients) in patients undergoing maxillary artery ligation.[122] External carotid artery ligation may still have advantages in the elderly or debilitated patient because it can be performed under local anesthesia.[121] Which vessels are ligated and the method of ligation will depend on the urgency of the situation and the surgeon's familiarity and results with the operation.

### Maxillary Artery Ligation

Seifert first described the transantral approach to the third division of the maxillary artery in 1928.[123] In 1935, Gergely studied this technique in cadavers and concluded it was the surgical procedure of choice for most cases of refractory epistaxis[124] but it was not until 1965 that the procedure was popularized by Chandler and Serrins.[125] It is currently the most widely used arterial ligation procedure for controlling posterior epistaxis. In some instances, bilateral maxillary artery ligation is required for unilateral bleeding because of cross-anastomoses from a dominant maxillary artery.[126]

Prior to the procedure, it is important to obtain a Waters' projection of the maxillary sinus to rule out significant anomalies (eg, hypoplasia) or pathology (eg, neoplasm) in the sinus. Through a standard gingivobuccal incision, the anterior wall of the maxillary sinus is exposed and removed with special care not to injure the infraorbital nerve. The posterior wall of the sinus is identified and a laterally based U-shaped mucosal flap elevated. Portions of the posterior wall are removed to gain exposure to the pterygopalatine fossa and the branches of the maxillary artery. It is possible to identify the sphenopalatine artery without opening the pterygopalatine fossa but this is technically difficult.[127] In most cases, the pterygopalatine fossa is opened and the branches of the maxillary artery are visualized with an operating microscope. Metal vascular clips are applied to ligate the blood vessels and it is recommended the clips be placed on all vessels as distally as possible since ligation of only the main trunk of the maxillary artery may allow retrograde flow through other branches.[12] An intranasal antrostomy under the inferior turbinate is generally placed along with a light vaseline gauze pack in the nose for 24 hours. It is not uncommon for mild bleeding following removal of the pack but this is generally of short duration (24 to 48 hours) and not severe.[12,119,128]

Recurrent severe epistaxis following maxillary artery ligation occurs in 5% to 15% of patients in most series. Factors contributing to these failure rates include the development of collateral circulation, failure to clip all of the vessels in the pterygopalatine fossa, incompletely closed vascular clips and bleeding from the ethmoid arteries.[129,130] Other factors associated with a higher rate of failure include advanced age, anemia, and a history of hypertension.[130] The failure rates for maxillary artery ligation compare favorably with those reported for conventional packing techniques. Wang and Vogel reported a failure rate of 14.3% with maxillary artery ligation compared to 26.2% with packing.[131] In addition, maxillary artery ligation was associated with fewer complications (40% versus 68%) and the average length of stay for patients treated by ligation was 2.2 days shorter than packing. Complications associated with maxillary artery ligation include hypoesthesia of the infraorbital nerve, persistent pain in the maxillary dentition, oroantral fistula, damage to sphenopalatine ganglion and vidian nerve, and total ophthalmoplegia.[132]

In addition to the transantral approach, Maceri and Makielski described an intraoral approach to ligation of the in-fratemporal portion of the maxillary artery.[133] This approach provides access to the first and second parts of the maxillary artery without opening the maxillary sinus and does not require a microscope. It can be used when the transantral approach is not feasible such as cases of sinus hypoplasia (eg, children), fracture, malignancy, or severe infection. The main criticism of this approach is that the site of ligation is more proximal than the transantral approach, with the greater potential for collateral revascularization and failure.

The intraoral approach is carried out under general anesthesia with an incision made in the upper gingivobuccal sulcus at the level of the second or third molar and continued inferiorly along the ramus of the mandible. The buccal fat pad is retracted medially or removed and the attachments of the temporalis muscle to the coronoid process of the mandible are identified. The temporalis muscle belly may need to be split and partially dissected from the mandible to gain access to the artery. Blunt dissection reveals the maxillary artery which is clipped or ligated and divided. There may be significant variation in the distance of the artery from the gingivobuccal mucosal incision site and the relationship of the artery to the pterygoid muscles.[134]

The most significant complications of the intraoral approach are cheek edema and trismus which can be quite severe and may take many months to resolve. Avoiding trauma to the muscles of mastication is important to minimize these complications.[134] Other potential complications include inferior alveolar nerve damage and infection of the infratemporal space.

### Ethmoid Artery Ligation

Ligation of the anterior ethmoid artery was first described by Kirchner in 1961.[135] The anterior ethmoidal artery supplies approximately 10% of the blood to the nasal mucosa and is generally larger and more dominant than the posterior ethmoidal artery. Ligation of the ethmoid arteries may be considered for persistent superior and anterior epistaxis and, in cases, where the source of bleeding cannot be well defined. It is frequently performed in combination with maxillary artery ligation. In many instances, the anterior ethmoidal artery is ligated without ligating the posterior ethmoidal artery because of the dominant blood supply through the anterior artery and the fear of injuring the optic nerve which is only 3 to 7 mm from the posterior ethmoidal artery.

The arteries are ligated before they leave the orbit through their respective foramina situated in the frontoethmoidal suture line. The arteries are identified through a curvilinear "Lynch" incision placed midway between the inner canthus and midline of the nose. The periosteum is incised and elevated to the lacrimal crest and the frontoethmoidal suture line is identified at the superior aspect of the lacrimal bone. The periosteum is elevated from the medial wall of the orbit (lamina papyracea) along the frontoethmoidal suture line. The anterior ethmoidal artery is located approximately 14 to 18 mm from the lacrimal crest and the posterior ethmoidal artery is approximately 10 mm posterior to this. The arteries are tied with suture or ligated with vascular clips. It is prudent to ligate the anterior artery first and re-examine the nose to see if the bleeding has stopped before considering the necessity of posterior ethmoidal artery ligation. In some cases, bilateral ethmoidal artery ligation is required.[125] Ligation of the ethmoidal arteries is generally associated with few complications but the potential complications, including intraorbital hematoma, extraocular muscle dysfunction, and blindness, are serious.[136]

### External Carotid Artery Ligation

External carotid artery (ECA) ligation is a relatively fast and simple procedure that can be done under local anesthesia without any special equipment.[137] It may be successful in reducing the capillary blood flow to the nasal mucosa in cases of refractory epistaxis, but there are major disadvantages to this procedure, including the significant potential for collateral blood supply to form distal to the ligation and the inability to embolize (see below) the maxillary artery following ligation of the ECA. Some authors have found ECA ligation in combination with anterior ethmoidal artery ligation to be a highly effective treatment to control refractory posterior epistaxis with no mortality or significant complications.[138] Waldron and Stafford reported control of epistaxis in 14 of 15 (93%) patients managed by ECA and anterior ethmoidal artery ligation.[137]

External carotid artery ligation is performed through a horizontal incision below the margin of the mandible. The incision crosses the anterior border of sternocleidomastoid muscle which is identified and retracted posteriorly exposing the carotid sheath. The ascending pharyngeal, superior thyroid, and lingual arteries are identified and the ECA is ligated distal to the superior thyroid artery. It is important to identify at least two branches of the ECA to avoid ligation of the internal carotid artery precipitating a stroke and possibly death of the patient. In addition, it is important to avoid injuring the vagus nerve or one of its branches, the hypoglossal nerve, the marginal mandibular nerve, or the sympathetic chain. A rare complication of complete facial paralysis thought to be secondary to either thrombosis or embolus obstructing the petrosal branch of the middle meningeal artery has been reported.[139]

### Septoplasty/Submucous Resection

Epistaxis from the anterior nose is usually easy to locate and effectively treated with either cauterization, packing, or a combination of the two. If there are anatomical or structural problems that impede easy access to the source of bleeding, then this anatomical obstruction may have to be dealt with surgically before gaining control of the bleeding site. The most common obstruction is a deviated nasal septum on the side of the bleeding. If it is not possible to place an effective anterior pack, a septoplasty or submucous resection is required to straighten the deformity before the packing can be placed. This usually requires a general anesthetic but it can sometimes be performed under local anesthesia.

Septal surgery has also been advocated for recurrent or severe epistaxis arising from the nasal septum. It is believed that elevating the mucosa off of the septal cartilage and bone between the perichondrium/periosteum and mucosa will disrupt the mucosal blood supply sufficiently to stop the epistaxis postoperatively. In addition, septoplasty and packing of the nose has been advocated as the first form of surgical therapy for patients with epistaxis refractory to conventional anterior and posterior packing. This has been shown to be an effective alternative to surgical ligation in many patients.[140]

## Endoscopic Cauterization

When the exact site of bleeding can be visualized in the nose, there is a higher likelihood of being able to stop the hemorrhage by local therapy. Fibreoptic nasal telescopes have greatly improved the ability to examine the posterior nose and nasopharynx and have been successfully employed to localize the source of bleeding in patients with posterior epistaxis. Various means of visualizing the posterior nose and nasopharynx have been used, including flexible[141–143] or rigid[144–148] nasal telescopes or an operating microscope.[96] Generally, when the bleeding vessel is identified, it is cauterized by one of several methods, including monopolar cautery, bipolar cautery,[151] or hot wire cautery.[96]

The technique has been found to be particularly useful during acute nose bleeds since it shortens the hospitalization and reduces the discomfort associated with nasal packing.[7] Suctioning helps to localize the bleeding site and aids cauterization of the bleeding site under direct vision.[143] The success rate with posterior endoscopic cautery approaches 90%.[95] Borgstein successfully treated 12 consecutive patients with posterior epistaxis using a flexible nasal telescope and cauterization under direct vision,[142] and O'Leary-Stickney et al. successfully treated five of six patients using rigid endoscopy.[144] Marcus reported good results in 27 patients with an insulated malleable suction electrocautery and a rigid endoscope.[143] The main complication is numbness of the palate, which develops in approximately 25% of patients and usually resolves or is not bothersome for most patients.[95]

In addition, it is possible to place vascular clips on the sphenopalatine artery and its branches endoscopically through the nose.[149,150] Stamm et al. treated 145 patients with severe posterior epistaxis by transnasal ligation of sphenopalatine artery branches in the nasal cavity.[150] The failure rate was 6.1%, and the authors felt that this technique significantly decreased patient morbidity compared with other methods of controlling epistaxis.

## Angiography and Embolization

Angiography is a well-established technique for viewing vascular anatomy including the carotid arterial system.[151] Digital subtraction angiography enhances the visible images of the blood vessels by subtracting out bone and soft tissues.[152] Angiography was first introduced to the management of epistaxis by Coel and Janon in 1972,[153] and in 1974, Sokoloff et al.[154] described the first case of embolization for intractable epistaxis.

Embolization takes advantage of the fine vascular detail seen by angiography to position a small catheter in the distal portions of bleeding vessels so that occluding substances can be placed.[155] There are many materials which have been used for embolization, including polyvinyl alcohol, absorbable gelatin sponge (Gelfoam), tissue glues, and coiled springs. The advantages of embolization over surgery are that it can be performed under local anesthesia, it generally occludes vessels more distally than ligation thereby reducing the risk of collateral blood supply, and it can reach surgically inaccessible areas. Angiography alone is indicated before surgical ligation if there is any history of carotid arterial disease (eg, transient ischemic attack, stroke, amaurosis fugax).[156]

Prior to embolization, bilateral evaluation of both the internal and external carotid arterial systems is important to identify the vascular base, the collateral circulation and rare arterial anastomoses.[157-160] A well-trained interventional neuroradiologist is essential to evaluate the patient for dangerous anastomoses between the internal and external carotid arteries or severe atheromatous disease that may contraindicate embolization. The branch of the external carotid artery primarily responsible for severe epistaxis is the maxillary artery. One or both maxillary arteries are embolized in patients with severe epistaxis not controllable by other means. The facial artery may also require embolization. The internal carotid blood supply to the nose through the ophthalmic artery and anterior and posterior ethmoidal arteries cannot be embolized except in exceptional circumstances because of the high risk of stroke and blindness. Moser et al. reported two cases of ophthalmic artery embolization for treatment of severe, refractory epistaxis.[161] One patient had a prosthetic eye and the second patient had vision sacrificed as a life-saving measure. In cases of intracavernous internal carotid artery aneurysms or caroticocavernous fistulae, detachable balloon occlusion[33,36,39,162,163] or copper-wire thrombosis[42] is required.

In experienced hands, the embolization success rate for severe or recurrent epistaxis, including repeat attempts, is in the range of 80% to 90%.[152,160,164,165] There are favorable[166] and unfavorable[160,165] reports as to the efficacy of embolization in treating patients with hereditary hemorrhagic telangiectasia. Following embolization, facial pain and trismus are common and are usually temporary side effects. Severe complications including hemiparesis,[164,167] facial nerve paralysis,[168,169] ophthalmoplegia,[170] and skin slough[160] are rare complications.

## Hereditary Hemorrhagic Telangiectasia (HHT)

The treatment of HHT is difficult and frustrating for both the patient and physician because most therapies are either ineffective or temporary. It is hard to make valid comparisons between the different medical and surgical treatment options because of the variable natural progression of epistaxis between patients, the difficulty in quantitating the epistaxis, and the fact that multiple therapies are often used which makes the assessment of each individual therapy difficult.[171] There are currently numerous medical and surgical treatments that have been proposed for managing the epistaxis associated with HHT. No single treatment has been proven universally effective.

### Medical Therapy for Hereditary Hemorrhagic Telangiectasia

Good hydration and humidification, avoidance of nasal trauma, and the use of nasal lubricants help reduce the frequency and severity of epistaxis in patients with HHT. Patients usually need iron supplementation and may require periodic blood transfusion to maintain an adequate hemoglobin level.

Some women with HHT experience an increase in the frequency and severity of epistaxis when there is a corresponding decrease in circulating estrogen (eg, following oophorectomy, postmenopause). Systemic or topical estrogen therapy is advocated by some authors but other studies fail to show any appreciable reduction in epistaxis.[172,173] Other authors have reported some success with aminocaproic acid[174] or intramucosal injections of sclerosing agents derived from maize.[175]

### Surgical Therapy for Hereditary Hemorrhagic Telangiectasia

The available surgical therapies include nasal packing, electrocauterization, laser photocoagulation, septodermoplasty, placement of various regional or free-tissue transfers, radiotherapy, arterial embolization, and arterial ligation. If a nasal pack is required to control acute hemorrhage, it is better to place packing material that is absorbable and does not require removal as this may further aggravate bleeding due to mucosal irritation and inflammation (see "Anterior Nasal Pack" and "Posterior Nasal Pack" sections above). Electrocauterization is effective for short-term control of a bleeding site but does not offer long-term control.

Laser photocauterization has been used for managing patients with HHT, but the efficacy has received mixed reviews. Some patients report less severe or frequent bleeding following laser treatment and many who have previously undergone a septodermoplasty report better control of their epistaxis and less morbidity with laser treatment. The laser is not effective for acute epistaxis but can be used immediately after electrical coagulation of a bleeding vessel. The carbon dioxide laser coagulates superficial lesions but deeper subepithelial arteriovenous malformations require the argon laser[176,177] or neodymium yttrium-aluminum-garnet (Nd-YAG) laser.[178–180] The Nd-YAG laser provides the deepest penetration but causes extensive surrounding tissue damage which may not be apparent at the initial laser treatment. Parkin and Dixon reported substantial improvement in eight patients treated with the Nd-YAG laser but the treatment had to be repeated every 4 to 6 months because of the development of new lesions.[178] Kluger et al. found the Nd-YAG laser was most useful in younger patients (< 50 years) with limited disease.[180]

The purpose of a septodermoplasty is to replace all of the telangiectatic mucosa with grafts of another material such as epidermis, dermis, oral mucosa,[171] human amniotic membrane,[181] or cultured epithelial sheets derived from the patients own buccal epithelium.[182] It is common to gain wide exposure to the septum and nasal cavity through an alar incision or in some cases through a more extensive incision along the nasofacial groove (lateral rhinotomy).[183] The mucosa is removed from the anterior half of the septum, nasal floor, and lateral nasal wall but the perichondrium with its blood supply is left intact. It is common to resurface the area with a split-thickness skin graft taken from the thigh. The graft is held in position with sutures anteriorly and carefully positioned packing. Most patients will continue to have epistaxis following septodermoplasty but it is usually less severe and frequent compared with the bleeding prior to the procedure. The telangiectasias usually grow back into the graft over a variable period of time. Other autografts have been used to resurface the nasal lining, including regional facial cutaneous flaps,[184] forehead myocutaneous flaps,[185] and microvascular radial forearm free flaps.[186]

Local intranasal radiation treatments (eg, brachytherapy) have been suggested as a useful modality in the management of refractory epistaxis in patients with HHT. Pohar et al. reported favorable results using intranasal brachytherapy in 43 patients given a single dose of radiation ranging from 15 to 35 Gy (median 30 Gy).[187] The dose given did not correlate with the control rate and the median time to significant epistaxis was 24 months (range 6 to 178 months). There were no major complications apart from septal perforation in four patients.

## Other Techniques for Control of Epistaxis

### Greater Palatine Foramen Block

A greater palatine foramen block can be used in difficult to control posterior epistaxis or for enhancement of local anesthesia when placing any type of nasal packing.[188] The greater palatine foramen is located in the hard palate and the corresponding canal runs in a posterosuperior direction to the pterygopalatine fossa where the maxillary artery and its branches to the posterior nasal cavity originate. It is possible to locate the greater palatine foramen in the hard palate and inject liquid material directly into the canal. The canal varies between 25 and 33 mm in length, and since the foramen rotundum lies 30 to 40 mm from the greater palatine foramen, the needle should be inserted no more than 25 mm into the greater palatine foramen to avoid intracranial or intraorbital injection. It is common to inject a solution containing xylocaine (1% or 2%) with epinephrine (1:100 000 to 1:200 000). The epinephrine will vasoconstrict the arteries but one of the main mechanisms of hemostasis appears to be volume compression since many liquids (eg, saline, sterile water, or glycerin) when injected alone seem to produce good hemostasis. Bharadwaj and Novotny treated 61 patients with posterior epistaxis by greater palatine injection with either 1% xylocaine without epinephrine (34) or sterile water (27).[189] Immediate hemostasis was obtained in 55 patients (90%) and recurrent bleeding occurred in 22 of these patients. All of the patients with recurrent bleeding responded to repeat injections and there were no serious complications.

## *Drugs*

Pharmacologic therapy for epistaxis is of limited value. Topical vasoconstrictors, such as cocaine or phenylephrine, are useful for slowing or stopping bleeding so the nose can be examined. In addition, topical thrombin may be useful in patients with clotting abnormalities.

DDAVP (1-desamino-8-D-arginine vasopressin) is a synthetic analog of vasopressin that decreases the bleeding time in patients with hemophilia A, von Willebrand's disease, and uremia. It is effective for rapid temporary correction of bleeding in these patients.[190–192] Glypressin (triglyclyl-lysine-vasopressin) is another drug similar to vasopressin but with fewer side effects and a longer duration of action. In one randomized controlled clinical trial, the intravenous administration of glypressin showed a statistically significant benefit compared with placebo in patients where no localized bleeding point could be visualized.[193] Topical glypressin has not been shown to be effective.[194] Antifibrinolytic agents are of no proven value.[195]

## *Cryotherapy*

Freezing the site of epistaxis has been used with reasonable success and a low complication rate to control both anterior and posterior epistaxis.[196–199] Cryotherapy is not commonly used to treat epistaxis because the technique is cumbersome, requires special equipment, and seems to be generally less predictable than other forms of management.

## Controversies

### *Nasopulmonary Reflex*

There is some controversy as to whether a nasopulmonary reflex exists, and, if it does, whether there is significance of this reflex in provoking cardiorespiratory problems in patients with nasal packing. Packing of the nose, particularly the nasopharynx, has been associated with hypoventilation, hypoxemia, cardiac arrhythmias, and cardiac arrest.

In 1968, Ogura and colleagues showed a decrease in pulmonary compliance in patients with nasal obstruction.[200] In 1971, Cassisi et al. showed a consistent lowering of $Po_2$ without significant alteration of $Pco_2$ in patients with posterior packing.[201] Jensen et al. monitored 12 patients for 3 days with bilateral anterior nasal packing after septoplasty and found a significant increase in the number and duration of nocturnal episodes of hypoxia during the first and second postoperative nights.[202] This contrasts with the recent study by Loftus et al. which did not find any significant drop in oxygenation in 19 patients with posterior packing monitored for more than 120 hours.[203] Two patients had desaturations to less than 90%—one in an actively bleeding patient and the other during a respiratory arrest in an alcoholic patient under sedation for delirium tremens. They felt these episodes of hypoxemia were more appropriately attributed to rebleeding or underlying medical problems than to primary oxygen status. Polysomnography was conducted by

Wetmore et al. on 12 patients with anterior and posterior nasal packing.[204] Ten patients (83%) showed evidence of obstructive sleep apnea with a mean apnea index of 29 (range 1 to 83), mean hypopnea index of 20 (range 9 to 33), and a lowest mean oxygen desaturation of 77% (range 17% to 91%). Ten of the 12 patients returned for follow-up polysomnograms after the packing had been removed and all showed improvement in their apnea index and lowest oxygen desaturation, although four patients still demonstrated at least mild obstructive sleep apnea.

The evidence suggests that there is a possibility of cardiorespiratory compromise in patients with nasal packing, particularly posterior packing. This may be multifactorial in origin with contributions from the nasopulmonary reflex, underlying cardiorespiratory disease, induced obstructive sleep apnea due to increased upper airway resistance, blood loss, and sedative drugs. Of all these possibilities, the induction of obstructive sleep apnea seems most tenable. Whatever the etiology, it is important to admit and properly monitor patients with posterior packing, particularly if they are elderly, demonstrate hypoxemia or hypercarbia, or have underlying cardiorespiratory disease.

*Initial Intervention*

Most patients with uncomplicated minor epistaxis from the anterior septum are easily managed by simple measures such as pressure, cauterization, and, in some cases, an anterior nasal pack. Nonetheless, variations exist in the way emergency departments manage patients with uncomplicated epistaxis. There are differences in the use of local anesthesia and nasal cauterization, the type of nasal pack used, whether patients are allowed to be sent home with a nasal pack in place, and whether patients are referred for otolaryngology follow-up.[5] In addition, the role of the emergency physician in treating these patients has been question by John et al.[205] They found that initially successful treatment by emergency physicians often failed

within 48 hours if the nose was actively bleeding and the bleeding site could not be visualized. They suggested this group be referred to an otolaryngologist on presentation.

The management algorithm for patients with more severe posterior epistaxis is controversial. Posterior nasal packing is commonly placed to tamponade the acute bleed. Some authors recommend "conservative management" and admit the patient to hospital, leaving the pack in place for 3 to 5 days.[81,206,207] If the packing fails to control the bleeding, other options are considered, such as surgical ligation,[208] embolization,[209] or repacking the nose under general anesthesia with or without septoplasty.[140] Even if the posterior pack was initially successful, others recommend early surgical ligation or embolization because of the approximate 25% failure rate with packing in addition to the morbidity, discomfort, and added length of stay associated with posterior nasal packing.[164] The choice of therapy will depend on many factors, such as the medical condition of the patient, the physician's experience, and the availability of interventional radiology. The cost of treatment may directly or indirectly influence the treating physician's behavior.[160,210]

## References

1. Doyle DE. Anterior epistaxis: a new nasal tampon for fast, effective control. Laryngoscope 1986;96:279–281.
2. Shaw CB, Wax MK, Wetmore SJ. Epistaxis: a comparison of treatment. Otolaryngol Head Neck Surg 1993;109:60–65.
3. Small M, Moran AG. Epistaxis and arterial ligation. J Laryngol Otol 1984;98:281–284.
4. Shaheen O. Studies of nasal vasculature and the problems of arterial ligation for epistaxis. Annals of the Royal College of Surgeons of England 1970;47:30–44.
5. Kotecha B, Cocks RA, Rothera MP. The management of epistaxis in accident and emergency departments: a survey of current practice. Arch Emerg Med 1990;7:35–41.
6. Mulbury PE. Recurrent epistaxis. Pediatr Rev 1991;12:213–217.

7. el-Silimy O. Endonasal endoscopy and posterior epistaxis. Rhinology 1993;31: 119–120.
8. Lucente FE. Thanatology: a study of 100 deaths. Trans Acad Ophthalmol Otolaryngol 1972;76:334–339.
9. International Congress of Anatomists: Nomina Anatomica (6th ed.). New York, NY: Churchill Livingstone; 1989: p. A54.
10. Lander MI, Terry O. The posterior ethmoid artery in severe epistaxis. Otolaryngol Head Neck Surg 1992;106:101–103.
11. Wentges RT: Surgical anatomy of pterygopalatine fossa. J Laryngol Otol 1975:89; 35–45.
12. Pearson BW, MacKenzie RG, Goodman WS. The anatomic basis of transantral ligation of the maxillary artery in severe epistaxis. Laryngoscope 1969;79:969–984.
13. Delpre G, Neeman A, Leiser A, et al. Deceptive epistaxis during gastroscopy (letter). Dig Dis Sci 1994;39:219.
14. Wolf M, Roth Y, Leventon G. Epistaxis mimicking upper gastrointestinal bleeding. J Fam Pract 1990;30:95–97.
15. Hutchison SM, Finlayson ND. Epistaxis as a cause of hematemesis and melena. J Clin Gastroenterol 1987;9:283–285.
16. Jackson KR, Jackson RT. Factors associated with active refractory epistaxis. Arch Otolaryngol Head Neck Surg 1988;114: 862–865.
17. Beran M, Petruson B. Occurrence of epistaxis in habitual nose-bleeders and analysis of some etiological factors. J Otorhinolaryngol Relat Spec 1986;48:297–303.
18. Nunez DA, McClymont LG, Evans RA. Epistaxis: a study of the relationship with weather. Clin Otolaryngol 1990;15: 49–51.
19. Stopa R, Schonweiler R. Causes of epistaxis in relation to season and weather status. HNO 1989;37:198–202.
20. Dimitroulis G, Steidler N. Massive bleeding following maxillofacial trauma. Case report. Aust Dent J 1992;37:185–188.
21. Sanderov B, Viccellio P. Fractures of the medial orbital wall. Ann Emerg Med 1988;17:973–976.
22. Ghorayeb BY, Kopaniky DR, Yeakley JW. Massive posterior epistaxis: a manifestation of internal carotid injury at the skull base. Arch Otolaryngol Head Neck Surg 1988;114:1033–1037.
23. Costantino PD, Russell E, Reisch D, et al. Ruptured petrous carotid aneurysm presenting with otorrhagia and epistaxis. Am J Otol 1991;12:378–383.
24. Teichgraeber JF, Russo RC. Treatment of nasal surgery complications. Ann Plast Surg 1993;30:80–88.
25. Tomasi M, Charpentier P, Lombard P, et al. Hemorrhagic complications of lower turbinectomy. Rev Laryngol Otol Rhinol (Bord) 1993;114:63–66.
26. Premachandra DJ, Bull TR, Mackay IS. How safe is submucosal diathermy? J Laryngol Otol 1990;104:408–409.
27. Kurata A, Kitahara T, Miyasaka Y, et al. Superselective embolization for severe traumatic epistaxis caused by fracture of the skull base. AJAR 1993;14:343–345.
28. Gelbert F, Reizine D, Stecken J, et al. Severe epistaxis by rupture of the internal carotid artery into the sphenoidal sinus. Endovascular treatment. J Neuroradiol 1986;13:163–171.
29. Wang AN, Winfield JA, Gucer G. Traumatic internal carotid artery aneurysm with rupture into the sphenoid sinus. Surg Neurol 1986;25:77–81.
30. Goleas J, Mihkael MA, Paige ML, et al. Intracavernous carotid artery aneurysm presenting as recurrent epistaxis. Ann Otol Rhinol Laryngol 1991;100:577–579.
31. Saim L, Rejab E, Hamzah M, et al. Massive epistaxias recurrent epistaxis. Ann Otol Rhinol Laryngol 1991;100:577–579.
31a.Saim L, Rejab E, Hamzah M, et al. Massive epistaxis from traumatic aneurysm of the internal carotid artery. Aust N Z J Surg 1993;63:906–910.
32. Isamat F. On post-traumatic intracavernous false aneurysms and arteriovenous fistulas. Acta Neurochir (Wien) 1987;85: 148–153.
33. Willinsky R, Lasjaunias P, Pruvost P, et al. Petrous internal carotid aneurysm causing epistaxis: balloon embolization with preservation of the parent vessel. Neuroradiology 1987;29:570–572.
34. Gallina E, Gallo O, Boccuzzi S, et al. Intracranial post-traumatic aneurysm of the internal carotid artery as cause of epistaxis: considerations of 2 cases. Acta Otorhinolaryngol Ital 1990;10:607–613.
35. Hollis LJ, McGashan JA, Walsh RM, et al. Massive epistaxis following sphenoid sinus exploration. J Laryngol Otol 1994; 108:171–173.
36. Han MH, Sung MW, Chang KH, et al. Traumatic pseudoaneurysm of the intracavernous ICA presenting with massive epistaxis: imaging diagnosis and endovascular treatment. Laryngoscope 1994; 104:370–377.

37. Hahn YS, Welling B, Reichman OH, et al. Traumatic intracavernous aneurysm in children: massive epistaxis without ophthalmic signs. Childs Nerv Syst 1990;6: 360–364.

38. Karamoskos P, Dohrmann PJ. Traumatic internal carotid artery aneurysm and massive epistaxis. Aust N Z J Surg 1989;59: 745–747.

39. Ghorayeb BY, Kopaniky DR, Yeakley JW. Massive posterior epistaxis. A manifestation of internal carotid injury at the skull base. Arch Otolaryngol Head Neck Surg 1988;114:1033–1037.

40. Liu MY, Shih CJ, Wang YC, et al. Traumatic intracavernous carotid aneurysm with massive epistaxis. Neurosurgery 1985;17:569–573.

41. Ildan F, Uzuneyupoglu Z, Boyar B, et al. Traumatic giant aneurysm of the intracavernous internal carotid artery causing fatal epistaxis: case report. J Trauma 1994; 36;565–567.

42. Ding MX. Traumatic aneurysm of the intracavernous part of the internal carotid artery presenting with epistaxis. Case report. Surg Neurol 1988;30:65–67.

43. Reddy K, Lesiuk H, West M, et al. False aneurysm of the cavernous carotid artery: a complication of transsphenoidal surgery. Surg Neurol 1990;33;142–145.

44. Romaniuk CS, Bartlett RJ, Kavanagh G, et al. Case report: an unusual cause of epistaxis: non-traumatic intracavernous carotid aneurysm. A case report with 12 year follow-up and review of the literature. Br J Radio 1993;66:942–945.

45. Wakabayashi T, Yasuoka Y, Kamei T. A case of bilateral nontraumatic internal carotid aneurysms presenting with recurrent massive epistaxis. Nippon Jibiinkoka Gakkai Kaiho 1991;94:1257–1264.

46. Chandy MJ, Rajshekhar V. Nontraumatic intracavernous carotid aneurysm presenting with epistaxis. J Laryngol Otol 1989; 103:425–426.

47. Sessions RB. Nasal hemorrhage. Otolaryngol Clin North Am 1973;6:727–744.

48. Wiggins P, McCurdy SA, Zeidenberg W. Epistaxis due to glutaraldehyde exposure. J Occup Med 1989;31:854–856.

49. Schwartz RH, Estroff T, Fairbanks DN, et al. Nasal symptoms associated with cocaine abuse during adolescence. Arch Otolaryngol Head Neck Surg 1989;115: 63–64.

50. Strumpf DA, Harrop P, Dobbin J, et al.

51. Fujisaki K, Shin T, Watanabe H, et al. Choanal bleeding due to nasopharyngitis. Auris Nasus Larynx 1986;13:169–176.

52. Guarisco JL, Graham HD. Epistaxis in children: causes, diagnosis, and treatment. Ear Nose Throat J 1989;68:522, 528–530, 532 passim.

53. Pace-Balzan A, Shankar L, Hawke M. Computed tomographic findings in atrophic rhinitis. J Otolaryngol 1991;20; 428–432.

54. Howard DJ. Life-threatening epistaxis in pregnancy. J Laryngol Otol 1985;99: 95–96.

55. Hansen L, Sobol SM, Abelson TI. Otolaryngologic manifestations of pregnancy. J Fam Pract 1986;23:151–155.

56. Bergua A, Vizmanos F, Monzon FJ, et al. Unavoidable epistaxis in the nasal infestation of leeches. Acta Otorhinolaryngol Esp 1993;44:391–393.

57. Golz A, Zohar S, Avraham S, et al.. Epistaxis caused by leeches. Harefuah 1989; 117:141–143.

58. Struyvenberg PA, van Boxel FA, Polderman AM. A leech as an unusual cause of epistaxis. Ned Tijdschr Geneeskd 1986; 130:791–792.

59. Robson AK, Barker CS, Whittet HB. Epistaxis as an unusual presentation of an antrochoanal polyp. J Laryngol Otol 1990; 104:643–644.

60. Lareo AC, Luce D, Leclerc A, et al. History of previous nasal diseases and sinonasal cancer: a case-control study. Laryngoscope 1992;102:439–442.

61. Johnson IJ, Campbell JB. Renal derived epistaxis. J Laryngol Otol 1993;107: 144–145.

62. Rubinstein AB, Arbit E. Intracranial meningiomas presenting with epistaxis—case report and literature review. J Otolaryngol 1985;14:248–250.

63. Gullane PJ, Davidson J, O'Dwyer T, et al. Juvenile angiofibroma: a review of the literature and a case series report. Laryngoscope 1992:102; 928–933.

64. Padgham ND, Parham DM. Haemorrhagic nasal nodules. Clin Otolaryngol 1993;18: 118–120.

65. Sheppard LM, Mickelson SA. Hemangiomas of the nasal septum and paranasal sinuses. Henry Ford Hosp Med J 1990;38: 25–27.

66. Parkin JD, Smith IL, O'Neill AI, et al. Mild

Massive epistaxis from nasal CPAP therapy. Chest 1989;95:1141.

bleeding disorders. A clinical and laboratory study. Med J Aust 1992;156:614–617.

67. Beran M, Stigendal L, Petruson B. Haemostatic disorders in habitual nose-bleeders. J Laryngol Otol 1987;101:1020–1028.

68. Kiley V, Stuart JJ, Johnson CA. Coagulation studies in children with isolated recurrent epistaxis. J Pediatr 1982;100: 579–581.

69. Denholm SW, Maynard CA, Watson HG. Warfarin and epistaxis—a case controlled study. J Laryngol Otol 1993;107:195–196.

70. Akama H, Hama N, Amano K. Epistaxis induced by a non-steroidal anti-inflammatory drug. J R Soc Med 1990;83:538.

71. McGarry GU. Drug-induced epistaxis. J R Soc Med 1990;83:812.

72. Watson MG, Shenoi PM. Drug-induced epistaxis? J R Soc Med 1990;83:162–164.

73. DiNardo LJ, Hendrix RA. The infectious and hematologic otolaryngologic complications of myelosuppressive cancer chemotherapy. Otolaryngol Head Neck Surg 1991;105:101–106.

74. Nossel HL. Disorders of blood coagulation factors. In: Petersdorf RG, Adams RA, Braunwald E, Isselbacher KJ, Martin JB, Wilson JD, Eds. *Harrison's Principles of Internal Medicine.* New York, NY: McGraw-Hill; 1983: pp. 1900–1909.

75. Poelmann AM, Aarnoudse JG. A pregnant woman with severe epistaxis: a rare manifestation of folic acid deficiency. Eur J Obstr Byn Reprod Biol 1986;23:249–254.

76. Rothstein SG, Schneider KL, Kohan D, et al. Emergencies in AIDS patients: the otolaryngologic perspective. Otolaryngol Head Neck Surg 1991;104:545–548.

77. Hift RJ, Bird AR, Sarembock BD. Acquired hypoprothrombinaemia and lupus anticoagulant: response to steroid therapy. Br J Rheumatol 1991;30:308–310.

78. Nossel HL. Clotting disorders. In: Petersdorf RG, Adams RA, Braunwald E, Isselbacher KJ, Martin JB, Wilson JD, eds. *Harrison's Principles of Internal Medicine.* New York, NY: McGraw-Hill; 1983: pp. 1894–1899.

79. Mittelman M, Ogarten U, Lewinski U, et al. Dipyridamole-induced epistaxis. Ann Otol Rhin Laryngol 1986;95:302–303.

80. Milam SB, Cooper RL. Extensive bleeding following extractions in a patient undergoing chronic hemodialysis. Oral Surg Oral Med Path 1983;55:14–16.

81. Kurien M, Raman R, Thomas K. Profuse epistaxis: an argument for conservative medical management. Singapore Med J 1993;34:335–336.

82. Janzen VD. Rhinological disorders in the elderly. J Otolaryngol 1986;15:228–230.

83. Weiss NS. Relation of high blood pressure to headache, epistaxis and selected other symptoms. N Engl J Med 1972;287: 631–633.

84. Shaheen OH. Arterial epistaxis. J Laryngol Otol 1975;89:17–34.

85. Plauchu H, de Chadarevian JP, Bideau A, et al. Age-related clinical profile of hereditary hemorrhagic telangiectasia in an epidemiologically recruited population. Am J Med Genet 1989;32:291–297.

86. Porteous ME, Burn J, Proctor SJ. Hereditary hemorrhagic telangiectasia: a clinical analysis. J Med Genet 1992;29:527–530.

87. AAssar OS, Friedman CM, White RI Jr. The natural history of epistaxis in hereditary hemorrhagic telangiectasia. Laryngoscope 1991;101:977–980.

88. McCaffrey TV, Kern EB, Lake CF. Management of epistaxis in hereditary hemorrhagic telangiectasia. Arch Otolaryngol 1977;103:627–630.

89. Stecker RH, Lake CF. Hereditary hemorrhagic telangiectasia: review of 102 cases and presentation of an innovation to septodermoplasty. Arch Otolaryngol 1965; 82:522–526.

90. Josephson GD, Godley FA, Stierna P. Practical management of epistaxis. Med Clin North Am 1991;75:1311–1320.

91. McGarry GW, Moulton C. The first aid management of epistaxis by accident and emergency department staff. Arch Emerg Med 1993;10:298–300.

92. Dost P, Polyzoidis T. Benefit of the ice pack in the treatment of nosebleed. HNO 1992;40:25–27.

93. Porter MJ. A comparison between the effect of ice packs on the forehead and ice cubes in the mouth on nasal submucosal temperature. Rhinology 1991;29:11–15.

94. Keen MS, Moran WJ. Control of epistaxis in the multiple trauma patient. Laryngoscope 1985;95:874–875.

95. Wurman LH, Sack JG, Flannery JV, et al. The management of epistaxis. Am J Otolaryngol 1992;13:193–209.

96. Nicolaides A, Gray R, Pfleiderer A. A new approach to the management of acute epistaxis. Clin Otolaryngol 1991;16:59–61.

97. Toner JG, Walby AP. Comparison of electro and chemical cautery in the treatment of anterior epistaxis. J Laryngol Otol 1990; 104:617–618.

98. Call WH. Control of epistaxis. Surg Clin North Am 1969;49:1235–1247.

99. Mabry RL. Management of epistaxis by packing. Otolaryngol Head Neck Surg 1986;94:412–415.

100. Reiter D, Alford E, Jabourian Z. Alternatives to packing in septorhinoplasty. Arch Otolaryngol Head Neck Surg 1989;115: 1203–1205.

101. Fairbanks DN. Complications of nasal packing. Otolaryngol Head Neck Surg 1986;94:412–415.

102. Pinczower E, Rice DH. Drug-induced dystonia and airway obstruction in a patient with nasal packing. Otolaryngol Head Neck Surg 1990;103:658–659

103. McGashan JA, Walsh R, Dauod A, et al. A comparative study of calcium sodium alginate (Kaltostat) and bismuth tribromophenate (Xeroform) packing in the management of epistaxis. J Laryngol Otol 1992;106:1067–1071.

104. Taylor MT. Avitene: its value in control of anterior epistaxis. J Otolaryngol 1980; 9:468–471.

105. Keen M. The Avitene pack: a new method to control epistaxis in a patient with poor platelet function. Laryngoscope 1986;96: 1411.

106. Heywood BB, Davis, RB, Yonkers AJ. The treatment of packing with porcine stripped packing. Trans Am Acad Ophthalmol Otolaryngol 1976;82:255–260.

107. Davis RB, Yonkers AJ, Heywood BB. Effects of a soluble fraction of porcine tissue on the aggregation of human blood platelets. Laryngoscope 1982;92:674–677.

108. Carr ME Jr, Gabriel DA. Nasal packing with porcine fatty tissue for epistaxis complicated by qualitative platelet disorders. J Emerg Med 1985;3:449–452.

109. Elwany S, Kamel T, Mekhamer A. Pneumatic nasal catheters: advantages and drawbacks. J Laryngol Otol 1986;100: 641–647.

110. McGarry GW, Aitken D. Intranasal balloon catheters: how do they work? Clin Otolaryngol 1991;16:388–392.

111. McFerran DJ, Edmonds SE. The use of balloon catheters in the treatment of epistaxis. J Laryngol Otol 1993;107:197–200.

112. Sadowsky AE, Leavenworth N, Wirtschafter JD. Compressive optic neuropathy induced by intranasal balloon catheter. Am J Ophthalmol 1985;99: 487–489.

113. Derkay CS, Hirsch BE, Johnson JT, et al. Posterior nasal packing. Are intravenous antibiotics really necessary. Arch Otolaryngol Head Neck Surg 1989;115: 439–441.

114. Cannon CR. Effective treatment protocol for posterior epistaxis : a 10-year experience. Otolaryngol Head Neck Surg 1993; 109:722–725.

115. Kersch R, Wolff AP. Severe epistaxis: protecting the nasal ala. Laryngoscope 1990; 100:1348.

116. Wareing MJ, Gray RF. Foley catheter fixation in posterior epistaxis. J Laryngol Otol 1993;107:1032–1033.

117. Cook PR, Renner G, William F. A comparison of nasal balloons and posterior gauze packs for posterior epistaxis. Ear Nose Throat J 1985;64:78–81.

118. Porras LF, Cabezudo JM, Lorenzana L, et al. Inadvertent intraspinal placement of a Foley catheter in severe craniofacial injury with associated atlanto-occipital dislocation: case report. Neurosurgery 1993; 33:310–312.

119. Montgomery WW, Reardon EJ. Early vessel ligations for control of severe epistaxis. In Snow JB, ed. *Controversy in Otolaryngology*. Philadelphia, Pa: W B Saunders Company; 1980: pp. 315–319.

120. Schaitkin B, Strauss M, Houck JR. Epistaxis: medical versus surgical therapy. A comparison of efficacy, complications and economic considerations. Laryngoscope 1987;97:1392–1396.

121. Cooke ET. An evaluation and clinical study of severe epistaxis treated by arterial ligation. J Laryngol Otol 1985;99: 745–749.

122. Spafford P, Durham JS. Epistaxis: efficacy of arterial ligation and long-term outcome. J Otolaryngol 1992;21:252–256.

123. Seifert A. Unterbinding der arteria maxillaris interna. Zeitsschr. f. Hals, Nasen U Ohrenseilk 1928;22:323–6.

124. Gergely Z. Transmaxillary ligature of the arteria interna (Seiffer's method). Acta Otolaryngol 1935;22:142–5.

125. Chandler JR, Serrins AF. Transantral ligation of the internal maxillary artery for epistaxis. Laryngoscope 1965;75:1151–5.

126. Premachandra DJ, Sergent RJ. Dominant maxillary artery as a cause of failure in maxillary artery ligation for posterior epistaxis. Clin Otolaryngol 1993;18:42–47.

127. Simpson GT II, Janfaza P, Becker GD. Transantral sphenopalatine artery ligation. Laryngoscope 1982;92:1001–1005.

128. Montgomery WW, Lofgran RH, Chasin

WD. Analysis of pterygopalatine surgery. Laryngoscope 1970;80:1190–1200.

129. Breda SD, Chol IS, Perksy MS, et al. Embolization in the treatment of epistaxis after failure of internal maxillary artery ligation. Laryngoscope 1989;99:809–813.

130. Metson R, Lane R. Internal maxillary artery ligation for epistaxis: an analysis of failures. Laryngoscope 1988;98:760–764.

131. Wang L, Vogel DH. Posterior epistaxis: comparison of treatment. Otolaryngol Head Neck Surg 1981;89:1001–1006.

132. Beall J, Scholl P, Jafek B. Total ophthalmoplegia after internal maxillary artery ligation. Arch Otolaryngol 1985;111: 696–698.

133. Maceri DR, Makielski KH. Intraoral ligation of the maxillary artery for posterior epistaxis. Laryngoscope 1984;94:737–741.

134. Stepnick DW, Maniglia AJ, Bold EL, et al. Intraoral-extramaxillary sinus approach for ligation of the maxillary artery: an anatomic study with clinical correlates. Laryngoscope 1990;100:1166–1170.

135. Kirchner JA, Yanagisawa E, Crelin ES Jr. Surgical anatomy of the ethmoidal arteries—a laboratory study of 150 orbits. Arch Otolaryngol 1961;74:382–7.

136. Couch JM, Somers ME, Gonzalez C. Superior oblique muscle dysfunction following anterior ethmoidal artery ligation for epistaxis. Arch Ophthalmol 1990;108: 1110–1113.

137. Waldron J, Stafford N. Ligation of the external carotid artery for severe epistaxis. J Otolaryngol 1992;21:249–251.

138. Hassard AD, Kirkpatrick DA, Wong FS. Ligation of the external carotid and anterior ethmoidal arteries for severe or unusual epistaxis resulting from facial fractures. Can J Surg 1986;29:447–449.

139. Prescott CA. An unusual complication of epistaxis. J Laryngol Otol 1988;102:176.

140. Cumberworth VL, Narula AA, Bradley PJ. Prospective study of two management strategies for epistaxis. J R Coll Surg Edinb 1991;36:259–260.

141. Premachandra DJ. Management of posterior epistaxis with the use of the fibreoptic nasolaryngoscope. J Laryngol Otol 1991;105:17–19.

142. Borgstein JA. Epistaxis and the flexible nasopharyngoscope. Clin Otolaryngol 1987;12:49–51.

143. Marcus MJ. Nasal endoscopic control of epistaxis—a preliminary report. Otola-

ryngol Head Neck Surg 1990;102: 273–275.

144. O'Leary-Stickney K, Makielski K, Weymuller EA Jr. Rigid endoscopy for the control of epistaxis. Arch Otolaryngol Head Neck Surg 1992;118:966–967.

145. Bingham B, Dingle AF. Endoscopic management of severe epistaxis. J Otolaryngol 1991;20:442–443.

146. McGarry GW. Nasal endoscope in posterior epistaxis: a preliminary evaluation. J Laryngol Otol 1991:105:428–431.

147. Wurman LH, Sack JG, Flannery JV Jr, et al. Selective endoscopic electrocautery for posterior epistaxis. Laryngoscope 1988;98:348–349.

148. Tolsdorff P. Hemostasis in the nose with bipolar suction and a coagulation probe under endoscopic control. Laryngol Rhinol Otol (Stuttg) 1985;64:394–398.

149. Sulsenti G, Yanez C, Kadiri M. Recurrent epistaxis: microscopic endonasal clipping of the sphenopalatine artery. Rhinology 1987;25:141–142.

150. Stamm AC, Pinto JA, Neto AF, et al. Microsurgery in severe posterior epistaxis. Rhinology 1985;23:321–325.

151. Rosnagle RS, Allen WE, Kier EL, et al. Use of selective arteriography in the treatment of epistaxis. Arch Otolaryngol 1980;106: 137–142.

152. Hicks JN, Vitek G. Transarterial embolization to control posterior epistaxis. Laryngoscope 1989;99:1027–1029.

153. Coel MN, Janon EA. Angiography in patients with intractable epistaxis. Am J Roentgenol Radium Ther Nucl Med 1972; 116:37–40.

154. Sokoloff J, Wickbom I, McDonald D. Therapeutic percutaneous embolization in intractable epistaxis. Radiology 1974;111: 285–287.

155. DeFilipp GJ, Steffey D, Rubinstein M, et al. The role of angiography and embolization in the management of recurrent epistaxis. Otolaryngol Head Neck Surg 1988; 99:597–600.

156. Welsh LW, Welsh JJ, Scogna JE, et al. Role of angiography in the management of refractory epistaxis. Ann Otol Rhinol Laryngol 1990;99:69–73.

157. Babu Manohar M, Sharp JF, Johnosn AP. Vertebro-carotid anastomosis as a cause of uncontrollable epistaxis. J Laryngol Otol 1994;108:247–248.

158. Lasjaunias P, Marsot-Dupuch K, Dovon D. The radio-anatomical basis of arterial em-

bolization for epistaxis. J Neuroradiol 1979;6:45–53.

159. Milczuk HA, Flint PW, Eskridge JM, et al. Quest for the aberrant vessel. Otolaryngol Head Neck Surg 1991;104:489–494.

160. Elden L, Montanera W, Terbrugge K, et al. Angiographic embolization for the treatment of epistaxis: A review of 108 cases. Otolaryngol Head Neck Surg 1994;111: 44–50.

161. Moser FG, Rosenblatt M, De La Cruz F, et al. Embolization of the ophthalmic artery for control of epistaxis: report of two cases. Head Neck 1992;14:308–311.

162. Simpson RK Jr, Harper RL, Bryan RN. Emergency balloon occlusion for massive epistaxis due to traumatic carotid-cavernous aneurysm. Case report. J Neurosurg 1988;68:142–144.

163. Crow WN, Scott BA, Guinto FC Jr, et al. Massive epistaxis due to pseudoaneurysm. Treated with detachable balloons. Arch Otolaryngol Head Neck Surg 1992; 118:321–324.

164. Vitek J. Idiopathic intractable epistaxis: endovascular therapy. Radiology 1991; 181:113–116.

165. Parnes LS, Heeneman H, Vinuela F. Percutaneous embolization for control of nasal blood circulation. Laryngoscope 1987;97:1312–1315.

166. Strutz J, Schumacher M. Uncontrollable epistaxis: angiographic localization and embolization. Arch Otolaryngol Head Neck Surg 1990;116:697–699.

167. Merland JJ, Melki JP, Chiras J, et al. The place of embolization in the treatment of severe epistaxis. Laryngoscope 1980;90: 1694–1704.

168. Metson R, Hanson DG. Bilateral facial nerve paralysis following arterial embolization for epistaxis. Otolaryngol Head Neck Surg 1983;91:299–303.

169. de Vries N, Versluis RJ, Valk J, et al. Facial nerve paralysis following embolization for severe epistaxis (case report and review of the literature). J Laryngol Otol 1986;100:207–210.

170. Jacobson DM, Pesicka GA. Transient superior oblique palsy following arterial ligation for epistaxis. Arch Ophthalmol 1991;109:320–321.

171. Siegel MB, Keane WM, Atkins JF Jr, et al. Control of epistaxis in patients with hereditary hemorrhagic telangiectasia. Otolaryngol Head Neck Surg 1991;105: 675–679.

172. Harrison DFN. Familial hemorrhagic tel-

angiectasia: 20 cases treated with systematic oestrogen. Q J Med 1964;33:25–27.

173. Tombleson PM. Local oestrogen for recurrent epistaxis caused by familial telangiectasia (letter). J R Coll Gen Pract 1988; 38:227.

174. Saba HI, Morelli GA, Logrono LA. Brief report: treatment of bleeding in hereditary hemorrhagic telangiectasia wit aminocaproic acid. N Engl J Med 1994;330: 1789–1790.

175. Borsik M, Herbreteau D, Deffrennes D, et al. Treatment of epistaxis in Rendu-Osler disease by intramucosal injection of ethibloc. Ann Otolaryngol Chir Cervicofac 1992;109:273–276.

176. Parkin JL, Dixon JA. Argon laser treatment of head and neck vascular lesions. Otolaryngol Head Neck Surg 1985;93: 211–216.

177. Haye R, Austad J. Hereditary hemorrhagic telangiectasia—argon laser. Rhinology 1991;29:5–9.

178. Parkin JL, Dixon JA. Laser photocoagulation in hereditary hemorrhagic telangiectasis. Otolaryngol Head Neck Surg 1981; 89:204–208.

179. Shapshay SM, Oliver B. Treatment of hereditary hemorrhagic telangiectasia by ND-YAG laser photo coagulation. Laryngoscope 1984;94:1554–1556.

180. Kluger PB, Shapshay SM, Hybels RL, et al. Neodymium-YAG laser intranasal photocoagulation in hereditary hemorrhagic telangiectasia: an update report. Laryngoscope 1987;97:1397–1401.

181. Zohar Y, Talmi YP, Finkelstein Y, et al. Use of human amniotic membrane in otolaryngologic practice. Laryngoscope 1987;97:978–980.

182. Milton CM, Shotton JC, Premachandran DJ, et al. A new technique using cultured epithelial sheets for the management of epistaxis associated with hereditary haemorrhagic telangiectasia. J Laryngol Otol 1993;107:510–513.

183. Goldsmith MM, Fry TL. Tips on septal dermoplasty. Laryngoscope 1987;97: 994–995.

184. Strauss M, Zohar Y, Laurian M. The management of severe recurrent epistaxis due to hereditary haemorrhagic telangiectasia using regional facial cutaneous flaps. J Laryngol Otol 1985;99:373–377.

185. Zohar Y, Sadov R, Shvili Y, et al. Surgical management of epistaxis in hereditary hemorrhagic telangiectasia. Arch Otola-

ryngol Head Neck Surg 1987;113: 754–777.

186. Bridger GP, Baldwin M. Microvascular free flap in hereditary hemorrhagic telangiectasia. Arch Otolaryngol Head Neck Surg 1990;116:85–87.

187. Pohar S, Mazeron JJ, Ghilezan M, et al. Management of epistaxis in Rendu-Osler disease: is brachytherapy effective? Int J Radiat Oncol Biol Phys 1993;27: 1073–1077.

188. Padrnos RE. A method for control of posterior nasal hemorrhage. Arch Otolaryngol 1968;87;181–183.

189. Bharadwaj VK, Novotny GM. Greater palatine canal injection: an alternative to the posterior nasal packing and arterial ligation in epistaxis. J Otolaryngol 1986;15: 94–100.

190. Brown OE. The use of desmopressin in children with coagulation disorders. Int J Ped Otolaryngol 1986;11:301–305.

191. Kobrinsky NL, Tulloch H. Treatment of refractory thrombocytopenic bleeding with 1-desamino-8-D-arginine vasopressin (desmopressin). J Pediatr 1988;112: 993–996.

192. Brown OE. The use of desmopressin in children with coagulation disorders. Int J Pediatr Otorhinolaryngol 1986;11: 301–305.

193. Vinayak BC, Birchall MA, Donovan B, et al. A randomized double-blind trial of glypressin in the management of acute epistaxis. Rhinology 1993;31:131–134.

194. Bende M, Pipkorn U. Topical terlipressin (Glypressin) gel reduces nasal mucosal blood flow but leaves ongoing nose-bleeding unaffected. Acta Otolaryngol (Stockh) 1990;110:124–127.

195. White A, O'Reilly BF. Oral tranexamic acid in the management of epistaxis. Clin Otolaryngol 1988;13:11–16.

196. Bluestone CC, Smith AC. Intranasal freezing for severe epistaxis. Arch Otolaryngol 1967;85:445–457.

197. Bluestone CD, Nixon VD. Intranasal freezing for severe epistaxis. Int Surg 1970:53; 11–15.

198. Hicks JN. Cryotherapy for severe posterior nasal epistaxis. Clinical and experimental study. Laryngoscope 1971;81: 1881–1902.

199. Chester WL. A substitute for the operation of plugging the posterior nares and at the same time applying pressure and cold to a large portion of the nasal tract. Br Med J 1984;1143.

200. Ogura JH, Unno T, Nelson JR. Baseline values in pulmonary mechanics for physiologic surgery of the nose: preliminary report. Ann Otol 1968;78:369–397.

201. Cassisi NJ, Biller HF, Ogura JH. Changes in arterial oxygen tension and pulmonary mechanics with the use of posterior nasal packing. Laryngoscope 1971;81: 1261–1266.

202. Jensen PF, Kristensen S, Juul A, et al. Episodic nocturnal hypoxia and nasal packs. Clin Otolaryngol 1991;16:433–435.

203. Loftus BC, Blitzer A, Cozine K. Epistaxis, medical history, and the nasopulmonary reflex: what is clinically relevant? Otolaryngol Head Neck Surg 1994;110: 363–369.

204. Wetmore SJ, Scrima L, Hiller FC. Sleep apnea in epistaxis patients treated with nasal packs. Otolaryngol Head Neck Surg 1988;98:596–599.

205. John DG, Alison AI, Scott DJ, et al. Who should treat epistaxis? J Laryngol Otol 1987;101:139–142.

206. Monux A, Tomas M, Kaiser C, et al. Conservative management of epistaxis. J Laryngol Otol 1990;104:868–870.

207. Schaitkin B, Strauss M, Houck JR. Epistaxis: medical versus surgical therapy: a comparison of efficacy, complications, and economic considerations. Laryngoscope 1987:97:1392–1396.

208. Wehrli M, Lieberherr U, Valavanis A. Superselective embolization for intractable epistaxis: experiences with 19 patients. Clin Otolaryngol 1988;13: 415–420.

209. Siniluoto TM, Leinonen AS, Karttunen AI, et al. Embolization for the treatment of posterior epistaxis. An analysis of 31 cases. Arch Otolaryngol Head Neck Surg 1993;119:837–841.

210. Bone RC. Epistaxis. In: Meyers AD, Eiseman B, eds. *Cost-effective Otolaryngology*. Ontario, Canada: BC Decker; 1990.

# 15

# Nasal Obstruction, Rhinorrhea, and Postnasal Drip

Helen M. Hollingsworth, M.D.
Richard S. Irwin, M.D.

## Introduction

Nasal obstruction, rhinorrhea, and post-nasal drip are nonspecific symptoms that may reflect inflammatory rhinitis, noninflammatory rhinitis, or structural abnormalities of the nasal passages, sinuses, or pharynx. These symptoms may occur alone or in combination.

Although these presenting complaints are nonspecific, an orderly evaluation starting with a history and physical examination and proceeding to an allergy evaluation, rhinopharyngolarynoscopy, radiographic studies, and blood tests for systemic illnesses, where indicated, will usually reveal the cause.

The purpose of this chapter is to review the pathogenesis of these symptoms individually, the diagnostic approach to elucidating the cause in a given patient, the diseases that should be considered in the differential diagnosis, and the specific treatment of these diseases that should result in resolution of the symptoms.

## Pathogenesis

### Mechanisms of Nasal Obstruction

The sensation of nasal obstruction may be variably reported by patients as stuffiness, congestion, or pressure or difficulty breathing through one or both nasal passages. This sensation may be caused by dilation of capacitance vessels in the nasal submucosa, edema of the mucosa, excess secretions in the nasal passages, cellular infiltration of the mucosa, and structural abnormalities.

The subjective sensation of obstruction is difficult to quantify and frequently does not correlate with the actual resistance to airflow. Therefore, patients may perceive nasal obstruction despite having excellent nasal patency, as in patients who have atrophic rhinitis following extensive resection of the turbinates. In contrast, other patients may not complain of nasal obstruction, despite having significant

From Irwin RS, Curley FJ, Grossman RF (eds): Diagnosis and Treatment of Symptoms of the Respiratory Tract. Armonk, New York, Futura Publishing Company, Inc., © 1997.

nasal mucosal edema or prominent nasal polyps on examination.

## Dilation of the Capacitance Vessels

Nasal patency is predominantly controlled by changes in congestion of a plexus of sinusoids located just beneath the submucosal glands.[1-3] Constriction and relaxation of these sinusoidal vessels is under sympathetic control. For instance, increased sympathetic discharge with exercise decreases the degree of nasal airflow resistance.[1,2] Similarly, sympathomimetic medications, such as the $\alpha$-adrenergic agent oxymetazoline, constrict these vessels and decrease nasal congestion.[4]

The degree of nasal airflow resistance normally alternates between the nasal cavities every 2 to 4 hours in 60% to 70% of the population.[2] This physiologic variation in nasal patency, or nasal cycle, is mediated by changes in congestion of the capacitance blood vessels in the submucosa of the middle and lower turbinates. Posture also influences the degree of vascular congestion, such that congestion increases in the supine position and in the dependent nares in the lateral recumbent position.

Vascular engorgement is an important feature of the immediate hypersensitivity reactions in the nose and is caused by release of certain mast cell and basophil mediators. This particular part of the allergic reaction in the nose can be reversed by topical application of oxymetazoline.[4]

## Nasal Mucosal Edema

The two most important causes of nasal mucosal edema are viral infections (eg, "common cold") and allergic rhinitis. The nasal manifestations of the common cold are felt to derive predominantly from dysautonomia caused by activation of cholinergic and noncholinergic-nonadrenergic nerves; pathological and cytological studies have shown little if any damage to the nasal mucosa.[5-7]

Following allergic activation, mast cell and basophil mediators, such as histamine, kinins, and eicosanoids, cause increased vascular permeability that, in turn, results in subepithelial mucosal edema.[3] This mucosal edema contributes to the sensation of nasal congestion, in addition to the above described distension of nasal venous sinusoids.

## Excess Secretions

Excess secretions are most likely to be perceived as causing nasal obstruction when they are thick and tenacious. The most common causes of this are infectious causes: viral upper respiratory infections and sinusitis. Other causes of obstruction, such as inflammatory infiltration and edema of the mucosa, may be accompanied by an increase in secretions, but the secretions are thin and watery and minimally contribute to obstruction. The pathogenesis of rhinorrhea is discussed further below.

## Cellular Infiltration

Following allergen-mediated activation of mast cells and basophils, many patients develop a late allergic response with recruitment of eosinophils, basophils, lymphocytes, and neutrophils to the nasal mucosa.[3,4] These recruited cells release their own cytokines and inflammatory mediators, prolonging the inflammatory response. The presence of these cells in the mucosa probably also contributes to the thickness of the mucosa and nasal airflow resistance.

Infiltrative processes, such as granulomatous inflammation in sarcoidosis, may present with nasal obstruction. A noncellular infiltrative process, myxedema in hypothyroid patients, can similarly cause nasal obstruction.

## Structural Abnormalities

Nasal obstruction can result from a variety of anatomical abnormalities and may

**Table I**
**Anatomical Abnormalities**
**and Space-occupying Lesions**

Choanal Atresia
Septal Deviation, Congenital, or Posttraumatic
Septal Spurs
Nasal Polyps
Synechiae After Nasal Trauma/Surgery
Granulomatous Disease
Saddle-nose Deformity*
Benign Tumors
Malignant Tumors
Concha Bullosa
Foreign Bodies
Meningocele
Hypertrophied Adenoids

* Saddle-nose deformity is typically a result of infection, immunologic disease, or malignancy.

be unilateral or bilateral. Table I provides a partial listing of structural abnormalities and space-occupying lesions that may cause nasal obstruction. Each of these will be considered in more detail in the "Differential Diagnosis" section.

## Mechanisms of Rhinorrhea

A variety of inflammatory and noninflammatory stimuli can increase the volume and alter the normal constituents of nasal secretions. For example, during the early phase of allergic inflammation, newly generated and preformed mediators are released by mucosal mast cells, glandular serous and mucous cells, goblet cells, and epithelial cells, causing vascular dilatation, increased vascular permeability, and increased secretion of mucous and glandular proteins.[1,8] Subsequent recruitment of basophils, eosinophils, lymphocytes, and neutrophils causes persistence of these effects. Histamine, an important mast cell and basophil mediator, produces a secretory response when instilled locally into the nose.[9] The response to histamine appears to result more from increased vascular permeability than from increased glandular secretion, based on analysis of protein content.[1]

Noninflammatory cholinergic stimulation via methacholine instillation or consumption of hot, spicy foods causes an increase in the volume of nasal secretions and a change in protein concentrations.[10] Protein analysis in these noninflammatory challenges suggests stimulation of glandular cells either directly via muscarinic receptors on submucosal glands (eg, methacholine) or indirectly via a nasal reflex arc from afferent nerve receptors in the mouth to submucosal glands in the nose (eg, hot, spicy foods).[1,10]

Increased vascular permeability has been demonstrated in experimental rhinovirus infection, suggesting that this may be the source of excess nasal secretions in the common cold.[7]

## Mechanisms of Postnasal Drip

Postnasal drip may be manifest clinically by the sensation of something "dripping" down the back of the throat, frequent throat-clearing implying the presence of abnormal secretions in the back of the throat, or cough. Patients may not be aware of postnasal drip, but careful examination of the posterior pharynx may reveal the presence of secretions or a cobblestone appearance on the posterior wall of the oropharynx. Postnasal drip can be caused by irritative processes above the pharynx (eg, allergic rhinitis, viral rhinitis, sinusitis, irritant rhinitis, gustatory rhinitis) that lead to excess nasal secretions which migrate along the nasal mucosa to the posterior pharynx.[11,12] Cigarette smoke can cause postnasal drip indirectly, by irritation of the nasopharynx, or directly, by irritation of the nasopharynx and/or oropharynx. Postnasal drip can also be caused by irritation coming from below the throat. For instance, gastroesophageal reflux provokes the sensation of postnasal drip through the irritant effect of gastric fluid refluxing to the pharynx.[13]

One interesting question is whether the specific constituents of the fluid affect the degree or type of symptoms in postnasal drip. For instance, in rhinovirus infections, a significant increase in kinins, but not histamine occurs.[7] The rise in concentration of kinins appears to correlate with severity of symptom scores, suggesting a causal relationship.[7] The irritative cough that frequently accompanies the common cold is similar to the angiotensin converting enzyme-induced cough that may also be mediated by kinins. Some patients with allergic rhinitis may complain more about postnasal drip and throat-clearing, but others may be troubled by an irritative cough, as well. Of note, kinins have been demonstrated in nasal secretions obtained during the early and late phases of experimental intranasal allergen challenge.[14]

Excessive secretions from the nose from nonirritative conditions (eg, vasomotor rhinitis) can also cause the sensation of postnasal drip. Fluid viscosity and volume may also play a role in the severity and type of associated symptoms.

The term "postnasal drip syndrome" is used to signify that a clinical problem is caused by an upper respiratory tract disease through the mechanism of postnasal drip.[11,15] Postnasal drip syndrome can, in turn, cause cough,[11,12,15,16] wheeze,[17] and dyspnea.[18]

## Diagnostic Approach

### Directed History and Physical Examination

The process of evaluating the cause of nasal congestion, rhinorrhea, and postnasal drip in any given patient should begin with a careful delineation of the time course of their symptoms and whether any association has been noted with seasonal pollen, home, work, hobby, or animal dander exposure.[19] Determining whether the patient has a family history of atopy is also important. This will set the stage for differentiating between allergic rhinitis, which is the most common type of chronic rhinitis, and the multiple nonallergic types of rhinitis.

Itchy eyes, nose, or palate are suggestive of an allergic cause. The onset of nasal symptoms with an upper respiratory tract

**Table II**
Physical Examination for Nasal Congestion, Rhinorrhea, and Postnasal Drip

General Appearance
  Allergic Shiners
  Oral Breathing
  Saddle-nose Deformity
  Throat clearing
  Sniffing
  Coughing
Tympanic Membranes
  Scarring
  Light Reflex
  Fluid
  Erythema
Eyes
  Crusting or Discharge
  Conjunctival Injection
  Giant Papillae
External Nose
  Deformity or Broadening
  Paranasal Tenderness
  Transverse Crease
Nasal Passages
  Patency of Nasal Antrum
  Septal Shape and Position
  Septal Spurs
  Nasal Secretions, Crusting
  Turbinates (size, shape, color)
  Polyps (unilateral, bilateral, size)
  Airflow
Oropharynx
  Odor
  Cobblestoning
  Scretions
  Erythema
Neck
  Lymph Nodes
  Thyroid
  Masses
Lungs
  Airflow
  Adventitial Sounds
Skin
  Atopic Dermatitis
  Other Eruptions Suggestive of Systemic Disease

infection and subsequent persistence suggests sinusitis. Other complaints, such as purulent nasal discharge, postnasal drip, cough, hyposmia, and paranasal pressure, are consistent with sinusitis, but not specific for it. Clear, watery secretions are associated with eosinophilic rhinitis, vasomotor rhinitis, cerebrospinal fluid (CSF) leaks, the onset of the common cold, and gustatory rhinitis. Fever is suggestive of infection or an inflammatory systemic illness, such as Wegener's granulomatosis. On the other hand, fever is present in only half of patients with sinusitis,[20,21] so its absence does not exclude the presence of sinusitis.

In addition, it is important to ascertain the severity of symptoms, realizing that most patients under-report nasal symptoms (eg, "doing well" may really mean using half a box of tissues a day instead of a full box). Quantitative questions may be more revealing than qualitative questions. Similarly, patients may not volunteer information about what remedies they have tried, but the diagnosis of rhinitis medicamentosa depends on knowing what over-the-counter nasal sprays and illicit drugs a patient may have used, as well as what medications a patient is taking for other medical problems.

A careful physical examination is the next step in evaluating nasal congestion, rhinorrhea, or postnasal drip.[19] Table II gives a list of features that a directed physical examination for evaluation of rhinitis symptoms ought to include. Transillumination of the paranasal sinuses is neither sensitive nor specific in the evaluation of sinusitis and is not included in the list.[22]

## Diagnostic Testing

A variety of tests and procedures are now available for evaluating the role of allergic inflammation, infiltrative diseases, sinus infection, and structural lesions in nasal symptoms (Table III). The findings of the detailed history and physical examination described above will determine which tests are most appropriate.

### Allergy Evaluation

**Allergy Skin Testing:** Of all the allergy tests available for evaluating rhinitis, skin test-

| **Table III** |
| :---: |
| Tests for Evaluating Rhinitis |

Allergy Assessment
   Serum IgE
   Allergy Skin Testing
   Allergy Radioallergosorbent Testing (RAST-IgE)
   Nasal Smear
   Nasal Provocation Challenge
   Nasal Lavage
Direct Visualization
   Mirror Examination
   Rhinolaryngoscopy
Imaging Studies
   Sinus X-rays
   Sinus CT Scan
   Sinus Magnetic Resonance Imaging
Functional Studies
   Rhinomanometry
   Nasal Flow-volume Loops
Miscellaneous
   Nasal Scraping/Biopsy
   Sweat Chloride Test

CT = computed tomography; RAST = radioallergosorbent testing.

ing to inhalants is probably the most useful and cost-effective.[23,24] Usually, a panel of inhalant allergens, composed of extracts of local pollens for the specific geographic area, dust mites, animal danders, feathers, molds, and cockroach, is developed. Standardized extracts that contain all of the important allergenic determinants present in native material are strongly recommended when they are available. Food allergens are rarely a cause of chronic rhinitis symptoms, so skin testing to foods is rarely indicated in this setting.

The advantages of allergy skin testing are (1) results are available quickly; (2) there is very minimal risk; (3) there are many years of experience with the technique and with correlating results with clinical presentation; (4) it is less expensive than radioallergosorbent (RAST) testing; (5) it can be used to identify a safe starting dose for immunotherapy; and (6) patients may be more inclined to follow through on environmental controls based on positive skin tests than on positive RAST.[25]

Prior to skin testing, patients need to be evaluated regarding presence of skin disease in the area to be used for testing and ingestion of medications that may interfere with testing (eg, $H_1$ and $H_2$ antihistamines, tricyclic antidepressants) or make testing hazardous (eg, beta blockers, monoamine oxidase inhibitors).[26] A validated technique for performing testing and recording results is also recommended.[24,26]

**Radioallergosorbent Testing:** Radioallergosorbent testing (RAST) can be used when skin testing is contraindicated because of skin disease or interfering medications.[23,25,27] Advantages of RAST include (1) there is less risk/discomfort to patient; (2) it is potentially easier to quantitate than skin test, although not true yet; (3) results are not affected by pharmacotherapy, obviating need to withdraw medication prior to testing; and (4) skin disease and psychiatric disturbances do not interfere with testing.[25]

Determination of total IgE is rarely helpful by itself,[19] except as a measure of disease activity in patients being treated for allergic fungal sinusitis.

**Nasal Cytology:** Nasal cytology[19,28,29] is easily obtained without discomfort to the patient by swabbing the nasal turbinate on both sides with a cotton-tipped applicator. The material obtained is then spread on a cytology slide and developed with Hansel's stain.[19,29] Cytologic evaluation of the nasal mucosa helps in the differentiation of the certain types of rhinitis. The presence of eosinophils suggests either allergic rhinitis or nonallergic rhinitis with eosinophils (NARES),[28,29] both of which are usually responsive to intranasal corticosteroids. A predominance of neutrophils suggests infection; basophilia suggests basophilic rhinitis.[29]

**Nasal Provocation and Nasal Lavage:** Nasal provocation challenge and nasal lavage have been very helpful in elucidating the mediators involved in early- and late-phase allergic responses in the nose, as well as the pathophysiology of viral and gustatory rhinitis. At this point, they remain research tools.[1,3,30-32]

## Rhinopharyngolaryngoscopy

Mirror examination has been used for years to examine the posterior nasopharynx and larynx, but requires skill and does not allow full visualization of the nasal passages. Fiberoptic rhinoscopy allows detailed visualization of the posterior two thirds of the nose which is not visible from the anterior nares. The procedure is brief and generally well tolerated by patients.[33,34] It is indicated particularly when nasal obstruction is persistent or unilateral.[33-35] One study has also reported the use of fiberoptic rhinoscopy in the diagnosis of sinusitis by identifying purulent material draining from one or more of the sinus ostia.[36] Interestingly, one subgroup of patients with positive rhinoscopy had negative sinus radiographs, but a high response rate to oral antibiotics.

## Ultrasonography

The technique of ultrasonography depends on transmission of low power, pulsed ultrasound waves into the sinus cavity by direct contact with the patient's face.[22] When the maxillary antrum is filled with fluid, the ultrasound waves are transmitted through the fluid and a strong echo is reflected off the posterior wall. Because ultrasound at this frequency does not transmit through air, no echo appears from the posterior wall of healthy, air-filled sinuses.

Unfortunately, study results have shown a poor predictive value of sinus ultrasound.[22] This is likely because of difficulty imaging sinuses other than maxillary and because the technique does not detect mucosal thickening well. Some practitioners find ultrasonography helpful in assessing the response of maxillary sinusitis to treatment.

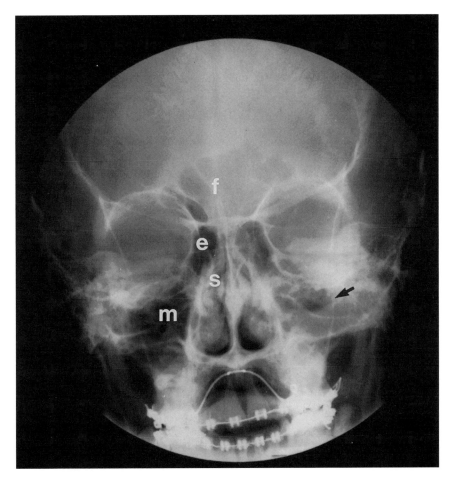

**Figure 1A.** Maxillary sinusitis. Caldwell projection during the standard multiview roentgeno-graphic examination of the paranasal sinuses in a 17-year-old patient with left maxillary sinusitis and periorbital cellulitis. There is an air-fluid level in the left maxillary sinus **(arrowhead)**. e = ethmoid sinus; f = frontal sinus; m = maxillary sinus; s = sphenoid sinus. Figure 1A to 1E reprinted from Jacobs TE, Irwin RS, Raptopoulos V. Upper respiratory tract infections in the critically-ill. J Intensive Care Med 1990;5:147 by permission of Blackwell Scientific Publications, Inc.

## Radiographic Evaluation

Using the four standard x-ray projections of the paranasal sinuses—occipito-frontal (Caldwell's projection)(Figure 1A), occipitomental (Waters' projection) (Figure 1B), lateral (Figure 1C), and submental vertex (axial) (Figure 1D)—is the traditional way of evaluating the sinuses for infection or tumors. Radiologic findings of sinusitis include an air-fluid level (Figures 1A to 1E), mucosal thickening of more than 5 mm in adults, and opacification (Figure 2).[20,37,38,39] In addition, other abnormalities of the upper airway such as enlarged adenoids may be found (Figure 3).

Studies to evaluate the accuracy of radiographic studies to identify infection documented by needle aspiration of the maxillary antra have been primarily of the occipitomental view. Sinus radiographs are predictive of a culture-positive maxillary antral aspirate in 70% to 80% of acute cases and more than 90% of chronic cases.[37–41]

On the other hand, computed tomog-

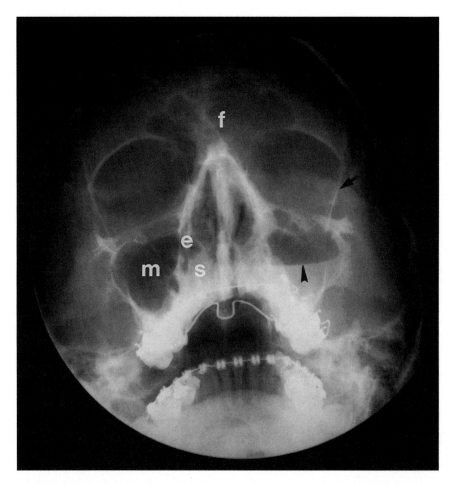

**Figure 1B.** Waters' projection during the standard multiview roentgenographic examination of the patient in Figure 1A. Note the air-fluid level in the left maxillary sinus **(arrowhead)**, as well as infraorbital soft-tissue swelling (arrow). e = ethmoid sinus; f = frontal sinus; m = maxillary sinus; s = sphenoid sinus.

raphy (CT) of the paranasal sinuses has certain advantages over standard radiographic evaluation of the sinuses. Usually, 4-mm sections are obtained in the coronal plane from the anterior frontal sinus wall to the posterior sinus wall.[42] Sometimes, 2 mm sections are used at the osteomeatal complex. Coronal cuts allow better visualization of the osteomeatal complex and identification of air-fluid levels. Axial cuts may be useful for evaluation of the posterior ethmoid or sphenoid sinuses or when dental artifact obscures coronal images.[42] Contrast is generally not necessary, unless tumor or vascular lesions are suspected.

Compared with CT scan of the sinuses, standard radiography may underestimate the presence or degree of sinus involvement, particularly in chronic sinusitis involving the ethmoid sinuses. Computed tomography provides a detailed picture of the osteomeatal complex, potentially elucidating a structural cause of recurrent or refractory sinusitis. For example, a concha bullosa (Figure 4), which may contribute to nasal obstruction or sometimes impinge on the osteomeatal complex, may be visualized on CT scan, but be missed on plain radiographs.

At this point no prospective studies

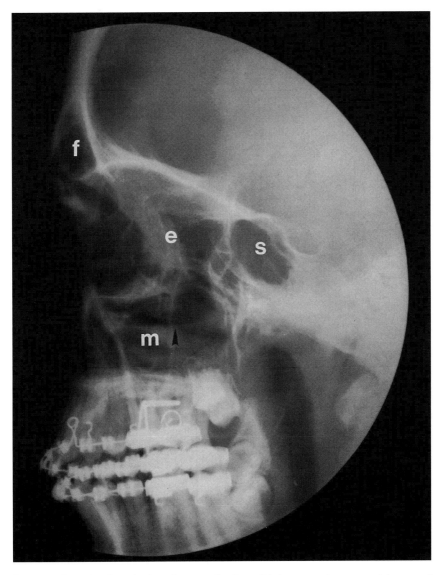

**Figure 1C.** Lateral projection during the standard multiview roentgenographic examination of the patient in Figure 1A. Note again the infraorbital soft-tissue swelling **(arrow)**. e = ethmoid sinus; f = frontal sinus; m = maxillary sinus; s = sphenoid sinus.

have been reported that compare standard sinus series radiography with CT scanning. In the outpatient setting, it seems reasonable to order standard radiography of the sinuses when the information is needed in 24 to 48 hours (eg, suspected acute sinusitis). On the other hand, if a definitive answer is desired regarding the presence of findings consistent with chronic sinusitis or structural causes of recurrent or chronic sinusitis, it seems more cost-efficient to obtain a CT scan. Future studies are needed to determine if CT is too sensitive a test and what its specificity is. Computed tomography of the sinuses is generally better than magnetic resonance imaging because it provides better imaging of bony structures.

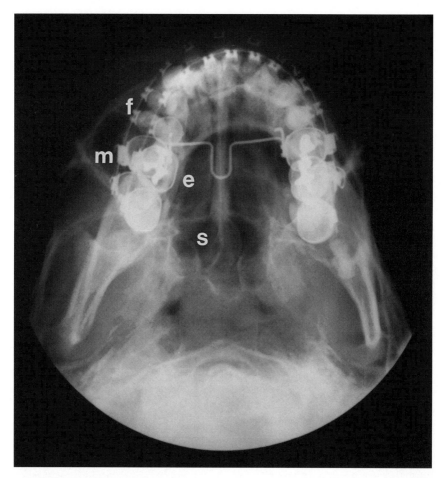

**Figure 1D.** Axial projection during the standard multiview roentgenographic examination of the patient in Figures 1A thru 1C. e = ethmoid sinus; f = frontal sinus; m = maxillary sinus; s = sphenoid sinus.

## Assessment of Nasal Airflow

Rhinomanometry, the measurement of nasal airway resistance, has been used predominantly in research studies to provide objective data about responses to nasal challenge or medication, but could be used in an office practice when objective measurements of nasal airflow are desired (eg, nasal allergen challenge, assessing response to nasal surgery).[19] Anterior rhinomanometry is simplest to perform, but results may be affected by deformation of the anterior nares by the instrument and by nasal cycling.[2] Posterior rhinometry does not have these disadvantages, but re-

quires more expensive equipment and more patient cooperation. Posterior rhinomanometry is helpful in assessing whether nasal airflow resistance is contributing to obstructive sleep apnea.[2]

Nasal flow-volume loops have also been used to study the pathophysiology of obstructive sleep apnea and may be preferable to rhinomanometry for this indication.[43,44]

## Nasal Biopsy

Nasal biopsy is required when the immotile cilia syndrome, immunologic con-

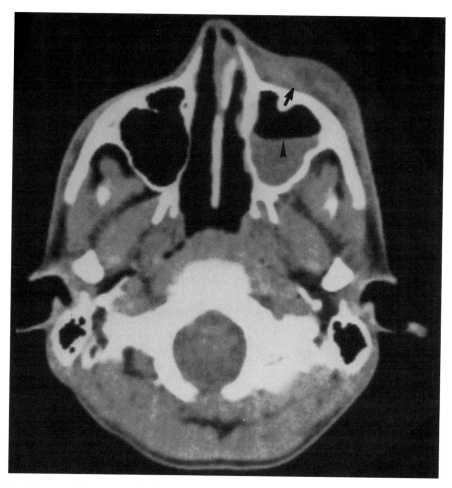

**Figure 1E.** Computed tomography (CT) scan was obtained in addition to the multiview roentgenographic examination in the patient in Figures 1A thru 1D to evaluate the extent of periorbital cellulitis. Note that both the air-fluid level in the left maxillary sinus **(arrowhead)**, as well as infraorbital soft-tissue swelling **(arrow)** are visible in the CT scan.

ditions (eg, Wegener's granulomatosis, Sjögren's syndrome, polymorphic reticulosis), sarcoidosis, or tumors are suspected. A sweat chloride test is used to diagnose cystic fibrosis. Serologic studies, such as the angiotensin-converting enzyme (ACE) level and antineutrophilic cytoplasmic antibody level, are helpful in the evaluation of sarcoidosis, Wegener's granulomatosis, and Churg-Strauss syndrome.

## Diagnostic Algorithms

Diagnostic algorithms for rhinorrhea, nasal obstruction, and postnasal drip appear in Figures 5A, 5B, and 5C. They incorporate directed history and physical examination with diagnostic testing in a systematic fashion.

## Differential Diagnosis

### Non-Infectious Causes of Rhinitis

*Inflammatory Rhinitis*

***Allergic Rhinitis:*** Allergic rhinitis usually has a childhood or adolescent onset and is

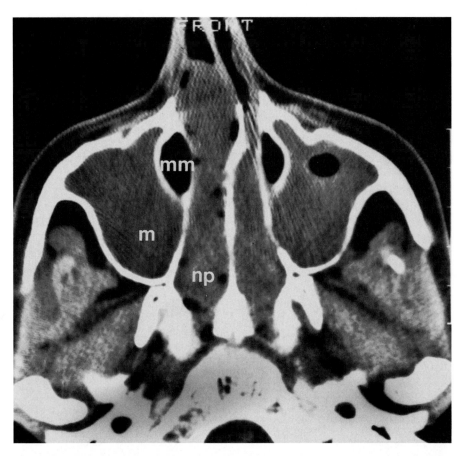

**Figure 2.** Nasal polyposis and pansinusitis. Computed tomographic scan of the paranasal sinuses in a 44-year-old patient with absent nasal airflow and anosmia. The nasal passages (np) are completely filled by extensive nasal polyps. The maxillary sinuses (m) are almost completely opacified. Intrasinus polyposis probably accounts for some of the soft tissue density filling the sinuses. mm = anterior portion of the middle meatus.

a manifestation of immediate hypersensitivity, mediated by allergen-specific IgE molecules on the surface of nasal mucosal mast cells.[30,32] Mast cell activation results in early- and late-phase release of mediators, which, in turn, causes vasodilation, edema, recruitment of eosinophils, basophils, neutrophils, and lymphocytes, as well as mucous gland stimulation.[1,30,32]

The allergens responsible for mast cell activation in the nose can be divided into those that cause seasonal symptoms (eg, tree, grass, ragweed, plantain, and sage pollens), perennial symptoms (eg, animal dander, feather bedding, dust mite, mold), or occupation-related symptoms (eg, animal dander, pharmaceutical agents, detergent enzymes). Although not a universal finding, itching of the eyes, nose, palate, and pharynx are more common with allergic than with nonallergic rhinitis.[45]

The nasal mucosa appears swollen and pale or bluish in color with clear secretions. The conjunctivae may be injected or granular-appearing. Other features of atopy, such as allergic shiners, nasal crease, Dennie's lines (infraorbital skin folds), and eczema, may also be noted. Skin tests are helpful in delineating which allergens are likely playing a role. Nasal smears reveal an eosinophilic infiltrate.[19,29]

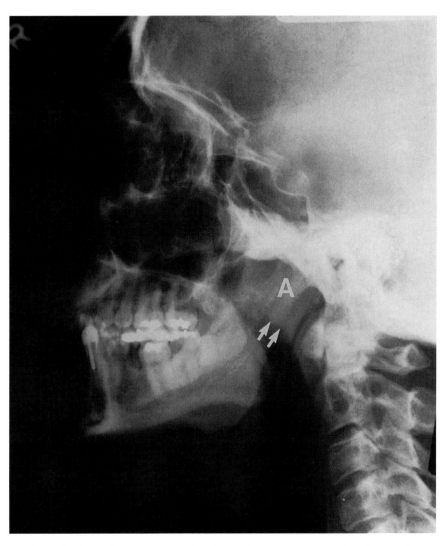

**Figure 3.** Enlarged adenoids causing nasal airflow obstruction. Lateral radiographic view of the paranasal sinuses and upper airway of a 27-year-old male patient. Sinuses appear clear, but adenoids (A) are enlarged, filling nasopharynx and posterior choanae of nose. The arrows point to the anterior margin of the adenoid tissue. Compare with Figure 1C. Nasal obstruction was relieved by adenoidectomy.

***Perennial Nonallergic Rhinitis:*** Perennial symptoms are frequently nonallergic.[28] One subset is nonallergic rhinitis with eosinophilia (NARES),[28,45,46] which has a later onset than allergic rhinitis and is characterized by perennial symptoms, negative allergy skin tests, and a negative family history of atopy. The pathogenesis is unknown, although the presence of eosinophils raises the possibility of non–IgE-mediated mast cell activation with release of chemotactic mediators for eosinophils. Watery rhinorrhea and sneezing are the predominant symptoms; itching is uncommon. The nasal mucosa may be unremarkable, erythematous or edematous, and pale/white. Serum IgE is normal. Nasal smears reveal eosinophilia.

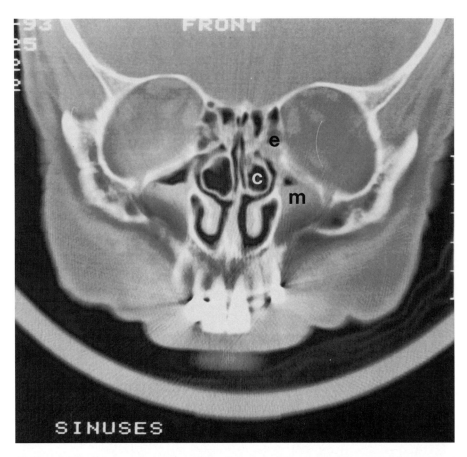

**Figure 4.** Concha bullosa and pansinusitis. Computed tomographic scan of a patient with a nonproductive cough for 6 months and intermittent postnasal drip. The maxillary sinuses (m) have air fluid levels. Opacities are noted in the ethmoid sinuses (e). Bilateral concha bullosa (c) are noted. The left osteomeatal complex is obliterated, but this appears to be caused by soft tissue, not the concha bullosa. The cough and postnasal drip resolved with a course of antibiotics and decongestants.

*Basophilic/Metachromatic Rhinitis:* A less common cause of perennial nonallergic rhinitis is basophilic/metachromatic rhinitis.[45] Rhinorrhea and nasal congestion are the usual complaints; pruritus is rare. As in eosinophilic nonallergic rhinitis, allergy skin tests are negative, there is no family history of atopy and the pathogenesis is unknown. Diagnosis is based on finding an increased number of basophils/metachromatic cells on the nasal smear.

*Atrophic Rhinitis:* The presentation of atrophic rhinitis is typically the subjective complaint of severe nasal obstruction despite patent nasal passages. Mucous secretions are frequently viscid and bacterial overgrowth in the absence of sinus infection may result in purulent secretions and a fetid odor.[45,47]

Atrophic rhinitis may be caused by aging, excessive surgical resection of nasal tissue, heavy exposure to cigarette smoke or other fumes, end-stage rhinitis medicamentosa, Wegener's granulomatosis, or midline granuloma. A history of nasal surgery, noxious exposures, or constitutional symptoms should be sought. The extent of any resection can be evaluated with rhinoscopy. A nasal biopsy showing keratin-

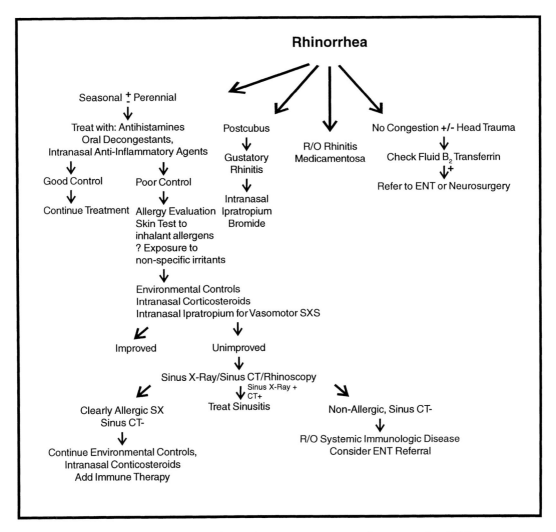

**Figure 5A.** Diagnostic algorithm for rhinorrhea. CT = computed tomography; ENT = ear, nose, and throat specialist; Sx = symptoms.

ized squamous epithelium is characteristic.[45]

*Immunologic Rhinitis:* Many of the systemic immunologic diseases affect the nasal passages, including Wegener's granulomatosis, Churg-Strauss syndrome, relapsing polychondritis, and Sjögren's syndrome. These diseases, as well as sarcoidosis and midline granuloma which are of unknown etiology, will be considered in this section. Frequently, the nasal symptoms are minor when viewed in the context of the other manifestations, but in some cases nasal symptoms may present prior to the onset of systemic disease.

In Wegener's granulomatosis, symptoms referable to the nose and sinuses are among the presenting manifestations two thirds of the time.[48–50] Nasal obstruction is the most common nasal complaint. Clear or purulent nasal discharge may also be noted. Initially, the nasal mucosa is edematous; as the disease progresses, the mucosa may become ischemic or ulcerated, leading to nasal crusting. Serous oti-

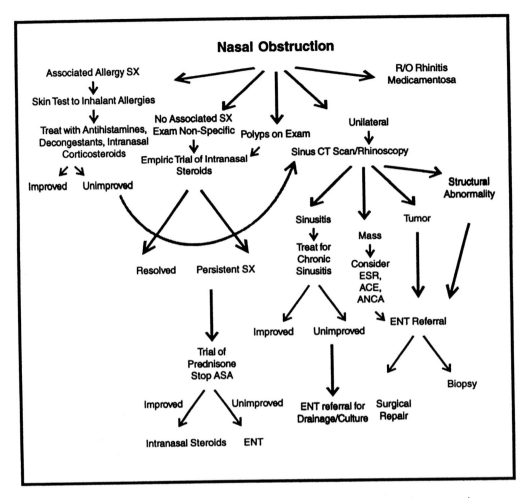

**Figure 5B.** Diagnostic algorithm for nasal obstruction. ACE = angiotensin-converting enzyme level; ANCA = antineutrophil cytoplasmic antibody; ASA = aspirin; CSF = cerebrospinal fluid; CT = computed tomography; ENT = ear, nose, and throat specialist; ESR = erythrocyte sedimentation rate; Sx = symptoms.

tis media may also be present. Destruction of cartilage and bone in advanced disease can lead to septal perforation and a saddle-shaped deformity of the nose. Proptosis may occur when there is extensive sinus involvement. Diagnostic evaluation should include biopsy of any ulcerations, sinus and chest radiographs, urinalysis, and measurement of serum antineutrophilic cytoplasmic antibodies (ANCA).[48–52] Antineutrophilic cytoplasmic antibodies are autoantibodies directed against constituents of polymorphonuclear leukocyte granules and monocyte lysosomes. Two different antibodies have been described, classic ANCA (C-ANCA) and perinuclear ANCA (P-ANCA). The C-ANCA reacts with a non-myeloperoxidase cytoplasmic component, a serine protease, and is highly associated with Wegener's granulomatosis (sensitivity greater than 75% during active disease).[52] The P-ANCA reacts predominantly with cytoplasmic myeloperoxidase and needs to be differentiated from antinuclear antibody (ANA) staining. Inclusion of P-ANCA increases the sensitivity for diagnosis of Wegener's to 90%.[52] Micro-

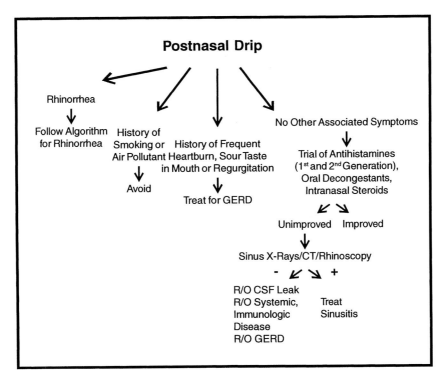

**Figure 5C.** Diagnostic algorithm for Postnasal drip. CSF = cerebrospinal fluid; CT = computed tomography; GERD = gastroesophageal reflux disease; Sx = symptoms.

scopic polyarteritis is more typically P-ANCA positive than C-ANCA.[52]

Despite the frequent involvement of the upper respiratory tract by Wegener's granulomatosis, roughly half of upper airway biopsy specimens show nonspecific changes.[50] The remainder show granulomas or vasculitis, but usually not both. When no ulcerations are visible, the yield may be even lower. Sinusitis seen radiographically may be due to active Wegener's granulomatosis or secondary bacterial infection, most commonly with *Staphylococcus aureus*. Sinus aspiration may be necessary to determine whether bacterial infection is present.[48]

Churg and Strauss described a syndrome of asthma, eosinophilia, vasculitis, and extravascular granulomas in 1951.[53] Paranasal sinus pain or tenderness and radiographic evidence of sinus opacification are frequent findings in patients with Churg-Strauss syndrome and are one of the six criteria for the diagnosis; the other criteria are asthma, eosinophilia greater than 10% on differential white blood cell count, mono- or polyneuropathy, non-fixed pulmonary infiltrates on chest radiography, and blood vessel biopsy with extravascular eosinophils.[54] Olsen described 32 patients with Churg-Strauss syndrome, 22 of whom had nasal symptoms and 8 of whom had severe nasal crusting with underlying pus.[55] The mucosa was described as being granular and friable. Several patients had pansinusitis, and two patients had septal perforations. Histologic studies revealed necrotizing granulomas and an intense eosinophilic infiltrate, but no vasculitis. Approximately 50% of patients with the Churg-Strauss syndrome are ANCA-positive (predominantly P-ANCA).[52]

Nasal involvement occurs in about 70% of patients with relapsing polychondritis.[48] Recurring bouts of nasal erythema and pain reflect inflammation of the nasal cartilage which eventually results in replacement of cartilage with fibrous tissue. With loss of the supporting structures, saddle-nosed deformity may result (49% of women, 10% of men).[48] Mucosal involvement, however, is rare. The diagnosis is based on the presence of cartilaginous involvement in two or more sites and histologic evidence of loss of basophilic staining of cartilage matrix, perichondral inflammation, cartilage destruction, and fibrosis.[48]

In addition to keratoconjunctivitis sicca and xerostomia, Sjögren's syndrome frequently results in severe nasal dryness and crusting.[48] Patients may complain of nasal obstruction and decreased sense of smell in addition to nasal dryness. The diagnosis is based on the presence of exocrine insufficiency, compatible serologic tests (eg, antibody titers to SS-A and SS-B antigens) and lymphocytic infiltration on nasal or labial biopsy.[48]

Nasal involvement in sarcoidosis is rare, approximately 4%, but may be a presenting manifestation.[48,56] Symptoms include nasal obstruction, anosmia, dryness, and crusting. Long-standing inflammation may eventuate in atrophic rhinitis. The appearance of the nasal mucosa is described as "pinhead-sized nodules with a hyperemic zone running together to form diffuse infiltrates."[48] A predilection for the septum and inferior turbinates may be noted.[57] Involvement of the nasal cartilage may cause saddle-nose deformities. Sarcoidosis may also cause nasopharyngeal mass lesions which arise in pharyngeal lymphoid tissue, usually in patients with extensive, generalized disease. Diagnosis rests on the histologic finding of noncaseating granulomas with negative special stains for microorganisms. Once a diagnosis has been established, serum ACE levels may be helpful in following disease activity.[58]

Midline granuloma, otherwise known as polymorphic reticulosis, was traditionally characterized as a disease with destructive lesions of the upper airway, nose, and midface without histologic evidence of vasculitis. Nasal congestion and sinusitis were reported to precede the appearance of destructive lesions by several months. Now, the question is being raised as to whether this is really a distinct pathologic process.[48] Spirochetal, fungal, mycobacterial, and protozoal infections, as well as Wegener's granulomatosis, sarcoidosis, carcinomas, and lymphomas may all cause midline destruction.[48] In addition, special T-cell markers have allowed identification of lymphoma in specimens which would otherwise have been called midline granuloma.[48,59] In evaluating patients with midline destructive processes, CT scan is helpful in delineating bony destruction. Biopsy of affected tissue should be performed and evaluated with lymphocyte-marker studies and special stains for micro-organisms, as well as cultures of biopsy specimens.

*Irritant-induced Rhinitis:* Rhinitis can also be caused by exposure to certain chemicals (eg, formaldehyde, nickel, chromate, chloramphenicol) and pollutants (eg, cigarette smoke, sulfur dioxide).[45] A careful occupational history for chemical and fume exposure, as well as questioning about active and passive cigarette smoke exposure, are important.

Most individuals experience mild dilation of the capacitance vessels during cold air exposure; however, certain sensitive individuals develop marked nasal congestion and rhinorrhea.[45] This phenomenon is included under inflammatory rhinitis because experimental cold air challenge in cold air–sensitive subjects has resulted in release of mast cell mediators into nasal secretions, albeit at a lower level than with antigen challenge.[31]

## Noninflammatory Rhinitis

**Rhinitis Medicamentosa:** Rhinitis medicamentosa can be caused by a variety of intranasal and systemic medications.[45] Prolonged use of intranasal vasoconstrictors and cocaine has been associated with severe rebound vasodilation. On examination, the nasal mucosa is usually fiery red, granular, and friable.[45] Complications in-

## Table IV
### Systemic Medications Associated with Rhinitis Medicamentosa

Reserpine
Hydralazine
Guanethidine
Methyldopa
Prazosin
Beta-blockers
Oral contraceptives
Tricyclic antidepressants
Acetylsalicylic acid
Cromolyn sodium
Beta-adrenergic agents
Angiotensin-converting enzyme inhibitors

clude sinusitis, otitis media, atrophic rhinitis, and nasal septal defects.

A list of systemic medications associated with rhinitis is given in Table IV.[60] The diagnosis should be suspected when nasal symptoms are temporally associated with initiation of one of these medications. A diagnostic trial of omitting the medication for 10 to 30 days should help in the evaluation. In a recent study, the median time for ACE inhibitor-induced cough to resolve after discontinuation of the drug was 26 days.[60a]

***Endocrinologic Rhinitis:*** Nasal congestion, postnasal drip, and "recurrent colds" are relatively common complaints in hypothyroid patients.[61] The nasal mucosa appears wet, edematous, and pale. Other findings suggestive of hypothyroidism, such as pretibial myxedema and delayed reflexes, should also be evident. Nasal biopsies show increased acid mucopolysaccharide and mucous gland proliferation. Thyroid function tests with an elevated thyroid stimulating hormone would confirm the diagnosis.

Rhinitis during pregnancy has many possible causes, the most common of which are allergic rhinitis, increased frequency of viral upper respiratory tract infections, increased frequency of bacterial sinusitis, and vasomotor rhinitis of pregnancy.[61] The latter is a nonspecific nasal congestion that usually develops in the second or third trimester and resolves within 5 days after delivery. Nasal vascular pooling related to the increased blood volume and, perhaps, progesterone-related vascular smooth muscle relaxation may contribute to nasal congestion.[61]

***Vasomotor Rhinitis:*** Patients with vasomotor rhinitis typically describe the sudden, unexpected onset of profound rhinorrhea, or nasal congestion. These symptoms are frequently described by patients with concomitant rhinitis from some other cause and improve with successful treatment of the underlying rhinitis. When it occurs as an isolated symptom, it is thought to be related to autonomic imbalance.[45] Nasal examination findings are nonspecific; watery rhinorrhea may be seen in patients with more secretory than congestive symptoms. Increased cholinergic tone or sensitivity is suggested by the effectiveness of ipratropium bromide in controlling vasomotor symptoms.

***Reflex-induced Rhinitis:*** Reflex-induced rhinitis [1,45] refers to vascular engorgement, glandular secretion, and sneezing caused by a variety of stimuli, including chilling of the body surface, change in position, strong odors, bright lights, sexual arousal, eating, and ingestion of alcoholic beverages. The degree of sensitivity to these stimuli varies from person to person. The symptoms may be nasal congestion, sneezing, or rhinorrhea. Usually, the onset is rapid and the symptoms are short-lived.[45]

The nasal mucosa may appear normal or edematous.

***Cerebrospinal Fluid Rhinorrhea:*** Leakage of cerebrospinal fluid (CSF) through a defect in the cribriform plate is another cause of rhinorrhea. Patients typically have a history of nasal or head trauma, although 10% of the time the leak may be precipitated by transient elevations in CSF pressure as with coughing, sneezing, or straining at stool.[62] The nasal discharge is watery and without associated nasal congestion. In addition to trauma, neoplastic disease and congenital abnormalities can cause CSF rhinorrhea.

The diagnosis is made by obtaining protein electrophoresis of the nasal secretions to test for presence of B2 transferrin (tau transferrin), a protein specific to CSF.[63] A quantitative glucose determination of nasal secretions greater than 30 mg/dL (1.7 mmol/L) is suggestive of CSF, but lower values do not rule out CSF leak.[63] The next step in the evaluation is localization of the leak using a procedure such as CT scanning with intrathecal metrizamide.[63]

## Infectious Causes of Rhinitis and Sinusitis

### Viral Nasopharyngitis

The common cold, viral nasopharyngitis, is the most common cause of acute nasal obstruction, rhinorrhea, sneezing, postnasal drip, and throat-clearing. Concomitant symptoms of fever, lacrimation, sore throat, hoarseness, and cough are variably present and help to differentiate this upper respiratory tract infection from allergic rhinitis or vasomotor rhinitis. Rhinovirus and adenovirus are frequently implicated, but influenza A, B, and C, parainfluenza, respiratory syncytial virus, coronavirus, herpes simplex virus, coxsackievirus, echovirus, *Mycoplasma pneumoniae* infection, *Chlamydia pneumoniae* infection, and Group A beta hemolytic streptococcal infection can present with the same clinical picture.

The symptoms are self-limited and usually resolve in 14 to 21 days unless complicated by bacterial sinusitis. An elegant series of CT studies of the sinuses during the common cold[64] has demonstrated frequent and varied involvement of the sinuses and their drainage passages. Eighty-seven percent of patients had abnormalities of one or both maxillary sinuses, most commonly radiopaque material interpreted as thick secretions because of the nonuniform nature of the density. In addition to the maxillary sinus findings, involvement of the ethmoid sinuses (65%), ethmoid infundibulum (77%), and sphenoid sinuses (39%) was frequent. Follow-up studies showed a lack of correlation between persistence or resolution of symptoms and objective findings on repeat CT, nasal airway resistance, and nasal blood flow. Although not evaluated in this particular study, acute bacterial sinusitis has been estimated to follow the common cold in 0.5%[65] to 5.0%[66] of patients.

### Sinusitis

Sinusitis is defined as being acute when symptoms of sinus infection persist no longer than 6 to 8 weeks or when fewer than four episodes of acute symptoms lasting 10 days occur per year. Acute sinusitis resolves with medical management, leaving no signs of significant mucosal damage.[67] Typical symptoms of acute infection are purulent nasal discharge, fever, paranasal pressure or discomfort, postnasal drip, and cough in the aftermath of the common cold. On exam, purulent secretions may be seen in the nasal passages, sometimes emanating from the middle meatus, as well as on the lateral wall of the oropharynx. The nasal mucosa may appear erythematous and edematous and airflow is frequently diminished. Frequently, the diagnosis is made on clinical grounds, based largely on the failure of symptoms to resolve 5 or more days after the onset of an upper respiratory tract infection. Sinus radiographs may also be obtained, especially if the patient is particularly ill and other complications of acute sinusitis are suspected (Figures 1A through 1E), or if confirmation of the diagnosis is wanted. Ultrasonography and transillumination are neither sensitive nor specific, but can be used to follow the course of therapy once a diagnosis has been made.

In adults with community-acquired, acute bacterial sinusitis, the most common infecting organisms are *Hemophilus influenzae*, *Streptococcus pneumoniae*,[40, 68,69] and, in children, *Moraxella (Branhamella) catarrhalis*.[21,70]

Recurrent, acute sinusitis is defined

as repeated episodes of acute sinusitis that resolve without significant mucosal damage.[67] When a patient has had more than three well-documented episodes of acute sinusitis in a year, it seems reasonable to evaluate that patient for predisposing factors such as allergic rhinitis, cigarette smoking, altered immunity, or structural abnormalities impairing sinus drainage.

Chronic sinusitis is defined as persistent sinusitis symptoms for longer than 8 weeks despite medical therapy combined with evidence of mucosal hyperplasia radiographically.[67] In adults, "chronic sinusitis" also refers to four or more episodes of acute sinusitis, each lasting at least 10 days, and CT evidence of mucosal thickening 4 weeks after medical therapy. In children, "chronic sinusitis" has been variably defined as sinusitis lasting longer than 3 weeks duration[70,71] or as either 12 weeks of persistent symptoms and signs or more than 5 episodes in a year in association with persistent changes on CT of the sinuses 4 weeks after medical therapy.[67]

Symptoms of chronic sinusitis are nonspecific; some patients complain only of cough and postnasal drip,[12,15,16] others will complain of nasal stuffiness, purulent nasal discharge, and postnasal drip.[67,72] Headache and facial pain are frequently absent.[72]

In adult, community-acquired chronic sinusitis, greater than 90% of surgically obtained specimens were culture positive; nearly 90% of these grew anaerobes.[41] The most common organisms isolated were anaerobic streptococci, *Bacteroides* species (mostly *melaninogenicus*), *Proprionibacterium* species (mostly *acnes*), α-hemolytic streptococci, and *Staphylococcus aureus*.[41] Similar evaluation in children has also shown a preponderance of anaerobes.[70,71] Noteworthy in both population groups is the significant number of β-lactamase–producing organisms, an important consideration for antibiotic selection.[37,41,69]

Several special circumstances give rise to infection with more unusual pathogens. Rhinocerebral mucormycosis, an invasive infection commonly caused by the *Rhizopus* species of fungi in the class Zygomycetes and order Mucorales is seen most often in patients with diabetes mellitus, acidosis, burns, chronic renal failure, cirrhosis, and immunosuppression.[74]

Other fungal infections, primarily with *Aspergillus* species, can be seen in normal hosts, but are usually invasive diseases of immunocompromised patients.[68,75,76] *Cryptococcus neoformans* can cause sinusitis with a high relapse rate and significant mortality in both immunocompetent and immunocompromised patients.[77] *Actinomyces* species,[74] *Candida* species,[78] and *Pseudoallescheria boydii*[68] have also been isolated from the sinuses, the latter in patients with acquired immunodeficiency syndrome (AIDS).

Allergic fungal sinusitis is a form of hypersensitivity reaction to fungal antigens in the sinus, usually in the absence of fungal invasion.[79,80] The typical features are a history of recurrent nasal polyps and asthma, in addition to radiographic evidence of pansinusitis.[79,80] Bony erosion may be seen radiographically.[79,80] The histologic diagnosis is made on mucinous material obtained surgically from the involved sinuses. Eosinophils, fungal hyphae, and Charcot-Leyden crystals are diagnostic; mycetomas, mucosal, and soft tissue invasion are not seen.[79] Serologic studies show an elevation in IgE specific to the fungus present, similar to the findings in allergic bronchopulmonary aspergillosis.[80]

## Fungal, Mycobacterial, and Treponemal Rhinitis

These unusual infections are only mentioned briefly, since a full discussion is beyond the scope of this review. In general, the nasal infection is a manifestation of disseminated disease.

Rhinosporidiosis, histoplasmosis, coccidioidomycosis, cryptococcosis, sporotrichosis, and blastomycosis can all cause mucosal infection of the nasal passages.[57] The nasal lesions are ulcerative, except for rhinosporidiosis which produces a polypoid nasal mass that may protrude from the nasal cavity.[57] Lepromatous leprosy involving the nasal passages has the picture of granulomatous infiltration of the mucosa similar to atrophic rhinitis. Ultimately, destruction and collapse of cartilage may develop.[57] *Mycobacterium tuberculosis* presents with nodular thickening of the septal mucosa and ventral septal perforation.[57] Tertiary syphilis also produces nodular and ulcerating lesions of the nasal mucosa with eventual cartilaginous and osseous destruction, if untreated. Gumma formation may present as an expanding lesion in the nasal cavity.[57]

## Gastroesophageal Reflux Disease

While gastroesophageal reflux disease (GERD) most likely causes pharyngeal irritation and postnasal drip directly, it may also stimulate the area reflexly via the vagus nerve.[13] Conceivably, GERD could also reflexly cause rhinorrhea and nasal stuffiness, but this remains to be determined. An in depth discussion of GERD can be found in Chapter 1, "Cough."

## Structural Lesions

When nasal congestion or obstruction is a predominant symptom, unilateral, or constant, the possibility of a structural lesion causing the symptom should be considered (Table I). A structural abnormality should also be considered when a patient with a known type of rhinitis does not respond appropriately to treatment. In children, choanal atresia can be a dramatic cause of nasal obstruction presenting at birth when bilateral or shortly after birth, if unilateral. Foreign bodies are not uncommon causes of obstruction in children. In adults, hypertrophied adenoids which have failed to regress, severe septal deviation, nasal polyps, and tumors may cause unilateral or, occasionally, bilateral obstruction.

Rhinoscopy and sinus CT are employed to differentiate among the diagnostic possibilities and to guide further evaluation and treatment.

## Nasal Polyps

Simple nasal polyps arise from the mucosa of the ethmoid sinuses and prolapse into the middle meatus where they can be seen as pale, gelatinous, almost translucent structures (Figures 6A and 6B). Occasionally, polyps may arise from the maxillary or sphenoid sinuses in which case they usually descend posteriorly into the antrochoanal space, the common space behind the nasal septum that both nasal cavities empty into. The mucosa of the turbinates can also undergo polypoidal changes.

Virtually all patients with nasal polyps have nasal blockage; 75% have hyposmia; 65% postnasal drip; 35% facial pain; and 25% ocular itching.[73] Symptoms suggestive of vasomotor rhinitis are common. Associated asthma is found in 30% of patients. On examination, patients frequently have a nasal sounding voice. Nasal polyps are usually bilateral and appear as rounded or raindrop-shaped semitranslucent masses. Depending on their size, polyps may be seen emanating from the middle meatus or prolapsing into the nasal valve, the space just anterior to the turbinates. Nasal polyps are insensitive to manipulation and rarely bleed.

Nasal polyps are uncommon in childhood, except as a manifestation of cystic fibrosis.[81] Other mucosal diseases such as the dysmotile cilia syndrome[81] and Young's syndrome (ie, azoospermia and sinopulmonary disease caused by abnormal mucociliary clearance, but with normal ciliary motility and structure and normal chloride transport)[81,82] have also been associated with nasal polyps in adults. In the general population, polyps usually develop after age 40 with a 2:1 male predominance. Approximately one third of patients with late onset asthma have been reported to have nasal polyps.[83] In these patients, the triad of asthma, nasal polyps, and aspirin hypersensitivity may be found.[81] Although the presence of degranulated mast cells and eosinophils in nasal polyps suggests an allergic cause, population studies have not shown an in-

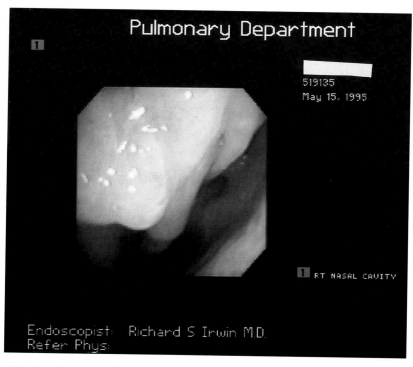

**Figure 6A.** Nasal polyp protruding into middle meatus. Simple polyp having the typical pale, gelatinous, almost translucent, tear drop appearance.

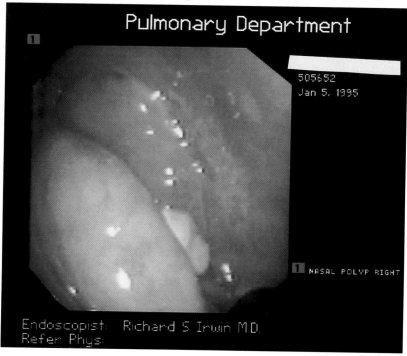

**Figure 6B.** Nasal polyp protruding into middle meatus. Polyp with pus at its inferior margin, suggesting that the polyp is preventing adequate drainage of bacterial sinusitis.

creased incidence of atopy among patients with nasal polyps.[83,84,85]

The histologic features of nasal polyps are similar to inflamed nasal tissue or the bronchial mucosa in severe asthma.[83] A respiratory epithelium overlies a thickened basement membrane with an edematous submucosa with a mixed cellular infiltrate, a few blood vessels, and little if any nervous tissue.[83] The constituents of the cellular infiltrate vary depending on the underlying disease: a striking eosinophilia in polyps of patients with aspirin-sensitive asthma, somewhat fewer eosinophils in polyps from patients with allergic rhinitis,[86] and a neutrophilic infiltrate in polyps from patients with nonallergic rhinitis.[87] The polyps of patients with cystic fibrosis typically have a thin basement membrane, a lack of eosinophils, and an increased amount of acid mucin.[83] Other cells found in the submucosa include plasma cells, small lymphocytes, and degranulated mast cells.

The edema fluid from polyps contains histamine, prostaglandins, leukotrienes, immunoglobulins, and other plasma proteins. The histamine levels are far higher than serum levels, consistent with local activation of mast cells.[83]

Microbiologic studies of polyp tissue have shown that polyps from patients with asthma grow a greater number and greater variety of aerobic bacteria than polyps from patients without asthma.[88] In addition, the number of infiltrating neutrophils appeared to correlate with the number of bacteria,[88] but was noted to vary from one field to another within a polyp. In several patients, a high neutrophil count was observed simultaneously with a high eosinophil count.

Although no clear pathogenetic mechanism has been outlined for nasal polyps, it seems likely that edema is caused by allergic, infectious, or irritant stimulation, possibly mediated by high levels of histamine causing capillary endothelial cell gaps.[81,83] Perhaps constriction by the narrow, bony sinus ostia, as well as the poor vascular supply impede resorption of the edema fluid. The interference with sinus drainage and impaired ciliary action may then contribute to bacterial invasion, sinusitis, and ongoing inflammation.[83] The high incidence of nasal polyps (49%) in patients with aspirin-sensitive asthma suggests possible mediation through arachidonic acid metabolism, but this is only speculative.[81]

Neoplasms, inverting papilloma (see "Tumors of the Nose, Sinuses, and Superior Pharynx" section later in the chapter), and hypertrophied, polypoid turbinates can all be mistaken for nasal polyps. If a presumptive polyp is friable, more firm than gelatinous, tender to manipulation, unilateral, or bleed spontaneously, an otolaryngologist should be consulted.[83]

### Rhinoscleroma

*Klebsiella rhinoscleromatis* is the causative agent of the chronic granulomatous disorder known as rhinoscleroma, the features of which have been reviewed by Colt and colleagues.[89] The nasal and oral mucous membrane are the most common sites of infection, but laryngotracheal and bronchial infection have also been described. This disease is endemic in areas of Eastern Europe, Asia, the Middle East, Central and South America, and Africa and may be seen in immigrants to the United States from these areas. Chronic rhinorrhea that may be mucopurulent and nasal congestion may persist for months. The disease may spread from an initial focus in the nose to the septum, sinuses, palate, vocal cords, and bronchus. Eventually, the indurated tissue takes on a woody consistency. The nasopharyngeal mucosa appears nodular. Radiography may reveal exuberant soft tissue in the nasal cavity, thickening of the nasal septum, sinusitis, and bony destruction. The endoscopic appearance is similar to papillomatosis, sarcoidosis, Wegener's granulomatosis, tuberculosis, fungal infections, and carcinoma. Diagnosis is made by culture and histologic examination of multiple biopsies. The characteristic histologic feature is Mikulicz's cell, a small histiocyte.[57] *K rhinocleromatis* should be seen in the

Mikulicz's cell and should be able to be cultured.

### Sinus Histiocytosis

Sinus histiocytosis with massive lymphadenopathy is a benign disorder that typically affects children and young adults and presents with prominent painless cervical lymphadenopathy. Roughly, a third of patients have extranodal disease most often in the upper respiratory tract, orbits, eyelids, and skin.[57] In the nasal cavity, diffuse mucosal infiltration or polyp formation may be found. Nasal obstruction is the most frequent symptom, but rhinorrhea and epistaxis may also be present. Involvement of the larynx and trachea may cause obstructive symptoms there.

The diagnosis is made by mucosal or lymph node biopsy. Characteristic features are the bland appearance of the histiocytes and the presence of phagocytosed lymphocytes.[57] The differential diagnosis would include malignant histiocytosis in which phagocytosed cells are typically red blood cells; malignant lymphoma which does not have lymphophagocytosis; histiocytosis X which has a greater number of eosinophils; and rhinoscleroma in which there should be typical Mikulicz's cells, and *K rhinoscleromatis* organisms.[57]

### Tumors of the Nose, Sinuses, and Superior Pharynx

**Benign Tumors:** Squamous papillomas are wart-like tumors that occur in the nasal vestibule and generally just cause local irritation.[90] Inverting papilloma (transitional cell papilloma) of the nose and sinus is histologically benign, but tends to spread to contiguous structures and to recur after excision. About 10% undergo malignant transformation.[90]

Adenomas, lymphangiomas, hemangiomas, and angiofibromas are all much less common.[90] Osteomas are found in the sinuses.[90,91] They grow very slowly and usually can be observed over time, if they do not cause pressure or obstruct the sinus. Chondromas usually involve the nasal septum. Angiofibromas occur in males around the time of puberty.[92] The presenting symptoms are marked epistaxis and nasal obstruction. Computed tomography is used to delineate the extent of the lesion.

**Malignant Tumors:** Squamous cell carcinoma is the most common malignant tumor of the nose and nasal sinuses.[93] The ethmoid region of the nose is the most common site of origin, although the cancer has usually spread by the time symptoms develop, making exact determination of the site of origin difficult.[93] Unilateral nasal obstruction, epistaxis, and broadening of the nasal bones are the most common manifestations.[90,93] Sinus involvement may cause facial pain or proptosis. Endoscopic visualization, biopsy, and plain radiographs or CT are needed for diagnosis and staging.

Metastases of adenocarcinoma, melanoma, cylindroma and sarcoma can present in the nasal passages, but are less common.[92] Lymphomas may also present in the nasal passages. Examples of this would be Burkitt's lymphoma and lethal midline granuloma.[49,92] Endoscopic visualization, CT, and biopsy are employed for diagnosis and staging.

## Treatment

### Non-infectious Causes of Rhinitis

#### Inflammatory Rhinitis

**Allergic Rhinitis:** The most important therapy for allergic rhinitis is avoidance. Dust mite control measures, removing sources of animal dander and feathers from the household, and wearing a mask at work are examples of important allergen avoidance interventions. Antihistamines and decongestants can be tried for symptomatic relief of nasal congestion, itching, and rhinorrhea caused by unavoidable allergen exposure.[30,94] Intranasal cromolyn sodium is well tolerated and side effects are rare.[32,94] However, more severe allergic rhinitis is frequently refractory to cromolyn sodium.[95] Topical beclomethasone,[32,95,96] flunisolide,[31] and budesonide[97] are all quite effective and, when used in recommended doses, do not appear to cause adrenal suppression.[30] An aqueous preparation of ipratropium bromide has been reported to decrease rhinorrhea in patients with perennial allergic rhinitis without significant adverse effects.[98]

When a patient presents with incapacitating symptoms of allergic rhinitis, a brief course of oral corticosteroids may be needed. Frequently, prednisone, 20 mg per day for 5 days, followed by intranasal corticosteroids, is sufficient to bring symptoms under control. If the combination of intranasal corticosteroids and oral antihistamine/decongestants does not provide adequate symptom relief for two allergy seasons, allergy immunotherapy should be considered to help control allergic rhinoconjunctivitis in future allergy seasons.[30]

**Perennial Nonallergic Rhinitis:** Topical intranasal corticosteroids are usually effective in reducing symptoms in nonallergic rhinitis with eosinophilia.[28,45] Oral antihistamines and decongestants may provide additional relief. In addition to the newer, nonsedating $H_1$ antihistamines, the older $H_1$ antihistamines should be tried, because they have both antihistaminic and anticholinergic effects. Ipratropium bromide has been shown to decrease watery rhinorrhea, but not nasal congestion.[99] At higher doses it can cause unacceptable nasal dryness and some systemic symptoms.

*Basophilic/Metachromatic Rhinitis:* Although not much is written about therapy of basophilic/metachromatic rhinitis, presumably both intranasal cromolyn and corticosteroids would be therapeutic, because of their mast cell/basophil stabilizing effects.

*Atrophic Rhinitis:* Treatment options for atrophic rhinitis have had limited success, but include topical steroids, antibiotics,

increased environmental humidity, saline sprays or irrigation, and implantation of bone chips.[45,47]

*Immunologic Rhinitis:* Corticosteroids and cyclophosphamide are the mainstays of treatment of Wegener's granulomatosis.[48,50] Surgery may be required for decompression if proptosis is present.[48,50] Corticosteroids are the treatment of choice for Churg-Strauss syndrome.[100] Patients who have refractory disease may need addition of cyclophosphamide.[100]

Milder cases of relapsing polychondritis may respond to nonsteroidal antiinflammatory agents; more severe cases have required high-dose corticosteroids and immunosuppressive agents.[48,101]

Treatment of the nasal dryness and sensation of nasal obstruction associated with Sjögren's syndrome is directed at moisturization.[48]

Mucosal disease caused by sarcoidosis can frequently be controlled with intranasal topical corticosteroids.[56] If these are ineffective or if cartilaginous involvement is present, systemic corticosteroids may help.[48,102]

Radiotherapy has been the treatment of choice for localized midline granuloma.[48] When the nasal biopsy reveals a specific infection, therapy should be directed to eradicate that organism. If a lymphoma or other tumor is responsible for the destructive process, specific therapy is indicated.

*Irritant Rhinitis:* When rhinitis is caused by irritant exposures, avoidance by changing occupation, wearing an appropriate mask, or stopping smoking should be recommended. Similarly, symptoms caused by cold air exposure can be reduced by wearing a mask or scarf.

## Noninflammatory Rhinitis

**Rhinitis Medicamentosa:** Rhinitis medicamentosa caused by overuse of intranasal decongestant medications is best managed by discontinuing the decongestant spray.

Frequently, an intranasal corticosteroid spray is needed to treat the nasal irritation caused by the decongestant spray and to treat the underlying cause of nasal congestion for which the patient was taking a decongestant.

When the cause of rhinitis medicamentosa is an oral medication, such as an antihypertensive agent or birth control pills, the inciting medication needs to be changed to an alternate choice.

***Endocrinologic Rhinitis:*** Treatment of nasal congestion related to hypothyroidism consists of thyroid replacement. Treatment of rhinitis symptoms in pregnancy carries the additional concern of avoiding harm to the developing fetus. Any medication should be carefully evaluated in terms of expected risks and benefits and the latest data about safety during gestation reviewed.[61]

***Vasomotor Rhinitis:*** If symptoms from vasomotor rhinitis are infrequent, no therapy is needed. Treatment of any concomitant cause of rhinitis, such as allergic rhinitis, may reduce the vasomotor symptoms. Otherwise, ipratropium bromide appears to be an effective form of treatment for vasomotor rhinitis,[103] perhaps suggesting increased cholinergic tone or sensitivity. Patients with refractory obstructive symptoms may benefit from turbinate reduction.[104]

***Reflex-induced Rhinitis:*** Because the symptoms of reflex-induced rhinitis tend to be short-lived, many patients prefer not to use medication. For patients who desire better control of their symptoms, medications with an anticholinergic effect, such as ipratropium bromide or first generation $H_1$ antihistamines, are helpful.[1,3]

***Cerebrospinal Fluid Rhinorrhea:*** While acute CSF rhinorrhea from trauma may spontaneously stop within 5 to 7 days, persistent CSF rhinorrhea from any cause requires surgical correction because of the risk of meningitis that complicates 25% to 50% of cases.[63,105]

## Infectious Causes of Rhinitis and Sinusitis

### Viral Nasopharyngitis

Treatment of the common cold is costly. Americans spend more than $1 billion per year on a variety of nonprescription remedies[106] and at least another $1.5 billion per year for physician-related expenses, including office visits, laboratory tests, and prescription medications.[106] Treatment can be considered in three categories: prevention, cure, and symptomatic relief.

For prevention, environmental measures would be likely to be beneficial if patients were to use them. Virucidal paper handkerchiefs with good personal hygiene have been shown to decrease transmission of experimental rhinovirus colds.[107] Inactivated rhinovirus vaccines have not been shown to offer protection and live attenuated vaccines have yet to be developed.[108] Daily, prophylactic use of interferon-$\alpha$ intranasal sprays for 7 days prevents approximately 80% of natural colds due to rhinovirus with an acceptable 10% risk of minor nasal bleeding.[108,109,110] Unfortunately, this therapy is only effective in preventing approximately 40% of all colds; those caused by viruses other than rhinovirus appear refractory. Vitamin C has also not proven effective as a preventive agent.[106]

Once the common cold is established, zinc gluconate lozenges may shorten it.[111] Further studies are needed to establish long-term safety of the lozenges and to confirm effectiveness. Enviroxime, a potent inhibitor of rhinoviruses *in vitro*, is poorly tolerated in clinical studies.[109] Vitamin C has not been found to abort the common cold.[106]

For symptomatic relief, medications with an atropinelike effect (eg, ipratropium bromide, first generation $H_1$ blockers) decrease rhinorrhea,[112,113] postnasal drip, and cough.[11] The newer, relatively nonsedating, second generation $H_1$ blockers are not effective in the common cold, because histamine does not participate in this illness. The first generation $H_1$ blockers are effective in the common cold because of their anticholinergic activity, not because of their antihistaminic effects.[114] Decongestants decrease nasal stuffiness.[106] Glycerol guaiacolate has not been shown to be beneficial.[115] The role of steam inhalation is unclear. The beneficial effects in one double-blind, randomized, placebo-controlled study[116] were not replicated by another.[117]

## Sinusitis

The treatment of viral sinusitis, as in the common cold, is symptomatic. When symptoms persist or start to worsen 5 days into the illness, acute bacterial superinfection should be suspected. At that point, decongestants and an antibiotic that will be effective against *H influenzae, Streptococcus* species and *M catarrhalis* in children should be prescribed.[69,70] Because of the emergence of beta-lactamase positive strains of *H influenzae*, ampicillin, and amoxicillin are no longer recommended for treatment of acute sinusitis, preferred choices are trimethoprim/sulfamethoxazole (TMP/SMZ), amoxicillin/clavulanate, loracarbef or cefuroxime[69] and clarithromycin.[117a,117b] While TMP/SMZ use may become limited by increasing resistance of *S pneumoniae* and lack of efficacy against Group A streptococci,[118] a recent prospective, randomized study showed that a 3-day course of TMP/SMZ was equally as effective as a 10-day course.[119] On the other hand, both groups had a 23% to 24% failure rate. For uncomplicated acute sinusitis, empiric therapy is appropriate, reserving sinus aspiration and culture for complicated or refractory cases.[68]

In chronic, community-acquired sinusitis, *S aureus* and anaerobes become more common pathogens. The antibiotics of choice, initially, are amoxicillin/clavulanate, loracarbef, or cefuroxime.[69,118] However, lack of response may necessitate a change in therapy to clindamycin or vancomycin, possibly guided by sinus aspirate cultures. Recommendations for the duration of therapy have varied, but a minimum of 3 weeks is preferred to ensure eradication of infection.[73,120] Many patients, particularly those with impaired drainage, altered immunity, or underlying illness (eg, cystic fibrosis, immotile cilia syndrome), will require longer courses.

Concomitant use of topical vasoconstrictors and oral decongestants are important to facilitate sinus drainage.[20,68,121] Guaifenesin is sometimes used in the hope of facilitating drainage, but no clear data exist to support this. Antihistamines may be helpful when allergic stimulation and consequent inflammation are impairing drainage. On the other hand, they may cause drying and inspissation of secretions when allergy is not playing a role. Topical corticosteroids are recommended to reduce inflammation in chronic sinusitis and shrink obstructing nasal polyps, when present.[73] Saline irrigation of the nasal passages is helpful when secretions are particularly thick or inspissated.

Indications for functional endoscopic sinus surgery include persistent sinusitis despite appropriate medical therapy, documented recurrent sinusitis with identifiable and related abnormalities of the osteomeatal complex and fungal sinusitis.[67,72,122]

## Fungal, Mycobacterial and Treponemal Rhinitis

Treatment of these infections should be directed at the specific infection with the assumption that the nasal findings are a manifestation of disseminated disease.

Allergic fungal sinusitis will need wide local debridement to provide adequate sinus aeration, followed by systemic corticosteroids.[79] Eventually, clinical improvement and normalization of serologic studies (total IgE, specific fungal IgE) should allow tapering of systemic corticosteroids and a change to ongoing therapy with intranasal corticosteroids.

## Gastroesophageal Reflux Disease

For guidelines on treating GERD, the reader is referred to Chapter 1, "Cough."

## Structural Lesions

Patients who have markedly enlarged turbinates causing nasal obstruction that is refractory to medical therapy may benefit from one of the turbinate reduction procedures.[104] The choices include electrocautery, cryosurgery, $CO_2$ laser, and submucosal resection.[104] The choice depends on whether the turbinate is enlarged by thickened mucosa that is not responsive to topical vasoconstrictors or enlarged turbinate bone and on the preferences of the otolaryngologist performing the procedure.

Severe septal deviation, septal spurs, and concha bullosa may require surgical treatment, if nasal obstruction is significant and clearly related to the structural abnormality.

### Nasal Polyps

Either inhaled or oral corticosteroids, as well as antibiotics for sinusitis, are the appropriate initial therapy. If nasal obstruction is severe, a 10-day tapering course of oral corticosteroids can be given, beginning with 50 mg of prednisone.[81] This should then be followed with intranasal beclomethasone,[73,81] flunisolide,[123] or budesonide.[124] Intranasal steroid injection has been used over the years, but carries the risk of steroid embolism to the retinal arteries with visual loss. [81]

When the polyps are quite large, respond poorly to intranasal corticosteroids, or are antrochoanal (arising from the maxillary or sphenoid antra and extending to the posterior opening between the nasal cavity and the nasopharynx), surgical polypectomy is appropriate. Simple polypectomy is usually sufficient, unless extensive pansinusitis is present, warranting more extensive surgery, such as sphenoethmoidectomy. Unfortunately, nasal polyps have a high recurrence rate, although postoperative intranasal corticosteroids appear to decrease recurrences.[84] Thus far, no clear evidence has accrued to suggest that more extensive surgery decreases the rate of recurrence.[125]

Patients with nasal polyps and asthma have a high incidence of acetylsalicylic acid (ASA) sensitivity which is manifested by profuse rhinorrhea, nasal congestion, and bronchoconstriction (Samter's triad).[126] Because the bronchoconstriction can be life-threatening, these patients should be counseled on how to avoid ASA. Other nonsteroidal anti-inflammatory drugs (NSAIDs) that are cyclo-oxygenase inhibitors may cause similar symptoms and should also be avoided. Patients who have a strong indication for taking ASA or NSAIDs can be desensitized to one of these medications by slowly increasing the dose of medication in a carefully monitored setting.[127] A subset of patients with rhinosinusitis who are aspirin-sensitive may experience an improvement in nasal symptoms with ASA desensitization.[128] A new medication that inhibits lipoxygenase has shown promise in inhibiting aspirin-sensitive asthma.[129]

### Rhinoscleroma

Prolonged (2 to 12 months), oral antibiotic treatment is usually effective for *Klebsiella rhinoscleroma.*[89] Antibiotics that have proven effective include: ampicillin, streptomycin, tetracycline, chloramphenicol, and TMP/SMZ. The antibiotic needs to be continued until complete resolution has occurred. Repeated cultures of biopsy specimens may be needed to ascertain whether bacteriologic cure has been effected.[89]

### Sinus Histiocytosis

Many types of therapy have been used to treat sinus histiocytosis, including excision, irradiation, antibiotics, corticosteroids, and antineoplastic chemotherapy.[57] Successful treatment with a combination of cyclophosphamide and prednisone has been reported.[57]

### Tumors

**Benign Tumors:** Squamous papillomas should be excised to relieve nasal obstruction and to be certain that the histology is benign because squamous cell carcinomas can have a similar appearance.[90,93] Inverting papilloma of the nose and sinus requires wide local excision, because it has a tendency to recur as well as to undergo malignant transformation.[90] Treatment of angiofibromas is usually a combination of angiographic embolization of feeding vessels and excision.[92]

***Malignant Tumors:*** Malignant tumors of the nose and sinuses, such as squamous cell carcinoma, usually require a combination of both radiation and surgical excision and sometimes chemotherapy.[90,92] Lymphomas are usually treated with specific chemotherapy based on the histologic type.

### References
_____

1. Raphael GD, Baraniuk JN, Kaliner MA: How and why the nose runs. J Allergy Clin Immunol 1991;87:457–467.
2. Schumacher. Rhinomanometry. J Allergy Clin Immunol 1989;83:711–718.
3. Kaliner M, Lemanske R. Rhinitis and asthma. JAMA 1992;268:2807–2829.
4. Naclerio RM. Allergic rhinitis. N Engl J Med 1991;325:860–869.
5. Winther B, Gwaltney JM Jr, Hendley JO. Respiratory virus infection of monolayer cultures of human nasal epithelial cells. Am Rev Respir Dis 1990;141:839–845.
6. Winthur B Gwaltney JM Jr. Mygind N, et al. Site of rhinovirus recovery after point inoculation of the upper airway. JAMA 1986;256:1763–1767.
7. Naclerio RM, Lichtenstein LM,, Kagey-Sobotka A, et al. Kinins are generated during experimental rhinovirus colds. J Infect Dis 1988;157:133–142.
8. Raphael GD, Igarashi Y, White MV, et al. The pathophysiology of rhinitis: V. Sources of protein in allergen-induced nasal secretions. J Allergy Clin Immunol 1991;88:33–42.
9. Raphael GD, Meredith, Baraniuk, et al. The pathophysiology of rhinitis: II. Assessment of the sources of protein in histamine-induced nasal secretions. Am Rev Respir Dis 1989;139:791–800.
10. Raphael GD, Druce HM, Baraniuk JN, et al. Pathophysiology of rhinitis. I. Assessment of the sources of protein in methacholine-induced nasal secretions. Am Rev Respir Dis 1988;138:413–420.
11. Curley FJ, Irwin RS, Pratter MR, et al. Cough and the common cold. Am Rev Respir Dis 1988;138:305–311.
12. Irwin RS, Curley FJ, French CL. Chronic cough: The spectrum and frequency of causes, key components of the diagnostic evaluation, and outcome of specific therapy. Am Rev Respir Dis 1990;141:640–647.
13. Cunningham ET, Ravich WJ, Jones B, et al. Vagal reflexes referred from the upper aerodigestive tract: An infrequently recognized cause of common cardiorespiratory responses. Ann Intern Med 1992;116:575–582.
14. Naclerio RM, Proud D, Togias AG, et al. Inflammatory mediators in late antigen-induced rhinitis. N Engl J Med 1985;313:65–70.
15. Irwin RS, Pratter MR, Holland PS, et al. Postnasal drip causes cough and is associated with reversible upper airway obstruction. Chest 1984;85:346–352.
16. Irwin RS, Corrao WM, Pratter MR. Chronic persistent cough in the adult: The spectrum and frequency of causes and successful outcome of specific therapy. Am Rev Respir Dis 1981;123:413–417.
17. Pratter MR,, Hingston DM, Irwin RS. Diagnosis of bronchial asthma by clinical evaluation: An unreliable method. Chest 1983;84:42–47.
18. Pratter MR, Curley FJ, Dubois J, et al. Cause and evaluation of chronic dyspnea in a pulmonary disease clinic. Arch Intern Med 1989;149:2277–2282.
19. Meltzer EO: Evaluating rhinitis: Clinical, rhinomanometric, and cytologic assessments. J Aller Clin Immunol 1988;82:900–908.
20. Johnson CM III, Gwaltney JM Jr. Sinusitis. In Schlossberg D, ed. *Infections of the Head and Neck.* New York, NY: Springer-Verlag; 1987: pp 81–89.
21. Rachelefsky GS. Sinusitis in children—diagnosis and management. Clin Rev Allergy 1984;2:397–408.
22. Slavin RG. The diagnosis and therapy of sinusitis and its complications. Insights in Allergy 1987;2:1–6.
23. American College of Physicians. Allergy testing. Ann Intern Med 1989;110:317–320.
24. American Academy of Allergy and Immunology Position Statement. Allergen Skin

Testing. J Allergy Clin Immunol 1993;92: 636–637.

25. American Academy of Allergy and Immunology. The use of in vitro tests for IgE antibody in the specific diagnosis of IgE-mediated disorders and in the formulation of allergen immunotherapy: Position statement. J Allergy Clin Immunol 1992; 90:263–267.

26. Noone S. Allergy Testing. In Emery L, Noone S, eds. *Ambulatory Care Nursing Policies and Procedures.* Frederick, Md: Aspen Publishers Inc; 1993: pp. XIII.3-XIII.14.

27. Smith SJ, Hendee WR. Testing for allergic disease. Ann Intern Med 1990;113:331.

28. Mullarkey MF. Eosinophilic nonallergic rhinitis. J Allergy Clin Immunol 1988;82: 941–949.

29. Lans DM, Alfano N, Rocklin R. Nasal eosinophilia in allergic and nonallergic rhinitis: Usefulness of the nasal smear in the diagnosis of allergic rhinitis. New Engl Allergy Proc 1989;10:275–280.

30. Norman PS. Allergic rhinitis. J Allergy Clin Immunol 1985;75:531–545.

31. Togias A, Naclerio RM, Proud D, et al. Studies on the allergic and nonallergic nasal inflammation. J Allergy Clin Immunol 1988;81:782–790.

32. Naclerio RM. The pathophysiology of allergic rhinitis: Impact of therapeutic intervention. J Allergy Clin Immunol 1988; 82:927–934.

33. Selner JC, Koepke JW. Rhinolarynoscopy in the allergy office. Ann Allergy 1985;54: 479–482.

34. Selner JC. Visualization techniques in the nasal airway: Their role in the diagnosis of upper airway disease and measurement of therapeutic response. J Allergy Clin Immunol 1988;82:909–916.

35. Schmacher MJ. Fiberoptic nasopharyngoscopy: A procedure for allergists? J Allergy Clin Immunol 1988;81:960–962.

36. Castellanos J, Axelrod D. Flexible fiberoptic rhinoscopy in the diagnosis of sinusitis. J Allergy Clin Immunol 1989;83: 91–94.

37. Daley CL, Sande M. The runny nose: Infection of the paranasal sinuses. Infect Dis Clin North Am 1988;2:131–147.

38. Evans FO, Sydnor JB, Moore WEC, et al. Sinusitis of the maxillary antrum. N Engl J Med 1975;293:735–739.

39. Salit IE. Diagnostic approaches to head and neck infections. Infect Dis Clin North Am 1988;2:35–55.

40. Hamory BH, Sande MA, Syndor A Jr. Etiology and microbial therapy of acute maxillary sinusitis. J Infect Dis 1979;139: 197–202.

41. Brook I. Bacteriology of chronic maxillary sinusitis in adults. Ann Otol Rhino Laryngol 1989;98:426–428.

42. Godley FA. Chronic sinusitis: An update. Am Family Phys 1992;45:2190–2199.

43. Williams AJ, Santiago S Jr. The nose and obstructive sleep apnea. Chest 1993;104: 993.

44. Shepard JW, Burger CD. Nasal and oral flow-volume loops in normal subjects and patients with obstructive sleep apnea. Am Rev Respir Dis 1990;142:1288–1293.

45. Zeiger RS. Differential diagnosis and classification of rhinosinusitis. In: Schatz M, Settipane GA, Zeiger RS, eds. *Nasal Manifestations of Systemic Diseases.* Providence, RI: Oceanside Publications; 1991: pp 3–20.

46. Enberg RN. Perennial nonallergic rhinitis: a retrospective review. Ann Allergy 1989; 63:513–516.

47. Hansen C. The oxena problem. Clinical analysis of atrophic rhinitis in 100 cases. Acta Otolaryngol 1982;93:461–464.

48. Falkoff RJ. Nasal manifestations of systemic immunologic diseases. In: Schatz M, Settipane GA, Zeiger RS, eds. Nasal Manifestations of Systemic Diseases. Providence, RI: Oceanside Publications; 1991: pp 21–33.

49. Batsakis JG. Wegener's granulomatosis and midline (nonhealing granuloma). Head Neck Surg 1979;1:213–222.

50. Fauci AS, Haynes BF, Katz P, et al. Wegener's granulomatosis: Prospective clinical and therapeutic experience with 85 patients for 21 years. Ann Intern Med 1983;98:76–85.

51. Nolle B, Specks U, Ludemann J, et al. Anticytoplasmic antibodies: their immunodiagnostic value in Wegener's granulomatosis. Ann Intern Med 1989;111:28–40.

52. Beer DJ. ANCAs aweigh. Am Rev Respir Dis 1992;146:1128–1130.

53. Churg J, Strauss L. Allergic granulomatosis, allergic angiitis, and periarteritis nodosa. Am J Path 1951;27:277–293.

54. Masi AT, Hunder GG, Lie JT, et al. The American College of Rheumatology 1990 criteria for the classification of Churg-Strauss syndrome (allergic granulomatosis and angiitis). Arthritis Rheum 1990; 33:1094–1100.

55. Olsen KD, Neel HB, DeRemee RA, et al.

Nasal manifestations of allergic granulomatosis and angiitis (Churg-Strauss syndrome). Otolaryngol Head Neck Surg 1980;88:85–89.

56. McCaffrey TV, McDonald TJ. Sarcoidosis of the nose and paranasal sinuses. Laryngoscope 1983;93:1281–1284.

57. Case records of the Massachusetts General Hospital. N Engl J Med 1981;305:1572–1580.

58. DeRemee RA, Rohrbach MS. Serum angiotensin converting enzyme activity in evaluating the clinical course of sarcoidosis. Ann Intern Med 1980;92:361–365.

59. Gaulard P, Henni T Marolleau J-P, et al. Lethal midline granuloma (polymorphic reticulosis) and lymphomatoid granulomatosis: Evidence for a monoclonal T-cell lymphoproliferative disorder. Cancer 1988;62:705–710.

60. Mabry RL. Rhinitis medicamentosa: The forgotten factor of nasal obstruction. South Med J 1982;75:817.

60a. Lacourciere Y, Brunner H, Irwin R, et al. Effects of modulators of the renin-angiotensin-aldosterone system on cough. J Hypertension 1994;12:1387–1393.

61. Incaudo GA, Schatz M. Rhinosinusitis associated with endocrine conditions: Hypothyroidism and pregnancy. In: Schatz M, Settipane GA, Zeiger RS, eds. Nasal Manifestations of Systemic Diseases. Providence, RI: Oceanside Publications; 1991: pp 53–61.

62. Shugar JMA, SOM PM, Eisman W, Biller JF. Nontraumatic cerebrospinal fluid rhinorrhea. Laryngoscope 1981;91:114–120.

63. Zlab MK, Moore GF, Daly DT, Yonkers AJ. Cerebrospinal fluid rhinorrhea: A review of the literature. Ear Nose Throat J 1992;71:314–317.

64. Gwaltney JM Jr, Phillips CD, Miller RD, et al. Computed tomographic study of the common cold. N Engl J Med 1994;330:25–30.

65. Dingle JH, Badger GF, Jordan WS Jr. *Illness in the Home: A study of 25,000 Illnesses on a Group of Cleveland Families.* Cleveland, Ill: Press of Western Reserve University; 1964:347.

66. Wald ER, Guerra N, Byers C. Upper respiratory tract infections in young children: duration and frequency of complications. Pediatrics 1991;87:129–133.

67. Kennedy DW. First-line management of sinusitis. Otolaryngol Head Neck Surg 1990;103:845–888.

68. Malow JB, Creticos CM. Nonsurgical treatment of sinusitis. Otolaryngol Clin North Am 1989;22:809–818.

69. Gwaltney JM Jr, Scheld WM, Sande MA, et al. The microbial etiology and antimicrobial therapy of adults with acute community-acquired sinusitis: A fifteen-year experience at the University of Virginia and review of other selected studies. J Allergy Clin Immunol 1992;90:457–462.

70. Wald ER. Microbiology of acute and chronic sinusitis in children. J Allergy Clin Immunol 1992;90:452–456.

71. Brook I. Bacteriologic features of chronic sinusitis in children. JAMA 1981;244:967–969.

72. Parsons DS, Phillips SE. Functional endoscopic surgery in children: A retrospective analysis of results. Laryngoscope 1993;103:899–903.

73. Slavin RG: Sinusitis in adults and its relation to allergic rhinitis, asthma, and nasal polyps. J Allergy Clin Immunol 1988;82:950–956.

74. Kaplan RJ. Neurologic complications of infections of the head and neck. Otolaryngol Clin North Am 1976;9:729–749.

75. Morgan MA, Wilson WR, Neel HB III. Fungal sinusitis in healthy and immunocompromised individuals. Am J Clin Pathol 1988;82:597–601.

76. Parnes LS, Brown DH, Garcia B. Mycotic sinusitis: A management protocol. J Otolaryngol 1989;18:176–180.

77. Choi SS, Lawson W, Bottone EJ, et al. Cryptococcal sinusitis: a case report and review of the literature. Otolaryngol Head Neck Surg 1988;99:414–418.

78. Dooley DP, McAllister CK. Candidal sinusitis and diabetic ketoacidosis: A brief report. Arch Intern Med 1989;149:962–964.

79. Waxman JE, Spector JG, Sale SR, et al. Allergic Aspergillus sinusitis: Concepts in diagnosis and treatment of a new clinical entity. Laryngoscope 1987;97:261–266.

80. Tsimikas S, Hollingsworth HM, Nash G. Aspergillus brain abscess complicating allergic Aspergillus sinusitis. J Allergy Clin Immunol 1994;94:264–267.

81. Settipane GA. Nasal polyps and systemic diseases. In: Schatz M, Settipane GA, Zeiger RS, eds. Nasal Manifestations of Systemic Diseases. Providence, RI: Oceanside Publications; 1991: pp 43–51.

82. Lau K, Lieberman J. Young's syndrome. An association between male sterility and bronchiectasis. West J Med 1986;144:744–746.

83. Slavin RG. Nasal polyps and sinusitis. In Middleton E, Reed CE, Ellis EF, et al., eds. *Allergy: Principles and Practice.* St. Louis, Mo: CV Mosby Co; 1988: pp 1291–1303.

84. Drake-Lee A, Lowe D, Swanston A, et al. Clinical profile and recurrence of nasal polyps. J Otolaryngol Otol 1984;98: 783–793.

85. Settipane G, Chafee F. Nasal polyps in asthma and rhinitis. J Allergy Clin Immunol 1977; 58:17–21.

86. Takasaka T, Kurihara A, Suzuki H, et al. The differentiation of polyps and their mucosal ultrastructure. Am J Rhinol 1990;4:159–162.

87. Drake-Lee A, Barker T, Thurley K. Nasal polyps II. Fine structure of mast cells. J Laryngol Otol 1984;98:285–292.

88. Dunnettte SL, Hall M, Washington JA, et al. Microbiologic analyses of nasal polyp tissue. J Allergy Clin Immunol 1986;78: 102–108.

89. Colt H G, Gumpert BC, Harrell JH. Tracheobronchial obstruction caused by Klebsiella rhinoscleromatis. Diagnosis, Pathologic features, and treatment. J Bronchol 1994;1:31–36.

90. DeWeese DD, Saunders WH, Schuller DE, et al. Nose and paranasal sinuses. In: De-Weese DD, Saunders WH, Schuller DE, et al., eds. *Otolaryngology-Head and Neck Surgery.* St. Louis, Mo: CV Mosby; 1988: pp 143–151.

91. Hall IS, Colman BH. Miscellaneous diseases affecting the sinuses. In: Hall IS, Colman BH, eds. *Diseases of the Nose, Throat and Ear.* New York, NY: Churchill Livingstone; 1987: pp 96–101.

92. Hall IS, Colman BH. Noninflammatory diseases of the pharynx. In: Hall IS, Colman BH, eds. *Diseases of the Nose, Throat and Ear.* New York, NY: Churchill Livingstone; 1987: pp 156–166.

93. Hall IS, Colman BH. Diseases of the nasal cavity. In: Hall IS, Colman BH, eds. *Diseases of the Nose, Throat and Ear.* New York, NY: Churchill Livingstone; 1987: pp 5–56.

94. Norman PS. Review of nasal therapy: update. J Allergy Clin Immunol 1983;72: 421–432.

95. Welsh PW, Stricker WE, Chu C-P, et al. Efficacy of beclomethasone nasal solution, flunisolide, and cromolyn in relieving symptoms of ragweed allergy. Mayo Clin Proc 1987;62:125–134.

96. Busse W. New directions and dimensions

97. Vanzieleghem MA, Juniper EF. A comparison of budesonide and beclomethasone diproprionate nasal aerosols in ragweed induced rhinitis. J Allergy Clin Immunol 1987;79:887–892.

98. Meltzer EO, HA Orgel, Bronsky EA, et al. Ipratropium bromide aqueous nasal spray for patients with perennial allergic rhinitis: A study on its effect on their symptoms, quality of life, and nasal cytology. J Allergy Clin Immunol 1992;90:242–249.

99. Kirkegaard J, Mygind N, Molgaard F, et al. Ordinary and high-dose ipratropium bromide in perennial nonallergic rhinitis. J Allergy Clin Immunol 1987;79:585–590.

100. Leavitt RY, Fauci AS. Pulmonary vasculitis. Am Rev Respir Dis 1986;134:149–166.

101. Michet CJ, McKenna CH, Luthra HS, et al. Relapsing polychondritis: Survival and predictive role of early disease manifestations. Ann Intern Med 1986;104:74–78.

102. Gordon WW, Cohn AM, Greenberg SD, et al. Nasal sarcoidosis. Arch Otolaryngol 1976;102:11–14.

103. Dolovich J, Kennedy L, Vickerson F, et al. Control of the hypersecretion of vasomotor rhinitis by topical ipratropium bromide. J Allergy Clin Immunol 1987;80: 274–278.

104. Fisher SR, Newman CE. Surgical perspectives on allergic airway disease. J Allerg Clin Immunol 1988;81:361–375.

105. Aarabi B, Leibrock LG. Neurosurgical approaches to cerebrospinal fluid rhinorrhea. Ear Nose Throat J 1992;71:300–305.

106. Lowenstein SR Parrino TA. Management of the common sold. Adv Intern Med 1987;32:207–234.

107. Dick EC, Hossain SU, Mink KA, et al. Interruption of transmission of rhinovirus colds among human volunteers using virucidal paper handkerchiefs. J Infect Dis 1986;153:352–356.

108. Douglas RG Jr. The common cold-relief at last? N Engl J Med 1986;314:114–115.

109. Douglas RM, Moore BW, Miles HB, et al. Prophylactic efficacy of intranasal alpha$_2$-interferon against rhinovirus infections in the family setting. N Engl J Med 1986;314:65–70.

110. Hayden FG, Albrecht JK, Kaiser DL, et al. Prevention of natural colds by contact prophylaxis with intranasal alpha$_2$-interferon. N Engl J Med 1986;314:71–75.

111. Eby GA, Davis DR, Halcomb WW. Reduction in duration of common colds by zinc

gluconate lozenges in a double-blind study. Antimicrob Agents Chemother 1984;25:20–24.

112. Borum P, Olsen L, Winther B, et al. Ipratropium nasal spray: A new treatment for rhinorrhea in the common cold. Am Rev Respir Dis 1981;123:418–420.

113. Gaffey MJ, Gwaltney JM Jr, Dressler WE, et al. Intranasally administered atropine methonitrate treatment of experimental rhinovirus colds. Am Rev Respir Dis 1987;135:241–244.

114. Irwin RS, Curley FJ, Bennett FM. Appropriate use of antitussives and protussives. Drugs 1993;46:80–91.

115. Kuhn JJ, Hendley JO, Adams KF, et al. Antitussive effect of guaifenesin in young adults with natural colds. Chest 1982;82:713–718.

116. Ophir D, Elad Y. Effects of steam inhalation on nasal patency and nasal symptoms in patients with the common cold. Am J Otolaryngol 1987;8:149–153.

117. Macknin ML, Mathew S, Medendorp SV. Effect of inhaling heated vapor on symptoms of the common cold. JAMA 1990;264:989–991.

117a. Karma P, Pukauder J, Penttila M, et al. The comparative efficacy and safety of clarithromycin and amoxicillin in the treatment of outpatients with acute maxillary sinusitis. J Antimicrobial Chemotherapy 1991;27, Suppl A:83–90.

117b. Dubois J, Saint-Pierre C, Tremblay C. Efficacy of Clarithromycin vs. Amoxicillin/Clavulanate in the treatment of acute maxillary sinusitis. ENT J 1993;72:804–810.

118. Wald ER. Antimicrobial therapy of pediatric patients with sinusitis. J Allergy Clin Immunol 1992;90:469–473.

119. Williams JW, Holleman DR, Samsa GP, et al. Randomized controlled trial of 3 vs 10 days of trimethoprim/sulfamethoxazole for acute maxillary sinusitis. JAMA 1995;273:1015–1021.

120. Friedman WH, Slavin RG. Diagnosis and medical and surgical treatment of sinusitis in adults. Clin Rev Allergy 1984;2:409–428.

121. Kern EG. Sinusitis J Allergy Clin Immunol 1984;73:25–31.

122. Josephson JS, Balwally AN. The functional endoscopic sinus surgery approach: Diagnosis and treatment of sinus disease in the allergic patient. Insights in Allergy 1992;7:1–5.

123. Drettner B, Ebbesen A, Nilsson M. Prophylactic treatment with flunisolide after polypectomy. Rhinology 1982;20:149–157.

124. Ruhno J, Anderson B, Denburg J, et al. A double-blind comparison of intranasal budesonide with placebo for nasal polyposis. J Allergy Clin Immunol 1990;86:946–953.

125. Mygind N. Nasal polyposis. J Allergy Clin Immunol 1990;86:827–829.

126. Samter M, Beers R. Intolerance to aspirin: Clinical studies and consideration of its pathogenesis. Ann Intern Med 1968;68:975–983.

127. Chiu JT. Improvement in aspirin-sensitive asthmatic subjects after rapid aspirin desensitization and aspirin maintenance (ADAM) treatment. J Allergy Clin Immunol 1983;71:560–567.

128. Lumry WR, Curd JG, Zeiger RS, et al. Aspirin-sensitive rhinosinusitis: The clinical syndrome and effects of aspirin administration. J Allergy Clin Immunol 1983;71:580–587.

129. Israel E, Fischer AR, Rosenberg MA, et al. The pivotal role of 5-lipoxygenase products in the reaction of aspirin-sensitive asthmatics to aspirin. Am Rev Respir Dis 1993;148:1447–1451.

# 16

# Anosmia

Renato Roithmann, M.D.
Yehudah Roth, M.D.
Philip Cole, M.D.
Jerry Chapnik, M.D.
Martin Hyde, M.D.

## Introduction

Most healthy persons have experienced impairment of olfactory acuity, commonly in the course of an upper respiratory infection. In the majority of cases, it is a brief episode with spontaneous recovery but there are individuals who suffer chronic, severe, and even complete loss of their olfactory sense from causes that vary widely between life-threatening and relatively innocuous. A dysosmia may provide the first symptom of an underlying disease. Estimates of the extent of chronic smell disorder in the general population vary, about 1% seems possible.[1]

An intact olfactory sense adds much to the quality of life. Its absence can lead to stress, depression, and even danger. Vitiated flavor diminishes enjoyment of food and can lead to disinterest and dietary complications. Lack of awareness of socially unpleasant odors of person or home can lead to ostracism, and unawareness of the odor of spoiled food or cooking gas can lead to disease and to death. The handicap deserves understanding and help from family and friends and from the medical practitioner to whom the problem is referred.

Diagnosis of smell disorders is complicated in many cases by the abundance of possible causing factors. Moreover, there are few major centers that specialize in management and research of olfactory problems to which a patient can be referred and dealt with in a practical manner.

Smell disorders can be classified into five categories according to the degree and type of symptoms:

I. Anosmia: total loss of sensitivity to all odors.
II. Hyposmia: decreased sensitivity to all odors.
III. Dysosmia (parosmia or cacosmia): smell distortion, or perception of an unpleasant odor when a normally pleasant odor is present or perception of odor in the absence of any odorants or olfactory stimulus, also named olfactory hallucination or phantosmia.
IV. Hyperosmia: increased sensitivity to all odors.

From Irwin RS, Curley FJ, Grossman RF (eds): Diagnosis and Treatment of Symptoms of the Respiratory Tract. Armonk, New York, Futura Publishing Company, Inc., © 1997.

V. Agnosmia: complete or partial inability to identify, classify, or differentiate an odor sensation verbally despite ability to recognize and distinguish between odorants.

The terms partial anosmia, partial hyposmia and partial hyperosmia may be used to describe forms of disturbed sensitivity to some, but not all odorants. Specific anosmia or hyposmia describes total or partial sense of smell to one or a very limited number of odorants.

Impaired olfaction can also be classified into three major types of loss according to the site of lesion: **transport loss** when there is disturbed access of a chemical stimulus to the smell receptors (mechanical obstruction); **sensory loss** when there is damage to the smell organs themselves (receptor cells); **neural loss** when there is damage to either the peripheral neural pathways that mediate smell transmission (olfactory nerves) or to the central olfactory pathways.[2,3]

## Anatomy and Physiology

Recognition of airborne particles is provided by olfaction and by the common chemical sense. Olfaction is transmitted by the receptors at the dendrite knobs of the bipolar olfactory neurons in the regeneratable olfactory neuroepithelium, located in the upper portion of the nasal cavity (Figure 1). From each olfactory knob a number of cilia protrude, immersed in mucus. Olfactory transduction is believed to occur mainly in those ciliated structures. Each olfactory neuron sends an axon that jointly forms the olfactory nerve,

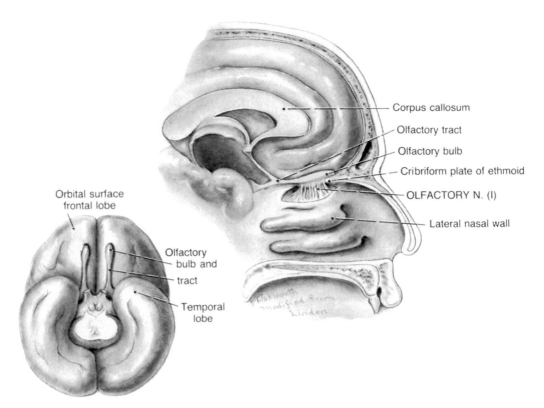

**Figure 1.** The olfactory nerve. Reprinted by permission of W.B. Saunders Company from Jacob SW et al. Structure and Function in Man 5th edition. Philadelphia, Pa: WB Saunders; 1982: p 285.

which, after penetrating the cribriform plate, reaches the olfactory bulb. The olfactory tracts pass along the base of the anterior fossa and enter the pyriform cortex. The odor information is subsequently widely distributed to cortical and subcortical locations.[5–8]

The olfactory transduction, coding, and cognition are complex processes that are not yet fully defined. Various amino acid G protein–linked receptors with different functional and neuromodulatory properties are involved in the process. Their mode of action is through triggering synthesis of second messengers, including cyclic adenosine monophosphate and inositol triphosphate, resulting in the opening of cation channels in the cellular membranes and subsequent creation of action potentials. Different activation by odorants of distinct groups of receptors is believed to generate patterns of neuronal activity that encode odor quality and quantity.[5,7–11]

The common chemical sense recognizes irritation or pungency. Its receptors are free trigeminal, glossopharyngeal, and vagal nerve endings dispersed all over the nasal mucosa, as well as in the cornea, conjuctiva, and oral mucosa. Those endings lie below the epithelium and are less accessible to incoming molecules than are the olfactory receptors. Many substances that create odor sensation can also evoke pungency, and these sensations might overlap in tested subjects.

Odor perception is highly dependent on the anatomy of the nasal air passages and airflow patterns and on individual attention, experiences, and development of personal hedonic codes within cultural restraints closely related to memory, as well as to taste and other pleasant or unpleasant associated sensations. It is also given to habituation upon closely repeated stimulations.[7,8,12,13]

## Etiology and Pathogenesis

The list of factors that cause or are associated with olfactory loss is large (Table I).[14–16] Aging, upper respiratory infections (URI), head trauma, and sinonasal disease are recognized as the most common causes of olfactory dysfunction (Table II).[8,15,17–20] A discussion of some of these causes follows.

## Aging

It is well-known that there is an age-related decrease in olfactory acuity.[21–25] The decline is more pronounced after the seventh decade of life; it varies between individuals and the rate of decline is odor-specific.[23,26] Males are more affected than females at all ages, and smokers are more affected than nonsmokers.[21] The cause is probably multifactorial and includes degenerative processes within the olfactory epithelium or central neural pathways, as well as an increased susceptibility to injury. There is a linear decline in the number of cells and in total olfactory bulb volume as accompaniments of aging.[27] Olfactory mucosa is gradually replaced by respiratory epithelium with aging.[23] Deterioration of cognitive ability and memory impairment in neurodegenerative disorders, such as Alzheimer's disease, Parkinson's disease, other systemic diseases, and their respective treatments may also play a role in the olfactory loss of the elderly.[28–33]

Taste impairment is also very common in the elderly, and it is suggested that it is related to olfactory loss.[20,34] Age-related changes in chewing and swallowing may worsen retronasal odor perception.[35,36]

## Upper Respiratory Infection

Various degrees of olfactory loss are very common in the course of URI. Fortunately, the dysfunction is usually transitory and complete recovery follows with resolution of mucosal inflammation and nasal airway patency. Olfactory neurons can be affected at the level of the epithelium, the bulb, or the central olfactory tracts,[17,37] and a small proportion of pa-

**Table I**
Olfactory Dysfunction: Possible Etiologic Categories

**Lesions of the nose/airway**
Structural Abnormality
  Deviated Septum
  Weakness of Alae Nasi
Nasal Polypi
Allergic Rhinitis
  Seasonal
  Perennial
Vasomotor Rhinitis
Atrophic Rhinitis
Chronic Inflammatory Rhinitis
  Syphilis
  Tuberculosis
  Sarcoidosis
  Scleroma
  Leprosy
  Wegener's Granulomatosis
  Midline Granuloma
Adenoid Hypertrophy
Sjögren's Syndrome
Hypertrophic Rhinitis
Rhinitis Medicamentosa

**Infections and Viral**
Influenza or Acute Viral Rhinitis
Acute Viral Hepatitis
Bacterial Rhinosinusitis
Bronchiectasis
Infected Teeth and Gums
Infected Tonsils
Others
  Fungal
  Rickettsial
  Microfilarial

**Nutritional/metabolic**
Vitamin Deficiency
  Vitamin A
  Vitamin $B_6$
  Vitamin $B_{12}$
Trace Metal Deficiencies
  Zn
  Cu
Protein Calorie Malnutrition
Total Parenteral Nutrition (without adequate replacement)
Cystic Fibrosis
Abetalipoproteinemia
Chronic Renal Failure
Cirrhosis of Liver
Gout
Whipple's Disease

**Neoplasms—Intracranial**
Osteomas
Olfactory Groove and Cribiform Plate Meningiomas
Frontal Lobe Tumors (esp. gliomas)
Paraoptic Chiasma Tumors
  Pituitary Tumors (esp. adenomas)
  Craniopharyngioma
  Suprasellar Meningioma
  Aneurysms
  Suprasellar Cholesteatoma
Temporal Lobe Tumors
Midline Cranial Tumors
  Parasagittal Meningiomas
  Tumors of the Corpus Callosum

**Neoplasms—intranasal**
Neuro-olfactory Tumors
  Esthesioneuroepithelioma
  Esthesioneuroblastoma
  Esthesioneurocytoma
  Esthesioepithelioma
Other Benign or Malignant Nasal Tumors
  Conductive Effect (eg, adenocarcinoma)
  Perceptive Effect (eg, schwannoma, neurofibroma)
  Nasopharyngeal Tumors with Extension
  Paranasal Tumors with Extension
  Leukemic Infiltration

**Neoplasms—carcinomas**
Lung
Gastrointestinal Tract
Ovary
Breast

**Neurologic**
Amyotrophic Lateral Sclerosis
Familial Dysautonomia
Refsum's Syndrome
Multiple Sclerosis
Parkinson's Disease
Progressive Supranuclear Palsy
Temporal Lobe Epilepsy
  Mesial Temporal Sclerosis (ammons horn sclerosis)
  Hamartomas
  Scars/previous Infarcts
Myasthenia Gravis
Retinitis Pigmentosa
Vascular Insufficiency and Anoxia
  Small Multiple Cerebrovascular Accidents
  Transient Ischemic Attacks
  Subclavian Steal Syndrome

*(continued)*

# Table I
## (*continued*)

Others
  Cerebral Abscess (esp. frontal or ethmoidal regions)
  Meningitis
  Syphilis
  Syringomyelia
  Paget's Disease
  Korsakoff's Disease
  Hydrocephalus
  Migraine

**Endocrine**
Adrenal Cortical Insufficiency—Addison's Disease
Congenital Adrenal Hyperplasia
Cushing's Syndrome
Hypothyroidism
Diabetes Mellitus
Primary Amenorrheas
  Chromatin Negative Gonadal Dysgenesis—Turner's Syndrome
  Hypogonadotropic Hypogonadism—Kallmann's syndrome
Hypergonadotropic Hypogonadism
Pseudohypoparathyroidism
Panhypopituitarism
Gigantism
Adiposogenital Dystrophy—Froelich's syndrome

**Congenital/hereditary Etiologies**
Syndrome of Hypogeusia and Hyposmia
Triad of:
  Submucous Cleft of Dorsal Hard Palate
  Facial Hypoplasia
Stunted Growth
"Red-Haired Disease" With Pigmentary Abnormality
Complete and Specific Anosmias of Genetic Origin
Bronchial Asthma
Multiple Lentigines Syndrome
Orbital Hypertelorism

**Trauma**
Most Common Proposed Mechanisms (1, Shearing of Olfactory Nerves; 2, Hemorrhage of the Basal Frontal Lobes and Bruising of the Olfactory Bulbs and Tracts)
Frontal Fracture (esp. fronto-ethmoidal fracture)
Occipital Contrecoup Injury
Nasal Fracture

**Drugs**
Adrenal Steroids (chronic usage)
Amino Acid Excess
  Histidine
  Cysteine
Anesthetics, Local
  Procaine HCl
  Cocaine HCl
  Tetracaine HCl
Anticancer Agents (eg, methotrexate)
Antihistamines (eg, chlorpheniramine maleate)
Antimicrobials
  Griseofulvin
  Lincomycin
  Streptomycin
  Tetracyclines
  Intranasal Tyrothricin
  Local Neomycin
  Neoarsphenamine
Antirheumatics
  Mercury or Gold Salts
  D-Penicillamine
Antithyroids
  Methimazole
  Propylthiouracil
  Thiouracil
Hyperlipoproteinemia Medications
  Clofibrate
  Cholestyramine
Intranasal Saline Solutions with:
  Acetylcholine
  Acetyl, β-methylcholine
  Menthol
  Strychnine
  Zinc sulfate
Opiates
  Codeine
  Hydromophone HCl
  Morphine
Psychopharmaceuticals (eg, psilocybin, LSD)
Sympathomimetics
  Amphetamine Sulfate
  Phenmetrazine Theoclate
  Fenbutrazate HCl
Others
  Antipyrine
  Oral ETOH
  Local Vasoconstrictors
  Cimetidine
  L-dopa

(continued)

## Table I
### (*continued*)

| Chemical Pollutants (gaseous) | Medical Intervention |
|---|---|
| Sulfuric Acid | Laryngectomy |
| Hydrogen Selenide | Rhinoplasty |
| Phosphorus Oxychloride | Anterior Craniotomy |
| Pepper and Cresol Mixture | Surgical Interruption of Olfactory Tract |
| Benzene | Frontal Lobotomy |
| Benzol | Temporal Lobotomy |
| Butyl Acetate | Paranasal Sinus Exenteration |
| Carbon Disulfide | Postanesthesia |
| Ethyl Acetate | Radiation Therapy |
| Ethyl Acrylate | Arteriography |
| Formaldehyde | Influenza Vaccination |
| Hydrazine | Maintenance Hemodialysis |
| Oil of Peppermint | Thyroidectomy |
| Trichloroethylene | Hypophysectomy |
| Hydrogen Sulfide | Adrenalectomy |
| Paint Solvents | Orchiectomy |
| Chlorine | Oophorectomy |
| Benzine | Gastrectomy |
| Nitrous Gases | |
| | **Psychiatric** |
| **Industrial Dusts (particulate)** | Schizophrenic Disorders |
| Coke/coal | Olfactory Reference Syndrome |
| Grain | Depressive Disorders |
| Silicone Dioxide | Hysteria |
| Spices | Malingering |
| Flour | |
| Cotton | **Others** |
| Paper | Presbyosmia |
| Cement | Physiologic Processes |
| Cadmium | Circadian Variation |
| Ashes | Menses |
| Lead | Pregnancy |
| Chromium | Idiopathic |
| Nickel | |
| Chalk | |
| Potash | |
| Iron Carboxyl | |

HCL = hydrogen chloride; LSD = lysergic acid diethylamide; ETOH = ethanol.

tients never recover their olfactory sense. The damage varies with patient susceptibility and with aggressiveness of the agent responsible for the URI episode, which is usually a virus.[38]

Electron microscopic and immunohistochemical studies clearly demonstrate damaged olfactory epithelium in such patients.[39] A reduction in the number of intact ciliated olfactory receptor neurons in cases of postviral olfactory dysfunction has been reported,[35] similar to changes observed after trauma (Figures 2, 3).[40] Olfactory epithelial damage was more pronounced in anosmic patients than in hyposmic ones.

Usually, these patients are unaware of any olfactory disorder preceding the URI episode, so a presumptive diagnosis of post-URI olfactory loss can be established by the temporal association between the dysfunction and the URI episode, if no other cause can explain it. Complete rhinologic evaluation to ex-

**Table II**
Incidence (%) of Etiologies of Olfactory Dysfunction

|  | *SUNY* | *CCCRC* | *UP* | *Mean* |
|---|---|---|---|---|
| Obstructive Nasal and Sinus Disease | 31 | 25 | 15 | 23 |
| Post-URI | 16 | 14 | 26 | 19 |
| Head Trauma | 18 | 11 | 18 | 15 |
| Toxins/Medications | 3 | 1 | 4 | 3 |
| Other | 19 | 25 | 16 | 21 |
| Idiopathic | 12 | 24 | 22 | 21 |
| Total | 100 | 100 | 100 | 100 |

SUNY = State University of New York; CCCRC = Connecticut Chemosensory Clinical Research Center; UP = University of Pennsylvania; URI = upper respiratory infection.

clude obstructive factors after the resolution of the URI episode is required to support the diagnosis.

Among patients with olfactory dysfunction, approximately 19% are post-URI (Table II). Females are more frequently affected (70%).[41] Older patients are more susceptible. Hyposmia is more common than anosmia, and other olfactory distortions such as phantosmia, may be present.

In addition to the local, virus-induced injuries noted above, the olfactory pathway may be a port of entry of infection to the central nervous system.

## Head Trauma

An average of 5.3% incidence of anosmia following head injury has been reported in a large trauma population. The estimated real incidence is greater, since cases of partial olfactory impairment may not be detected.[34] There is a positive correlation between the severity of head injury and the likelihood of olfactory loss,[42,43] but minor injuries also can cause permanent damage. Occipital trauma may be more likely to produce anosmia than frontal trauma.[44]

There are three possible mechanisms of injury in posttraumatic anosmia: transport olfactory loss by deformity of the nasal cavity, sensory olfactory loss by shearing of olfactory nerves at the cribri-

form plate which is considered the most common injury, and neural olfactory loss by damage to olfactory brain centers. Posttraumatic olfactory epithelium shows reduced numbers of receptor cells and degenerate cells.[35,45–47] Axon tangles may be found in the vicinity of the basement membrane (Figure 3), which is postulated to be regenerated axons that failed to reach the olfactory bulb and make central synaptic connections due to fibrosis and scar tissue at the cribriform plate.

The prognosis for smell recovery following traumatic loss is poor.[48] The high degree of suspicion necessary for diagnosis in these cases is facilitated when a temporal relationship between the injury and olfactory loss (usually anosmia) is clearly established by the history. Olfactory tests help to determine the extent of sensory loss and to monitor outcome.

## Transport Losses (Sinonasal Disease)

Various degrees of olfactory impairment can result from blockage of airflow to the olfactory region of the nose. In these cases, in which odorants cannot reach the olfactory epithelial region, obstruction plays an important role.[49] The most prevalent cases of olfactory transport loss are caused by mucosal swelling associated with the common cold. The incidence of olfactory loss in cases of nasal and paranasal sinus disease may be as high as 31%

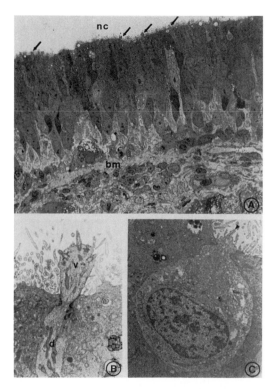

**Figure 2.** Electron photomicrographs of olfactory biopsy specimens from a normosmic volunteer. **A:** Low-power view (×970) revealing epithelium, basement membrane (bm), lamina propria, olfactory vesicles of ciliated receptor cells (arrows), and nasal cavity (nc). **B:** High-power view (×15 838) of a ciliated receptor cell dendrite (d) and olfactory vesicle (v). **C:** High-power view (×10 690) of a microvillar cell. Note the microvilli at apical surface (arrowhead). Reprinted by permission of Raven Press from Strahan RC et al.[40]

(Table II). Structural obstruction, commonly nasal polyps and edema resulting from chronic inflammation, can block the olfactory cleft (Figure 4). Disturbed nasal airflow patterns, mucus alterations, infection, inflammatory products, and stretching of the olfactory neurons by edema may all be involved.[50–55] Fluctuation of olfactory acuity is common in sinonasal patients, especially those with allergic rhinitis, and treatment, mainly with topical steroids, can improve olfaction. Exercise, heavy lifting, or showering may produce a temporary relief of symptoms due to reflex nasal mucosal decongestion.[56]

Septal deviations are found frequently during routine otolaryngologic examination, but our clinical experience does not reveal olfactory complaints in these patients unless there is complete obstruction of the nasal airway. Improvement in olfactory identification postseptorhinoplasty was found only in patients who initially presented with extreme septal deviation.[57]

Nonallergic rhinitis and nasal tumors also can cause olfactory impairment. There is evidence that obstructive adenoid hypertrophy is associated with decreased sense of smell in children that is corrected by adenoidectomy.[58] Laryngectomized patients often complain of loss of smell function,[59] probably due to decreased nasal airflow,[60] but studies have failed to demonstrate a significant correlation between measurements of nasal airflow and olfactory sensitivity in either healthy volunteers or in patients.[55,61]

## Medications and Toxic Exposures

The list of medications, toxic chemicals, and pollutants associated with temporary or permanent olfactory dysfunction is long (Table I). Olfactory damage may result from a single acute exposure or more frequently from chronic or repeated exposures to such agents. Fortunately, drugs cause olfactory impairment in only a small number of patients for whom they are prescribed (Table II). Since many of these drugs are taken for treatment of diseases that in themselves are associated with olfactory loss (eg, cancer, hypothyroidism, hypertension, diabetes), it is difficult to establish a cause-effect relationship. Therefore, the diagnosis of a drug-related olfactory loss is one of exclusion in the majority of cases and can be better established retrospectively in patients who recover their olfactory function after cessation of the medication.

The effects of pollutants vary from slight irritation of the nasal mucosa to permanent olfactory impairment.[62–67] Var-

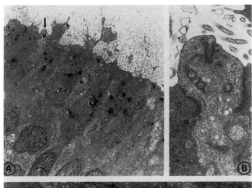

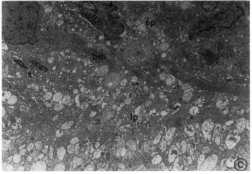

**Figure 3.** Electron photomicrographs of olfactory biopsy specimens from a patient with posttraumatic anosmia. **A:** Low-power view (×2888) of olfactory neuroepithelium demonstrating receptor cell vesicles (*v*) that lack cilia. **B:** Higher power view (×23 000) of receptor cell vesicle indicated by arrow in photo to left. Cilia were absent in this section and all adjacent sections. **C:** View (×7290) of proliferation of axon tangles within the epithelium (ep) and lamina propria (lp). bm = basement membrane. Reprinted by permission of Raven Press from Strahan RC et al.[40]

ious degrees of olfactory neuroepithelial damage, from metaplasia to focal necrosis, can result from chronic exposure to these agents.[68] Current and previous smokers demonstrate a dose-related impairment of odor identification.[69] Passive smokers may also be affected.[56] Gradual improvement in the smell function seems to follow cessation of smoking.

## Congenital Anosmia

Patients in this category have never experienced olfactory sensation, and it is difficult for them to understand the concept of odor.[70] Congenital anosmia is found in association with other anomalies, as in cases of Kallmann's and Turner's syndromes, but it occurs more commonly (80%) as an isolated finding.[71-73] A familial tendency is suggested by a dominant inheritance pattern and incidence of the abnormality is more frequent in females.[74] A common pathophysiologic basis for congenital anosmia has not been established but immature olfactory epithelium that appears unable to connect with the olfactory bulb has been demonstrated in a few patients.[70,71,75-77] In most of these patients, taste and the common chemical sense are intact and, because they have never been aware of odors, they seem less disturbed by their deficit than do patients with acquired anosmia.

## Neoplasms

This category includes both benign and malignant tumors that originate in or involve the nasal cavities, such as squamous-cell carcinoma, adenocarcinoma, inverted papilloma, esthesioneuroblastoma, juvenile angiofibroma, and intracranial tumors (eg, meningiomas, frontal lobe gliomas, pituitary tumors, temporal lobe tumors). The presence of olfactory impairment with unilateral nasal, ophthalmologic or neurologic symptoms of pain, epistaxis, nasal obstruction, rhinorrhea, visual loss, or headache should raise suspicion. Depending on their location and size, intranasal tumors can restrict airflow to the olfactory cleft and produce a transport olfactory loss or they can cause direct damage to the cribriform plate and the olfactory epithelium. The presence of lesions of this nature must be sought in all olfactory impaired patients. Advances in imaging techniques not only enable precise delineation of intranasal and intracranial tumors to be made, but also may assist in establishment of a diagnosis.[78,79]

## Endocrine and Metabolic Disorders

Several endocrine and metabolic disorders are associated with olfactory dysfunction (Table I).

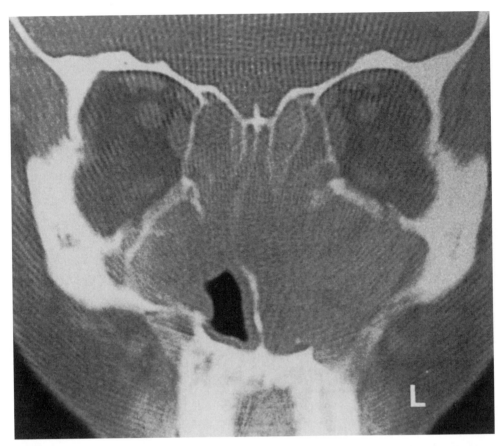

**Figure 4.** Coronal computed tomography scan demonstrating polyposis in nasal cavity and the maxillary and anterior ethmoid sinuses. Reprinted by permission of Martin Dunitz Ltd and JB Lippincott Co.[50]

### Acute and Chronic Liver Disease

About a third of patients suffering from acute viral hepatitis[80] or alcoholic liver disease[81,82] have abnormal detection and recognition of odorants. The mechanism of olfactory impairment associated with liver disease is unknown, but vitamin A and zinc deficiencies have been suggested, and recovery from chemosensory dysfunction has been reported following liver transplantation.[30]

### Diabetes Mellitus

Both taste and olfactory functions are affected in diabetic patients. Olfactory dysfunction might result from vasculopa-

thy and degenerative complications rather than neuropathy.[83–85]

### Hypothyroidism, Pseudohypoparathyroidism, and Adrenal Insufficiency

Thyroid, parathyroid, and adrenal diseases affect smell and taste function in some patients.[86,87] Patients with pseudohypoparathyroidism may have a reduction in both olfactory and taste sensations (type 1a) or they may not (type 1b).[88]

## Neurologic Disorders

Olfactory auras are common in temporal lobe epilepsy, and seizure disorders may generate olfactory distortions (parosmia, phantosmia).[89,90] It has been speculated that impaired olfaction, that can appear as the first symptom of Alzheimer's and Parkinson's diseases,[29,30] could reflect structural and biochemical damage to neurons of the olfactory epithelium, the anterior olfactory nucleus, the olfactory tubercule, and the olfactory cortex. Indeed, olfactory epithelial biopsy may be employed as a diagnostic measure in these cases.

Olfactory dysfunction can appear as an early sign of central nervous system involvement in HIV–infected patients.[91] The finding might be explained by the loss of neurons in the superior frontal gyrus that has been shown to be as great as 38% in patients with AIDS.[92]

## Psychiatric Disorders

The clinical spectrum of depression and hallucinations may include olfactory complaints. A psychiatric evaluation should be considered in patients if olfactory hallucinations are suspected in order to avoid a misdiagnosis of idiopathic anosmia and to enable an appropriate therapeutic approach to be made.[93] Although the mechanism of psychiatric impairment has not been clearly elucidated, it has been suggested that since schizophrenic patients can exhibit olfactory loss,[94,95] it may be related to alterations at the lymbic system.

## Iatrogenic Causes

Nasal surgery, frontal surgical approaches to the skull base, or temporal lobe surgery that is performed for treatment of intractable epilepsy might traumatize the olfactory pathway and result in partial or total loss of olfaction.[96,97] The overall patients' risk of anosmia from nasal surgery is low (1.1%).[98] Furthermore, it has been shown that olfactory losses following nasal procedures are usually temporary and complete recovery of olfactory function can be anticipated in the majority

of patients.[57] Endoscopic sinus surgery for chronic sinusitis and nasal polyposis is usually followed by improvement of olfaction.[99–101] Olfactory biopsy has manifested no discernible adverse effect on the ability to smell, when performed under endoscopic guidance and with appropriate instrumentation.[39,102]

Radiation therapy for head and neck tumors, such as nasopharyngeal carcinomas and pituitary adenomas, has been found to profoundly affect the sense of smell for lengthy periods of time.[103]

## Idiopathic

There are anosmic patients in whom a thorough evaluation does not provide an acceptable explanation for their condition. These patients are usually in the young- to middle-aged group and in good health.[8] In some cases, atypical olfactory epithelium may be demonstrated.[104]

## Diagnostic Approach

### Diagnostic Strategy

A detailed medical history, a careful physical examination, and olfactory testing, complemented as indicated by imaging and other specialized investigations, should be undertaken in all cases of anosmia. Olfactory tests are particularly important to objectively assess and to quantify the symptoms. The information provided by the evaluation may help the clinician to differentiate between transport, sensory, and neural losses. Determination of the site of the lesion restricts the number of possible causes of the disorder and may help to establish an etiologic diagnosis.[105]

Transport loss is frequently found in the acute phase of viral and bacterial rhinitis and in allergic and nonallergic rhinitis. It can be caused by intranasal structural abnormalities resulting from nasal valve collapse, septal deviations, intranasal and nasopharyngeal tumors, nasal polyps, ostiomeatal complex disease, and scarring in the olfactory area by nasal trauma or surgery.

Sensory loss results from viral infection, chemical exposure, radiation therapy to the head, medications affecting cell turnover, intranasal or central nervous system tumors with extension to the cribriform plate, iatrogenic causes secondary to sinonasal surgery, and aging.

Neural loss can be a consequence of head or maxillofacial trauma, tumors of the anterior cranial fossa, neurosurgical procedures, congenital disorders, neurotoxic medications, or aging. Since it may be impossible to differentiate clearly between sensory and neural losses, the term "sensorineural loss" may be useful.

## Medical History

Clinical evaluation of anosmia begins with a thorough history. Some of the most important points to be clarified are the nature and duration of the complaint, whether the loss is total or partial, whether it is for all odorants or only specific ones, and if it is an existing yet disturbed sense of olfaction. Further points to be established are when the disorder was first noticed, olfactory function prior to the loss, any relationship with facial or head trauma, nasal or craniofacial surgery, or infection, and whether there has been use of specific medication, exposure to chemical agents or irradiation. Time may be another important clue—Was the onset sudden as in cases of infection or trauma or was it gradual as in cases of tumor, nasal polyps, or systemic disease? Improvement is common with resolution of infection or withdrawal from exposure to toxic agents. Symptoms fluctuate in cases of chronic rhinitis and in drug-related conditions.

The presence of associated symptoms of epistaxis, nasal obstruction, rhinorrhea, or facial pain should be explored. Intranasal tumors are usually accompanied by unilateral nasal symptoms. Parosmia is a common consequence of nasal infection, and phantosmia may occur in psychiatric disorders and epilepsy. Neurologic symptoms and signs of visual dysfunction, headache, facial sensation changes, and depression should be taken into account and evidence of systemic disease, drug abuse, excessive tobacco and alcohol consumption, dietary deficiencies, radiation exposure, or familial history of olfactory-related disorders should be considered. Taste disorders are a common accompaniment of olfactory disorders, and they may originate from loss of the olfactory component of flavor or from direct loss of taste sensation. Response to previous treatments, such as local or systemic steroids, zinc, vitamins, or intranasal surgery, should be noted.[8,14,56,106-108]

## Physical Examination

Nasal cavities and paranasal sinuses deserve special attention because of the prevalence of sinonasal pathology in patients with olfactory impairment and because appropriate medical or surgical treatment of transport losses offer a good chance of improvement. Examination must include external inspection for deformities and scars and anterior rhinoscopy before and after topical decongestion of the nasal mucosa. Further examination by flexible fiberoptic or rigid telescope ensures a precise visualization of the superior and posterior areas of the nose, the olfactory cleft, the paranasal sinus ostia, the posterior choanas and the nasopharynx. It is important to note mucosal changes, the character of the secretions, structural abnormalities of the nasal valve, deviation or perforation of the septum, turbinate atrophy or hypertrophy, ostiomeatal complex abnormalities, and intranasal or nasopharyngeal masses.

A complete evaluation of neighboring structures is essential, and it should include evaluation of the eyes, ears, teeth, gums, tongue, pharynx, and neck. In addition, a thorough neurologic examination is mandatory.

## Olfactory Testing

Tests of olfaction aim to determine an individual's ability to recognize an odorant, to detect threshold concentrations, to define how strong or pleasant the stimuli are, and to differentiate it from other stimulants. The tests are potentially useful for monitoring progression of disease and are powerful tools for medicolegal purposes. Several methods have been suggested to assess olfaction, but only a few have gained relative popularity.

Open-bottle tests using containers of common odorants are easy to prepare and to perform. Classically, such a test employs three bottles, two contain a blank and one contains the odorant (ie, vanilla for olfactory stimulation and ammonia for common chemical sense stimulation). The detection ability is tested by having the subject select the odorant-containing bottle. Threshold can be assessed by a multistep, forced-choice test for one or several odorants in ascending concentrations, determining threshold values for odor (or pungency) detection or recognition.[7,8,67,109–111]

Another popular evaluation method employs a scratch-and-sniff booklet containing several microencapsulated standard odorants. This semiquantitative method tests smell identification or recognition. It measures mainly olfactory acuity rather than distortion, and it is dependent on the vigor of the scratch and on the way the sample is positioned in front of the nose. This test is simple, self-administered, portable, can be mailed to the test subject, and, most importantly, is consistent and has been found to be useful in the clinical setting.[5,7,8,68,110]

There are several modifications to these methods, as well as additional estimates of odor intensity and pleasantness, that are not discussed here.[5–8,109] Because controlled stimuli (known and constant relative concentrations of gas and liquid phases in the sample, and a standardized airstream) are important, especially for threshold determinations, some olfactometers have a limited (mainly research) availability and use. Other attempts to obtain machine-assisted measurements of olfaction, by magnetic resonance imaging (MRI) and positron-emission tomography, have so far yielded little benefit.[7,8]

Because hyposmic patients commonly complain of taste disorders, taste function may sometimes be evaluated as well. There are standardized methods to assess taste thresholds, magnitude, and pleasantness, similar in principle to smell tests. Taste evaluation is usually easier to perform than olfactory tests, and it offers the patient some practice at this type of sensory testing as a prelude to assessment of smell function.[7]

## Olfactory-Evoked Potentials

Evoked potentials (EP) are now widely used clinically in otolaryngology,[112] opthalmology, and neurology.[113] The most common applications are as objective tools to measure sensory acuity or discrimination ability and to explore the location of lesions affecting sensory pathways.

Typically, a series of many auditory, visual, or somatosensory stimuli is presented, and computer averaging that is time-locked to the stimuli, extracts the minute EP signal from concurrent, spontaneous electrophysiologic "noise" (eg, EEG or myogenic activity). Both the EP and noise are registered by skin electrodes placed over nerve tracts or on the head.

Gross potentials can originate throughout the entire sensory pathway from receptor to cerebral cortex. They may appear as a complex waveform lasting up to several hundred milliseconds, but usually, specific EP components (eg, receptor, brainstem, cortical) are focused upon by using particular stimulus patterns and electrode placements.

Clinical inferences are usually based on EP presence or absence, magnitude, latency, and wave-shape, all of which can reflect receptor and pathway function. Complex electrode arrays and computer analysis allow scalp topographic mapping of EP and can reveal the location and activity of both cortical and deep intracranial sources.[114] Recently, sensitive magnetometers have been used to detect the magnetic analogs of EP (evoked magnetic fields [EMF]) associated with ionic flow, giving further, objective information about events in cerebral cortex.[115]

Receptor (mucosal) and cerebral EP to olfactory stimuli were first recorded many years ago.[116–118] Their clinical application was first reported in the early 1970s,[119,120] but progress has been severely limited by difficulty in generating the accurately-timed sequences of controlled stimuli needed for time-locked averaging to succeed and by rapid olfactory response adaptation to repeated stimuli, in contrast to other stimulus modalities.

Over the last decade several groups, particularly in Germany, have developed the required stimulus control techniques.[121,122] Coupled with standard equipment for EP analysis, these stimulation systems have made it more practicable to investigate olfactory EP and explore their clinical applications (Figure 5).

Research to date has revealed that chemosensory EP elicited by stimulating the nasal mucosa include both truly olfactory and chemosomatosensory responses. Some stimuli, such as carbon dioxide, are odorless but excite nociceptors innervated by the trigeminal nerve. Others, such as vanillin, are exclusively olfactory stimuli. Many odorants excite both systems concurrently, especially at high concentrations. EP studies are now refining the distinctions and interactions between these different excitations, and EP measures correlate usefully with subjective reports of sensation disorders in a variety of pathologies, including Kallmann's syndrome, parkinsonism, head injury, and upper respiratory infection.[123]

Instrumentation for olfactory EP measurement is not yet widely available, but rapid advances can be expected. Olfactory EP are already yielding a better understanding of olfactory mechanisms, as well as objective confirmation of anosmia, quantification of hyposmia and parosmia, and differential diagnosis of end-organ and central pathway dysfunction.[122–124] Soon, these techniques may emerge as an important, practical complement to anamneses and existing formal psychometric methods.

## Imaging

Computed tomography (CT) and MRI are important in the evaluation of olfactory disorders, in order to rule out intracranial pathology when the diagnosis is not clear. CT is indispensable for identification of sinonasal disease that may not be detected rhinoscopically, and it is an essential prerequisite for endoscopic surgery (Figure 6), important for evaluating neighboring orbital structures, the optic nerves, the internal carotid arteries, the cribriform plate, and the anterior cranial fossa.[79,125,126]

Although standard radiographic views (plain films) of the nasal cavities and paranasal sinuses may have a screening merit, they are of limited value in the diagnosis and assessment of chronic, recurring sinus infection. They are inadequate for evaluation of the ethmoidal air cells, the upper two thirds of the nasal cavity, the infundibulum, the middle meatus, and the frontal recess. MRI, due to its superior soft tissue resolution, facilitates diagnosis and delineation of tumors and fungal infections, but does not depict the osseous sinus walls and ostia adequately[127] (Figure 7).

Imaging may also demonstrate other disorders associated with olfactory loss, such as unsuspected trauma to the cribriform plate and skull base, congenital anomalies (eg, encephalocele, fibro-osseous lesions), Paget's disease, central nervous system lesions, or areas of central nervous system atrophy that follow a stroke or result from Alzheimer's disease or from multiple sclerosis.[128]

## Nasal Airflow and Patency Studies

Rhinometry is employed for objective assessment of the nasal airway. Acoustic rhinometry measures cross-sectional areas and volumes of the lumen at different points in the nose and detects obstructions (Figure 8). Rhinomanometric measurements of transnasal airflow and pressure, although not directly related to olfactory function, can detect abnormal nasal

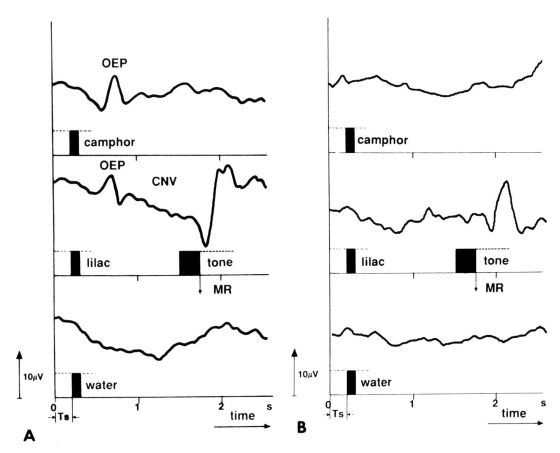

**Figure 5.** Olfactory evoked responses: **A:** Normal olfaction. Olfactory evoked potentials (OEP) and contingent negative variation (CNV) records. OEP is evoked by camphor and lilac stimuli, while CNV develops after the lilac when a second, confirmatory stimulus is expected. Manual reaction (MR) terminates potentials. Control stimulation with water was negative. **B:** Anosmia. Neither OEP nor CNV are recorded. Confirmatory noise presented after lilac evoked only auditory response. While the potential use of evoked responses is demonstrated, their associations with expectations and noise are shown as well. $Ts$ = transport time (seconds). Reprinted by permission of Annals of Otology, Rhinology and Laryngology from Auffermann H et al. Ann Otol Rhinol Laryngol 1993;102:8.

airflow and the severity, side, approximate site, and mucovascular component of obstructions that might be associated with olfactory disorders.[61,129–134]

## Laboratory Tests

Because many systemic conditions affect olfaction, several auxillary tests such as blood evaluation, hepatic, renal and brain function, metabolic and endocrine assessment, allergy, and malignancy screening, should be considered.

## Olfactory Mucosal Biopsy

Olfactory mucosal biopsy followed by histological, immunohistochemical, and ultrastructural studies have provided better understanding of human olfactory structure and function in health and disease[35,39,110,135] and may be of diagnostic

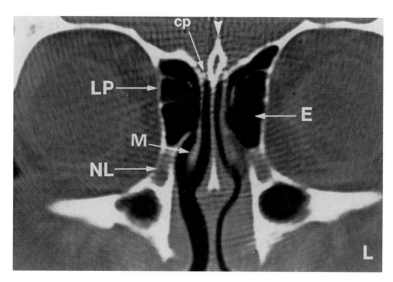

**Figure 6.** Coronal computed tomography through the anterior ethmoids and adjacent structures. *LP* = lamina papyracea; *NL* = nasolacrimal duct; *cp* = cribriform plate; *M* = middle turbinate; *E* = ethmoid cell; *arrowhead* = crista galli. Reprinted by permission of The Journal of Otolaryngology.[125]

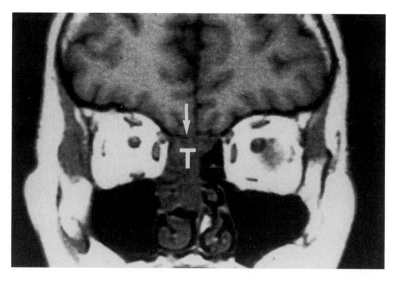

**Figure 7.** Coronal magnetic resonance (T1) scan demonstrating esthesioneuroblastoma (T) arising from the roof of the nasal cavity invading the ethmoid complex. Reprinted by permission of Martin Dunitz Ltd and JB Lippincott Co.[50]

value. It may be important to collect multiple samples from a single subject because of the uneven distribution of olfactory cells, the variable distribution of olfactory epithelium among multiple patches of respiratory epithelium, and the various stages of olfactory receptor cell structure due to continuous turnover.[22] Developments in instrumentation have enabled precise human olfactory biopsy to be per-

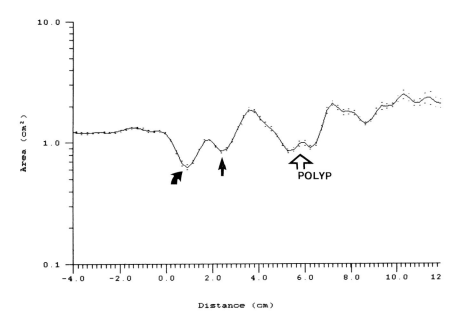

**Figure 8.** Acoustic rhinometric print out. Curved arrow shows the entrance of the nasal valve (ostium internum) and straight arrow shows the anterior end of the inferior turbinate at the piriform aperture (isthmus nasi).

formed with no discernible changes in olfactory function.[40,102] Although specific epithelial changes have been described in postviral infection, posttraumatic anosmia and congenital anosmia, more studies are necessary to better define the diagnostic information provided by this technique.

## Evaluation Management

As outlined in the previous sections, the evaluation of a patient with smell disorder may be a complicated process, and requires employing versatile measures. A suggested diagnostic algorithm is summarized in (Table III).

## Treatment

Although significant advances have been made in the understanding of pathophysiological mechanisms and in techniques for diagnosis of olfactory function in health and disease, current therapeutic alternatives are limited. There are no therapies of proven efficacy for treatment of sensorineural loss. Successful management of nasal or paranasal sinus disease that produces a transport olfactory loss can however restore olfactory function. Therapy in such a case is directed towards relief of nasal obstruction or infection. Medical treatments include antihistamines, decongestants, cromoglycate, topical and systemic steroids, and antibiotics and will help patients in varying degrees depending on the cause, severity, and stage of their disease.[136] Systemic steroids are effective in improving olfaction in patients with nasal polyposis but anosmia often returns on cessation of therapy and the risk of significant systemic side effects during administration and withdrawal contraindicate long-term use of this form of medication.[137] Few studies have assessed the effects of topical steroids in improving olfactory function in cases of allergic rhinitis not associated with either obstructive nasal polyps or chronic sinusitis with ostiomeatal complex obstruction.[138] Some topical steroid preparations produce

**Table III**
Evaluation Management
for Smell Disorders

1. History
   Smell Ability Prior to Loss
   Hyposensation or Distortion of Perception
   Possible Associated Taste Disorders
   Sinonasal Disease and Therapy
   Medications and Toxic Exposure
   Head Trauma
   Upper Respiratory Infections
   Neurologic Disorders
   Metabolic and Endocrine Diseases
   Psychological Problems
   Neoplastic Disease
   Congenital/Familial
2. Physical Examination
   Nose
   Head and Neck
   Neurologic Examination
3. Olfactory Testing
   Detection
   Identification
   Evoked Potentials
   Possible Taste Evaluation
4. Imaging
   CT, MRI
5. Nasal Airflow and Patency Studies
6. Auxillary Tests
   Laboratory Tests
   Olfactory Mucosal Biopsy

CT = computed tomography; MRI = magnetic resonance imaging.

drying of the mucosa but most are considered safe for the long-term use, with the exception of dexamethasone.[139,140]

Sinus surgery, especially functional endoscopic surgery,[141,142] is widely used for the management of chronic or recurring sinus infections that persist despite appropriate medical and conventional surgical treatment. It is considered effective treatment for recurrent sinusitis secondary to nasal polyposis and for the correction of a concha bullosa, a large ethmoidal bulla or a laterally displaced uncinate process, which are common anatomic variants that predispose to sinusitis and to transport olfactory loss. Many patients experience improved olfactory acuity after surgical treatment,[99,101] especially when topical

steroids are used to reduce the recurrence rate. The multifactorial etiology of chronic sinusitis and nasal polyopsis is probably associated with recurrences observed in some patients despite appropriate medical and surgical treatment.[143]

Currently there are no specific medical therapies that alter the course of postviral anosmia, but several patients recover olfactory function spontaneously to various degrees and over differing periods of time.

Recovery following head trauma is less probable, and it is not possible to predict prognosis. A time course of recovery as long as 5 years following head injury has been reported.[34] Although no specific treatment is indicated, an encouraging and reassuring attitude is certainly justified.

There is little evidence to support therapeutic benefit in the use of vitamin A or zinc in anosmic patients,[56,70,144,145] and side effects of these measures are not uncommon.[146]

Topical application of cocaine to the olfactory area has been reported to produce positive results in the treatment of phantosmia,[147] but these results could not be substantiated by other investigators.[2,148] Successful surgical management of phantosmia has been reported in a few patients[8,148] in whom a full-thickness portion of the olfactory epithelium was excised from the cribriform plate. Recovery may have been due to removal of diseased neurons from the olfactory area. This technique might avoid the anosmia that follows olfactory bulbectomy. The treatment of dysosmia and phantosmia related to sinonasal disease should follow the principles previously described.

An essential component of the management of anosmic patients is to reassure those in whom there is no serious threat to life. Although, in many cases, a thorough investigation might fail to determine a specific diagnosis, it is important for the caregiver to show concern for the problem and to discuss it realistically with the patient. Special precautions for personal safety, such as installation of smoke detectors at home, use of electrical rather than gas appliances, and paying attention to the risk of spoiled foods, should be advised. Dietary advice is very important because of the potentially negative influence of anosmia on the flavor of food, which affects intake in many patients. Self-reporting of dietary patterns can identify factors responsible for notable weight changes and be of use as a screening questionnaire to find those who require counselling.[108] Individualized counselling to increase the appeal of foods through flavor fortification[149] and accentuation of non-chemosensory properties, such as texture, appearance, and temperature, can help patients with sensorineural olfactory loss. Friends and family members should cooperate and advise the patient in personal and domestic matters of unpleasant odors and use of unsuitable perfumes.

## Summary

In this chapter, the authors have attempted to provide a practical guide for clinicians concerned with management of patients who complain of olfactory problems.

The importance of a careful history is emphasized, and appropriate examinations and investigations are discussed. Contemporary methods of diagnostic imaging and nasal endoscopy are of particular value.

Fortunately, many acute hyposmias and anosmias recover spontaneously, and many chronic cases associated with structural and mucosal obstructions have a favorable prognosis in response to current therapeutic measures. Antibiotics, steroids, and surgery have extended the clinician's armamentarium in the treatment of these distressing conditions. Yet, there are patients whose prognosis for recovery of olfaction is unfavorable and for whom there is no current treatment, especially for those who have sustained neurological damage.

In addition to the employment of technological advances in therapy and avoidance of unnecessary treatment, a sympathetic appreciation by the clinician of the patient's affliction, realistic prognostication, and wise advice concerning such practical matters as diet and safety contribute substantially to patient care.

## References

1. Report of the Panel on Communicative Disorders to the National Advisory Neurological and Communicative Disorders and Stroke Council. Washington, DC: National Institutes of Health, 1979. NIH Publ. No. 79.1914, pp. 319.

2. Kimmelman CP. *Disorders of Taste and Smell.* Washington: American Academy of Otolaryngology—Head and Neck Surgery Foundation, Inc. 1986.

3. Snow JBJ, Doty RL, Bartoshuk LM, et al. Categoriazation of chemosensory disorders. In: Getchell TV, Doty RL, Bartoshuk LM. Snow JBJ, ed. Smell and Taste in Health and Disease. New York, NY: Raven Press, 1991:445–447.

4. Jacob SW, Francone CA, Lossow WJ. *Structure and Function in Man.* Philadelphia, Pa: WB Saunders Company; 1982: 285.

5. Berglund B, Lindvall T. Olfaction. In: Proctor DF, Andersen I, eds. *The Nose: Upper Airway Physiology and the Atmospheric Environment.* Amsterdam, Elsevier; 1982:279–305.

6. Takagi SF. *Human Olfaction.* Tokyo: University of Tokyo Press; 1989.

7. Henkin RI. Evaluation and treatment of human olfactory dysfunction. In: English GM, ed. *Otolaryngology. Vol. 2.* Philadelphia, Pa; Harper & Row; 1993:chap 5.

8. Leoplod DA. Physiology of olfaction. In: Cummings CW, Frederickson JM, Harker LA, Krause CJ, Schuller DE, eds. *Otolaryngology—Head and Neck Surgery.* St. Louis, MO: Mosby; 1993:640–664.

9. Farbman AI. *Cell Biology of Olfaction.* Cambridge University Press, Cambridge, Mass; 1992.

10. Anholt RRH. Molecular aspects of olfaction. In: Serby MJ, Chobor KL, eds. *Science of Olfaction.* New York, NY: Springer-Verlag; 1992:51–79.

11. Getchell TV, Su Z, Getchell ML. Mucous domains: microchemical heterogeneity in the mucociliary complex of the olfactory epithelium. In: Marsh J, Goode J, eds. *The Molecullar Basis of Smell and Taste Transduction. Ciba Foundation Symposium 179.* Chichester: Wiley; 1993:27–50.

12. Stoddart DM. *The Scented Ape: The Biology and Culture of Human Odour.* Cambridge, Mass: Cambridge University Press; 1990.

13. Engen T. *Odor Sensation and Memory.* New York, NY: Praeger; 1991.

14. Feldman JI, Wright HN, Leopold DA. The initial evaluation of dysosmia. Am J Otolaryngol 1986;7:431–444.

15. Doty RL, Bartoshuk LM, Snow Jr JB. Causes of olfactory and gustatory disorders. In: Getchell TV, Doty RL, Bartoshuk LM, Snow JBJ, eds. *Smell and Taste in Health and Disease.* New York, NY: Raven Press; 1991:449–462.

16. Schiffman SS. Taste and smell in disease. I. N Engl J Med 1983;308:1275–1279.

17. Leopold DA, Hornung DE, Youngentob SL. Olfactory loss after upper respiratory infection. In: Getchell TV, Doty RL, Bartoshuk LM, Snow JBJ, eds. *Smell and Taste in Health and Disease.* New York, NY: Raven Press; 1991:731–734.

18. Leopold DA. Olfactory function and disorders. In: BJ Bailey, ed. *Head and Neck Surgery—Otolaryngology.* Philadelphia, Pa: JB Lippincott Company; 1991:254.

19. Goodspeed RB, Gent JF, Catalanotto F. Clinical evaluation results from a taste and smell clinic. Postgrad Med 1987;81:251–260.

20. Deems DA, Doty RL, Settle G, et al. Smell and taste disorders, a study of 750 patients from the University of Pennsylvania Smell and Taste Center. Arch Otolaryngol Head Neck Surg 1991;117:519–528.

21. Doty R, Shaman P, Applebaum SL, et al. Smell identification ability: changes with age. Science 1984;226:1441–1443.

22. Murphy C. Cognitive and chemosensory influences on age-related changes in the ability to identify blended foods. J Gerontol 1985;40:47–52.

23. Paik SI, Lehman MN, Seiden AM, et al. Human olfactory biopsy: the influence of age and receptor distribution. Arch Otolaryngol Head Neck Surg 1992;118:731–738.

24. Russel MJ, Cummings BJ, Profitt BF, et al. Life span changes in the verbal categorization of odors. J Gerontol 1993;48:P49–P53.

25. Ship JA, Weiffenbach JM. Age, gender, medical treatment, and medication effects on smell identification. J Gerontol 1993;48:M26–M32.

26. Wysoki CJ, Gilbert AN. The National Geographic smell survey: effects of age are heterogenous. Ann NY Acad Sci 1989;561:12–28.

27. Bhatnagar KP, Kennedy RC, Baron G, et al. Number of mitral and cells and the bulb volume in the aging human olfactory bulb: a quantitative morphological study. Anat Rec 1987;218:73–87.

28. Stevens JC, Cain WS. Age-related deficiency in the perceived strength of six odorants. Chemi Sens 1985;10:517–529.

29. Doty RL. Influence of age and age-related diseases on olfactory function. Ann NY Acad Sci 1989;561:76–86.

30. Doty RL. Olfactory dysfunction in neurodegenerative disorders. In: Getchell TV, Doty RL, Bartoshuk LM, Snow JBJ, eds. *Smell and Taste in Health and Disease.* New York, NY: Raven Press; 1991:735–752.

31. Deems RO, Friedman MI, Friedman LS, et al. Clinical manifestations of olfactory and gustatory disorders associated with hepatic and renal disease. In: Getchell TV, Doty RL, Bartoshuk LM, Snow JBJ, eds. *Smell and Taste in Health and Disease.* New York, NY: Raven Press; 1991:805–816.

32. Feldman JI, Murphy C, Davidson TM, et al. The rhinologic evaluation of alzheimer's disease. Laryngoscope 1991;101:1198–1202.

33. Corwin J. Assessing olfaction: cognitive and measurement issues. In: Serby MJ, Chobor KL, eds. *Science of Olfaction.* Springer-Verlag; Berlin; 1992:335–354.

34. Stevens JC, Bartoshuk LM, Cain WS. Chemical senses and aging. Chem Sens 1984;9:167–179.

35. Costanzo RM, Becker DP. Smell and taste disorders in head injury and neurosurgery patients. In: Meiselman HL, Rivlin RS, eds. *Clinical Measurements of Taste and Smell.* New York, NY: MacMillan Publishing Company; 1986:565–578.

36. Moran DT, Jafek BW, Eller PM, et al. Ultrastructural histopathology of human olfactory mucosa. Microscopy Research and Technique 1992 23:103–110.

37. Ojeda VJ, Archer M, Robertson TA, et al. Necropsy study of the olfactory portal of entry in herpes simplex encephalitis. Med J Austral 1983;1:79–81.

38. Mott AE, Leopold DA. Disorders in taste and smell. Med Clin North Am 1991;75:1321–1353.

39. Yamagishi M, Nakano Y. A re-evaluation of the classification of olfactory epithe-

lia in patients with olfactory disorders. Eur Arch Otorhinolaryngol 1992;249:393–399.

40. Strahan RC, Jafek BW, Moran DT. Biopsy of the olfactory neuroepithelium. In: Getchell TV, Doty RL, Bartoshuk LM, Snow JBJ, eds. *Smell and Taste in Health and Disease.* New York, NY: Raven Press; 1991:703–709.

41. Hendriks APJ. Olfactory dysfunction. Rhinology 1988;26:229–251.

42. Costanzo RM, Zasler N. Head trauma. In: Getchell TV, Doty RL, Bartoshuk LM, Snow Jr JB, eds. *Smell and Taste in Health and Disease.* New York, NY: Raven Press; 1991:711–730.

43. Van Damme PA, Freihofer HP. Disturbances of smell and taste after high central midaface fractures. J Craniomaxillofac Surg 1992;20:248–250.

44. Sumner D. Post-traumatic anosmia. Brain 1964;87:107–120.

45. Hasegawa S, Yamagishi M, Nakano Y. Microscopic studies of human olfactory epithelia following traumatic anosmia. Arch Otorhinolaryngol 1986;243:112–116.

46. Jafek BW, Eller PM, Esses BA, et al. Posttraumatic anosmia: ultrastructural correlates. Arch Neurol 1989;46:300–304.

47. Yamagishi M, Okazoe R, Ishizuka Y. Olfactory mucosa of patients with olfactory disturbance following head trauma. Ann Otol Rhinol Laryngol 1994;103:279–284.

48. Keane JR, Baloh RW. Posttraumatic cranial neuropathies. Neurol Clin 1992;10:849–867.

49. Leopold DA. The relationship between nasal anatomy and human olfaction. Laryngoscope 1988;98:1232–1238.

50. Shankar L, Evans K, Hawke M, Stammberger H. *An Atlas of Imaging of the Paranasal Sinuses.* London: Martin Dunitz and JB Lippincott Co.; 1994:169.

51. Church JA, Bauer H, Bellanti JA, et al. Hyposmia associated with atopy. Ann Allergy 1978;40:105–109.

52. Loury MC, Kennedy DW. Chronic sinusitis and nasal polyposis. In: Getchell TV, Doty RL, Bartoshuk LM, Snow JBJ, eds. *Smell and Taste in Health and Disease.* New York, NY: Raven Press; 1991:517–528.

53. Apter AJ, Mott AE, Cain WS, et al. Olfactory loss and allergic rhinitis. J Allergy Clin Immunol 1992;90:670–680.

54. Henkin RI. Allergic rhinitis. N Engl J Med 1992;326:576–577.

55. Cowart BJ, Flynn-Rodden K, McGeady SJ, et al. Hyposmia in allergic rhinitis. J Allergy Clin Immunol 1993 91:747–751.

56. Seiden AM, Duncan HJ, Smith DV. Office management of taste and smell disorders. Otolaryngol Clin North Am 1992;25:817–835.

57. Goldwyn RM, Shore S. The effects of submucous resection and rhinoplasty on the sense of smell. Plast Reconstr Surg 1968;41:427–432.

58. Ghorbanian SN, Paradise JL, Doty RL. Odor perception in children in relation to nasal obstruction. Pediatrics 1983;72:510–516.

59. DeBeule G, Damste P. Rehabilitation following laryngectomy: the results of a questionnaire study. Br J Disord Commun 1972;7:141–147.

60. Doty RL, Frye R. Influence of nasal obstruction on smell function. Otolaryngol Clin North Am 1989;22:397–411.

61. Eccles R, Jawad MSM, Morris S. Olfactory and trigeminal thresholds and nasal resistance to airflow. Acta Otolaryngol (Stockh) 1989;108:268–273.

62. Schiffman SS. Drugs influencing taste and smell perception. In: Getchell TV, Doty RL, Bartoshuk LM, Snow JBJ, eds. *Smell and Taste in Health and Disease.* New York, NY: Raven Press; 1991:845–850.

63. Cometto-Muniz JE, Cain W. Influence of airborne contaminants on olfaction and the common chemical sense. In: Getchell TV, Doty RL, Bartoshuk LM, Snow JBJ, eds. *Smell and Taste in Health and Disease.* New York, NY: Raven Press; 1991:765–785.

64. Schiffman SS, Nagle HT. Effect of environmental pollutants on taste and smell. Otolaryngol Head Neck Surg 1992;106:693–700.

65. Schiffman SS, Gatlin CA. Clinical physiology of taste and smell. Annu Rev Nutr 1993;13:405–436.

66. Cometto-Muniz JE, Cain W. Efficacy of volatile organic compounds in evoking nasal pungency and odor. Arch Environ Health 1993;48:309–314.

67. Commetto-Muniz JE, Cain WS. Sensory reactions of nasal pungency and odor to volatile organic compounds: the alkylbenzenes. Am Ind Hyg Assoc J 1994;55:811–817.

68. Schwartz BS, Doty RL, Monroe C, et al. Olfactory function in chemical workers exposed to acrylate and methacrylate vapors. Am J Pub Health 1989;79:613–618.

69. Frye RE, Schwartz BS, Doty RL. Dose-related effects of cigarette smoking on olfactory function. JAMA 1990;263: 1233–1236.

70. Leopold D, Hornung DE, Schwob JE. Congenital lack of olfactory ability. Ann Otol Rhinol Laryngol 1992;101:229–236.

71. Jafek BW, Gordon AS, Moran DT, et al. Congenital anosmia. Ear Nose Throat J 1990;69:331–337.

72. Spetzler RF, Herman JM, Beals S, et al. Preservation of olfaction in anterior craniofacial approaches. J Neurosurg 1993;79: 48–52.

73. Caviness Jr VS. Kallmann's syndrome—beyond "migration." N Engl J Med 1994;326:1775–1777.

74. Singh N, Grewal MS, Austin JH. Familial anosmia. Arch Neurol 1970;22:40–44.

75. Douek E, Bannister LH, Dodson HC. Recent advances in the pathology of olfaction. Proc Roy Soc Med 1975;68:467–470.

76. Schwob JE, Leopold DA, Mieleszko Szumowski KE, et al. Histopathology of olfactory mucosa in Kallmann's syndrome. Ann Otol Rhinol Laryngol 1993;102: 117–122.

77. Jafek BW, Murrow B, Johnson EW. Olfaction and endoscopic sinus surgery. Ear Nose Throat J 1994;73:548–552.

78. Kern RC, Mathog RH. Neoplasms of the nose and paranasal sinuses. In: Getchell TV, Doty RL, Bartoshuk LM, Snow JBJ, eds. Smell and Taste in Health and Disease. New York, NY: Raven Press; 1991: 599–620.

79. Li C, Youssem DM, Doty RL, et al. Neuroimaging in patients with olfactory dysfunction. AJR 1994;162:411–418.

80. Henkin RI, Smith FR. Hyposmia in acute viral hepatitis. Lancet 1971;1:823–826.

81. Garret-Laster M, Russel RM, Jacques PF. Impairment of taste and olfaction in patients with cirrhosis: the role of vitamin A. Human Nutr: Clin Nutr 1984;38C: 203–214.

82. Shear PK, Butters N, Jernigan TL, et al. Olfactory loss in alcoholics: correlations with cortical and subcortical MRI indices. Alcohol 1992;9:247–255.

83. Settle RG. The chemical senses in diabetes mellitus. In: Getchell TV, Doty RL, Bartoshuk LM, Snow JBJ, eds. Smell and Taste in Health and Disease. New York, NY: Raven Press; 1991:829–843.

84. Weinstock RS, Wright HN, Smith DU. Olfactory dysfunction in diabetes mellitus. Physiol Behav 1993;53:17–21.

85. Le Floch JP, Le Lievre G, Labroque M, et al. Smell dysfunction and related factors in diabetic patients. Diabetes Care 1993; 16:934–937.

86. Henkin RI, Bartter FC. Studies on olfactory threshold in normal man and in patients with adrenal cortical insufficiency: the role of adrenal cortical steroids and of serum sodium concentration. J Clin Invest 1966;45:1631–1639.

87. Mackay-Sim A. Changes in smell and taste function in thyroid, parathyroid, and adrenal diseases. In: Getchell TV, Doty RL, Bartoshuk LM, Snow JBJ, eds. Smell and Taste in Health and Disease. New York, NY: Raven Press; 1991: 817–827.

88. Weinstock RS, Wright HN, Spiegel AM, et al. Olfactory dysfunction in humans with deficit guanine nucleotide-binding protein. Nature 1986;322:635–636.

89. Bancard J, Talairach J. Clinical semiology of the frontal lobe seizures. Adv Neurol 1992; 57:3–58.

90. Luciano D. Partial seizures of frontal and temporal region. Neurolog Clin 1993;11: 805–822.

91. Brody D, Serby M, Ettene N, et al. Olfactory identification deficits in HIV infection. Am J Psychiatry 1991;148:248–250.

92. Everall IP, Lutheral PJ, Lantos PL. Neuronal loss in the frontal cortex in HIV infection. Lancet 1991;337:1119–1121.

93. Levenson JL. Dysosmia and dysgeusia presenting as depression. Gen Hosp Psychiatry 1985;7:171–173.

94. Serby M, Larson P, Kalkstein D. Olfactory sense in psychoses. Biol Psychiatry 1990; 28:830.

95. Wu J, Buchsbaum MS, Moy K, et al. Olfactory memory in unmedicated schizophrenia. Schizophr Res 1993;9:41–47.

96. Jones-Gotman M, Zatorre RJ. Olfactory identification deficits in patients with focal cerebral excision. Neuropsychologia 1988;26:387–400.

97. Fiser A. Changes of olfaction due to aesthetic and functional nose surgery. Acta otorhino-laryngologica Belg 1990;44: 457–460.

98. Kimmelman CP. The risk to olfaction from nasal surgery. Laryngoscope 1994; 104:981–968.

99. Seiden AM, Smith D. Endoscopic intranasal surgery as an approach to restoring olfactory function. Chem Senses 1988;13: 736.

100. Yamagishi M, Hasegawa S, Suzuki S, et

al. Effect of surgical treatment of olfactory disturbance caused by localized ethmoiditis. Clin Otolaryngol 1989;14:405–409.

101. Hosemann W, Goertzen MD, Wohlleben R, et al. Olfaction after endoscopic endonasal ethmoidectomy. Am J Rhinol 1993; 7:11–23.

102. Lanza DC, Deems DA, Doty RL, et al. The effect of human olfactory biopsy on olfaction: a preliminary report. Laryngoscope 1994;104:837–840.

103. Ophir D, Guterman A, Gross-Isseroff R. Changes in smell acuity induced by radiation exposure of the olfactory mucosa. Arch Otolaryngol Head Neck Surg 1988; 114:853–855.

104. Yamagishi M, Nakamura H, Hasegawa S, et al. Immunohistochemical examination of olfactory mucosa in patients with olfactory disturbance. Ann Otol Rhinol Laryngol 1990;99:205–210.

105. Snow Jr JB. Differential diagnosis of transport and sensorineural chemosensory disorders. In: Getchell TV, Doty RL, Bartoshuk LM, Snow JBJ, eds. Smell and Taste in Health and Disease. New York, NY: Raven Press; 1991:469–470.

106. Snow Jr JB, Doty RL, Bartoshuk LM. Clinical evaluation of olfactory and gustatory disorders. In: Getchell TV, Doty RL, Bartoshuk LM, Snow JBJ, eds. *Smell and Taste in Health and Disease.* New York, NY: Raven Press; 1991:463–467.

107. Kimmelman CP. Clinical review of olfaction. Am J Otolaryngol 1993;14:227–239.

108. Mattes RD, Cowart BJ. Dietary assessment of patients with chemosensory disorders. J Am Diet Assoc 1994;94:50–56.

109. Zusho H, Asaka H, Okamoto M. Diagnosis of olfactory disturbance. Auris-Nasus-Larynx 1981;8:19–26.

110. Doty RL. Psychophysical measurement of odor perception in humans. In: Laing DG, Doty RL, Breipohl W, eds. *The Human Sense of Smell.* Berlin: Springer, 1991: 95–134.

111. Cain WS, Cometto-Muniz JE, deWijk RA. Techniques in the quantitative study of human olfaction. In: Serby MJ, Chobor KL, eds. *Science of Olfaction.* New York, NY: Springer-Verlag; 1992:279–308.

112. Hyde M. Auditory evoked potentials. In: Alberti P, Ruben R, eds, *Otologic Medicine and Surgery, Vol 1.* New York, NY: Churchill Livingstone; 1988:443–486.

113. Regan D. Human brain electrophysiology: evoked potentials and evoked magnetic fields in science and medicine. New York, NY: Elsevier; 1989.

114. Scherg M. Fundamentals of dipole source potential analysis. In: Grandori F, et al., eds. *Auditory Evoked Magnetic Fields and Electric Potentials. Advances in Audiology, Vol. 6.* Basel: Karger; 1990: 40–69.

115. Hari R. The neuromagnetic method in the study of the human auditory cortex. In: Grandori F, et al. eds. *Auditory Evoked Magnetic Fields and Electric Potentials. Advances in Audiology,* Vol. 6. Basel: Karger; 1990:222–282.

116. Finkenzeller P. Gemittelte EEG-Potentiale bei olfaktorischer Reizung. Pflugers Arch Ges Physiol 1966;292:76–80.

117. Allison T, Goff W. Human cerebral evoked responses to odorous stimuli. Electroencephalogr Clin Neurophysiol 1967;23:558–60.

118. Osterhammel P, Terkildsen K, Zilstorff K. Electro-olfacto-grams in man. J Laryngol 1969;83:731–3.

119. Geisen M, Mrowinski D. Klinische Untersuchungen mit einem Impulsofaktometer. Arch Klin Exp Ohren Nasen Kehlkopfheilkunde 1970;196:377–380.

120. Herberhold C. Computer-Olfaktometrie mit getrenntem Nachweis von Trigeminus- und Olfaktoriusreaktion. Arch Klin Exp Ohren Nasen Kehlkopfheilkunde 1972;202:394–397.

121. Kobal G, Hummel T. Olfaction: chemosensory evoked potentials in patients with olfactory disturbances. Rhinology 1988;26(suppl):1–18.

122. Aufferman H, Gerull G, Mathe F, et al. Olfactory evoked potentials and contingent negative variation simultaneously recorded for diagnosis of smell disorders. Ann Otol Rhinol Laryngol 1993;102: 6–10.

123. Kobal G, Hummel T. Olfactory evoked potentials in humans. In: Getchell TV, Doty RL, Bartoshuk LM, Snow JBJ, eds. *Smell and Taste in Health and Disease.* New York, NY: Raven Press; 1991:255–275.

124. Evans WJ, Kobal G, Lorig TS, et al. Suggestions for collection and reporting of chemosensory (olfactory) event-related potentials. Chem Senses 1993;18:751–756.

125. Roithmann R, Shankar L, Hawke M, et al. CT imaging in the diagnosis and treatment of sinus disease: A partnership between the radiologist and the otolaryngologist. J Otolaryngol 1993;22:253–260.

126. Zinreich SJ, Kennedy DW, Rosenbaum

AE, et al. Paranasal sinuses: CT imaging requirements for endoscopic surgery. Radiology 1987:163:769–775.

127. Zinreich SJ. Imaging of chronic sinusitis in adults: X-ray, computed tomography, and magnetic resonance imaging. J Allergy Clin Immunol 1992;90:445–451.

128. Kimmelman CP. Medical imaging of smell and taste disorders. In: Getchell TV, Doty RL, Bartoshuk LM, Snow JBJ, eds. *Smell and Taste in Health and Disease.* New York, NY: Raven Press; 1991: 471–479.

129. Hilberg O, Jackson AC, Swift DL, et al. Acoustic rhinometry: evaluation of nasal cavity geometry by acoustic reflection. J Appl Physiol 1989;66:295–303.

130. Cole P. The respiratory role of the upper airways: a selective clinical and pathophysiological review. St Louis, Mo: Mosby 1993.

131. Grymer LF, Illum P, Hilberg O. Septoplasty and compensatory inferior turbinate hypertrophy: a randomized study evaluated by acoustic rhinometry. J Laryngol Otol 1993;107:413–417.

132. Cole P, Roithmann R. Rhinomanometry: clinical applications. In: Gershwin ME, Incado G, eds. *Diseases of the Sinuses: a Comprehensive Textbook of Diagnosis and Treatment.* Totowa-NJ: Humana Press, Inc. 1996 (In press).

133. Roithmann R, Cole P, Chapnik J, et al. Acoustic rhinometry in the evaluation of nasal obstruction. Laryngoscope 1995; 105:275–281.

134. Roithmann R, Cole P, Chapnik J, et al. A correlative study of acoustic rhinometry, nasal resistance and the sensation of nasal patency. J Otolaryngol 1994;23:454–458.

135. Moran DT, Carter RI. Jafek BW. Electron microscopy of human olfactory epithelium reveals a new cell type: the microvillar cell. Brain Res 1982;253:39–46.

136. Kennedy DW. First-line management of sinusitis: a national problem? Otolaryngol Head Neck Surg 1990;103:845–888.

137. Mott AE. Topical corticosteroid therapy for nasal polyposis. In: Getchell TV, Doty RL, Bartoshuk LM, Snow JBJ, eds. *Smell*

*and Taste in Health and Disease.* New York, NY: Raven Press; 1991:553–572.

138. Scott AE. Medical management of taste and smell disorders. Ear Nose Throat 1989;68:386–392.

139. Sahay JN, Ibrahim NBN, Chatterjee SS, et al. Long-term study of flunisolide treatment in perennial rhinitis with special reference to nasal mucosal histology and morphology. Clin Allergy 1980;10: 451–457.

140. Holopainen E, Malmberg H, Binder E. Long-term follow-up of intranasal beclomethasone treatment: a clinical and histological study. Acta Otolaryngologica 1982;386:270–273.

141. Stammberger H. Endoscopic endonasal surgery—concepts in treatment of recurring rhinosinusitis. Part I. Anatomic and pathophysiologic considerations. Otolaryngol Head Neck Surg 1986;94:134–136.

142. Stammberger H. Endoscopic endonasal surgery—concepts in treatment of recurring rhinosinusitis. Part II. Surgical technique. Otolaryngol Head Neck Surg 1986; 94:147–156.

143. Kennedy DW. Prognostic factors, outcomes and staging in ethmoid sinus surgery. Laryngoscope 1992;102(Part 2): 1–18.

144. Duncan RB, Briggs M, Wellington NZ. Treatment of uncomplicated anosmia by vitamin A. Arch Otolaryngol 1962;75: 36–44.

145. Henkin RL, Schecter PJ, Friedewald WT, et al. A double blind study of the effects of zinc sulfate on taste and smell dysfunction. Am J Med Sci 1976;272:285–299.

146. Fosmire GJ. Zinc toxicity. Am J Clin Nutr 1990;51:225–227.

147. Zilstorff K. Olfactory disturbances: diagnosis and treatment. ORL Digest 1972; 37–43.

148. Kaufman MD, Lasiter KR, Shenoy BV. Paroxysmal unilateral dysosmia: a cured patient. Ann Neurol 1988;24:450–451.

149. Schiffman SS, Warwick ZS. Flavor enhancement of foods for the elderly can reverse anorexia. Neurobiol Aging 1988;9: 24–26.

# 17

# Craniofacial Pain

Allan S. Gordon, M.D.
David Mock, D.D.S.

## Introduction

Headache and orofacial pain are ubiquitous and multidimensional. In a telephone survey, Linet et al.[1] found that 57.1% of males and 76.5% of females reported a significant headache within the previous 4 weeks. Locker[2] found that, in a population of noninstitutionalized patients over the age of 50, 37.2% reported oral or facial pain in the previous 4 weeks. One need only stroll along the aisles of a local pharmacy and observe the plethora of headache remedies. It indicates the prevalence of this complaint. It is now well recognized that pain in this region, particularly chronic pain, is a complex, multifactorial sensation, possibly involving multiple processes and structures, including the teeth, oral mucosa, jaws, temporomandibular joints, orofacial muscles, sinuses, nose, pharynx, eyes, and ears. The pain may also be a symptom of a recognized neurological, vascular, or metabolic disease. Pain can be referred from intracranial lesions, from the cervical spine, or even more distant sites. Emotional and psychiatric disorders can also precipitate or exacerbate craniofacial pain. Hence, the diagnosis and management of the patient often

requires a multidisciplinary approach, including dental and medical practitioners with collaboration between the appropriate disciplines.

Appropriate health care must be diagnosis-driven, and this is nowhere more problematic than in the craniofacial complex. If the source or reason for the patient's complaint is not readily apparent, he or she suffers additional distress by being sent from one practitioner to the next with considerable repetition of investigative procedures and also suffers disillusionment. This constant stream of referral, self-referral, coming, and going is often called the craniofacial pain "merry-go-round." In many cases, the protracted course of the pain, combined with the investigation and frustration on the part of both the patient and health practitioners, aggravates and complicates the situation. Invasive attempts at treatment can further complicate the patient's presentation. In difficult cases, there are four considerations in the evaluation of a patient presenting with craniofacial pain. It is important to identify predisposing factors, precipitating factors, perpetuating factors, and protective mechanisms adopted by the patient in an attempt to minimize the pain

From Irwin RS, Curley FJ, Grossman RF (eds): Diagnosis and Treatment of Symptoms of the Respiratory Tract. Armonk, New York, Futura Publishing Company, Inc., © 1997.

and/or related dysfunction. (Dr. Jon Hunter, personal communication).

It is beyond the scope of this chapter to deal with all aspects of craniofacial pain. Indeed textbooks are written about craniofacial pain and headache (see Neurologic Clinics, November 1990; Medical Clinics of North America, May 1991; Wolff's Headache; and other textbooks referred to in this chapter). Instead, dentoalveolar causes, disorders related to the temporomandibular apparatus, and the most common neurological disorders will be discussed. Pain arising from diseases of the eyes, ears, nose, sinuses, throat, and mouth are covered elsewhere in this text. This chapter will not discuss serious intracranial pathology. such as subarachnoid hemmorhage, subdural hematoma, space occupying lesions, or raised intracranial pressure as causes of craniofacial pain, nor will it discuss meningitis or other causes of meningeal irritation. Lastly, it will not discuss temporal arteritis, other "vascular" headaches, or posttraumatic headache.

## Diagnosis

### History

Despite the monumental advances made in the past few decades in diagnostic imaging and laboratory investigation, a complete and competent patient history is still the most valuable tool in the diagnosis of craniofacial pain. Although potentially tedious, the patient must be allowed to describe the onset, development of the symptoms, and any associated trauma or events.

He or she must be asked to indicate the sites of the symptoms manually, rather than just by description. Patients often have a different understanding of their anatomy than the clinician. For example, it is not unusual for a patient to describe pain in the "jaw joints" only to indicate the angle of the mandible or the temple. Daily variations in the symptoms or their relationship to jaw function, stress, or other activity should be questioned. The duration of the pain, its severity, and pos-

sible triggers should be pursued and any associated limitation of mandibular movement or noises emanating from the temporomandibular joints should be noted. If the patient describes multiple symptoms, such as facial pain and headaches, the temporal relationship of these could be significant. Similarly, the patient should be asked about any other associated features, such as photophobia, phonophobia, and nasal or sinus symptoms. These might suggest a migrainous disorder. Although the policy of always assuming one disease is usually applicable, the possibility of more than one unrelated disorder must also be considered. If the patient complains of any loss or alteration of sensation, the patient should again be asked to manually outline the region, and if confirmed on clinical examination, a space occupying lesion must be ruled out.

Noting other possibly related symptoms such as tinnitus, vertigo, or perceived hearing loss may also suggest a direction for further investigation. Any sleep disturbance, change in libido, anhedonia, or loss of appetite, energy, memory, or concentration may suggest an emotional or psychiatric component to the patient's complaints. Often, questioning the patient about his or her predominant mood will open a floodgate of valuable information. Parafunctional habits, such as bruxism, teeth-clenching or nail-biting, may also contribute to the patient's symptoms, although excessive emphasis on these prevalent habits is a common error.

Comparing the patient's evaluation of the magnitude of impact of their craniofacial symptoms on their normal life functioning to the clinical findings can also be useful. Finally, the patient's previous treatment and their response should be noted. This can avoid wasting time pursuing either a diagnosis that can be discounted or a treatment doomed to failure. In addition, the patient's medication history might suggest that at least some of their complaints are drug-related or iatrogenic.

There are certain danger symptoms that should alert the clinician that a more serious medical or neurological condition is present. These symptoms include changes in the pattern of headache or facial pain; "the worst headache I ever had"; measurable worsening of headache or pain over a defined period of time; changes in cognition; new onset in an elderly patient; a history of trauma, neck stiffness, fever and other systemic complaints; the complaint of facial, bulbar, or limb weakness; sensory symptoms; diplopia; vertigo; or associated medical diseases. In these situations, a complete neurological evaluation is indicated.

All practitioners should carry out a preliminary and cursory psychological evaluation, such as described herein. If psychological factors or disorders are suggested, appropriate referrals should be made. One must be very cautious in labeling individuals as having "functional" or "psychosomatic" disorders without appropriate corroborating opinions and/or evidence as such labels are subsequently difficult to eliminate.

## Physical Examination

The initial evaluation of a patient can be divided into two phases: orofacial and neurological. These should not be considered independently but in concert.

### Orofacial Examination

The evaluation begins as the patient enters the examining room. The patient's gait and posture, as well as any evidence of facial swelling or asymmetry should be noted.

The clinical examination begins with the palpation of the temporomandibular joints and facial/masticatory musculature. Grading the tenderness to pressure is valuable in evaluating its significance. High-grade (grade III) tenderness is readily apparent by the patient's immediate, marked avoidance reaction; whereas, mild tenderness (grade I) requires the patient to ponder momentarily when questioned about soreness. Moderate tenderness (grade II)

falls somewhere between these two responses. The facial aspect of the joints can be located by applying the fingers to the face anterior to the ears bilaterally and having the patient open and close the mouth (Figure 1). Pressure should also be applied to the posterior aspect of the joints, via the external auditory meatus, to evaluate tenderness in the posterior capsule and ligaments (Figure 1). The masseter, sternomastoid, and temporalis muscles can also be palpated extraorally (Figures 2 and 3). Tenderness should be recorded in the superior, middle, and inferior aspects of the masseter and the anterior, middle, and posterior aspects of the temporalis. Intraorally, the coronoid attachment of the temporalis can be found by running one finger up the anterior ramus of the mandible, (Figure 3) and the zygomatic attachment of the masseter by applying pressure laterally below the zygoma (Figure 2). The lateral pterygoid region is evaluated by applying pressure with one finger in the posterior buccal sulcus adjacent to the second and third maxillary molar teeth (Figure 3).

Having the patient open and close their mouth with the tips of the fingers over the temporomandibular joints facilitate detection of clicks or crepitus. Whether these are audible or palpable and whether they occur on opening and/or closing should be recorded to assist in determining their significance. A reciprocal click may suggest a self-reducing disc displacement.

The range of mandibular movement should also be recorded, particularly mandibular opening. The normal range is quite variable but extreme limitation may be significant. Similarly, deviation of the mandible on opening or an inability to move the mandible laterally in a relatively symmetrical fashion may suggest unilateral muscle spasm or physical obstruction of movement. The clinician must also consider the possibility that the patient is guarding movement to avoid pain. Any pain on mandibular movement and its site should also be recorded. Intraorally, the general state of the patient's dentition should be evaluated, particularly the level

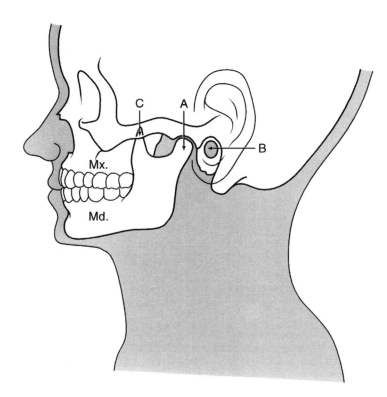

**Figure 1.** Diagrammatic representation of the lateral skull. (a) Condylar head of the mandible, palpable facially in front of the external auditory meatus. (b) Anterior wall of the auditory canal. Pressure in the direction of the arrow is transmitted to the posterior aspect of the temporomandibular joint, including the posterior capsule and attachment of the disk. (c) Coronoid process of the mandible, to which the anterior fibres of the temporalis muscle attach. mx = maxilla; md = mandible.

of dental maintenance, missing teeth, or obvious dental disease. The occlusion should also be examined, concentrating on whether it appears functional or not. It is also important to ensure that no oral lesions are overlooked and palpation of the major salivary glands is advisable.

If any dental abnormalities are detected or suggested by the history, dental sensitivity to percussion and/or pressure can be evaluated. Selective anesthesia is also useful to determine the significance of dental disease. If the history suggested any alteration of sensation, this also can be examined with a pin or needle, following the distribution of the appropriate cranial nerves.

The need for radiographic examination can be evaluated at this point. Particularly, the need for dental radiographs, including a panoramic view (Figure 4), should be considered. Technetium bone scans are a sensitive means of detecting dentoalveolar disease, not visible on routine radiographs, or active arthritis (Figure 5). Where a temporomandibular disorder is suspected, tomograms may be useful to examine for disorders or changes in the articular bony surfaces. Arthrography, an invasive procedure, and magnetic resonance imaging (MRI) have also been proven useful in the evaluation of the internal anatomy and dynamics of the temporomandibular joint; however, the necessity for their routine use is questionable.[3]

## Neurological Examination

A neurological examination, if required, should be performed by a physi-

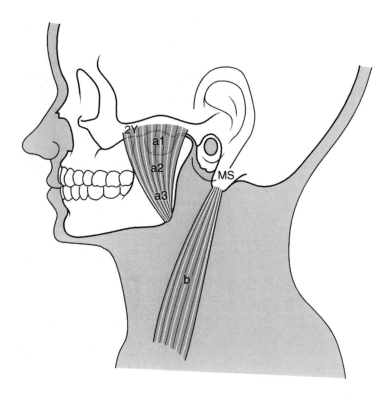

**Figure 2.** Diagrammatic representation of the lateral skull. **A:** Masseter muscle, extending from the zygomatic process of the maxilla (zy) to the angle of the mandible: a1 = superior; a2 = middle; a3 = inferior. **B:** Sternomastoid muscle, extending from the mastoid process (ms) to the clavicle.

cian and, other than the cursory procedures mentioned above, are not within the expertise of a dental practitioner. Physicians, on the other hand, must perform such an examination. We will herein only emphasize those aspects of the neurological assessment most pertinent to the patient presenting with craniofacial pain. This includes assessment of level of consciousness, mental status, language and speech; and cranial nerves I to XII—particularly funduscopic exam, pupils, and eye movements, muscle of mastication and muscles of facial expression, facial sensation, hearing, and the bulbar functions. In addition evaluation of the motor system, primary and secondary sensory abnormalities, deep tendon reflexes, plantar responses, coordination and gait, and cervical and lumbar spine examination is necessary. Danger signs include change in consciousness, cognition and language;

spasticity, and other focal motor or sensory findings that may suggest a hemispheric lesion; abnormal eye movements and nystagmus; limb or gait ataxia; asymmetrical reflexes and Babinski responses; papilledema and pupillary asymmetry; and neck stiffness. A progressive change or deterioration in neurological function always suggests an organic process. Lastly the presence of systemic findings or other disease processes should always suggest the presence of a structural neurological disease.

*Laboratory Testing*

Other testing including neurophysiological testing, such as electroencephalography (EEG), electromyography (EMG), nerve conduction studies, multimodal sensory evoked response testing, and ves-

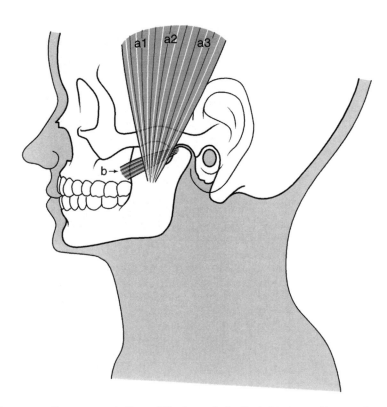

**Figure 3.** Diagrammatic representation of the lateral skull. **A:** Temporalis muscle: a1 = anterior; a2 = middle; a3 = posterior. **B:** Lateral pterygoid muscle extends from the pterygoid plates to the condylar head and capsule of the temporomandibular joint, deep to the mandible.

tibular function testing, should be performed together with imaging techniques including computed tomography (CT) scanning, single photon-emitting computerized tomography (SPECT), and MRI. These are carried out in order to determine the location and cause of the neurological process.

### Diagnostic Approach to Chronic Craniofacial Pain

This can be found in algorithmic form in Figure 6.

## Differential Diagnosis, Pathogenesis and Treatment: A Practical Classification of Craniofacial Pain

The utility of any classification system depends on its applicability to the clinical situation and its effect on patient care. Attempts to classify headache and facial pain have tended to reflect the particular field of interest of the author(s). The Craniofacial Pain Research Unit at Mount Sinai Hospital (CFPRU), of which the authors of this chapter are affiliated, is composed of health practitioners from various fields (Anaesthesiology, Dentistry, Neurology, Otolaryngology, Psychiatry). We suggest an applied classification, expanded and modified after the IHS Classification[4] and incorporating the suggestions of Solomon and Lipton[5] and Kudrow[6,7] (Table I).

### Dentoalveolar Pain

Dental disease is the most common cause of orofacial pain. In most cases the source of the pain is apparent and treat-

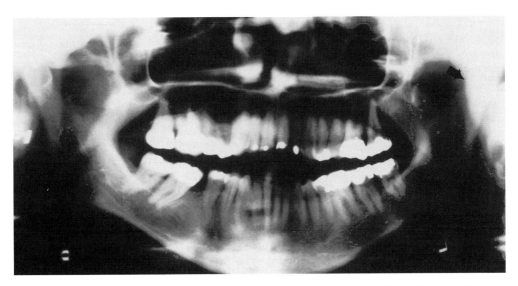

**Figure 4.** A panoramic radiograph of the maxilla and mandible. The left condylar neck is hyperplastic **(arrows)**, as compared to the right.

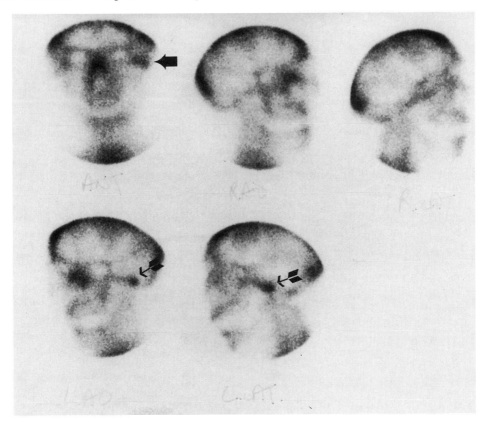

**Figure 5.** Technetium bone scan demonstrating increased uptake, suggestive of active arthritis of the left temporomandibular joint **(arrows)**.

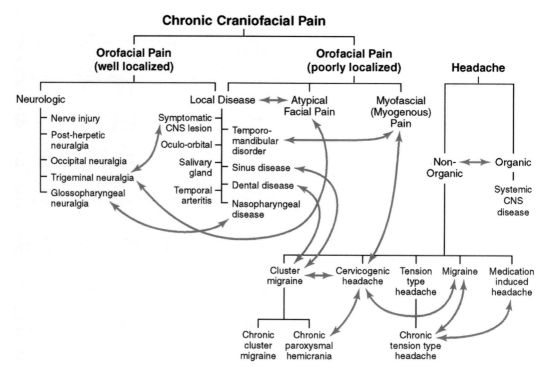

**Figure 6.** Diagnostic algorithm for chronic craniofacial pain. Arrows indicate common diagnostic dilemmas. CNS = central nervous system; TMD = temporomandibular disorders.

ment can be administered without delay. Even in cases where an orofacial pain is poorly localized, a dental cause should be the first consideration. The sensory innervation of the teeth and supporting structures is supplied by branches of the trigeminal nerve, V2 the maxilla, and V3 the mandible. The human dentition consists of 28 teeth (excluding third molars or "wisdom teeth"), suspended in supportive alveolar bone by a periodontal ligament. Dental pain may originate from either the teeth themselves, the periodontal structures, or the alveolar bone.

## Pulpal Pain

Pain of pulpal origin is often poorly localized by the patient.[8,9] The dental pulp occupies the center of the tooth, surrounded with dentin, with tubules containing processes of the odontoblasts within parallel tubules. The cell bodies of the odontoblasts line the dentinal wall of the pulp and the remainder consists of rather primitive mesenchymal tissue, blood vessels, and nerve fibers. The exterior of the tooth is covered by enamel. Whereas the latter is insensitive, any stimulus to the odonoblastic processes or the dental pulp will elicit pain. At times, the patient cannot even identify whether the pain is maxillary or mandibular. Since the sensory capability of the dental pulp, for clinical purposes, is almost entirely nociceptive, any stimulus at threshold levels will elicit pain. Thus, even thermal stimulation of exposed dentine or root surfaces will elicit a painful response. A tooth with an inflamed pulp can be identified by a disproportionate response to otherwise non-noxious stimulation, such as heat or cold. Electrical stimulation can also be used clinically, although the interpretation of fine distinctions in the level of stimulation required to elicit a response is po-

**Table I**
A Practical Classification of Craniofacial Pain

I. Dentoalveolar Pain
  a. Pulpal
  b. Periodontal and Alveolar
II. Pain Arising from the Temporomandibular Joint and Related Apparatus (TMD)
  a. Intra/Peri-articular
  b. Musculo-ligamentous
  c. Combination of a. and b.
III. Pain Arising from Diseases of the Eyes, Ears, Nose, Sinuses, Throat, and Mouth
IV. Pain of Neurological Origin
  1. Migraine
    a. Migraine Without Aura
    b. Migraine With Aura
    c. Migraine Equivalents
    d. Complicated Migraine
  2. Tension-type headache
    a. Episodic
    b. Chronic
    c. Chronic Daily Headache Syndrome
  3. Mixed Tension-Vascular Headache
  4. Medication-Induced Headache
  5. Cluster Migraine
    a. Episodic Cluster
    b. Chronic Cluster
      i) Unremitting from onset (primary)
      ii) Evolved from episodic (secondary)
    c. Chronic Paroxysmal Hemicrania
  6. Temporal Arteritis
  7. Vascular Headache
    a. Subarachnoid Hemorrhage
    b. Intracerebral Hemorrhage
    c. Cerebral Ischemia
    d. Hypertension
  8. Due to Raised Intracranial Pressure, Traction, or Inflammation
  9. Cranial Neuralgias, Nerve Trunk Pain, and Deafferentation Pain
    a. Persistent (Not Tic-like) Pain of Cranial Nerve Origin
      i) Compression or distortion of cranial nerve origin
      ii) Demyelination of cranial nerves
      iii) Infarction of cranial nerves
      iv) Inflammation of cranial nerves
        a. Herpes Zoster
        b. Postherpetic neuralgia
        c. Other
    b. Cranial Neuralgias
      i) Trigeminal neuralgia
        a. Primary (idiopathic) trigeminal neuralgia
        b. Secondary trigeminal neuralgia
          — Primary intracranial tumors
          — Secondary tumors
          — Multiple sclerosis
          — Vascular malformations (ie, aneurysm)
        c. Special types
          — Posttraumatic trigeminal neuralgia
          — Cluster-tic syndrome
      ii) Glossopharyngeal neuralgia
      iii) Occipital neuralgia
      iv) Other including nerve injuries
    c. Central Causes
      i) Anaesthesia dolorosa
      ii) Thalamic pain
      iii) Atypical facial pain (AFP)
        a. Primary AFP (possibly exacerbated by a dental or surgical procedure)
        b. Secondary AFP
          — Precipitated by dental treatment or orofacial surgery
          — Posttraumatic
        c. Associated with migraine or TMD
        d. Burning Mouth Syndrome
  10. Posttraumatic Headache (PTH)
    a. Acute PTH
    b. Chronic PTH
  11. Cervicogenic Headache
  12. Miscellaneous Headache

tentially fraught with error. The most valuable tool in identifying pulpal pain is the detection of a cause, such as, a recent large restoration, dental caries, or a fracture. At times, the cause is not readily apparent. If the caries is beneath a restoration or the tooth has been cracked without separation of the parts, it may be overlooked. Acute pulpal pain may vary from a hypersensitivity to severe acute pain, but will usually be exacerbated by thermal change. Occasionally, an acute pulpitis may progress into a chronic state producing a lower grade pain and often decreased pulpal sensitivity. In the latter case, the pain may disappear completely, only to recur with subsequent injury. Often the pain will remit once the pulp of the tooth dies and not recur until the periodontium or alveolar bone is involved. Where the patient cannot even isolate whether the pain is maxillary or mandibular, selective local anaesthesia may be helpful.

### Periodontal and Alveolar Pain

Unlike pulpal pain, periodontal pain is usually well localized and the patient can indicate the site. Periodontal pain can originate from a primary periodontal problem; however, in most cases it is the result of progression from a necrotic tooth pulp, producing an apical periodontitis. In these cases, there is not usually any significant reaction to thermal change but the offending tooth will be acutely tender to percussion or often even pressure. Thus, the patient will complain of pain on eating or even closing their teeth together. They may also claim that the tooth feels elevated in its socket, resulting from the accumulation of pus or edema in the apical periodontal tissues. With time, the infection will involve the alveolar bone at the tooth apex and an apical abscess may result. The symptoms of the latter are similar to those of an apical periodontitis; however a spreading infection may follow.

Primary periodontal pain may result from trauma, dental manipulation, localized periodontitis, or even a foreign body embedded between the teeth. A fractured tooth can also result in a localized, painful periodontal lesion, even if the tooth has been devitalized by endodontic treatment. In many instances, the cause may not be readily apparent, even though the patient can quite precisely localize the site.

Some discomfort can be associated with eruption of teeth and, although this is anticipated in childhood, it is unexpected later in life when the third molars erupt. If a tooth is prevented from complete eruption or impacted, the follicle may become infected resulting in a pericoronitis. Similarly, the flap of mucosa overlying a par-

tially erupted tooth may become inflamed giving rise to an operculitis. Either of these situations will also result in pain. The pain may be localized to the site of inflammation or may refer to adjacent structures. Thus, pain from an impacted third molar may refer to the opposite arch, maxillary sinuses, temporal region, or ear. Inflammation from the region of an impacted mandibular third molar can involve the attachment of the masseter muscle resulting in spasm and pain. Occasionally, infection from a mandibular third molar will track back into the pterygomandibular space resulting in trismus and oropharyngeal pain.

## Temporomandibular Disorders

The temporomandibular disorders (TMD) are a poorly understood complex of clinical problems involving the temporomandibular joints (TMJ), associated structures, and related musculature.[10] Initially described by Costen[11] as a single syndrome of pain in the region of the ear, tinnitus, dizziness, and dysphagia, it is now understood to be a collection of musculoskeletal disorders with similar and often overlapping symptomatology. Costen related the symptoms to occlusal disorders; however, it is now understood that the cause is usually multifactorial, including predisposing, precipitating, and perpetuating factors. The patient's symptoms can originate from articular soft tissues, bone, the muscles of mastication, or various combinations. At present, there is no evidence to support the hypothesis that these conditions are necessarily progressive, and there is considerable evidence supporting the concept that they often remit without or despite treatment. This has unfortunately led to false reinforcement of the efficacy of various treatment modalities based on anecdotal evidence. The need for therapy therefore should be based on a detailed clinical history and a careful clinical examination, understanding that most patients will improve with minimal or no treatment. A corollary to this conclusion is that, in most cases, the treatment should not result in any irreversible changes to the patient's anatomy or dental function.

Symptoms of a TMD include pain in the TMJ and craniofacial-cervical region. The pain is often described as a dull, steady pain with severe exacerbations. The pain can also masquerade as temporal headache, ear ache, or posterior auricular pain. The patient also may give a history of a bothersome clicking, popping, or grating noise in the TMJ. This is often accompanied by limitation of mandibular movement or a "locking" of the jaw. Additional complaints may include occlusal instability, jaw fatigue, and difficulty in chewing, yawning, or talking. The pain can be aggravated by chewing, extensive talking, hard exercise, clenching, and other oral parafunctional habits, and it may be alleviated by rest, limitation of mandibular movement, or analgesics.

Clinical examination usually reveals tenderness to pressure over the TMJ and/or the muscles of mastication. Clicking or crepitus may be audible or palpable emanating from the TMJ with movement and there may be demonstrable limitation of mandibular movement. Generally, movement of the mandible will elicit pain. Although the patient may complain of a hearing loss or altered sensation, none will usually be demonstrable.

Various etiologic factors have been implicated but none have been identified unambiguously or conclusively. As noted earlier, it is generally accepted that the cause of TMD is generally multifactorial. From the history and examination, predisposing factors—such as a nonfunctional occlusion, congenital or developmental malformations, alterations of the periarticular or intra-articular soft tissue or articular degenerative changes, and arthritides—may be discovered.

Patients with TMD, particularly those with an apparently related history of trauma, have a multiplicity of complaints. They may have diffuse muscle pain and have symptoms and signs suggestive of fibromyalgia.[12] These patients complain of diffuse myalgia, have specific tender fibrositic points, a sleep disturbance, and depression. They may also complain of poor memory, altered appetite and libido, and fatigue. They are often unable to work and seem more disabled than one would expect given the nature of their trauma.

The precipitating event could be anything from a prolonged dental appointment to direct physical trauma. Temporomandibular disorders are often encountered subsequent to a less direct traumatic event or associated with other musculoskeletal injury, such as in a motor vehicle accident. A chronic posttraumatic TMD is often refractory to treatment, conservative or otherwise, and can be associated with an increased incidence of neuropsychological deficits, reminiscent of a mild traumatic brain injury.[13,14] Perpetuating factors can include the various predisposing factors, psychological or psychiatric disorders, or parafunctional habits.

A number of techniques have been proposed as diagnostic aids for use in patients suspected of having a TMD. These include sonography, EMG, ultrasound, and various jaw-tracking devices. There is not sufficient evidence to support their application in the clinical evaluation of such patients.[15–18] In fact, there may be a risk of misdirecting the patient's management.

Ideally, treatment or management of a disease or disorder is directed by a specific diagnosis and an understanding of the etiology. In this case, management has to be empirical because of the heterogeneous nature of the TMDs, the multifactorial etiology, and the absence of scientifically corroborated treatment modalities. Generally, initial treatment is symptomatic. This consists of reassurance of the patient, jaw exercises and/or physical therapy, and analgesics. Where the patient's symptoms appear to be primarily muscular in origin, moist heat application and muscle relaxants can be prescribed. On the other hand, if the patient's symptoms seem to originate from the TMJs themselves, local application of ice and nonsteroidal anti-inflammatory drugs may be preferable. Intra-articular injections of steroids may be useful where one of the arthritides is indicated; whereas, intramuscular trigger point injections can be considered where specific muscular trigger points can be demonstrated. Tricyclic antidepressants have been shown to be useful in the management of many chronic pain situations as well. The possible inter-relationship between some TMDs and a sleep disorder is presently under investigation.

Rest is a fundamental component of TMD management. Generally, voluntary resting of the mandible by avoidance of tough chewy foods and avoiding wide opening is adequate. Rarely, interarch wiring or elastics are necessary, and care must be exercised to avoid dental damage. Intraoral occlusal appliances may assist in controlling the influence of predisposing or perpetuating factors such as parafunctional habits or malocclusion. An interocclusal stabilizing appliance provides a balanced occlusion without interferences and avoids any irreversible alteration of the dentition. Appliances that reposition the mandible are, at best, rarely indicated and risk producing irreversible changes in the patient's dentition. It has been suggested that where such an appliance is used and the patient's symptoms have been reduced, the device should be slowly adjusted to return the mandible to its normal position. The relationship between dental occlusion and TMDs is inconclusive and, more significantly, there is no compelling evidence to support the routine adjustment of occlusion in its treatment.[19,20]

Psychological and behavioral techniques may be useful adjuncts to treatment to assist the patient by providing coping skills. Where indicated by the patient's history, psychiatric assessment and/or treatment may be valuable to control predisposing or perpetuating factors.

Surgical intervention is indicated for specific articular disorder; however, even in these cases, the influence of other perpetuating or predisposing factors may complicate the recovery and outcome. The American Association of Oral and Maxillofacial Surgeons has suggested the following criteria for candidates for temporomandibular joint surgery:[21]

(1) documented TMJ internal derangement or other structural joint disorders with appropriate imaging;

(2) positive evidence to suggest that the symptoms and objective findings are a result of a structural disorder;

(3) pain and/or dysfunction of such magnitude as to constitute a disability to the patient;

(4) prior unsuccessful nonsurgical treatment;

(5) prior management to the extent possible, of bruxism, oral parafunctional habits, other medical or dental conditions, and other contributing factors that may affect the outcome of surgery;

(6) patient consent after a discussion of potential complications, goals to achieve, success rate, timing, postoperative management, and alternative approaches including no treatment.

Surgical management may include arthrocentesis, arthroscopy, or open arthrotomy, with soft and/or hard tissue alteration.

A team approach to these patients is necessary in order to be successful, since they have complaints involving many different systems.

## Atypical Facial Pain

Atypical facial pain (AFP) is defined as a persistent, chronic facial pain that does not fulfill the criteria of trigeminal neuralgia or other cranial neuralgias. It is not associated with objective neurological, craniofacial, or dental findings and often presents with a nonanatomical distribution. It has been known as phantom tooth pain,[22,23] atypical odontalgia,[24] atypical facial neuralgia,[23] migratory odontalgia,[5] and the wandering tooth syndrome.[25]

Frazier and Russell first differentiated these patients from those with trigeminal neuralgia in 1924.[25] Since then, it has been extensively studied and, because it is often a diagnosis of exclusion, it lends itself to abuse.

The cause of AFP is uncertain. Deafferentation is suspected in some cases of repeated nerve injury or trauma, resulting in central neuronal hyperactivity.[26,27] There appears to be a patient susceptibility factor, predisposing these patients to a chronic pain syndrome. In the view of the members of the Craniofacial Pain Research Unit, those individuals with recurrent headache, previous chronic pain syndrome or affective or somatoform disorders seem to be more susceptible to the development of AFP (personal communication). Investigations examining neuropsychological parameters and sleep disorders as well as some of the other factors mentioned are currently underway.

Patients with AFP complain of constant, burning or boring, deep and poorly defined pain, in contrast to trigeminal neuralgia, which is characterized by localized, lancinating, spasmodic pain with trigger zones. Women predominate and, although the average age is between 40 and 50, the age can range from 20 to 70 with a bimodal distribution.[28,29] Patients may present with symptoms suggestive of dental pain involving one or several teeth either sequentially or concurrently. The pain may cross the midline and is often not anatomically consistent. It may appear simultaneously in multiple quadrants.

When the patient's pain has a throbbing character, migraine may be suspected. Tender cervicofacial musculature may suggest an associated myofascial pain. Dental disease is often suspected first, leading to needless dental restorations, endodontic treatment, and extractions usually resulting in aggravation and perpetuation of the patient's pain.[28,30] In some cases, the pain is precipitated by a dental or surgical procedure or facial trauma (secondary AFP). There are often associated, possibly predisposing and perpetuating, affective disorders, somatization, and other personality disturbances, as well as disordered sleep.[28,31,32] Further research is indicated to determine whether these are primary or secondary to the chronic pain syndrome.

Classifying these patients is a challenge. A practical classification is suggested in Table I. Loeser[33] suggests that there are four types of unilateral AFP patients. The first type is associated with sensory findings and nerve damage after either sinus or dental surgery, trauma, or after surgery for a trigeminal neuralgia. In-

clusion of this kind of patient in an AFP group is questionable because there is clear-cut nerve injury. The second type progresses insidiously, eventually showing signs of a trigeminal neuropathy. A deep, basal neoplasm or infection is often demonstrated and therefore classification as a "secondary" trigeminal neuralgia seems most appropriate. The third have cluster/vascular components and likely should be classified with those conditions. The fourth type occurs without antecedent and the patient complains of a burning, constant, and usually circumscribed pain and fits more closely with the presentation classically encountered and described above. This classification does not relate the dental and other precipitating or exacerbating procedures to the condition. Clearly, other types of objective parameters need to be delineated to adequately classify and understand these conditions. As in other chronic craniofacial syndromes, the patient's ultimate disorder often seems to be the result of a relatively innocuous precipitating event in a predisposed patient. The patient's symptoms are then perpetuated by other psychological or physiological factors including multiple dental and other interventions.

The AFP patient presents a difficult challenge for both diagnosis and management. A collaborative, multidisciplinary approach is essential with the combined expertise of dentists and neurologists necessary. Psychiatric evaluation is more effective and accepted if it is a part of the early assessment, rather than a late referral, after all other diagnostic and therapeutic procedures have proven fruitless. When indicated, an otolaryngological or ophthamalogical consultation is also useful. Structural or neurological disease must be ruled out by clinical examination and appropriate imaging. Speculative dental treatment is contraindicated. Panoramic dental views, SPECT bone scans of facial bones, CT scans, and MRI are also useful when indicated.

These patients have a peculiar and often unique presentation. They are often angry about their treatment history (frequently with justification). They have peculiar responses to placebo "anaesthetic" injections[34] and, in a recently completed study in our center (G. Swartz et al. In preparation) designed to test the efficacy of treating their pain with parenteral administration of calcitonin, AFP patients responded with disproportionate and vigorous nausea and vomiting. They generally have little insight into their problem and are demanding of solutions, while blaming previous treating practitioners for their dilemma. They often document their treatment and the various practitioners that they have seen, arriving with a lengthy, detailed chronicle.

The patients are generally not compliant with their medications. Tricyclic amines, such as amitryptiline or nortryptiline,[5,24] may offer relief but patients often discontinue the medication prematurely.[34] Analgesics are commonly ineffective[35] and nonsteroidal anti-inflammatories, at best, may give temporary relief. In our experience, carbamazepine and valproic acid are of limited value in this condition and nonpharmacological treatments also tend not to be helpful.[35] Neurosurgical procedures, including nerve block and "tic" surgery, are usually counterproductive.[35] A conservative multidisciplinary approach, employing tricyclics in modest doses, is recommended.

## Burning Mouth Syndrome

There are a variety of known conditions that can result in a generalized or localized burning sensation of the oral mucous membranes. These include nutritional deficiencies, endocrinopathies, xerostomia, anemias, and superficial candidiasis.[36] In turn, some of these are secondary to other diseases and disorders. Unfortunately, in most cases, no organic basis for the patient's complaints is apparent. In these cases, the condition is referred to as a burning mouth syndrome. Although we have classified it under AFP, many would give it a separate designation and we are describing it separately. When the burning is localized, a local irritant can be implicated. For example, an abundance

of calculus on the lingual aspect of the mandibular incisor teeth can produce a sensitivity and burning of the tip of the tongue. Alterations of sensory perception have been demonstrated in patients with this syndrome.[37-39]

Any reduction in the quantity or change in the quality of saliva can result in a burning sensation of the oral mucosa. With increasing age, there is such a change and thus an accompanying oral discomfort. Destruction of salivary gland tissue is a component of the triad of Sjögren's syndrome, along with a loss of lacrimation and a collagen disease, such as rheumatoid arthritis or lupus erythematosis. A variety of drugs in common use also affect salivation and, hence, can cause a burning mouth as a secondary effect. This is particularly noticeable with the antidepressants and antihypertensives.

After a thorough investigation has failed to elucidate an underlying organic basis for the patients complaint, all that remains is a diagnosis of idiopathic burning mouth syndrome. Some have linked this with AFP and others have speculated that it is a manifestation of depression or other psychological disorders.[40,41] In reality, this symptom can likely result from a wide spectrum of organic and inorganic disorders; however, many cases will still remain idiopathic. Although often responsive to antidepressant therapy,[39] some cases can only be treated symptomatically.

## Trigeminal Neuralgia

There are few human conditions more tormenting than the sharp, severe, jabbing pains of trigeminal neuralgia (TN) or tic douloureux. Long known as a severely painful condition affecting an older population, the patients are subject to numerous attempts at surgical and medical treatment, yet are frequently misdiagnosed.

Primary TN commonly manifests after the age of 50. Although it can present in the third or fourth decade, these cases are notable. An early onset should always suggest the possibility of a secondary TN and therefore another disorder sought. Females are usually cited as being slightly more often affected than males, 3 : 2 according to Solomon and Lipton.[5] However, Loeser[33] suggests that the incidence may be equal. An attack is classically unilateral with the right side being more commonly affected than the left. The condition clearly respects anatomical boundaries, affecting one or more branches of the fifth cranial nerve (V1, V2, V3). The third (mandibular) division or V3 is most commonly involved, with the second (maxillary) or V2 and the first (ophthalmic) or V1 following respectively. Simultaneous involvement of V2 & V3 is also quite common. The condition is never simultaneously bilateral but in 3% of cases it can affect both sides during different attacks.

The pain is electriclike or shocklike, of short duration and spasmodic, generally causing the patient to wince or eliciting an avoidance reaction. At times, a series of lancinating pains come together in a staccatolike manner. The attacks can be stereotyped. There may be pain-free periods between attacks and occasionally months or years can intervene. Trigger spots are common in the scalp, nostril, cheek, face, upper lip, teeth or gums. The patient usually complains that even lightly touching these areas, such as with a hairbrush, a wisp of cotton, a jet of cold air, a washcloth, a toothbrush or a razor, will trigger the pain. Talking or kissing can induce a spasm of pain. Some patients refuse to wash or shave the affected part of their face or brush their teeth. Presentation in an older person with poor dentition may lead to the mistaken diagnosis of dental disease causing unnecessary dental treatment or extraction. A constant pain prodrome has been reported, and may complicate the early diagnosis.[42] Sometimes patients complain of a constant burning, background with superimposed ticlike bursts.

Increasingly there have been reports of variants. Alberca and Ochoa[43] describe a cluster-tic syndrome with features of cluster headache and TN, and Shankland[44] discusses typical and atypical trigeminal neuralgia, a variation not included in the classifications to date.

When there is an accompanying sensory alteration or other cranial nerve abnormality, a primary cause should be sought. Schwannomas, meningiomas, and multiple sclerosis should be considered. A recent Mayo Clinic study of approximately 3000 patients revealed that 10% had a tumor.[45] The authors recall a case of carcinoma of the maxillary sinus presenting as TN-like spasmodic facial pain. Quite often structural lesions present with trigeminal neuropathic pain which is more constant, often associated with sensory loss, and which does not share all the spasmodic features of TN.[46] Dental disease may mimic TN and TN may present as dental pain. Rarely cases are seen which begin after dental trauma. Atypical facial pain can usually be differentiated by the characteristics of the pain. When pain is induced by chewing, disorders of the TM joint apparatus must be considered.

Jannetta[47,48] has suggested that TN results from compression of the trigeminal nerve root by an adjacent artery or other vascular lesion with continuous pulsation leading to secondary changes and spontaneous discharges. The superior cerebellar artery may compress the rostral component of the nerve producing V2 and V3 pain. The anterior inferior cerebellar artery may compress the caudal and posterior portion of the nerve producing V1 pain. This theory has been supported by Hamlin and King.[49] Recently, Ochoa et al.[50] reported a case of basilar artery ectasia associated with TN.

Ratner et al.[51] and Shaber and Krol[52] have popularized the concept of a peripheral cause of TN with jaw microinfections leading to localized nerve damage and deafferentation. Central theories suggest hyperactivity in the trigeminal nucleus and reverberating circuits centrally, like epilepsy.[53–55]

Pagni[55] presents a unifying theory which suggests that TN is a type of sensory reflex epilepsy. The posterior root is damaged or distorted by a vessel or compressed by another lesion producing demyelination and/or microneuromas. This chronic damage leads to ectopic impulses and afterdischarges which kindle spontaneous impulse generation in the gasserian ganglion and an epileptic subliminal focus in the trigeminal nucleus which induces "seizures" of pain in the gasserian ganglion and the trigeminal nucleus.

Careful neurological examination is mandatory to exclude sensory loss or other alterations suggestive of a primary lesion or disease. Similarly, careful dental and sinus examination is also necessary, including enlisting the aid of imaging techniques. Cheng et al.[45] confirmed the clinical impression of a high incidence of structural lesions.

The mainstay of medical treatment is carbamazepine controlling symptoms in 70% to 80% of those treated.[56] In fact, if there is no initial response to this drug, the diagnosis should be reconsidered. Occasionally, however, a nonspecific response to carbamazepine may occur.[57] Lithium and carbamazepine have been used to treat tic cluster.[58] Epstein and Marcoe[59] proposed the use of topical capsaicin intraorally. When carbamazepine is used, monitoring of liver function is mandatory. Diphenylhydantoin is usually considered a second- or third-line drug.[35] Baclofen is helpful[60] at times, as is valproate[61] and pimozide.[62] In refractory cases, combinations of drugs may have to be enlisted.[35] Opiates, nonsteroidal anti-inflammatories, and analgesics are minimally effective in pain control.

Nerve blocks are sometimes used as is peripheral avulsion, but most surgeons prefer percutaneous radiofrequency gangliolysis.[63] This works well and the pain is relieved for quite some time. Unfortunately anaesthesia is invariable. Rarely, a particularly painful and difficult to manage combination of continuous pain and anaesthesia in the affected nerve (anaesthesia dolorosa) may ensue. This condition is most likely due to deafferentation and denervation hypersensitivity.[5] Glycerol injection has become popular[64] in the European literature, but at times long-lasting relief of symptoms is not forthcoming.[65] Jannetta[48] popularized suboccipital craniotomy with microvascular decompression. Sindou and Mertens[66] reported a 91% cure rate in TN with this procedure. Loeser[33] suggested an 85% suc-

cess rate with a 0.5% mortality rate using this therapeutic modality. Acupuncture treatment needs to be subjected to rigorous review[67] since the current literature does not contain many well controlled studies.

## Glossopharyngeal Neuralgia

Glossopharyngeal neuralgia (GN) or ticlike pain in the distribution of the ninth cranial nerve is much less common than TN but results in symptoms similar to TN in the tonsillar fossa, the back of the tongue, or into the ear or jaw.[35] The pain also may be constant with ticlike features superimposed. Triggers include eating, swallowing, yawning, or talking but are not necessary for the pain to occur. Occasionally syncope may occur.[68] The condition responds to carbamazepine but not as well as in trigeminal neuralgia. Surgical intervention is more difficult and could include sectioning of the root of the ninth cranial nerve, microvascular dissection, or thermocoagulation.[66] Careful otolaryngologic examination is necessary to rule out local pathology. The posterior fossa and base of the skull should be imaged to exclude glomus tumors and other structural lesions.

## Occipital Neuralgia

This condition has been increasingly recognized as a cause of occipital head pain.[35,69] The pain can be paroxysmal, beginning in the suboccipital region and extending toward the vertex. At times, the pain can be referred anteriorly in a migraine-type pattern. There may be an aching discomfort that persists between attacks. There is sensory loss or dysesthesia in the distribution of the greater or lesser occipital nerves as well as localized tenderness. The condition, which is assumed to be due to an entrapment, is often relieved by nerve block.[70] It must be differentiated from migraine, tension-type headache, and structural lesions at the cervicomedullary junction and from cervico-genic headache (see below). Cervical spine radiographs and imaging of the cervi-comedullary junction by MRI are recom-mended.

## Nerve Injury

A particularly disabling pain is pro-duced by injury to the trigeminal nerve or its branches. This is not unexpected after severe facial trauma but it is also common following surgical interventions. In our clinic, we have seen numerous cases of in-fraorbital nerve injuries after Caldwell-Luc or other sinus surgery,[71] inferior alve-olar nerve injury after lower third molar extraction[72,73] and lower quadrant end-odontic procedures, or maxillary branch injuries with upper quadrant dental proce-dures. These patients have anatomically correct hypesthesia, hyperesthesia, and severe pain, often defying conservative management. The etiology of the pain re-lates to the complications of nerve injury including deafferentation, neurogenic in-flammation, and sympathetic hyperactiv-ity.[74] Loeser[75] discusses, at length, such deafferentation pain. Treatment is gener-ally difficult. Various surgical approaches including removal of neuromas and nerve graft on postsurgical inferior alveolar inju-ries are available.[76,77] Generally speaking, treatment is symptomatic and includes drug therapy (tricyclics, antiepileptics) or analgesics. Various neurostimulatory techniques can also be attempted as can acupuncture treatment; however, these treatments are rarely successful in control-ling the severe pain attributed to nerve in-jury.

## Cluster Migraine (Cluster Headache)

Cluster migraine refers to a group of painful disorders known by many other names, including migrainous neuralgia,[78] greater superficial petrosal neuralgia,[79] Horton's neuralgia,[80,81] and cluster head-ache.[82] Initially assumed to be fairly ste-reotypical, a classification has been de-rived to describe certain subtypes, modified after the IHS classification (Table I).[4,6,7] Although called cluster mi-graine they are really quite a different dis-order and classified separately.

The etiology and pathophysiology of cluster migraine is interesting. It was ini-tially thought to be a vascular vasodilatory problem mediated by histamine;[81] how-ever, more recently, it has been postulated that a primary neuronal discharge through the trigeminal system[83] mediated by sub-stance P[84] is responsible. This is sup-ported by the fact that somatostatin, a sub-stance P inhibitor, reduces cluster attacks.[85] Other possibilities include auto-nomic dysfunction to explain the pupil-lary and lacrimation findings. One inter-esting observation is the circadian evidence suggesting hypothalamic in-volvement,[7] mediated through serotoner-gic neurons. Kudrow[86] postulated a dis-turbance of autoregulation of blood flow secondary to carotid body dysfunction, leading to the use of oxygen therapy. Trauma has occasionally predisposed pa-tients to cluster headache. There is a school that advocates cavernous sinus in-flammation as a cause.[84] Sleep apnea has been linked to some cases of cluster.[87,88]

The typical feature of episodic cluster is, as the name implies, the clustering of attacks during periods lasting between 2 weeks and 3 months, separated by remis-sions of at least 14 days, but usually sev-eral months.[89] Kudrow[90] suggested that the prevalence rate of cluster headache in men is between 0.4% and 1%. Typical epi-sodic cluster is a disease which predomi-nates in men by 5 to 7:1, as opposed to migraine, which is more common in women. Usually, it begins in the third or fourth decade, but there is a wide age range, with a peak incidence from 40 to 49 in men, and 60 to 69 in women.[91]

Episodic cluster is the most common variety with attacks occurring for periods lasting 7 days to 1 year, separated by pain-free periods lasting 14 days or more. Two such bouts are necessary to confirm the di-agnosis according to Mathew,[92] although the IHS classification states that five typical headaches meeting the criteria would suffice. It is a lifetime disease with relatively low remission rates.[93,94] In some the diagnosis is simple, but in others the presentation is deceptive and one almost backs into it.

The typical history is that of a middle-aged male awakening at night with severe pain in and above the eye or in the temple, sometimes after having consumed some alcohol the evening before. The eye tears profusely, usually there is sweating of the forehead, and ipsilateral nasal stuffiness. The pain crescendos over 10 to 15 minutes and becomes unbearable. It is always unilateral during an attack. During a cluster, the same eye is invariably affected. Even in subsequent clusters, the contralateral side is only occasionally affected.

The pain is a searing or boring pain, in the eye, or slightly above or below it. At times the pain extends into the maxilla or even the teeth with a dental presentation. An unsuspecting dental practitioner may try dental treatment with potentially disastrous results. The pain may sometimes be experienced in the suboccipital region or in the neck near the angle of the jaw. The patient may writhe in pain and feel his eye is being pushed out. The eye may become red and tear. The examiner may notice Horner's syndrome with miosis, ptosis, and anhidrosis.

The symptoms can last for an hour or more (rarely 2 to 3 hours) and then disappear. They may recur once or several times, usually at the same time, suggesting a circadian disturbance.[87] Nocturnal pain is classical. The patient may become quite agitated during the attack.

Clustering is suggested by the episodic pains occurring several days in a row for several days, weeks, or months without let up. Pain-free periods may occur for months or even years. It is said that the onset is more common in the spring or fall. Alcohol is a common precipitant as is nitroglycerin.

Emotional factors are less important as a stressor than in migraine. Graham[95] described these individuals as being timid with dependency needs whereas Friedman[96] called them "ambitious, proficient,

goal-oriented, hard-driving, compulsive but insecure and lacking in self-confidence." In general, it is difficult to be certain of any predominant personality type in this kind of headache.

There is a variant called chronic cluster migraine. These patients either, de novo, or after a series of attacks, lack periods of remission, do not respond as well to treatment, and have a large number of attacks frequently. By definition the attacks must go on for at least a year. These people's lives are consumed by the illness as they are constantly awaiting the next dreaded headache. They have had a series of less than successful treatments, and have usually suffered socioeconomic hardship. Sometimes, they lapse into drug-seeking behavior.

The chronic paroxysmal hemicrania variety occurs more commonly in women. These attacks are brief (15 minutes), recurrent, frequent (5 to 20 per day), and respond dramatically to indomethacin.[6,7] Sometimes these episodes can be precipitated by head movement.[89]

The differential diagnosis for cluster migraine includes glaucoma and other ocular lesions, orbital and retro-orbital lesions, migraine, trigeminal neuralgia, pituitary tumors, carotid aneurysm, and dental, sinus, and cervical spine disease. The patient should be evaluated with these conditions in mind and appropriate investigations undertaken. Dental presentations are common. The sinuses and retro-orbital areas are commonly imaged. A residual Horner's syndrome is another cause for concern suggesting the presence of an intrathoracic lesion as well, although the lack of anhidrosis is more suggestive of a very distal lesion near the orbit.

Treatment of the acute attack could include ergotamine,[97] dihydroergotamine,[98] sumatriptan,[99] acetylsalicylic acid (ASA), acetaminophen, certain nonsteroidal anti-inflammatories, and opiates. Oxygen inhalation can provide short-term relief.[100] In view of the reported linkage between sleep apnea and cluster migraine, diagnosis should be considered and, if present, treated.[87] Dihydroergotamine and sumatriptan take 30 minutes to become effective. By that time the attack may be over, negating their practical value. If the patient is willing to self-administer these drugs, or if the new proposed intranasal preparations are successful,[101,102] this would be a practical approach. Analgesics, anti-inflammatories, and narcotics are difficult when attacks are so frequent. Dihydroergotamine is also used by some for up to 72 hours in order to terminate the attack, requiring hospitalization.

Because of the diificulties mentioned, we usually recommend oxygen therapy, if practical, or ergotamine, recognizing that the attack may be over before the medication begins to work. Because of this, we often use Decadron (16 mg/day) for 1 week with tapering doses over the following 10 days; however, the dose may have to be extended for more than a week leading to side effects. These include weight changes, avascular necrosis, gastrointestinal disturbance, and others.

There are other prophylactic drugs as well. Kudrow[103] advocated lithium carbonate but, in our experience, it has not been quite as effective, unless combined with other agents such as corticosteroids. Methysergide can be effective, particularly early in the course[92] but patients usually express concern about the potential fibrotic and other side effects. Antimigraine agents such as calcium-channel blockers[98] have also been used. Of these, flunarizine has been most effective in our hands. Kudrow[7] suggests combining daytime verapramil, a calcium channel blocking agent, with nighttime ergotamine to break the cycle. Sodium valproate has also been used with some success.[104]

One specific difficulty in deciding about treatment modalities and how long to treat relates to the spontaneous remission that occurs in this condition. Therefore, one has to consider withdrawing treatment after 1 or 2 pain-free weeks. If the drug has been effective, the pain may recur upon withdrawal. If not, the drug is not necessary and should be withdrawn. For chronic cluster headache, one is reluctant to consider corticosteroids and, in some cases, neurosurgical intervention may be necessary including radiofrequency trigeminal gangliorhizolysis,[105] which is effective but is associated with postoperative facial numbness.

## Acute Herpes Zoster and Postherpetic Neuralgia

The varicella zoster virus may produce two very painful neuropathic pain syndromes: the acute herpes zoster skin and mucosal lesions known as shingles and the difficult, chronic pain condition known as postherpetic neuralgia (PHN).

Herpes zoster or shingles is a reactivation of the varicella zoster virus usually contracted as chicken pox during childhood. The virus appears to lay dormant in the trigeminal, geniculate, and dorsal root ganglia for many years and for various reasons, becomes activated later in life. This can occur in immunocompromised individuals (eg, those suffering from AIDS or lymphoma) or it may occur in the elderly with no known immunological disturbance but in whom cell-mediated immunity may have lessened.[106] When reactivation occurs, the virus migrates down the sensory nerve fibers producing skin and/or mucosal vesicles in a dermatomal distribution.

In 10% to 15% of people affected by acute herpes zoster, the trigeminal nerve is involved.[5] Eighty percent of these involve the first division of the trigeminal nerve, involving the forehead and the eye (ophthalmic herpes zoster). This can involve the extraocular nerves as well. The other common presentation is known as the Ramsay Hunt syndrome in which facial palsy is seen associated with vesicles involving the ear, the external canal, and sometimes the skin inferior or anterior to the canal (fifth cranial nerve), and the eighth cranial nerve as well producing vertigo and auditory symptoms. Here, the virus is postulated to lay dormant in the geniculate ganglion.[107]

Pre-eruptive pain is common up to 2 to 3 days before the blisters appear. Juel-Jensen and MacCallum[108] state that this pre-eruptive phase may last up to 3 weeks.

The acute phase is very painful in the area involved with a constant burning, gnawing pain, superimposed upon by a burst of shock-like, brief, tic-like pains. These are distributed through the dermatome. There may be areas of anesthesia and hyperesthesia around the vesicles. In most cases, after a few weeks, the vesicles heal leaving scars, and the pain disappears. In a small percentage, 9% according to Ragozzino et al.[109] and 14.3% according to Hope-Simpson,[110] another kind of pain may develop subsequently. This is known as postherpetic neuralgia. Cobo et al.[111] suggest that 52% of patients with herpes zoster ophthalmicus have PHN with 22% presenting by 1 year. Acyclovir is said to lessen the time course of acute herpes zoster,[112] but not to lessen the appearance of postherpetic neuralgia.[113] Bilora et al.[114] found that younger patients fared better with acyclovir. Huff et al.[115,116] suggested a deceased incidence of PHN with acyclovir and, recently Hoang-Xuan et al.,[117] in a series of patients with ophthalmic herpes, found fewer complications and more rapid healing with acyclovir. Watson et al.[118] stated "the bulk of evidence to date provides reasonable support for the use of moderate doses of a corticosteroid, such as prednisone (60 mg daily), at the outset of shingles in the nonimmunocompromised patient, with gradual reduction over 2 weeks." Others suggest there is no benefit in prescribing prednisone specifically for the prevention of PHN.[119]

Most authors would not define the persisting pain as PHN unless it lasts for 3 months[120] or 6 months.[75] In their classical study, Watson et al.[120] noted that 47 of 208 patients with postherpetic neuralgia had trigeminal involvement. Sixty five percent of the entire group were women but he concluded that this reflected the usual predominance of women alive in the older age group. Fifty percent of patients with herpes zoster at 60 years and 75% at 70 years develop PHN at 1 month after the rash. Watson[121] states that 5% of patients with all types of Zoster have pain at 3 months and 3% have severe pain at 1 year. Observations by Cobo et al.[111] suggest that

the trigeminal nerve may act differently from other neurological disturbances.

Postherpetic pain is similar to the acute symptom with a constant, severe background pain and superimposed tic-like spasms. There may be other sensations as well. Watson et al.[118] describe hyperesthesia, dysesthesia, or allodynia in the areas involved. The scars may be anesthetic, but there may be persisting areas of hypoesthesia or hyperesthesia inside and outside the area of scarring. Commonly this occurs in the forehead or around the ear in cranial PHN. The pain may be described as burning, gnawing, stabbing, shooting, and sharp. Physical activity and emotional factors may lead to exacerbation of the pain. This can be incapacitating, particularly in an older patient.

The acute pain is caused by the virus invading the ganglion, nerve root, and nerve, producing a hemorrhagic inflammation. Rarely leptomeningeal and parenchymal involvement can occur. Later, fibrosis can be found in the ganglion, nerve root, and nerve. Some pathologic studies have demonstrated dorsal column involvement lasting as long as 9 months. The persisting pain may be associated with a relative loss of peripheral large fibers with persistence of smaller substance P containing smaller fibers.[118] Central deafferentation is said to be responsible for much of the persisting pain, but peripheral factors are likely important as well.[120]

Treatment is very difficult. The mainstay of treatment is the tricyclic group of antidepressants, particularly amitriptyline in doses of approximately 75 mg per day,[122] although side effects (dizziness, dryness, weight gain) and, in older people, cardiological effects are of concern. Chlorprothixene may be effective[123] but only in doses higher than 100 mg.[124] Other suggested treatment approaches have recently been reviewed by Rowbotham.[125] Topical capsacian applied locally can reduce the pain,[118] although its use is awkward and patients object to the burning sensation particularly around the eyes. Nerve blocks,[126] topical aspirin,[127,128] acupuncture,[129] transcutaneous electrical nerve stimulator (TENS),[130] topical local anesthetic,[131] and Emla cream[132] have been tried with some success. Sympathetic blockade has also been advocated.[133] Fortunately, the symptoms gradually lessen with time. Since there is central deafferentation, producing more distal lesions, would be ineffective. Therefore, permanent nerve block, and most of the surgical procedures used to treat TN, should not be used.

## Cervicogenic Headache

The term "cervicogenic headache" refers to a specific kind of headache arising from the cervical spine.[134] The concept that cervical spine disease may be a source of significant headache is relatively novel[135–137] and was the topic for discussion at the first North American Cervicogenic Headache Conference which took place in Toronto in September 1995. Classically,[138] it has been taught that degenerative disease of the cervical spine results in local neck pain and stiffness; radicular pain, numbness, and weakness; and signs and symptoms of a cervical myelopathy with arm and leg weakness, spasticity, paresthesia and sensory loss, and neurogenic bladder symptoms.[139] The concept of referred occipital head pain was accepted but the idea of cervical source pain being referred to the ipsilateral eye and forehead was a relatively new concept in the West.[138] Nonetheless, in the early 1980's the European literature made considerable reference to cervical spine source headache.[135,139]

Edmeads[139] emphasized the similarities between migraine without aura and cervicogenic headache. Diagnostic criteria, including specific radiologic criteria, have recently been defined for cervicogenic headache.[4,135] For example, at least one of the following radiologic findings involving the cervical spine are necessary for the diagnosis: (1) movement on flexion/extension of the cervical spine; (2) abnormal posture; or (3) fractures, congenital abnormalities, bone tumors, rheumatoid, arthritis and/or other pathology. The nature of pain arising from cervical spondylosis is

closer to a tension-type headache. Sjaastad et al.[136] showed that 5 out of 55 patients with radiologic cervical spondylosis noted headaches similar to tension-type headache. By contrast, radiologic abnormalities may not be necessary for the diagnosis. Fredrikson et al.[140] found no specific radiologic abnormalities in their 11 females with cervicogenic headache.

One must differentiate headache arising from the cervical spine and the fairly specific syndrome of cervicogenic headache. The condition known as cervicogenic headache has been defined as a unilateral headache, without side shift, beginning in the posterior aspect of the head but ultimately spreading anteriorly to the frontal region or eye.[135] The pain is characterized by rather mild and protracted pain episodes, followed by the pain chronicity, with an undulating course. Women are affected far more frequently than men. There may be a history of whiplash trauma.[137] Clinical examination[135] reveals a decreased range of motion of the cervical spine. There may be localized point tenderness in the suboccipital region and occasionally light pressure on the tender muscle nodule may trigger pain shooting into the ipsilateral eye. The pain can be accompanied by photophobia, lacrimation, and nausea suggesting migraine.[134] Ipsilateral shoulder and occasional arm pain may also accompany the headaches, and attacks may be precipitated mechanically through neck movement. Patients often prefer to wear a cervical collar to restrict lateral movement.

Both migraine and cervicogenic headache may have associated nausea, vomiting, photophobia, and/or phonophobia, but only cervicogenic headache is associated with a decreased range of motion, mechanical precipitation of pain by movement or by local pressure on C-2 or the greater occipital nerve, ipsilateral shoulder and arm pain, and unilaterally without side shift.[141]

In treating patients with this condition, it is found that anesthetic blockade of the greater occipital nerve results in decreased frontal pain, even though the frontal or supraorbital area has not been anesthetized. The convergence of the trigeminal nucleus (descending tract of V) and the input from the upper cervical nerve roots (via the substantia gelatinosa) has been postulated as being responsible for the referred pain.[142] Cervical nociceptive input thus may lead to neuronal hyperactivity in the substantia gelatinosa and then in the nucleus caudalis of V. Nociceptive input from C-1 to C-3 nerves would produce headache. Blocking the input would lead to lessening pain anteriorly. Thus blocking the greater occipital nerve is more effective than blocking the supraorbital nerve in reducing cervicogenic headache but not migraine without aura or tension type headache.[143]

Schoenen and Maertens de Noordhout[89] caution that cervicogenic headache, like chronic tension-type headache, although triggered initially by peripheral mechanisms, may in its chronic form be caused by central dysfunction.

The differential diagnosis of cervicogenic headache includes occipital neuralgia (local sensory loss and no frontal radiation), atlantoaxial subluxation, posterior fossa lesions, as well as migraine without aura and tension-type headache. Of 5520 patients with headache in a 1993 study by Pfaffenrath and colleagues,[144] 13% of patients had cervicogenic headache with a significant number having migraine, tension-type headache, or some other chronic headache condition.

Analgesics and nonsteroidal anti-inflammatories as well as cyclobenzaprine can provide some relief as does local physiotherapy and biofeedback. However, more specific therapy may be necessary. Kehr et al.[145] reported an 87% success rate with uncoforaminectomy. Greater occipital nerve block is quite helpful in this condition and, if this relief is only temporary, neurolysis can be carried out.[143] C-2 and C-3 facet joint block is also undertaken as well as supraorbital nerve block with local anesthetic and corticosteroids.[146] Bovim and colleagues[147, 148] reported that C-2 and C-3 facet blockade was effective in 9 of 14 patients with cervicogenic headache. It has been suggested that. in "benign" conditions, other more invasive surgical treatment including cordotomy, Drez lesions (dorsal root entry zone), gangliectomy, and rhizolysis should be avoided.[149] With the exception of facet rhizotomy, the ablative modalities have little role in so-called "benign" chronic cervical pain syndrome.

Nerve block techniques have been used for less differentiated pain conditions as well. Anthony[70] reported that 184 of 500 patients with idiopathic headache responded to greater occipital nerve block. Cronen and Waldman[150] described the use of cervical steroid epidural block to relieve intractable tension-type headache. Gawal and Rothbart[151] also reported on the management of headache and cervical pain with occipital nerve block. These patients are subject to "whiplash" and all the pain and cognitive disturbances involved in a posttraumatic syndrome and may not be pure examples of cervicogenic headache. Because it is only part of a therapeutic milieu for these complicated patients, "nerve block therapy" requires rigorous critical evaluation before it can be widely applied.

## Tension-type Headaches

Headache is a common disorder. The overall lifetime headache vulnerability has been estimated to be over 90% with 6.1% of males and 14% of females reporting four or more headaches in the previous month.[152] Lance et al.[153] estimated that 40% of patients referred to a headache clinic were referred because of tension headache. Diamond[154] estimates that 80% of headache patients patients seen either by the family physician or the generalist suffer from muscle contraction or tension headaches.

Most people are familiar with ordinary "tension-type headaches" during which they feel a tight band around the head, or tense, tender muscles in the occipital, temporal, or frontal regions. This headache was originally known as "tension headache" because it was thought to be associated with increased muscle tension. This name was abandoned because it implied that stress or anxiety was causing the pain. "Muscle contraction headache," another term that was used, implies sustained muscle contraction, but clearly this is not always present. A third common name is "psychogenic headache," but psychogenic disorders have not been demonstrated in all patients with this syndrome. Other names include "stress headache," "psychomyogenic headache," and "ordinary headache."[89,152]

Essentially there are two variants of tension-type headache (TTH): episodic and chronic.[154] The IHS classification further subclassifies the episodic and chronic tension-type headache by the presence or absence of pericranial tenderness—a differentiation not included here since it may not be relevant to clinical presentation, pathogenesis of pain, or response to therapy.[155]

The typical history of episodic tension-type headache includes a late afternoon onset, a sensation of a tight band or cap around or on the head, a sense of heaviness in the head, or a pressing or nonpulsating, tightening feeling. Some individuals complain of a viselike band around the head. It can occur at other times of the day as well. The headache is of mild to moderate severity and most people are able to work through it. The pain is usually bilateral but 10% are unilateral. The pain can be felt in the occipital, temporal, or frontal regions. The scalp may feel very tender and some individuals can point to a particularly troublesome spot. These headaches are not usually aggravated by walking stairs or similar physical activity. Nausea, vomiting, and photophobia should be absent but the presence of only one of these does not exclude the diagnosis. The headache lasts from 30 minutes to 7 days. These headaches can manifest themselves in relation to stress, emotional conflicts, or fatigue. If the patient has had at least 10 of these and has fewer than 180 days per year of headache, then the term episodic tension-type headache is applicable.[4] There are often behavioral symptoms including anxiety, depression, poor sleep, and behavioral difficulties. Because patients with episodic tension headache may have unilateral pain, anorexia, nausea, or photophobia, the differential diagnosis may

include migraine without aura, temporal arteritis, and organic brain disease.

Chronic tension-type headache is similar in most respects but occurs more than 180 days per year. It is more likely to be linked to a serious emotional disorder such as depression.[154] Individuals with chronic TTH often have overlapping factors that complicates the diagnosis and terminology. These factors include excessive medication use and dependency, associated migraine or vasular headache, myofascial pain (particularly associated with trauma), and cervical spine dysfunction.

The term "chronic daily headache" was previously used to describe the above patients. The terminology was excluded by the IHS classification, although recently it has been reactivated.[156–158] Some authors are loathe to accept the exclusion of chronic daily headache from the IHS classification.[159] A modified classification of chronic daily headache, after Silberstein[152] and Silberstein et al.[158] is suggested in Table II. We will continue to use the term chronic TTH in these discussions.

It was said that neurophysiologically TTH could be differentiated from migraine,[153] particularly by excessive EMG activity indicating heightened reflex motor activity and muscle contraction.[154] More recently, it has been suggested that there is a continuum between migraine and tension-type headache and that the pathophysiology is the same.[160] Thus, migraine is "transformed" into chronic daily headache when the headaches become so

---

**Table II**
Classification of Chronic Daily Headache

I. Primary Chronic Daily Headache
  a. Transformed Migraine
  b. Chronic Tension-type Headache
  c. New Daily Headache
  d. Hemicrania Continua
II. Secondary Chronic Daily Headache
  a. Posttraumatic Headache
  b. Cervical Spine Disorders
  c. Headache with Vascular Disorder and Nonvascular Intracranial Disease

frequent and severe that they are almost constant and lose their pulsatile features.[161,162] This usually occurs 8 to 10 years after onset as periodic migraine. There is an increased incidence of depression, sleep disturbance, and analgesic dependency. Over 90% of females and 84% of males had a close family member with headache and a higher than expected incidence history of substance abuse, alcoholism. and depression.[156] Solomon et al.[159] determined that 50% of patients with chronic daily headache in their population also had drug dependency. Alternately, some patients develop interparoxysmal headache, that is constant pain between the migraines. Many patients referred to our Craniofacial Pain Research Unit with daily headache have internal derangements of the TMJ or associated myofascial pain, with intraoral and extraoral tender muscle points. In fact, patients referred to the dental side by community dentists as TMJ problems and to the neurologists by family physicians as "tension headaches" are often interchangeable, suggesting many overlapping features and similarities. Cervical spine x-rays of patients with chronic tension-type headache show straightening and low set shoulders,[163] indicating significant overlap in pathophysiology and symptoms.

Evaluation of these patients with episodic and chronic tension-type headaches involves a very careful history emphasizing the temporal development of symptoms; a detailed inquiry into the characteristics of the symptoms; documentation of previous treatment including medication intake; an appreciation of the social milieu including job history and family/spousal issues; the presence or absence of compensation issues including work and motor vehicle accidents; and other psychosocial and interpersonal relationship factors. In addition to the standard general evaluation looking for systemic disease and the neurological evaluation, the physician must evaluate the dental occlusion and temporomandibular apparatus, the cervical spine, and various trigger and tender points. Glaucoma should be considered and, as well, the temporal arteries should

be palpated, thinking of temporal arteritis. Investigations depend upon a number of factors, including length of time the headache has been present, any significant change in headache pattern, or the presence of neurological findings. Dental factors are often overlooked and the patient should be evaluated for bruxism, intraoral pathology, and a TMD. A team approach involving predominantly neurology and dentistry is useful, as is a diagnostic questionnaire, in the evaluation of the patient.[164] Psychologic inquiries are made and the psychiatrist should be consulted liberally and early in the investigation, looking for anxiety states, depression, and somatization disorders. If there is any suggestion of sinus or nasopharyngeal disease, otolarygological consultation is essential. Imaging is carried out where indicated.

Tension headache is not simply the result of painful contraction of the extracranial musculature because the patient is tense. Botulinum toxin injections, which would be expected to provide temporary muscular paralysis, does not reduce pain.[165] Numerous studies have failed to correlate muscle contraction recorded by surface EMG with pain.[166,167] Richman and Haas[168] recently reported that continuous, chronic tension-type headache was unaffected by two hours of frontalis and trapezius relaxation. Moreover, pericranial muscle tenderness does not correlate with headache.

The question arises as to whether the pain is secondary to, and a reflection of, a central phenomenon. Increasingly it has been suggested that migraine and tension headache are part of a continuum.[169] Migraine is considered to be related to a central neuronal disturbance residing in the brainstem and hypothalamus regions involving alterations in ascending or descending serotonergic or monoaminergic systems.[170] Moskowitz[171] emphasizes a trigeminovascular system disturbance in migraine. Perhaps this is triggered centrally. Tension headache, therefore, would have a similar underlying pathophysiology or at least the same system may be abnormally set. Serotonin, which is implicated in migraine, is thought to be important in the cause of tension-type headaches.[172] A recent study suggested that changes in serotonin preceded the vascular and muscular changes of migraine and tension-type headache.[173] Genetics may predispose the patient to tension-type headache, with multiple precipitating factors including head trauma, infection, severe emotional despair, and the use of analgesics and ergots. Stressful life events, particularly minor daily hassles,[174] also play an important perpetuating role.

Many different treatment methods have been suggested. For episodic, relatively infrequent TTH, remedies include over-the-counter analgesics such as ASA or acetaminophen; in some individuals rest and in others exercise; stress reduction; nonsteroidal anti-inflammatories; and judicious use of muscle relaxants. In chronic TTH, excessive analgesic use may be counterproductive, facilitating a medication-induced headache (see section below). Relaxants such as diazepam and barbiturate-containing compounds are to be avoided except, perhaps, briefly in an acute situation, since drug dependency may become a problem. Tricyclics such as amitriptyline or doxepin can relieve pain, anxiety, and a sleep disturbance and are often very helpful. Tizanidine was recently found to alleviate chronic tension-type headache[175,176] but is not available in North America for this use. Adding a beta blocker such as propranolol can also be effective in preventing the withdrawal migraines that occur if analgesic is reduced or the migraines commonly associated with mixed chronic TTH. Valproate may be effective in weaning patients.[177,178] Manna and colleagues demonstrated that fluvoxamine decreases chronic headache as well.[179]

Psychiatric intervention is occasionally necessary but usually for diagnostic purposes and to suggest treatment.[180] Biofeedback or various forms of relaxation therapy can be used despite some negative reports.[168] Physical therapy, particularly to the cervical spine and tender muscle points, is effective.[181] Patients in our Unit have reported impressive relief with vigorous physical exercise. Trigger point injection therapy also appears to reduce pain. Recently, there has been a popular trend towards repeated cervicotrigeminal nerve blocks,[143] but this therapeutic approach requires scientific validation. If there is a temporomandibular concern, conservative treatment is recommended such as an occlusal stabilizing appliance, analgesics, and physical therapy.

Treatment of chronic TTH patients, particularly those with drug dependency issues and medication-induced headache, is quite complex and time intensive. Patients often improve on the basis of the personality, drive, and enthusiasm of the treating health care professional. It may require in-hospital management to wean patients off their analgesics, ergot compounds, and relaxants. At times, antimigraine therapy is not only indicated with beta blockers and methysergide, but also valproate. In addition to the drug management, many centers require their patient to sign a contract with the treating team that can involve various aspects of behavior modification, an exercise program, and a rigid selection of drugs.

## Medication-induced Headache

While there are drugs such as nitroglycerin, nifedipine, and indomethacin that are known to cause headaches in certain individuals, the purpose of this section is to discuss drug-induced headache resulting from medications initially used for headache relief. Many of these patients begin with TTH or migraine that then change into medication-induced headache.

There are basically two groups of drugs fulfilling these criteria, the ergots and analgesics. Steiner et al.[182] estimated that 10% of patients referred to a headache clinic suffer this problem. It occurs after exceeding a minimum daily dose of the drug for more than 3 months. The headache is chronic and occurs virtually daily, disappearing about 1 month after cessation of the offending drug.

The ergots, specifically ergotamine tartrate, are particularly culpable.[183,184] Instead of taking ergotamine, at the most once or twice a week as one might expect given a normal migraine pattern, the drug is used on a regular basis either daily or almost daily to prevent headache.[185] In these situations, oral ergot dosage is more than 2 mg per day and rectal dosage is greater than 1 mg per day. The patient finds that if he or she misses a day, a headache will ensue. In an attempt to prevent this, patient might be taking up to 10 mg per day rather than 10 mg per week. Occasionally the same pattern is seen but with a considerably smaller, but regular dose. Stopping the medication results in headache with associated nausea, vomiting, diarrhea, restlessness, and insomnia. Later prophylactic medications that were relatively ineffective suddenly become effective.

The diagnosis becomes apparent when there is a recurring migrainelike headache, at least 2 to 3 times a week responsive selectively to ergotamine, while refractory to other symptomatic preventive medications.[184] The headache is diffuse, pulsating and distinguished from migraine by an absent attack pattern and/or associated symptoms. Pascal and Berceani[186] have successfully treated these individuals on an outpatient basis by using naproxen as a substitute.

Overuse of analgesics is associated with increased headaches and decreased effect of prophylactic agents.[187,188] In fact, it might take up to a 12-week washout period to reregulate the nociceptive systems.[189] The culpable medications include ASA, acetaminophen, barbiturates, caffeine, or codeine-containing compounds. One must be suspicious of analgesic headache in cases in which the patient is taking more than 50 gm of ASA (or the analgesic equivalent), more than 100 tablets of an analgesic preparation, or one or more narcotic analgesics. Analgesic headaches are characterized by sleep abnormalities, tolerance to medication, withdrawal symptoms, headache improvement after withdrawal of symptomatic medications, and/or nullification of the benefit of daily

headache. Women are more commonly afflicted. Drug-seeking behavior may ensue and the patient becomes very anxious. Walker et al.[190] reported on an increasing prevalence of analgesic rebound headache in a community hospital.

The medication-induced headache dosages for these kinds of drugs varies and there may be individual susceptibility.[191] These headaches occur only in the headache-susceptible population. When analgesics are taken for other reasons, rebound does not occur. There is presumed to be a downregulation of an already suppressed pain system, involving either endorphins, norepinephrine, or serotonin. Elevated 5-HT receptor levels in these patients have been demonstrated in these patients.[192]

Kudrow[187] described withdrawal reactions that may require short hospitalization because of the nervousness, restlessness, nausea, headache, diarrhea, and even withdrawal seizures for those on barbiturates. Rothrock et al.[178] have shown that valproate, as may sumatriptan, may be a drug useful for severe specific migraines.[177]

Management requires a "multimodal" approach involving discontinuation of the drug, breaking the cycle with IV dihydroergotamine, initiating prophylactic treatment, behavioral therapy, provision of information about the medications and their effects, and a continuity of care.[184]

As a treating physician, it can be difficult to avoid such entanglement with a patient and even more difficult to extricate oneself. Nonetheless, this is an increasingly common type of headache requiring constant vigilance. The overlap between this syndrome and the chronic daily headache or chronic tension-type headache syndromes can present a challenging clinical problem.[193]

## Migraine Headaches

Migraine is a very common, yet misunderstood disease.[194] Far more than just recurring episodes of very painful headaches, it is a complex disorder involving not just the brain but the eye, the autonomic nervous system, and many other organs, producing myriad symptoms and signs.

The prevalence varies from study to study. A recent report of a group of Italian medical students gives a migraine prevalence of 6.9% and a tension-type headache prevalence of 14.3%.[195] Edmeads et al.[160] recently reported a survey of Canadian adults in which 16.3% suffered migraine. A Finnish study yielded a prevalence of 10.1%.[196] Rasmussan and colleagues,[197, 198] in a Danish study, reported a prevalence of 15% of those surveyed between the ages of 25 to 64. Migraine without aura is more than twice as common as migraine with aura. Females are more commonly affected by migraine except for prepubertal boys and girls.[199] The male:female ratio in migraine without aura is 1:7 and is 1:2 in migraine with aura.[197] Solomon[199] gives a figure of one male for every three females after puberty. Migraines are more disabling, more painful, and longer in duration than any other kind of headache. Females report more disability with headache than do males.[200] Women also find that pregnancy has a variable effect on their migraine.[201]

Migraine is commonly said to run in families. Diamond[202] reports a 70% family history of headache in migraine patients. Some migraineurs have parents, grandparents, siblings, and children (more commonly female) with a history of headache. There are also twin studies that are suggestive of a genetic influence as well, but this remains controversial. There is no clear-cut pattern of either dominant or recessive inheritance. It may be an example of a multigene disorder where exogenous, environmental factors come together to interact with a genetic abnormality.

What was called common migraine or sick headache is now referred to as migraine without aura. These attacks, which last from 4 to 72 hours, share certain features under the IHS[4] classification. They rarely occur more than once a week and most patients have fewer than two per month. The head pain should be unilateral, throbbing, or pulsating. The intensity of the pain is moderate to severe, enough to inhibit daily activities. The headaches may be aggravated by walking up stairs or other routine physical activity. They may become bilateral and they may change from side to side, from attack to attack. Usually nausea, vomiting, photophobia, or phonophobia is present. The patient may go into a dark room with a cold towel or washcloth. Interestingly, 10% to 15% may have premonitory symptoms of mood swings,[194] (particularly euphoria), bursts of energy, anorexia, bloating, food-craving, or yawning. During the episode, patients may appear pale, sick, and sweaty with tender, pulsating temporal arteries. Similarly, afterwards there may be fatigue and polyuria.

Classical migraine is now termed "migraine with aura." The auras usually precede the headache by 15 to 30 minutes. Some 90% of these auras are visual.[199] These auras can include scotomas, blind spots and hemianopsia; flashing lights and visual fortifications; and metamorphosis or changes in form, size, or position. Aphasias, hemianesthesias, and hemiplegias are much less common as auras but may be seen in "complicated migraine" where these neurological symptoms may persist. In other ways these headaches are similar to migraine without aura, headache, and postheadache phases. Rarely, the auras come during or after the headache (interposed migraine). There is a variant of migraine with aura known as "basilar artery migraine," seen usually in young women when the aura suggests involvement of the vertebral-basilar system.[194] Symptoms can include quadriplegia, diplopia, vertigo, loss of consciousness, paresthesia, and ataxia. Lower half headache or "facial migraine" is uncommon and can include throbbing pain in the eye, cheek, mandible, or dental pain but otherwise has all the features of migraine. This can sometimes be misdiagnosed as dental disease.

There is an interesting variant called "acephalgic migraine" or migraine without headache in which transient, focal, strokelike symptoms occur in a migraine predisposed individual without the normal accompanying headache.[194] Common complaints include monocular blindness, scintillating scotomata, or paresthesiae of the face, arm, and/or leg. These are common in young women, particularly those in various stages of pregnancy. These patients, just like patients with migraine with aura, should be evaluated for other causes of stroke including cardiac-source embolism, coagulation disturbances, atheroembolic disease, vasculitis, and fibromuscular hyperplasia. There are a number of migraine equivalents seen mainly in children including cyclical vertigo, recurring abdominal pains, and car sickness.

There are a number of commonly accepted triggers[194] for migraine including insomnia; oversleeping; fatigue; stress and anxiety; mental effort; phases of the menstrual cycle, particularly "menstrual migraine"; bright lights; and oral contraceptives. The relation to foods, such as nitrates, tyramine-containing cheeses, citrus fruit and red wine, is more problematic.[203] Weather changes, particularly drops in barometric pressure, are commonly cited by patients as being important.

The theories of pathogenesis have varied over the years from vascular to neurogenic.[204] Likely some combination is accurate. The pathophysiology is complicated and can be only briefly considered. Moskowitz[171,205] promoted the "trigeminal vascular system" as the final common pathway. This explanation is a novel one as it forces a paradigm shift in the way we think of the function of a sensory nerve. The trigeminal nerve innervates the major pain sensitive structures particularly the large cerebral arteries in the circle of Willis, the dural vessels, and the major venous sinuses. In close approximation are sympathetic nerve twigs and parasympathetic fibers. Antidromic activation of these trigeminal fibers, presumably originating from cell bodies in the spinal nucleus of V in the upper spinal cord, leads to release of neuropeptides such as substance P,[206] calcitonin gene-related peptide,[207] and neurokinin A.[208] These neuropeptides are carried along unmyelinated C fibers.[205] This release may be modulated by 5-HT$_1$ receptors acting presynaptically. The neuropeptides lead to neurogenic inflammation (including also prostaglandins and bradykinin), vasodilatation, and platelet and mast cell aggregation. This causes sensitization and stimulation of trigeminal nociceptive fibers and orthodromic conduction back to the brainstem upper cervical cord where the substantia gelatinosa and nucleus caudalis of V interact. Pain is referred to the peripheral territory of V1 and the superior cervical roots because of convergence of visceral and somatic afferents in the brain stem.

Controversy has surrounded the vasospastic theory, whereby the aura is said to be due to cerebral hypoperfusion and is postulated to precede and lead to hyperperfusion. Oleson[188] did demonstrate focal hypoperfusion over the cortical area which was said to be responsible for the aura symptoms. Cerebral hyperperfusion was demonstrated later in the attack but not linked with headache. Oleson[209] demonstrated normal cerebral perfusion in migraine without aura; whereas, Bes and Fabre[210] found diffuse or focal hyperperfusion unrelated to headache intensity and localization. Currently cerebral vasospasm has not been clearly linked to central nervous system symptoms.

Lauritzen[211] has provided indirect evidence to support Leao's[212] theory of spreading cortical depression rather than ischemia producing neurological symptoms. Evidence that it occurs in humans is lacking. It has been suggested that the certain activity reductions observed with magneto-encephalography[213] or the unilateral reductions of alpha activity seen with topical EEG mapping[214] is related to spreading depression.

Other factors must also be considered in the pathophysiology of this disorder. A deficiency of serum magnesium may be related to altered cerebral blood flow or serotonin.[215] Three modes of involvement for serotonin have been suggested: there are 5-HT$_1$ receptors in the central gateways (eg, substantia gelatinosa), serotonergic fibers project to the cortex, and there are 5-HT$_1$ receptors on the major blood vessels.[173] Ferrari[216] reported neurotransmitter changes in blood and there is a long history of platelet disturbances.[217] Increased globulin levels in migraine have also been noted, implying a humoral immunity problem.[218]

Schoenen and Maertens de Noordhout[89] referred to Welch,[219] Edmeads,[220] and Lance[221] and suggested the following unified theory of causation: "migraine, both with and without aura, can be regarded as a constitutional, perhaps genetically determined, hypersensitivity of the brain and trigeminovascular system to external (triggers) and internal stimuli." Lance[222] expanded upon this. In his view, migraine is a neurovascular reaction to sudden change in the internal or external environment. Each individual has a hereditary "migrainous threshold" with the degree of susceptibility depending upon the balance between excitation and inhibition at various levels of the nervous system. In migraine, there is an unstable trigeminovascular reflex with a segmental defect in the pain control pathway permitting an excessive discharge of part of the spinal nucleus of V and its thalamic connections in response to excessive afferent input or cortical drive. The end result is the interaction of brain stem and cranial blood vessels, with afferent impulses from the latter creating the pulsating characteristics of the pain. Diffuse projections from the locus ceruleus project to the cortex producing oligemia and spreading depression. Thus, there is an interconnection between the trigeminovascular system and spreading depression.

Treatment can be divided into nonpharmacologic and pharmacologic.[223] A detailed history is necessary to identify possible trigger factors including foods or drugs to be avoided.[194,203] An assessment of personality, and work, family, and personal stressors is also key. Diamond[202] wrote, "Based upon my own clinical experience, I would concur with the work of Wolff . . . who reviewed the Rorschach records of migraine patients and found a tendency to rigidity, perfectionism, intolerance, obsessive-convulsive features . . . ." Although this may overstate the problem, psychological difficulties are often present in migraineurs. Stress management and psychological management

may be helpful and biofeedback can be useful to teach some of these individuals principles of relaxation and awareness of stress and their body. Some individuals find exercise classes, meditation, and yoga as helpful means of controlling anxiety. Acupuncture and other modalities have all been tried with some success.[224]

To treat the acute pain, most people get by with simple analgesics including ASA and acetaminophen with or without codeine. Unfortunately excessive use of these drugs may lead to medication-induced headache. Oral naproxen is recommended by Raskin[225] and Teves et al.[226] Davis et al.[227] have shown a 74% response rate to parenteral ketorolac, a drug that Kumar also recommends.[228] Ergotamine tartrate is recommended particularly by suppository[222] or through other routes.[223] Sumatriptan, a 5-HT$_{1D}$ receptor blocker, is expensive but works quite effectively by mouth. More severe headaches may require parenteral sumatriptan.[89,229] Dihydroergotamine is commonly given parenterally, particularly in refractory migraine.[230,231] Weisz[232] reported on the effectiveness of home administration of dihydroergotamine in chronic recurrent migraine. Chlorpromazine given parenterally is also effective[233] although hypotension commonly occurs. Nasal sprays are being developed for sumatriptan and for dihydroergotamine.[101,102] Opiates may have to be used in severe cases. Metoclopramide or domperidone, given parenterally, reduces nausea and gastroenterological symptomatology and allows the use of simple analgesics such as ASA orally, even during severe headaches. Naproxen has been useful in treating acute migraines[226] as has tolfemic acid, a drug not available in Canada, although it has been used prophylactically as well.[234,235] Klapper and Stanton[236] report that dihydroergotamine and metoclopramide are more effective than meperidine and an antiemetic. Trying to sleep for a few minutes in a dark room is good symptomatic treatment. Nefedipine is used successfully to abort acute attacks.[237]

A recent trend, starting in Europe but

now established in North America, is the use of nerve blocks. Anthony[70] reported on the use of greater occipital nerve blocks stating that 48% of patients in his large series of with migraine responded to greater occipital nerve block.

When there are recurring headaches, prophylactic medications are considered. Most of the agents that are effective have a response rate approximating 70%. Beta blockers, particularly propranolol,[223,235] are well tolerated and effective, although thery may react adversely with ergotamine.[238] Metropolol[224] and nadolol are used quite successfully.[223] The calcium channel blocker of choice is flunarazine[238] but this can occasionally result in bouts of severe depression.[203,223] The drug is recommended by the Medical Letter[223] but has not yet been released in the United States.[203] Nifedipine and other blockers such as verapramil are also recommended.[223,231] Tolfonemic acid may be used in this way.[235] Serotonin blocking agents such as methysergide and pizotylene are also effective,[223] although the former may cause internal fibrosis. Valproate has been recommended by Raskin[225] and others.[239] Tricyclics such as amitriptyline are helpful when there is anxiety, depression, or a sleep disorder. Ziegler et al.[240] reported that amitriptyline significantly decreases the severity, frequency, and duration of migraines, whereas propranolol impacts only upon the severity. In general these prophylactic agents are reserved for when there are several bad bouts of headaches over a period of a few weeks.

## Conclusion

It is apparent that the diagnosis and management of patients presenting with craniofacial or orofacial pain is complex, crossing classical professional and intraprofessional boundaries. These conditions are a common cause of pain and disability, striking major portions of the labor force and the population at large. Diagnosis is obviously an important aspect of the ultimate treatment and, therefore, a multidisciplinary and collaborative approach is recommended.

## References

1. Linet MS, Stewart WF, Celentano DD, et al. An epidemiological study among adolescents and young adults. JAMA 1989; 261:2211–2216.
2. Locker D. The burden of oral disorders in a population of adults. Community Dental Health 1992;9:109–124.
3. Romanelli GG, Harper R, Mock D, et al. Evaluation of Temporomandibular joint internal derangement. J Orofacial Pain 1993;7:254–261.
4. Olesen J. Headache Classification Committee of the International Headache Society. Classification and diagnostic criteria for headache disorders, cranial neuralgias, and facial pain. Cephalgia. 1988; 8(suppl 7):90–96.
5. Solomon S, Lipton RB. Facial Pain. Neurol Clin 1990;8:913–928.
6. Kudrow L. Cluster headache: new concepts. Neurol Clin 1983;1:369–383.
7. Kudrow L. Diagnosis and treatment of cluster headache. Med Clin North Amer 1991;75:579–594.
8. Mitchell DF, Tarplee RE. Painful pulpitis: a clinical and microscopic study. Oral Surg Oral Med Oral Pathol 1960;13: 1360–1370.
9. Glick DH. Locating referred pulpal pains. Oral Surg Oral Med Oral Pathol 1962;15: 613–623.
10. McNeill C, Mohl ND, Rugh JD, et al. Temporomandibular disorders: diagnosis, management, education and research. J Am Dent Assoc 1990;120:253–263.
11. Costen JB. A syndrome of ear and sinus symptoms dependent upon disturbed function of the temporomandibular joint. Ann Otol 1934;43:1–15.
12. McCain GA. Fibromyalgia: a myofascial syndrome. In: Wall PD, Melzack R, eds. Textbook of Pain. Edinburgh: Churchill Livingstone;1994:474–494.
13. Romanelli GG, Mock D, Tenenbaum HC. Characteristics and response to treatment of posttraumatic temporomandibular disorder: A retrospective study. Clin J Pain 1992;8:6–17.
14. Goldberg M, Mock D, Ichise M, et al. Assessment of neuropsychological deficit in

posttraumatic TMD. J Dent Res 1994;73: 18.

15. Widmer CG, Lund JP, Feine JS. Evaluation of diagnostic tests for TMD. J Calif Dent Assoc 1990;18:53–60.

16. Mohl ND, McCall WS, Lund JP, et al. Devices for the diagnosis and treatment of temporomandibular disorders: Part I. Introduction, scientific evidence, and jaw tracking. J Prosthet Dent 1990;63:198–201.

17. Mohl ND, Lund JP, Widmer CG, et al. Devices for the diagnosis and treatment of temporomandibular disorders: Part II. Electromyography and sonography. J Prosthet Dent 1990;63:332–336.

18. Mohl MD, Ohrback RK, Crowe HC. Devices for the diagnosis and treatment of temporomandibular disorders: Part III. thermography, ultrasound, electrical stimulation and EMG biofeedback. J Prosthet Dent 1990;63:472–477.

19. Seligman DA, Pullinger AG. The role of intercuspal occlusal relationships in temporomandibular disorders: A review. Journal of Craniomandibular Disorders, Facial and Oral Pain 1991;5:96–106.

20. Seligman DA, Pullinger AG. The role of functional occlusal relationships in temporomandibular disorders: A review. Journal of Craniomandibular Disorders, Facial and Oral Pain 1991;5:265–279.

21. Dolwick MF, Heffez L, Roser SM. 1992, Temporomandibular joint surgery. In: Parameters of Care and Maxillofacial Surgery: A Guide for Practice Monitoring and Evaluation. J Oral Maxillofacial Surg 1992;50(Suppl 2):121–143.

22. Marbach JJ. Phantom tooth pain. J Endodont 1978;4:362–372.

23. Marbach JJ, Hulbrock J, Hohn C, et al. Incidence of phantom tooth pain: an atypical facial neuralgia. Oral Surg Oral Med Oral Pathol 1982;53:190–193.

24. Rees RT, Harris M. Atypical odontalgia. Brit J, Oral Surg 1979;16:212–218.

25. Frazier CH, Russell EC. Neuralgia of the face. An analysis of seven hundred and fifty four cases with relation to pain and other sensory phenomena before and after operation. Arch Neurol Psychiatry 1924; 11:557–563.

26. Sessle BJ. Dental deafferentation can lead to the development of chronic pain. In: Oro-Facial Pain and Neuromuscular Dysfunction: Mechanisms and Clinical Correlates. Klineberg I, Sessle BJ. eds, Oxford: Pergamon 1985:115–129.

27. Sessle BJ. 1992, Neurobiology of facial and dental pain. In: Sarnat BC, Laskin DM eds. The Temporomandibular Joint: A Biological Basis for Clinical Practice. Fourth Edition Philadelphia: WB Saunders 1992: 124–142.

28. Mock D, Frydman W, Gordon AS. Atypical facial pain: a retrospective study. Oral Surg Oral Med, Oral Pathol 1985;59: 472–474.

29. Sharav Y. Orofacial Pain. In: Wall PD, Melzack R eds. *Textbook of Pain*. 3rd Edition. London: Churchill Livingstone; 1994:563–582.

30. Remick RA, Blasberg B, Barton J, et al. Ineffective dental and surgical treatment associated with atypical facial pain. Oral Surg Oral Med, Oral Pathol 1983;55: 355–358.

31. Remick RA, Blasberg B, Campos PE, et al. Psychiatric disorders associated with atypical facial pain. Can Psychiatr Assoc J 1983;28:178–181.

32. Feinmann C, Harris M, Cawley R Psychogenic facial pain: presentation and treatment. Br Med J 1984;288:436–438.

33. Loeser JD. Tic douloureux and atypical facial pain. In: Wall PD, R Melzack R, eds. *Textbook of Pain*. 3rd Edition. Edinburgh: Churchill Livingstone; 1994:699–710.

34. Galli G, Gordon A, Shandling M, et al Diagnostic and prognostic features of atypical facial pain: A pilot study. American Academy of Orofacial Pain Meeting, 1993.

35. Dalessio DJ. The Major Neuralgias in Wolff's Headache and Other Head Pain. Ed Donald J. Dalessio, Oxford University Press, New York, Oxford 1987; Ch 15: 266–288.

36. Zegarelli D J. Burning mouth: An analysis of 57 patients. Oral Surg Oral Med Oral Pathol 1984;58:34–38.

37. Grushka M, Sessle BJ, Howley TP. Psychophysical evidence of taste dysfunction in burning mouth syndrome. Chem Senses 1986;11:485–498.

38. Grushka M, Sessle BJ, Howley TP. Psychophysical assessment of tactile, pain and thermal sensory functions in burning mouth syndrome. Pain 1987;28:169–184.

39. Mott AE, Grushka M, Sessle BJ,. Diagnosis and management of taste disorders and burning mouth syyndrome. Dent Clin North America 1993;37: 33–71

40. Schoenberg B. Psychogenic aspects of the burning mouth. NY State Dent J 1967;33: 467–473.

41. Harris M. Psychogenic aspects of facial pain. Brit Dent J 1974;136:199–202.
42. Mitchell RG. Pre-trigeminal neuralgia. Br Dent J 1980;149:167–170.
43. Alberca R, Ochoa JJ. Cluster tic syndrome. Neurology 1994;44:996–999.
44. Shankland WE. Trigeminal neuralgia: typical or atypical. Crania 1993;11:108–12
45. Cheng TM, Cascino TL, Onofrio BM. Comprehensive study of diagnosis and treatment of trigeminal neuralgia secondary to tumour. Neurology 1993;43:2298–2302.
46. Burchiel KJ. 1993, Trigeminal neuropathic pain. Acta Neurochir 1993; 58(Suppl):145–149.
47. Jannetta PJ. Arterial compression of the trigeminal nerve at the pons in patients with trigeminal neuralgia. J Neurosurg 1967;26:159–162.
48. Jannetta PJ. Microsurgical approach to the trigeminal nerve for tic doloreux. Prog Neurolog Surg 1976;7:180–200.
49. Hamlin PJ, King TT. Neurovascular compression in trigeminal neuralgia: a clinical and anatomical study. J Neurosurg 1992;76:948–954.
50. Ochoa JJ, Alberca R, Canadilla S, et al. Cluster-tic syndrome and basilar artery ectasia: a case report. Headache 1993;33:205–206.
51. Ratner EJ, Person P, Kleinman DJ, et al. Jawbone cavities and trigeminal and atypical facial neuralgias. Oral Surg Oral Med Oral Pathol 1979;48:298–308.
52. Shaber EP, Krol AJ. Trigeminal Neuralgia—a new treatment concept. Oral Surg Oral Med Oral Pathol 1980;49:286–293.
53. Calvin WH, Loeser JD, Howe JF. A neurophysiological theory for the pain mechanism in trigeminal neuralgia. Pain 1977; 3:147–154.
54. Fromm GH. Trigeminal neuralgia and related disorders. Neurol Clin 1989;7: 305–320.
55. Pagni CA. The origin of tic doloreux: a unified view. J Neurosurg Sc 1993;37: 185–94.
56. Crill WE. Drugs years later: carbamazepine. Ann Int Med 1973;79:844–847.
57. Mock D, Noyek A, Gordon A, Marko J. Sinus pain responsive to Tegretol. Oral Surg Oral Med Oral Pathol 1982;54: 640–641.
58. Pascal J, Berciano J. Relief of cluster tic by the combination of lithium and carbamazepine. Cephalgia 1993;13:205–206.
59. Epstein JB, Marcoe JH. Topical application of capsaicin for treatment of oral neuropathic pain and trigeminal neuralgia. Oral Surg Oral Med Oral Pathol 1994;7: 135–140.
60. Fromm GH, Terrence CF. Comparison of L-baclofen and racemic baclofen in trigeminal neuralgia. Neurology 1987;37: 1725–1728.
61. Peiris JB, Perera GL, Devendra SV, Lionel ND. Sodium valproate in trigeminal neuralgia. Med J Australia 1980;2:278.
62. Lechin F, vander Dijs B, Lechin MB. Pimozide therapy for trigeminal neuralgia. Arch Neurol 1989;46:960–963.
63. Sweet WH. Percutaneous methods for the treatment of trigeminal neuralgia and other faciocephalic pain: comparison with microvascular decompression. Sem Neurol 1988;8:272–279.
64. Hakansson S. Trigeminal Neuralgia treated by injection of glycerol into the trigeminal cistern. Neurosurg 1981;9: 638–646.
65. Fardy MJ, Zakrzewska JM, Patton DW. Peripheral surgical techniques for the management of trigeminal neuralgia—alcohol and glycerol injection. Acta Neurochire (Wien) 1994;129: 181–184.
66. Sindou M, Mertens P. Microsurgical vascular decompression (MVD) in trigeminal and glosso-pharyngeal neuralgia: A 20 year experience. Acta Neurochir Suppl 1993;58:168–170.
67. Rosenkopf KL. Current concepts concerning the diagnosis and treatment of trigeminal neuralgia. Cranio 1989;7: 312–318.
68. Metheetrairut C, Brown DM. Glossopharyngeal neuralgia and syncope secondary to neck malignancy. J Otolaryngology 1993;22: 18–20.
69. Lord SM, Barnsley L, Wallis BJ, Bodguk N. Third occipital nerve headache: a prevalance study. J Neurol Neurosurg Psych 1994;57:1187–1190.
70. Anthony M. Headache and the greater occipital nerve. Clin Neurol Neurosurg 1992;94:297–230.
71. Walsted A, Raaschin HD, Bonding P. Surgical treatment of chronic maxillary sinusitis: report of a new surgical technique and an evaluation of traditional surgery. Ugeski Laeger 1989;151: 2802–2805.
72. Pogrel MA, Kaban LB. Injuries to the inferior alveolar nerve and lingual nerves. J Calif Dent Assoc 1993;21:50–54.
73. Swanson AE. Incidence of inferior alveolar nerve injuries in mandibular third

nerve molar surgery. J Can Dent Assoc 1991;57:327–328.

74. Fields HI. Nerve injury. The Annual Meeting of the American Academy of Oro-Facial Pain, Scottsdale, Arizona, Feb 1993.

75. Loeser JD. Definition of, etiology, and neurologic assessment of pain originating in the nervous system following deafferentation. In: Bonica JJ, Lindblom U, Iggo A. eds. *Advances in Pain Research and Therapy, Vol 5.* New York, NY: Raven Press, 1983:701.

76. Evans GR, Crawley W, Dellon AL. Inferior alveolar nerve grafting: an approach without intermedullary fixation. Ann Plast Surg 1994;33: 221–224.

77. Jones RH, Microsurgical repair of nerves injured during third molar surgery. Aust Dent J 1992;37: 253–61.

78. Harris W. Neuritis and Neuralgia. London, Oxford University Press 1926.

79. Gardner WJ, Stowell A, Dutlinger R. Resection of the greater superficial petrosal nerve in the treatment of unilateral headache. J Neurosurg 1947;4:105–114.

80. Horton BT, MacLean AR, Craig WM. A new syndrome of vascular headache: Results of treatment with Histamine: Preliminary report. Mayo Clin Proc 1939;14: 257–260.

81. Horton BT. Histamine cephalgia. Lancet 1952;7:92–98.

82. Kunkle EC, Pfeiffer JB Jr, Wilhoit WM et al. Recurrent brief headaches in "cluster" pattern. Trans Am Neurol Assoc 1951;77: 240–243.

83. Moskowitz M. Pain mechanisms underlying vascular headache. Rev Neurol 1989; 145:181–193.

84. Hardebo JE. The involvement of the trigeminal substance P neurons in cluster headache. An hypothesis. Headache 1984;24:294–304.

85. Geppetti P, Brocchi A, Caleri D, et al. Somastatin for cluster headache attacks. In: Pfaffenrath V, Lundberg P O Sjaastad O eds, *Updating in Headache.* Berlin: Springer-Verlag; 1985: 302–305.

86. Kudrow L. A possible role of the carotid body in the pathogenesis of cluster headaches. Cephalgia 1983;3:241–247.

87. Buckle P, Kerr P, Kryger M. Nocturnal cluster headache associated with sleep apnea. A case report. Sleep 1993;16: 487–489.

88. Kudrow L. The pathogenesis of cluster headache. Curr Opin Neorol 1994;7: 278–282.

89. Schoenen J, Maertens de Noordhout A Headache. In: Wall P, Melzack R eds. *Textbook of Pain*, 3rd Edition. London: Churchill Livingstone; 1994: 495–521.

90. Kudrow L. Cluster headaches. In: Blau JN, ed. *Migraine: Clinical and Research Aspects.* Baltimore, Md: Johns Hopkins University Press; 1987:113.

91. Swanson JW, Yanagihara F, Steng PE, et al. Incidence of cluster headache: a population based study in Olmstead County, Minnesota. Neurology 1994;44:433–437.

92. Mathew NT. Advances in Cluster Headache. Neurol Clin 1990;8:867–890.

93. Pearce JM. Natural history of cluster headache. Headache 1993;33:253–256.

94. Ekbom K. Pattern of cluster headaches with a note on the relation to angina pectoris and peptic ulcer. Acta Neurol Scand 1970;46:225–237.

95. Graham JR. Cluster headache. Headache 1972;11:175–185.

96. Friedman AP, Mikropoulos HE. Cluster headache. Neurology 1958;8:653–663.

97. Ekbom KA. Ergotamine tartrate orally in Horton's "histamine cephalgia" (also called Harris' "ciliary neuralgia"). Acta Psychiatr Scand 1947;46(Suppl):106–113.

98. Campbell JK. Diagnosis and treatment of cluster headache. J Pain Symptom Manage 1993;8: 155–164.

99. The Sumatriptan Cluster Headache Study Group: Treatment of acute cluster headache with sumatriptan. New Engl J Med 1991;325: 322–326.

100. Kudrow L. Response of cluster migraine to oxygen inhalation. Headache 1981;21: 1–4.

101. Ziegler D, Ford R, Kriegler J, et al. Dihydroergotamine nasal spray for the acute treatment of migraine. Neurology 1994; 44: 447–453.

102. Salonen R, Ashford F, Dahlof C, et al. Intranasal sumatriptan for the acute treatment of migraine. International Intranasal Study Group J Neurol 1994;44: 447–453.

103. Kudrow L. Lithium prophylaxis for chronic cluster headache. Headache 1977;17:15–18.

104. Hering R, Kuritsky A. Sodium valproate in the treatment of cluster headache: An open clinical trial. Cephalgia 1989;9: 195–198.

105. Mathew NT, Hurt W. Percutaneous radiofrequency trigeminal gangliorhizolysis in

intractable cluster headache. Headache 1988;28:328–331.

106. Harnisch JP. Zoster in the elderly: clinical, immunologic, and therapeutic considerations. J Am Ger Soc 1984;32: 789–793.

107. Aleksic SN, Budzelowich GN, Lieberman AN. Herpes zoster oticus and facial paralysis (Ramsay Hunt Syndrome). Clinicopathologic study and review of the literature. J Neurol Sci 1973;20:149–159.

108. Juel-Jensen BE, MacCallum FO. *Herpes simplex varicella and zoster*. Philadelphia, Pa: J B Lipincott; 1972.

109. Ragozzino MW, Melton LJ, Kurland LT, et al. Population based study of herpes zoster and its sequelae. Medicine 1982; 21:310–316.

110. Hope-Simpson RE. Post herpetic neuralgia J Royal Coll Gen Pract 1975;25: 571–575.

111. Cobo M, Fowlkes GN, Liesegang T, et al. Observations on the natural history of H. Zoster ophthalmicus. Curr Eye Res 1987; 6:195–199.

112. Murakawa K, Ishimoto E, Nama K, et al. Clinical investigation of 200 patients with acute Herpes Zoster—factors influencing treatment of herpetic pain. Masui Jap J Anaesthesiol 1989;38:1597–6041.

113. Wood MJ, Johnson RW, McKendrick MW, et al. A randomized trial of acyclovir for 7 or 21 days with or without prednisolone for the treatment of acute herpes zoster. New Eng J Med 1994;330:896–900.

114. Bilora F, Genovese R, Presotto F, et al. Herpes zoster and post-herpetic neuralgia. Comparison between elderly patients and young adults treated with acyclovir. Minerva Med 1994;85:333–337.

115. Huff JC, Beam B, Balfour HH Jr, et al. Trearment of Herpes Zoster with oral acyclovir. Am J Med 1988;85: 89–89

116. Huff JC, Drucker JL, Clemmen A, et al. Effect of oral acyclovir on pain resolution in Herpes Zoster: a reanalysis. J Med Virol 1993;1(Suppl) 93–96.

117. Hoang-Xuan T, Buchi E, Herbort CP, Denis J, Frot P, Thenault S, Pouliquen Y. Oral acyclovir for herpes zoster ophthalmicus. Ophthamol 1992;9:1062–1070.

118. Watson CP, Evans RJ, Watt VR. Postherpetic neuralgia and topical capsaicin. Pain 1988;33:333–340.

119. Calza AM, Schmid E, Harms M. Systemic corticosteroids do not prevent post-herpetic neuralgia. Dermatol 1992;184: 314–316.

120. Watson CPN, Morsehead C, Van der Kooy D, et al. Postherpetic neuralgia postmortem. Pain 1988;34:129–138.

121. Watson CP. Postherpetic Neuralgia. Neurol Clin 1989;7:231–248.

122. Watson CP, Evans RJ, Reed K, et al. Amitriptyline versus placebo in post herpetic neuralgia. Neurol 1982;32:670–673.

123. Farber GA, Burks JW. Chlorprothixene therapy for herpes zoster neuralgia. South Med J 1974;67:808–812.

124. Nathan PW. Chlorprothixene (Tarasan) in post-herpetic neuralgia and other severe chronic pains. Pain 1978; 5:367–371.

125. Rowbotham MC. Treatment of post-herpetc neuralgia. Semin Dermatol 1992;11: 218–25.

126. Tubaki T, Fukui J, Tanaka O, et al. Early treatment of H. Zoster with nerve block is extremely important in patients with herpetic pain. Sangyo Ika Daigaku Zasshi 1987;9:45–51.

127. King RB. Concerning the management of pain associated with herpes zoster and of postherpetic neuralgia. Pain 1988;33: 73–78.

128. King RB. Topical ASA in chloroform and the relief of pain due to herpes zoster and post-herpetic neuralgia. Arch Neurol 1993;50:1046–53.

129. Coughlan CJ. Herpes zoster treated by acupuncture. Cent Afr J Med 1992;38: 466–467.

130. Woolf CJ, Thompson JW. 1994, Stimulation Fibre-induced Analgesic Transcutanous Electrical Nerve Stimulation (TENS) and Vibration. In: Wall PD, Melzack R eds. *Textbook of Pain*. 3rd Edition, London: Churchill Livingstone; 1994: 1191–1208.

131. Rowbotham MC, Fields HL. Topical lidocaine reduces pain in post-herpetic neuralgia. Pain 1989;38:297–302.

132. Stow PJ, Glynn CJ, Mino B. EMLA cream in the treatment of postherpetic neuralgia: Efficacy and pharmacokinetic profile. Pain 1989;39:301–5.

133. Winnie AP, Hartwell PW. Relationship between time of treatment of acute herpes zoster with sympathetic blockade and prevention of post herpetic neuralgia: Clinical support for a new theory of the mechanism by which sympathetic blockade provides therapeutic benefits. Reg Anesth 1993;18:277–282.

134. Sjaastad O. Cervicogenic Headache. In: Dalessio DJ, ed. *Wolff's Headache and Other Head Pain*. New York, NY and Ox-

ford: Oxford University Press; 1987: 402–406.

135. Sjaastad O. The headache of challenge for our time: cervicogenic headache. Funct Neurol 1990;5:155–158.

136. Sjaastad O, Fredrikson TA, Pfaffenrath V. Cervicogenic headache: Diagnostic criteria Headache 1990;30:25–26.

137. Evans RW. Some observations on whiplash injuries. Neurol Clin 1992;10: 957–7.

138. Brain WR, Northfeld DWC, Wilkinson M. The neurological manifestations of cervical spondylosis. Brain 1952;75: 187

139. Edmeads J. The cervical spine and headache. Neurol 1988;38:1874–78.

140. Fredrikson TA, Fougner R, Tangerud A, et al. Cervicogenic headache. Radiologic investigation concerning headache. Cephalgia 1989;9:39–46.

141. Sjaastad O, Bovim G. Cervicogenic headache. The differentiation from common migraine. An overview. Funct Neurol 1991;6:93–100.

142. Bogduk N. The anatomical basis for cervicogenic headache. J Manip Physiol Th 1992;15:67–70.

143. Bovim G, Sand T. Cervicogenic headache, migraine without aura and tension-type headache. Diagnostic blockade of greater occipital and supraorbital nerves. Pain 1992;51:43–48.

144. Pfaffenrath V, Isler H, Ekbom K. Chronic daily headache Cephalgia 1993;13(Suppl 12): 66–67.

145. Kehr P, Lang G, Jung FM. Uncusektomie und Uncoforaminectomie nach Jung. Langenbecks Arch Chir 1976;341: 111–125.

146. Barnsley L, Lord S, Bodguk N. Comparative local anesthetic blocks in the diagnosis of cervico-zygapophyseal joint pain. Pain 1993;55:99–106.

147. Bovim G, Berg R, Dale LG. Cervicogenic headache: anesthetic blockade of cervical nerves C2–5 and facet joint C2-C3. Pain 1992;49:315–320.

148. Bovim G, Fredrikson TA, Stolt-Neilsen A, et al. Neurolysis of the greater occipital nerve in cervicogenic headache. A follow-up study. Headache 1992;32:175–179.

149. Wetzel FT. Chronic benign cervical pain syndrome. Surgical considerations. Spine 1992;17:367–374.

150. Cronen MD, Waldman SD. Cervical steroid epidural nerve block in the palliation of pain secondary to intractable tension-type headache. J Pain Symptom Manage 1990;5:379–381.

151. Gawal M, Rothbart P. Occipital nerve block in the management of headache and cervical pain. Cephalgia 1992;12:9–13.

152. Silberstein SD. Tension-type headaches. Headache 1994;34:82–87.

153. Lance JW, Curran DA, Anthony M. Investigation into the mechanism and treatment of chronic headache. Med J Aust 1965;2:909–914.

154. Diamond S. Muscle Contraction Headache. In: Dalessio DJ, ed. *Wolff's Headache and Other Head Pain.* New York, NY and Oxford: Oxford University Press; 1987:172–189.

155. Schoenen J, Gerard P, De Pasqua V, et al. Multiple clinical and paraclinical analyses of chronic tension-type headache associated or unassociated with disorder of pericranial muscles. Cephalgia 1991;11: 135–139.

156. Saper JR. Daily chronic headache. Neurol Clin 1990;8:891–901.

157. Silberstein SD. Tension-type and chronic daily headache. Neurol 1993;43:1644–1649.

158. Silberstein SD, Lipton RB, Solomon S, Mathew NT. Classification of daily or near daily headache. Proposed revisions to IHS criteria. Headache 1994;34:1–7.

159. Solomon S, Lipton RB, Niew LC. Evaluation of chronic daily headache-comparison to chronic TTH. Cephalgia 1992;12: 365–368.

160. Edmeads J, Findley H, Tugwell P, et al. Impact of migraine and tension-type headache on life-style, consulting behaviour, and medication use: a Canadian population survey. Can J Neurol Sci 1993; 20:131–137.

161. Mathew NT. Prophylaxis of migraine and mixed headache: A randomized control study. Headache 1981;21:105–109.

162. Mathew NT. Transformed migraine. Cephalgia 1993;13 (Suppl 12):78–83.

163. Nagasawa A, Sakalibara T, Takahashi A. Roentgenographic findings of the cervical spine in tension-type headache. Headache 1993;33:90–95.

164. Hapak L, Gordon A, Locker D, et al. Differentiation between musculoligamentous, dento-alveolar and neurologically based craniofacial pain with a diagnostic questionnaire. J Orofacial Pain 1994;8:350–356.

165. Zwart JA. Tension-type headache: Botuli-

num toxin paralysis of temporal muscles. Headache 1994;34:458–462.

166. Budzynski TH, Stoyva JM, Adler CS, et al. EMG biofeedback and tension headache; a controlled outcome study. Psychosom Med 1973;35:484–496.

167. Vaughan R, Pall MI, Haynes SN. Frontalis EMG response to stress in subjects with muscle contraction headaches related to mental effort. Headache 1977;17:733–737.

168. Richman JL, Haas DC. Continuous tension-type headache unaffected by two hours of frontalis and trapezius relaxation. Headache 1994;34:458–462.

169. Featherstone HJ. Migraine and muscle contraction headaches: a continuum. Headache 1984;25:194–198.

170. Raskin NH. Headache. 2nd Edition. New York, NY: Churchill Livingstone; 1988.

171. Moskowitz MA. Neurobiology of vascular head pain. Ann Neurol 1984;6:157–168.

172. Kunkel RS. Diagnosis and treatment of muscle contraction (tension type) headaches. Med Clin North Amer 1991;75:595–603.

173. Marcus DA. Serotonin and its role in headache pathogenesis and treatment. Clin J Pain 1993;9:159–167.

174. DeBenedittis G, Lorenzetti A. The role of stressful life events in the persistence of primary headache: major events vs daily hassles. Pain 1992;51:35–42.

175. Fogelholm R, Murros K. Tizanidine in chronic tension-type headache: a placebo controlled double blind cross-over study. Headache 1992;32:509–513.

176. Nakashima K, Tumura R, Wang Y, et al. Effects of tizanidine administration on exteroceptive suppression of temporalis muscle in chronic tension-type headache. Headache 1994;34:455–7.

177. Mathew NT, Ali S. Valproate in the treatment of persistent chronic daily headache. An open label study. Headache 1991;31:71–74.

178. Rothrock JF, Kelly NM, Brody ML. A differential response to treatment with divalproex sodium in patients with intractable headache. Cephalgia 1994;Ch 6: 87–111.

179. Manna V, Bolino F, Di Cicco L. 1994. Chronic tension type headache, mood depression, and serotonin: theraputic effects of fluvoxamine and mianserine. Headache 1994;34:44–49.

180. Dalessio DJ. Some reflections on the etiologic role of depression in head pain. Headache 1968;8:28–31.

181. Vernon H, Steinman I, Hagino C. Cervicogenic dysfunction in muscle contraction headache and migraine: a descriptive study. J Manipulative Physiol Ther 1992; 15:418–429.

182. Steiner TJ, Couturier EGM, Catarci T, et al. Social aspects of drug abuse in headache. Functional Neurol 1992;6(suppl 7): 11–14.

183. Saper JR, Jones JM. Ergotamine tartrate dependency: features and possible mechanisms. Clin Neuropharmacol 1986;9: 244–256.

184. Mathew NT. Drug-induced headache. Neurol Clin 1990;8:903–912.

185. Lance JW. Mechanisms in Management of Headache. Boston, Mass: Butterworth; 1982.

186. Pascal J, Berceani S. Daily chronic headache in patients with migraine induced by abuse of ergotamine-analgesia. Neurology 1993;8:212–215.

187. Kudrow L. Paradoxical effects of frequent analgesic abuse. In: Critchley M, Friedman A, Gorini S, Sicuteri F, eds. Advances in Neurology, Vol 33. New York, NY: Raven Press; 1982: 335.

188. Isler H. Migraine treatment as a cause of chronic migraine. In: Rose FC, ed. Advances in Migraine Research and Therapy. New York: Raven Press 1982: 159–164.

189. Rapoport AM, Weeks RE, Sheftell FD, et al. The "analgesic washout period": a critical variable in the evaluation of headache treatment efficacy. Neurol 1986; 36(suppl 1):100–101.

190. Walker J, Parisi S, Olive D. Analgesic rebound headache in a community hospital. South Med J 1993;86:1202–5.

191. Schoenen J, Lenarduzzi P, Sianard-Gainko J. Chronic headaches associated with analgesics and/or ergotamine abuse: a clinical survey of 434 consecutive outpatients. In: Rose FC, ed. New Advances in Headache Research. London: Smith Gordon; 1989:255–259

192. Hering R, Gleva V, Pattichis K, et al. 5-HT levels in migraine patients with migraine induced headache. Cephalgia 1993;13: 410–412.

193. Diener HC. A personal view on the classification and definition of drug dependent headache. Cephalgia 1993;13(Suppl-12): 68–71.

194. Ziegler DK. The Treatment of Migraine. In: Dalessio DJ, ed. Wolff's Headache and Other Head Pain. New York, NY and Ox-

ford: Oxford University Press; 1987; Ch 6: 87–111.

195. Monteiro JM, Matos E, Calheiros JM. Headache in medical school students. Neuroepidemiol 1994;13:103–107.

196. Honkasalo ML, Keprio J, Heikkila K, et al. A population based survey of headache and migraine in 22,809 adults. Headache 1994;33:403–412.

197. Rasmusan BK, Oleson J. Migraine with aura and migraine without aura: an epidemiological study. Cephalgia 1992;12: 221–228.

198. Rasmussan BK, Jensen R, Schroll M, et al. Interrelations between migraine and tension-type headache in the general population. Arch Neurol 1992;49:914–918.

199. Solomon S. Migraine diagnosis and clinical symptomatology. Headache 1994;34: S8–12.

200. Stewart WF, Shecter A, Lipton RB. Disability, pain intensity and attack frequency and duration. Neurology 1994;44:S24–29.

201. Chen TC, Levitan A. Headache recurrence in pregnant women with migraine. Headache 1994;34:107–110.

202. Diamond S. Migraine headaches. Med Clin North Amer 1991;75:545–566.

203. Monro J, Carini C, Brostoff J. Migraine is a food allergic disease. Lancet 1984;2: 719–721.

204. Sicuteri F. Migraine, a central biochemical dysnociception. Headache 1986;16: 145–149.

205. Moskowitz MA. Basic mechanisms in vascular headache. Neurol Clin 1990;8: 801–815.

206. Liu-Chen LY, Mayberg M, Moskowitz MA. Immunohistochemical evidence for a substance P-containing trigeminovascular pathway to pial arteries in cats. Brain Res 1983;268:162–166.

207. McCulloch J, Uddman R, Kingman TA, et al. Calcitonin gene related peptide: functional role in cerebrovascular regulation. Proc Natl Acad Sci 1986;83:5731–5735.

208. Saito K, Greenberg S, Moskowitz MA. Trigeminal origin of beta-preprotachykinin products in feline pial blood vessels. Neurosci Lett 1987;76:69–73.

209. Oleson J. Cerebral blood flow in migraine with aura. Pathologie et Biologie 1992;40: 318–324.

210. Bes A, Fabre N. D'ebit sanguine cerebral et migraine sans aura. Pathologie et Biologie 1992;40:325–331.

211. Lauritzen M. Spreading depression and migraine. Pathologie Biologie 1992;40: 332–337.

212. Leao AA. Spreading depression of activity in cerebral cortex. J Neurophysiol 1944;7:359–390.

213. Barkley GL, Tepley N, Simkins RT, et al. Neuromagnetic findings in migraine. Preliminary findings. Cephalgia 1990;10: 171–176.

214. Schoenen J. Clinical neurophysiology studies in headache: a review of data and pathophysiological hints. Funct Neurol 1992;7:191–204.

215. Mauskop A, Altura BT, Cracco RO, et al. Deficiency in serum ionized magnesium but not total magnesium in patients with migraine. Possible role of Ica2 and /Img2 ratio. Headache 1993;33:1358–1360.

216. Ferrari MD. Biochemistry of migraine. Pathologie Biologie 1992;40:287–292.

217. Ollat H, Garruchaga JM. Agonistes et antagonistes de la serotonine et migraine. Pathologie Biologie 1992;40:305–312.

218. Shimomura T, Araga S, Kowa H, et al. Immunoglobulin kappa/lambda ratios in migraine and tension-type headache. Jap J Psychiatr Neurol 1992;46:721–726.

219. Welch KMA. Migraine, a biobehavioural disorder. Arch Neurol 1987;44:323–327.

220. Edmeads J. Migraine—disease or syndrome? Pathologie Biologie 1992;40: 279–283.

221. Lance JW. The pathophysiology of migraine: a tentative synthesis. Pathologie Biologie 1992;40:355–360.

222. Lance JW. Current concepts of migraine pathogenesis. Neurol 1993;43:S11–15.

223. Drugs For Migraine. The Medical Letter 1995;37: 17–20

224. Hesse J, Mogelvang B, Simonsen H. Acupuncture vs. metroprolol in migraine prophylaxis: a randomized trial of trigger point inactivation. J Intern Med 1994;235: 451–456.

225. Raskin NH. Modern pharmacotherapy of migraine. Neurol Clin 1990;8:857–866

226. Teves TA, Steiffler M, Korczyn AD. Naproxen sodium versus ergotamine tartrate in the treatment of acute migraine attacks. Headache 1992;32: 280–282.

227. Davis CP, Tuve DR, Schaffer NC, et al. Ketorolac as a rapid and effective treatment of migraine headache: evaluation by patients. Amer J Emerg Med 1993;11: 573–575.

228. Kumar KL. Recent advances in acute management of migraine and cluster

headache. J Gen Intern Med 1994;9: 339–348.

229. The Subcutaneous Sumatriptan International Study Group: Treatment of migraine attacks with sumatriptan. New Engl J Med 1991;325: 316–325.

230. Mathew NT, Reuveni U, Perez F. Transformed or evolutive migraine. Headache 1987;27:102–106.

231. Scott AK. Dihydroergotamine: a review of its use in the treatment of migraine and other headaches. Clin Neuropharmacol 1992;15;289–296.

232. Weisz MA, el-Raheb M, Blumenthal HJ. Home administration of IM dihydroergotamine for the treatment of acute migraine headache. Headache 1994;34:371–373.

233. Lane PL. Comparative efficacy of chlorpromazine and meperidine with dimenhydrinate in migraine headache. Ann Emerg Med 1989;18:360–365.

234. Hansen PE. Tolfonemic acid in acute and prophylactic treatment of migraine: a review. Pharmacol Toxicol 1994;75(Suppl 2);81–82.

235. Kjaergard Rasmussan MJ, Holt Larsen B, et al. Tolfonemic acid vs propranol in the prophylactic treatment of migraine. Acta Neurol Scan 1994;89:446–450.

236. Klapper JA, Stanton J. Current emergency treatment of severe migraine headache, Headache 1993;33:560–562.

237. Hoffert MJ, Scolz MJ, Kantor R. A double blind controlled study of nifedipine as an abortive treatment in acute attacks of migraine with aura. Cephalgia 1992;12: 323–324.

238. Medical Letter Handbook of Adverse Drug Interactions 1995:138.

239. Mathew NT, Saper JR, Silberstein SD, et al. Migraine prophylaxis with divalproex sodium. Arch Neurol 1995;52:281–286.

240. Ziegler DK, Hurwitz A, Preskorn S, et al. Propranolol and Elavil in the prophylaxis of migraine. Pharmacokinetic and therapeutic effect. Arch Neurol 1993;50:25–30.

# Index

621